# CULTURE AND MENTAL HEALTH

A comprehensive textbook

# CULTURE AND MENTAL HEALTH

## A comprehensive textbook

EDITED BY KAMALDEEP BHUI & DINESH BHUGRA

**Kamaldeep Bhui** MBBS, BSc (Pharmacology), MSc (Epidemiology), MSc (Mental Health Studies),
FRCPsych, MD, Dip Clin Psychotherapy
Professor of Cultural Psychiatry and Epidemiology
Barts and The London School of Medicine and Dentistry
Queen Mary University of London
and Honorary Consultant Psychiatrist
East London and City Mental Health Trust
London, UK

**Dinesh Bhugra** MBBS, MRCPsych, MPhil, MSc (Sociology), MA (Social Anthropology), FRCPsych, PhD
Head
Cultural Psychiatry Section
Institute of Psychiatry, London
and Honorary Consultant Psychiatrist, Maudsley Hospital
London, UK

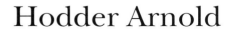

## Hodder Arnold

A MEMBER OF THE HODDER HEADLINE GROUP

First published in Great Britain in 2007 by
Hodder Arnold, an imprint of Hodder Education and a member of the Hodder Headline Group,
338 Euston Road, London NW1 3BH

http://www.hoddereducation.com

Distributed in the United States of America by
Oxford University Press Inc.,
198 Madison Avenue, New York, NY10016
Oxford is a registered trademark of Oxford University Press

Hodder Headline's policy is to use papers that are natural, renewable and
recyclable products and made from wood grown in sustainable forests.
The logging and manufacturing processes are expected to conform to the
environmental regulations of the country of origin.

Whilst the advice and information in this book are believed to be true and
accurate at the date of going to press, neither the author[s] nor the publisher
can accept any legal responsibility or liability for any errors or omissions that
may be made. In particular (but without limiting the generality of the preceding
disclaimer), every effort has been made to check drug dosages; however it is still
possible that errors have been missed. Furthermore, dosage schedules are
constantly being revised and new side-effects recognized. For these reasons the
reader is strongly urged to consult the drug companies' printed instructions
before administering any of the drugs recommended in this book.

*British Library Cataloguing in Publication Data*
A catalogue record for this book is available from the British Library

*Library of Congress Cataloging-in-Publication Data*
A catalog record for this book is available from the Library of Congress

ISBN    978-0-340-81046-0

1 2 3 4 5 6 7 8 9 10

Commissioning Editor: Serena Bureau/Philip Shaw
Project Editor: Layla Vandenbergh/Clare Patterson
Production Controller: Karen Tate
Cover Design: Nichola Smith
Indexer: Laurence Errington

Typeset in 10/12 pts Minion by Charon Tec Ltd (A Macmillan Company), Chennai, India
www.charontec.com
Printed and bound in Malta

What do you think about this book? Or any other Hodder Arnold title?
Please visit our website at www.hoddereducation.com

# Contents

# About the editors

**Kamaldeep Singh Bhui** is Professor of Cultural Psychiatry and Epidemiology at Barts and The London Medical School, Queen Mary University of London, and Consultant Psychiatrist at East London and City Mental Health Trust. He qualified in medicine at the United Medical Schools of Guy's and St Thomas' (UMDS), where he later worked as a research associate and research fellow. He completed his psychiatry training at the Maudsley Hospital, and his MD at the Institute of Psychiatry as a Wellcome Trust Fellow, investigating common mental disorders among Punjabi and English primary care attendees. He completed a BSc in pharmacology at University College London, and an MSc in epidemiology at the London School of Hygiene and Tropical Medicine, after an MSc in mental health studies and a diploma in clinical psychotherapy both at UMDS. His training as a psychoanalytic psychotherapist was at the British Association of Psychotherapy.

His research interests include social exclusion and environmental effects on health, with a specific focus on health services research, the integration of anthropological and epidemiological research methods, and investigations of risk factors such as cultural identity, explanatory models of mental disorders, geographical mobility and racism among immigrant and refugee populations. His clinical work has involved working in community psychiatry, specifically assertive outreach teams with severely mentally ill people, and more recently with homeless people in London. He is now working in a psychotherapy service in Tower Hamlets, with a key role in training and education.

Kamaldeep Singh Bhui is practising psychoanalytic psychotherapist, and Consultant Psychiatrist in Psychotherapy in East London and City Mental Health Trust, Director of MSc Transcultural Mental Healthcare at Queen Mary, Chair, the Transcultural Special Interest Group of the Royal College of Psychiatrists, Founding Board Member and Co-chair of the Scientific Committee of the World Association of Cultural Psychiatry, President Elect for the Psychiatry Section of the Royal Society of Medicine, Fellow of the Royal College of Psychiatrists, and founding Co-Director of the CARE International Foundation. He teaches and examines medical undergraduate and multi-disciplinary postgraduate students.

**Dinesh Bhugra** received his undergraduate training at the Armed Forces Medical College, Poona University, India, his general psychiatric training at Leicester University where he obtained his MPhil and higher psychiatric training on the Bethlem and Maudsley SR Rotation Scheme. He attained further degrees in Sociology (MSc) and Social Anthropology (MA) in London and a PhD in 1999. In 1994 he was appointed Senior Lecturer and Honorary Consultant at the Institute of Psychiatry and appointed to Chair of Mental Health and Cultural Diversity in 2002. He heads the Section of Cultural Psychiatry and is developing training materials for teaching cultural formulations.

As Honorary Consultant at the Maudsley Hospital, he runs clinical services in couple, relationship and sex therapy. His main research interests are psychosexual medicine, cross-cultural psychiatry, schizophrenia, pathways into psychiatric care, deliberate self-harm and primary care. He is co-author/editor of 14 books, the most recent of which are volumes on *Culture and Self-Harm* (Psychology Press) and *Handbook of Psychiatry* (Byword Viva).

# Contributors

**Oyedeji Ayonrinde** MBBS, MRCPsych, MSc
Bethlem Royal Hospital, South London and Maudsley NHS
Trust, London, UK

**Goffredo Bartocci** MD
Psychiatrist and Psychoanalyst, Former Professor at the
University of Turin and Head of the Rome Transcultural
Psychiatry Unit. President Elect of the World Association of
Cultural Psychiatry and Chair of the Italian Institute of
Transcultural Mental Health

**Simon Dein** MRCPsych, PhD
Senior Lecturer in Anthropology and Medicine, University
College London, UK, and Editor, *Mental Health, Religion and
Culture*

**Ruth DeSouza** Dip Nurs, Grad Dip Adv Nurs Pract, MA
Centre Co-ordinator/Senior Research Fellow, Centre for Asian
and Migrant Health Research, National Institute for Public
Health and Mental Health Research, AUT University, Auckland,
Aotearoa/New Zealand

**Marjolein van Duijl** MD
Psychiatrist, Programme Coordinator Psychotrauma, Lentis,
Mental Health Organization Groningen, and Researcher, Rob
Giel Research Center, Department of Psychiatry, University of
Groningen, The Netherlands

**Daniel Fekadu** MD, MRCPsych
Department of Child Psychiatry, Institute of Psychiatry, King's
College London, UK

**KWM Fulford** DPhil, FRCP, FRCPsych
Professor of Philosophy and Mental Health, University of
Warwick; Honorary Consultant Psychiatrist, University of Oxford;
Co-Director, Institute for Philosophy, Diversity and Mental Health,
University of Central Lancashire; Special Adviser for Values-
Based Practice, Department of Health, London; and Editor, PPP

**Isaak Ya Gurovich** MD
Deputy Director, Moscow Research Institute of Psychiatry,
Russia

**Cecil G Helman** MBChB, FRCGP, Dip.Soc.Anthrop.
Professor of Medical Anthropology, School of Social Sciences
and Law, Brunel University, and Senior Lecturer, Department of
Primary Care and Population Sciences, Royal Free and
University College Medical School, University College London,
UK

**Ernest Hunter**
Regional Psychiatrist, Queensland Health, and Adjunct
Professor, North Queensland Health Equalities Promotion Unit,
School of Population Health, University of Queensland,
Australia

**Gerard Hutchinson**
Psychiatry Unit, Department of Clinical Medical Sciences, The
University of the West Indies, Trinidad and Tobago

**Karen Iley** RN, BSc (Hons) Health Studies, MSc Sociology, Health and
Healthcare
Lecturer in Adult Nursing, University of Salford, UK

**Mario Incayawar** MD, MSc, DESS
Director, Runajambi (Institute for the Study of Quichua
Culture and Health), Otavalo, Ecuador
Former Henry R Luce Professor in Brain, Mind, and Medicine:
Cross-Cultural Perspectives, Claremont Colleges, California, USA

**Rachel Jenkins** MD(Cantab), FRCPsych, Dist FAPA, FFOHM
Director, WHO Collaborating Centre, Institute of Psychiatry,
London; Visiting Professor, London School of Hygiene and
Tropical Medicine, London, UK

**Murad M Khan**
Professor, Department of Psychiatry, Aga Khan University,
Karachi, Pakistan

**Pius A Kigamwa** MBChB (Nrb), MMed(Psych) (Nrb)
Lecturer, Department of Psychiatry, College of Health
Sciences, University of Nairobi, Kenya

**Robert Kohn** MD
Associate Professor, Brown University Department of
Psychiatry and Human Behavior, Butler Hospital,
Rhode Island, USA

**Valery Krasnov** MD
Director, Moscow Research Institute of Psychiatry, Russia

**Nemu Lallu**
Ministry of Health, New Zealand

**Paul Chi Wai Lam** ROT (HK), PhD
Occupational Therapist, Hong Kong Housing
Society, Elderly Resources Centre, Hong Kong, China

**Christoph Lauber** Dr Med
Psychiatrist, Senior Lecturer, Psychiatric University Hospital,
Zurich, Switzerland

**Keith Lloyd** MD, MSc(Econ), MSc, FRCPsych
Professor of Psychological Medicine, University of Wales
Swansea, UK

**James Nazroo** MBBS, BSc (Hons), MSc, PhD, FFPH
Professor of Sociology, School of Social Sciences, University of
Manchester, UK

**Roger MK Ng** MBChB, MSc (Birm), MRCPsych (UK), FHKCPsych, FHKAM
(Psychiatry), ACT
Specialist in Psychiatry; Certified Cognitive Therapist, and
Senior Medical Officer, Department of Psychiatry, Kowloon
Hospital, Hong Kong, China

**Anna N Nguithi** MBChB (Nrb), MMed(Psych) (Nrb)
Consultant Psychiatrist, Upper Hill Medical Centre, Nairobi, Kenya

**Frank G Njenga** MD, FRCPsych
Consultant Psychiatrist, Upper Hill Medical Centre, Nairobi,
Kenya

**Michael Odenwald** Dr rer nat, Dipl Psych
Researcher, Department of Psychology, University of Konstanz,
Germany; Clinical Researcher, Schizophrenia Research Ward,
University of Konstanz and Centre for Psychiatry Reichenau,
Germany; Clinical Researcher, Psychological Research and
Outpatient Clinic for Refugees, University of Konstanz,
Reichenau, Germany

**Ahmed Okasha** MD, PhD, FRCP, FRCPsych, FACP(Hon)
Director, World Health Organization Collaborating Center for
Research and Training in Mental Health, Institute of Psychiatry,
Ain Shams University, Cairo, Egypt

**Gbenga Okulate** MB ChB, FMCPsych, FWACP
Nigerian Army Reference Hospital, Yaba, Lagos, Nigeria

**Charles Pace**
Senior Lecturer in Social Work, University of Malta, Malta

**Vikram Patel**
Reader in International Mental Health and Wellcome Trust
Senior Clinical Research Fellow in Tropical Medicine, London
School of Hygiene and Tropical Medicine, UK

**Rajendra Pavagada** DPM, MD
Consultant Psychiatrist, Department of Psychiatry, Counties
Manukau DHB, Auckland, New Zealand

**Veronica Pearson** BSocSci (Econ) Hons, MSc, CQSW, DPhil
Professor, Department of Social Work and Social
Administration, The University of Hong Kong, Hong Kong, China

**Albert Persaud** MRIPHH
Co-Founder and Director of the Centre for Applied Research
and Evaluation (CARE) International Foundation, London, UK

**Martin Prince**
Professor of Epidemiological Psychiatry, Section of
Epidemiology, Health Services Research Department, Institute
of Psychiatry, King's College London, UK

**Omar Rahman**
Professor of Demography and Executive Director, Centre for
Health, Population and Development, Independent University,
Bangladesh

**Beverley Raphael** AM, MBBS, MD, FRANZCP, FASSA, FRCPsych, HonMD
(Newcastle, NSW)
Professor of Population Mental Health and Disasters,
University of Western Sydney, and Professor of Psychological
Medicine, Australian National University, Australia

**Zoë K Reed** BSc
Executive Director, South London and Maudsley NHS
Foundation Trust, UK

**Wulf Rössler** MedDip, Psych
Professor of Clinical and Social Psychiatry, University of
Zurich, and Clinical Director, Psychiatric University Hospital
'Burghölzli', Zurich, Switzerland

**David Sallah** PhD, MSc, B ed, RN
Professor of Mental Health, Director of Research, Ethics and Consultancy, School of Health, University of Wolverhampton UK; Director, Centre for Health and Social Care Improvement, University of Wolverhampton, UK, and National Director, Black and Minority Ethnic Mental Health Programme, Care Services Improvement Partnership and National Institute for Mental Health in England, Department of Health, UK

**Anand Satyanand**
Governor General, New Zealand

**Derrick Silove** MB ChB (Hons I), FRANZCP, MD
Director, School of Psychiatry, University of New South Wales and Professor of Psychiatry, Centre for Population Mental Health Research, Sydney South West Area Health Service, Australia

**Tobias Schmitt** Dipl Psych
Psychological Research and Outpatient Clinic for Refugees, University of Konstanz, Germany

**Zachary Steel** MPsychol (Clinical), BA (Hons)
Senior Lecturer and Clinical Psychologist, Center for Population Mental Health Research, School of Psychiatry, University New South Wales, Sydney, Australia

**Athula Sumathipala**
Clinical Researcher, Institute of Psychiatry, King's College London, UK

**Leslie Swartz** MSc (Clin Psych), PhD
Professor of Psychology, Stellenbosch University, South Africa, and Honorary Research Associate, Human Sciences Research Council, South Africa

**Suraj B Thapa**
Researcher, Institute of Psychiatry and Department of International Health, University of Oslo, Norway

**Nasir Warfa** MSc, PhD
Lecturer in Transcultural Psychiatry, Centre for Psychiatry, Queen Mary's School of Medicine and Dentistry, University of London, UK

**Kim Woodbridge**
Operational Manager, Adult Mental Health Service, Milton Keynes Primary Care Trust, UK

**Ka Chee Yip** MBBS, FHKCPsych, FHKAM (Psychiatry), MRCPsych (UK)
Medical Superintendent, Kowloon Psychiatric Observation Unit, Consultant Psychiatrist and Chief of Service, Department of Psychiatry, Kowloon Hospital, Hong Kong Special Administrative Region, China

**Li Zhanjiang**
An Ding Hospital, Beijing, China

# Foreword

*Norman Sartorius*

'J'ai vu des Francais, des Italiens des Russes mais quant à l'Homme je déclare ne jamais l'avoir rencontré de ma vie',[1] wrote Joseph de Maistre in his *Soirées de Saint-Petersbourg* in 1821. It would be difficult to find a more succinct description of one extreme of the continuum of opinions about the importance of culture for the definition of a human being, a continuum that ranges from the belief that humans are entirely defined by the culture in which they grow and live to the denial that cultural differences exist.

The definitions of mental health could also be arranged on a continuum that starts with the definition of mental health as the absence of mental illness to the definition that completely disregards the presence of mental illness. From this point of view, mental health (and health in general) is seen as a dimension of human existence compatible with the presence of mental illness and impairment. The consequence of the acceptance of one extreme or the other of the definitions of mental health has a variety of practical implications. If we accept that mental health is defined by the absence of mental illness, it is psychiatry as an organized body of practitioners that will have the principal role in the improvement of mental health because it is supposed to play the key role in the treatment of mental illness. If mental health is seen as a capacity to cope with distress and excessive stress, and other correlates of mental disorders, it is again psychiatry that has a leading role. However, this time psychiatry will not be the principal actor but the discipline that provides knowledge and leadership in programmes of prevention of mental disorders. A definition of mental health as a state of balance within oneself and between oneself and the environment would place the responsibility for the development of strategies that could enhance mental health in the camp of philosophers, theologians and educators, and wider society.

Wisely, the editors of this volume avoided the trap of trying to define their subject too narrowly: instead of dwelling on special cultural factors that could have an impact on mental health or dwelling on possible advantages or disadvantages of different definitions of mental health they steered their textbook into the territory of transcultural or cultural psychiatry where they are joining the venerable tradition of authors such as H.B.M. Murphy, K.W. Bash, T.A. Lambo, P.M.Yap, A. Kiev, A. Leighton, J. Murphy, W. Tseng and others. These authors searched for (and applied) insights from anthropology, sociology, the epidemiology of mental disorders in different countries, philosophy and other disciplines. Such a comprehensive approach aims to improve the practice of psychiatry and the care for people with mental illness and their families all over the globe in a manner that is compatible with their local cultural contexts.

In the second part of the volume, the editors have assembled an array of experts that reads like a *Debrett's Peerage* list or *Gotha* of International and Cultural Psychiatry. As one would expect, this range of experts deliver an amazingly rich description of mental disorders and psychiatry in different parts of the world; the more one reads their contributions the more obvious it becomes

---

[1] "I have seen Frenchmen, Italians, Russians but as far as the Human is concerned I declare that I have never met one during my life".

that it is important to have a textbook on culture and mental health using a comparative paradigm. The knowledge assembled by these experts and their respective disciplines shows that human beings at first glance do not differ all that much in the types and courses of illness. However, close scrutiny does show differences in the ways distress is expressed, interpreted and remedied, and in the form of programmes for mental health care and improvement. Noticing differences resulting from local cultural contexts and belief systems, and cultural determinants of the expressions of distress, and uptake of treatments, warrants better evidence on which to base interventions and care programmes. Varying degrees of progress towards mental health programmes are demonstrated. Historical and cultural attitudes towards mental illness vary between countries and continents, as does the amount of information and knowledge about the mental health of populations.

The book before you is a harmonious presentation of theoretical issues and practical problems relevant to mental health care produced by meshing the knowledge from scientific disciplines. There are precise descriptions of the form of mental disorders and of programmes of care for people with mental illness in different parts of the world. We should be profoundly grateful to the editors for the efforts that they have made to offer this splendid opus to us.

*Norman Sartorius*
*January 2007*

# Acknowledgements

The Editors thank Lisa Kass for assistance with reference formatting, local editors and authors for their expertise and enthusiasm, service users for sharing their distress and experiences, and our families for sharing our vision of learning and knowledge as a means to a better and more just society.

## Chapter 7

Dr J Brincat, Professor M Therese Camilleri Podesta, Dr D Cassar, Dr Ruth Farrugia, Ms Miriam Gauci, Mr Manuel Mangani, Dr G Muscat Azzopardi and Dr Ray Xerri for their enlightening discussion and clarifications.

Peggy Lu and Leon Lee, Chinese Mental Health Association in UK, for translating the section on China.

## Chapter 8

Arthur Battram for early discussions and help in formulating thinking.

## Chapter 12

Professor V Ababkov for very valuable information on the history of Russian psychiatry, especially from the St Petersburg division.

## Chapter 14

This chapter is reprinted with kind permission from Dave Jago, Royal College of Psychiatrists. Originally published as Okasha, A. 2004: Focus on psychiatry in Egypt. *British Journal of Psychiatry* 185, 266–72.

## Chapter 19

Miss Sioui Maldonado Bouchard for her assistance in reviewing the quality of the English language.

## Chapter 27

Dr WH Lo, consultant psychiatrist in charge of the Hong Kong Mental Health Service from 1974 to 1990, for providing some of the information on the past psychiatric service.

## Chapter 29

Dr Liang Ju of the Guangzhou Federation of the Disabled and Ms Chui Chi, a retired senior cadre of the Bureau of Civil Affairs, Guangzhou for permitting her to interview them extensively for this chapter. 'We have worked together for many years and it can be truly said of them that they made a difference.'

# Abbreviations

AAAPA — Association of Allied African Psychiatrists and Associations
ACC — Accident Compensation Corporation
ACT — assertive community treatment
ADHD — attention deficit hyperactivity disorder
AESOP — Aetiology and Ethnicity in Schizophrenia and Other Psychoses
AHDSOO — Asset and Health Dynamics Study of the Oldest Old
AIDS — acquired immune deficiency syndrome
AI-SUPERPFP — American Indian Service Utilization, Psychiatric Epidemiology, Risk and Protective Factors Project
BSE — bovine spongiform encephalopathy
CALD — culturally and linguistically diverse
CAREC — Caribbean Epidemiology Centre
CBCL — Child Behavior Checklist
CCHS — Canadian Community Health Survey
CDI — Child Depression Inventory
CFA — Confirmatory Factor Analysis
CIDI — Composite International Diagnostic Interview
CIDI-PC — primary care version of the Composite International Diagnostic Interview
CIDIS — Composite International Diagnostic Interview Simplified

CIDI-SF — Composite International Diagnostic Interview – short form
CIS-R — Clinical Interview Schedule
CMD — common mental disorders
CME — continuing medical education
COHRED — Commission on Health Research for Development
DALYs — disability adjusted life years
DAO — Duly Authorised Officer
DDNOS — dissociative disorders not otherwise specified
DHBs — District Health Boards
DIS — Diagnostic Interview Schedule
DISC-IV — Diagnostic Interview Schedule for Children
DSM-IV — *Diagnostic and Statistical Manual of Mental Disorders,* fourth edition
DSS — Demographic and Surveillance System
ECA — Epidemiological Catchment Area Study
ECT — electroconvulsive therapy
EMHS — Ethiopian Mental Health Society
ENUSP — European Network of (ex-)Users and Survivors of Psychiatry
EPA — Ethiopian Psychiatrists Association
EU — European Union
EUFAMI — European Federation of Associations of Families of Mentally Ill People
FECCA — Federation of Ethnic Community Councils of Australia

| | | | |
|---|---|---|---|
| GDP | gross domestic product | NSF | National Service Framework |
| GNP | gross national product | OECD | Organization for Economic Cooperation and Development |
| GPs | general practitioners | | |
| HIV | human immunodeficiency virus | PAHO | Pan American Health Organization |
| ICD-10 | *International Classification of Diseases, 10th revision* | PBI | Parental Bonding Interview |
| ICMR | Indian Council of Medical Research | PCA | Principal component analysis |
| | | PHOs | primary health organizations |
| ILO | International Labour Organization | PPGHC | Psychological Problems in General Health Care |
| IMF | International Monetary Fund | PSE | Present State Examination |
| INDEPTH | International Network of Field Sites with Continuous Demographic Evaluation of Populations and their Health in Developing Countries | PTSD | post-traumatic stress disorder |
| | | QPMA | Questionnaire for Psychiatric Morbidity in Adults |
| | | QMPI | Questionário de Morbidade Psiquiátrica Infantil |
| IPS | individual placement support | QOL | quality of life |
| IRPCs | Immigration Reception and Processing Centers | SADS | Schedule for Affective Disorders and Schizophrenia |
| IRT | Item Response Theory | SDQ | Strength and Difficulties Questionnaire |
| IT | information technology | | |
| MAPSS | Mexican American Prevalence and Services Survey | SEIFA | Socio-Economic Indexes for Areas |
| MHA | Mental Health (Compulsory Assessment and Treatment) Act 1992 | SRQ-20 | Self-Report Questionnaire (20-item version) |
| | | SSAGA | Semi-Structured Assessment for the Genetics of Alcoholism |
| NCS | National Comordity Study | | |
| NCS-R | National Comordity Study Replication | SSRI | selective serotonin reuptake inhibitors |
| NESARC | National Epidemiologic Survey on Alcohol and Related Conditions | TAPS | Team for the Assessment of Psychiatric Services |
| | | TCA | tricyclic antidepressants |
| NGO | non-governmental organization | TPVs | Temporary Protection Visas |
| NHANES | National Health and Nutrition Examination Survey | UM-CIDI | University of Michigan Composite International Diagnostic Interview |
| NHANES-III | Third National Health and Nutrition Examination Survey | UN | United Nations |
| NHS | National Health Service | UNDP | United Nations Development Programme |
| NIMHE | National Institute for Mental Health in England | WPA | World Psychiatrists Association |
| NLAES | National Longitudinal Alcohol Epidemiologic Survey | YLDs | years lived with disability |
| NPHS | National Population Health Survey | | |

# Editors' introduction

## Kamaldeep Bhui and Dinesh Bhugra

## INTRODUCTION

*Culture and Mental Health: A Comprehensive Textbook* sets out both basic and advanced theoretical, philosophical and clinical foundations for teachers and students, practitioners and policy-makers. This textbook builds on national and international policy and service knowledge; doing this and retaining clinical and practice relevance, informed by research, is not an easy task. The authors reveal their local worlds, including their everyday practice, with the aspiration to improve the quality of mental health care to diverse cultural groups. Outside the specialist centres of excellence, there is little information and few training opportunities in culture and mental health care. For most countries routine data on mental health episodes and the epidemiology of mental illness by racial, ethnic and cultural group are lacking. It is often difficult to discern, and rarely confirmed, whether the influence of culture on the expression and management of mental distress follows universal and predictable patterns irrespective of the culture or the country of interest.

Social stratification is often proposed to explain all ethnic and racial variations in prevalence,

experience and outcomes of mental illness. This position, if taken to one extreme, excludes and negates the role of ethnicity and cultural influences (see Karlson and Nazroo, 2002).

A further factor that hinders the collation of more knowledge and data is disquiet that just by studying cultures there is potential to generate inequalities and act in a racist and discriminatory manner. We consider this an irrational feeling as data require explanation; by proposing to expose inequalities of care experiences by race or ethnic group or culture, we maintain that service providers, policy-makers and practitioners can then address the causes of inequalities in an informed and mature manner. We contend that knowledge is essential, and data are necessary to monitor patterns and degrees of inequity. Where inequity has been demonstrated, this cannot be tackled without regular repeated measures of the progress towards a more fair system of care.

Where there is no routine information, this means that clinical care is not guided by evidence, but by individual clinical experience(s), perceptions, and interests. This can result in inferences about the role of culture; these inferences often take an essentialist and stereotypical perspective on cultural groups, and often conflate race, migrant and ethnic group status, and ignore the separate role of more subtle subcultural and social influences. In the absence of data, cultural values, prejudices and stereotypes abound, and may dominate decision-making around health practice and service development.

There are few resources both for the newly qualified practitioner and the experienced specialist, the undergraduate and postgraduate, and for the practitioner, policy-maker and service manager who all wish to improve their knowledge about culture and mental health care. This textbook aims to address this gap, and to take readers through the stages of evolving their understanding about the role of culture in mental health, wellbeing and about innovation in care practices.

## CULTURE AND MENTAL HEALTH: A BRIEF HISTORY

The term 'culture and mental health care' is used as a generic term to capture this field of study. 'Cultural psychiatry' is sometimes misunderstood to only be of relevance to medically qualified practitioners and psychiatrists; however, we consider that the term is much broader and embraces aspects of mental health care to diverse populations by a diverse workforce, diverse in ethnic and cultural origins and professional training. Therefore, in this textbook, the term cultural psychiatry is also used to reflect a broad subject that encompasses a wide range of mental health care practices, actors and actions which lead to recovery.

A newsletter called *Transcultural Research in Mental Health Problems* (Editorial, 1956) was produced by the Departments of Psychiatry and of Anthropology at McGill University in Canada. This marked the start of a new field within psychiatry called 'transcultural psychiatry', now often called cultural psychiatry. Cultural psychiatry originally had four broad aims (Mead, 1959). First, it would be a framework within which cross-cultural comparisons could be made. Second, it would offer a forum within which the knowledge gained in one part of the world could be made available to other parts of the world. Third, it would provide an overarching institutional framework within which the mental health aspects of various international programmes could be integrated and harmonized. Fourth, it would allow global mental health problems to be considered at a global level, bringing together relevant authorities from around the world.

This textbook addresses these formative ambitions, and emphasizes culture as a subject of interest in its full complexity, rather than only from a positivistic scientific perspective that is removed from the shades of grey and nuances of the everyday lives of people coping with distress and misfortune. Since the beginning of the cultural psychiatry movement, other related subjects have been more openly debated, perhaps taking aspects of cultural psychiatry and developing them for specific audiences and peoples. Thus spiritual psychiatry or religious aspects of mental health care are now acknowledged to be important in the everyday care of people, and in understanding resilience and promoting recovery. A field of study called critical psychiatry has re-emerged to challenge and shape the nature of mental health care, in order to reveal underlying power relationships and potential unhealthy aspects of practice and the organization of services. A significant development is the due emphasis now given to international psychiatry. These fields of enquiry have much to do with cultural psychiatry, and may even have been given impetus by the growth of cultural psychiatry and its challenges to universalistic use of knowledge and technology without due emphasis to cultural contexts. Some aspects of race, ethnicity and culture, as understood by anthropologists and cultural psychiatrists, are not always retained in research studies and publications from international psychiatry. International psychiatry may not easily acknowledge issues such as racism and prejudice, and how these shape therapeutic relationships. Psychiatry, and by inference international psychiatry, without attention to cultural variables that take account of beliefs, attitudes, service users' views and local ethnography of the cultural fabric of societies, risks becoming a psychiatry of other peoples rather than of our people, or a psychiatry of aliens rather than being about the lives of understood people (Tseng, 2001).

## A NEW TEXTBOOK

Cultural psychiatry is now firmly embedded in conventional mental health policy and practice in the UK and USA, Australia and New Zealand, and is growing in influence in other countries and societies around the world (Bains, 2005). Witness to this expansion of interest and recognition is the World Association of Cultural Psychiatrists' inaugural meeting held in Beijing in 2006. This development urges a clearer conceptualization of what constitutes cultural psychiatry and the subject of culture and mental health care.

Our investigations of the relationship between culture and mental health span some 20 years of work at the University of London's Institute of Psychiatry and Centre for Psychiatry at Barts and The London Medical School. When we committed ourselves to this subject in the late 1980s, in the UK at least, cultural or transcultural psychiatry was not a well-known subject. There were few textbooks or guides for clinicians, irrespective of seniority, experience and professional discipline. The few exceptions were textbooks such as *Transcultural Psychiatry* (Cox, 1986), and later *Aliens and Alienists* (Littlewood and Lipsedge, 1987), and *Rethinking Psychiatry: From Cultural Category to Personal Experience* (Kleinman, 1988). Since then, other volumes have been added, for example, *Mental Health Service Provision for a Multicultural Society* (Bhui and Olajide, 1998), the authoritative *Handbook of Cultural Psychiatry* and the *Clinicians' Guide to Cultural Psychiatry* (Tseng, 2001, 2004), and *Cross Cultural Psychiatry: A Practical Guide* (Bhugra and Bhui, 2001).

Cultural psychiatry in the UK and USA has also investigated the role of racism at an individual and institutional level, but not as a public health issue or organizational factor in public services. More specific analyses of racism in mental health care were provided by Fernando (1995; Fernando *et al.*, 1999) and in *Racism and Mental Health* (Bhui, 2002).

These textbooks provide a wealth of learning and knowledge but most are written for specialists, or those with a special interest, or relate to a specific nation, or sets of problems, and do not always embrace policy, service organization and delivery, clinical practice, and illness behaviour in the context of the local cultural fabric of a society. In order to reach a state of preparedness to effectively use such books, there is a need for the evolution of some cultural competency or (cap)ability to understand indigenous or culturally 'emic' perspectives as having virtue and value. As such there is a need to move from culturally destructive, to culture-blind, to culturally competent to culturally proficient cycles of learning, practice and research. There is also a need to understand policy, service organization, workforce and cultural contexts as well as the more focused clinical practice issues between a patient and health professional or a healer and a sufferer.

## CULTURE AND MENTAL HEALTH: A COMPREHENSIVE TEXTBOOK

*Culture and Mental Health: A Comprehensive Textbook* addresses these multiple perspectives. There are two main sections: Part 1: Basic Sciences and Part 2: World Experts.

In the Basic Sciences section leaders in specific fields of study present a summary of the key theories and background literature that is necessary to understand the new and still emerging field that examines the role of culture in the expression and management of mental distress: religious studies, epidemiology, sociology, anthropology, health services research and policy, management studies, philosophy and ethics, legal studies, psychology and psychopathology. There is also an historical account of culture-bound syndromes, the authenticity of which, in the opinion of the editors, has been overemphasized.

The World Experts section presents historical, service development, policy and epidemiological information about local issues of relevance in regions of the world: Russia, East Asia (Hong Kong and China), Africa (Egypt, Ethiopia, Kenya,

Somalia, Nigeria and South Africa), South Asia (India, Pakistan, Bangladesh and Sri Lanka), New Zealand, Australia, the USA and Canada, Latin America, Europe, and the Caribbean Islands.

The juxtaposition of chapters from countries around the world offers a unique opportunity to compare and contrast, synthesize and conceptualize new solutions to improve mental wellbeing. We took a regional approach to ensure that a wide range of countries and peoples from across the globe were included. There are inter-regional and inter-country patterns of similarity and difference, and areas of practice, policy, law and health service provision where comparison can be made.

## BASIC SCIENCES IN CULTURAL PSYCHIATRY

There is now an emphasis on multidisciplinary training, practice and research on the role of culture, race and ethnicity in the genesis and alleviation of distress. This means that a nurse, social worker or psychologist may be a lead clinician. Service users will be working closely with professionals from a wider range of disciplines. Forms of knowledge must span across professional boundaries, and cultural psychiatry must incorporate forms of knowledge from diverse disciplines. The evolution of culture and mental health as a clinical practice, research and policy discipline must embrace other relevant disciplines such as philosophy (Chapter 5), laws (Chapter 7), epidemiology (Chapter 4), sociology (Chapter 3), health services research and policy (Chapter 9), management studies (Chapter 8), psychology and psychopathology (Chapter 10), religious studies (Chapter 6) and anthropology (Chapter 4).

A dated expression of cultural psychiatry is found in textbooks as a list of culture-bound syndromes; these are the only aspect of cultural psychiatry that has entered general psychiatric textbooks and professional examinations. In Chapter 11 Lloyd critiques the notion of culture-bound syndromes, and gives them a more appropriate place in studies of mental health care (Sumathipala *et al.*, 2004). However, we have not given a detailed history of

cultural psychiatry, for which readers are referred to Bains (2005). Bains asserts that the alliance between anthropology and psychiatry was strengthened by the 'prevailing idealism, optimism and the bridging language of psychodynamic theory' (Bains, 2005, p. 144). Psychodynamic and psychotherapeutic models and insights are often invoked in this textbook, but we have not here pursued a comprehensive account of culture and psychotherapy, which is now also becoming a subject area undergoing a re-visioning from theoretical, technical and philosophical positions (see Moodley and Palmer, 2006).

## WORLD EXPERTS

Fukuyama (1992) argues that modernity itself has inflicted a world of multiple post-modern visions, something that becomes evident on reading this volume. Culturally influenced identities, predominantly collective or individual, or traditional or liberal, may be threatened when there is a meeting of diverse religious and cultural groups with different and sometimes conflicting values. Some suggest that war and hostile conflict will diminish with time, and that even where wars now exist, these are a direct consequence of a clash of cultures and identities, and that this is the threat to future prosperity and social cohesion in all societies (Lieber and Weisberg, 2002).

If cultural values do emerge as the only domain of future conflict and negotiation and political action, it is indeed necessary to be equipped with knowledge about cultures, and their influence on wellbeing in a wider sense. The role of understanding culture and mental health care become greater than a health care issue. Indeed, at the time of writing there is overt conflict in the Middle East and in Africa; economic inequity, unequal access to knowledge and political influence and a lack of mutual trust and understanding are argued to contribute. Terrorism itself has been voiced as being born of social and religious exclusion, and conflicts of values and cultures that are not effectively managed with sensitivity, courtesy and deep understanding. Studies of culture and mental health are therefore not only of health care relevance, but unearth social and political issues to which a thoughtful analysis of culture and conflict may contribute (see Bhui, 2002).

The World Experts section attempts to provide a global view to map and enrich the collective understanding of the genesis of mental distress, and how it is shaped and managed in diverse cultural, racial, national and of course global settings. The compilation of chapters from countries is not random, nor exhaustive, but aims to capture the best data available over the world. These chapters illustrate and reveal why nation, race, culture and ethnic group are important variables in mental health practice, policy and research for all populations. Authors were selected on the basis of the existence of data (quantitative and qualitative) for a chosen geographical region, and for the presence of skilled expertise in that region to capture the complexities of the local subject matter from a diverse range of disciplines and theoretical frameworks. The geographical areas chosen illustrate some of the generalities of mental health care in its cultural and cross-cultural context, alongside specific issues of local relevance.

Universalistic assumptions in a book on mental health would enable a tidy, template-driven and comparative statement about each nation as if epidemiological and health service data from each country are indeed comparable in all aspects. Each world expert provides data or universalistic information, where this exists, alongside examples of local ethnography and in-depth analyses of local care priorities. However, each chapter also acts as 'text' in its own right, carrying and conveying sentiments, presumptions, assumptions and the historical, political and health premises that have shaped the current policy and status of mental health care in each country. Readers have to read not only the raw information, but also the nature in which mental health care is discussed, the emphases given to culture, and the historical integration of cultural psychiatry (and psychology, nursing, social work, etc.), with routine practice, research and policy.

Readers will find incisive accounts of tribes, languages, racial groups and cultural settings; indigenous folk categories of illness and diagnosed conditions are compared across continents.

Diverse cultural flux in any land emerges from indigenous and immigrant influences during the histories of each nation. It is clearly not possible to place the 'whole world in a single volume', to represent each and every country, and every language and every tribe or subcultural group; in addition there cannot be a neat symmetry about what information is available for each country, as the epidemiological data, the ethnographic explorations, and availability of mature maps of policy and practice vary from country to country.

In part this variability reflects variation of effort, as well as patchy and inconsistent interest from the global health and social care community; the degree of shared historical, political and colonial interest between any one country and another Western, and often richer and developed country, has also been influential. More information is available from the UK, the USA, New Zealand and Australia, than perhaps from Kenya, South Africa or Nigeria. This division in knowledge about health care economies is gradually being diminished as the World Health Organization, World Psychiatric Association, World Association of Cultural Psychiatry, and other national and international bodies discern and pursue the need for better knowledge and more active management of global mental health.

The pace and commitment to map mental health needs in any one country also varies from country to country due to its allocated priority in relation to other local health and social priorities that face each nation; the variation is also in part influenced by the culturally determined perceptions of what constitutes mental illness. Japan has, for example, given greater credence to the existence of depression since the high suicide rates were noted there. Prior to this depression was not as widely acknowledged and was greatly stigmatized. It is evident that as infectious disease has been better tackled in the developed world, noncommunicable diseases have increased as a cause of mortality. These patterns will be replicated in the developing world as incident infectious disease diminishes. This progress is expected to accompany a reduction in levels of poverty, social exclusion and mortality, with expected increases in quality of life and life expectancy. The HIV epidemic challenges this vision, and is a key priority in many countries, but especially in the developing world. For the developing world, HIV, poverty, and gender and class inequality are relevant to mental health and wellbeing. The challenge for professionals is to address mental health care in diverse cultural contexts, but also to retain the authentic flavour of how cultures are lived at a local level, and not let the issues emerging from local cultures be lost simply because they are not found to be sufficiently relevant in all countries or in a sufficient number of countries. The World Health Organization states that depression will be a major cause of disability and life lost through disability. Ways of coping with depression, engaging local carers, spiritual and religious and complementary sectors of health care, may improve recovery (see Chapters 4, 13, 15, 16 and 18).

There are global trends showing higher suicide rates in young people (Wasserman *et al.*, 2005). Could this be due to the cultural and developmental challenges facing young people (Bhui *et al.*, 2005)? What would a culturally appropriate and sensitive response in each of these countries look like? Cultural transitions and acculturation, something that is often discussed as being of relevance to migrants, is of importance to all cultural groups living in our ever smaller world. Cultural adaptations take place within villages, towns, regions and countries following migration and geographical mobility; however, global migration and mass movement of people from one culture to another challenges health providers in economic and service terms, but also in the philosophical realms: what constitutes mental health care and mental disorder? Writings from New Zealand, South Africa, Hong Kong and Africa, and by Odenwald and van Duijl, Lloyd, Prince and Helman all challenge conventional health professionals' notions of mental disorder, contrasting these professionalized accounts against those from traditional healers and their indigenous healing practices.

Recent critiques and well-conducted studies have demonstrated that interventions that are not expensive are necessary in the developing world, and that, paradoxically, these actually have important implications in the developed world (Araya *et al.*,

2006). Perhaps just as solutions applied to the developing countries need to take account of cultural issues, so do those in the developed world. Indeed, a focus on culture and mental health care in the developing world seems to be facilitating a re-conceptualization of the role of culture in the developed world's health care economies. Tackling the cultural implications for mental health care will, through respectful understanding, (a) ensure more effective take-up of treatment, (b) tackle stigma, (c) reduce inequalities, (d) eradicate institutionalized practices and policies that are actually producing inequalities, and (e) improve recovery technologies. Omitting the cultural variable risks failure of recovery.

We hope the volume inspires practitioners, providers, policy-makers and researchers to progress their learning in this area. There is a need for a textbook that captures principles and practices, offers examples and data where they exist. The best textbooks are read, engage, beguile and excite a reader. We hope readers find the writings as stimulating and thought-provoking as did the editors.

## REFERENCES

Araya, R., Flynn, T., Rojas, G., Fritsch, R. and Simon, G. 2006: Cost-effectiveness of a primary care treatment program for depression in low-income women in Santiago, Chile. *American Journal of Psychiatry* 163, 1379–87.

Bains, J. 2005: Race, culture and psychiatry. A history of transcultural psychiatry. *History of Psychiatry* 16, 139–54.

Bhugra, D. and Bhui, K. 2001: *Cross Cultural Psychiatry: A Practical Guide*. London: Arnold.

Bhui, K. 2002: *Racism and Mental Health*. London: Jessica Kingsley.

Bhui, K. and Olajide, D. 1998: Cultural competence and the law of mental health. In *Mental Health Service Provision for a Multi-Cultural Society*. London: Saunders.

Bhui, K., Stansfeld, S., Head, J., Haines, M., Hillier, S., Taylor, S., Viner, R. and Booy, R. 2005: Cultural identity, acculturation, and mental health among adolescents in east London's multiethnic community. *Journal of Epidemiology and Community Health* 59, 296–302.

Cox, J.L. 1986: *Transcultural Psychiatry*. London: Croom Helm.

Editorial 1956: *Transcultural Research in Mental Health Problems* 1 (April).

Fernando, S. 1995: *Mental Health in a Multi-Ethnic Society.* London: Routledge.

Fernando, S., Ndegwa, D. and Wilson, M. 1999: *Forensic Psychiatry, Race and Culture.* London: Routledge.

Fukuyama, F. 1992: *The End of History and the Last Man.* New York: Free Press.

Karlson, S. and Nazroo, J. 2002: Relation between racial discrimination, social class, and health among ethnic minority groups. *American Journal of Public Health* 9, 624–31.

Kleinman, A. 1988: *Rethinking Psychiatry: From Cultural Category to Personal Experience.* New York: Free Press.

Lieber, R. and Weisberg, R.E. 2002: Globalization, culture and identities in crisis. *International Journal of Politics, Culture, and Society* 16, 273–96.

Littlewood, R. and Lipsedge, M. 1987: *Aliens and Alienists.* London: Routledge.

Mead, M. 1959: Mental health in the world perspective. *Transcultural Research in Mental Health Problems* 6 (July).

Moodley, R. and Palmer, S. 2006: *Race, Culture and Psychotherapy: Critical Perspectives in Multicultural Practice.* London: Routledge.

Sumathipala, A., Siribaddana, S.H. and Bhugra, D. 2004: Culture-bound syndromes: the story of dhat syndrome. *British Journal of Psychiatry* 184, 200–9.

Tseng, W.S. 2001: *Handbook of Cultural Psychiatry.* San Diego: Academic Press.

Tseng, W.S. 2004: *Clinicians' Guide to Cultural Psychiatry.* San Diego: Academic Press.

Wasserman, D., Cheng, Q. and Jiang, G.X. 2005: Global suicide rates among young people aged 15–19. *World Psychiatry* 4, 114–20.

# BASIC SCIENCES

# Anthropology and its contributions

## Cecil G Helman

## WHAT IS ANTHROPOLOGY?

Anthropology is one of the building blocks of modern cultural psychiatry. From the Greek word meaning 'the study of man', it has been described in the *British Medical Journal* as 'the most scientific of the humanities and the most humane of the sciences' (Editorial, 1980). Its aim is the holistic study of humankind – its origins, religions, economies, social and political organizations, languages, artefacts and art. Modern anthropology has several branches (Keesing and Strathern, 1998). Physical anthropology, or human biology, is the study of the evolution of the human species, and of the reasons for the diversity of present-day human populations. It utilizes the techniques of archaeology, palaeontology, serology and studies of primate behaviour and ecology, to understand human pre-history. Material culture deals with the physical artefacts of humanity, both present and past, and includes studies of the arts, agricultural implements, musical instruments, weapons, clothing and tools of different populations, and all other forms of technology they use to control, exploit and enhance their social or natural environments. Social and cultural anthropology both deal with the comparative study of present-day human societies, but there are differences in emphasis between these two approaches. In the UK the dominant approach is social anthropology, which emphasizes the social dimensions of human life. It sees people as social animals, organized into groups that regulate and perpetuate themselves, and thus it is a person's experience as a member of society that shapes his or her view of the world. In this perspective 'culture' is seen as one of the ways that human beings organize and legitimize their society, and provides the basis for its social, political and economic organization. In the USA, by contrast, cultural anthropology focuses more on the systems of symbols, meanings and ideas that comprise a culture, and of which social organization is just an expression. In practice, these transatlantic differences in emphasis provide valuable and complementary perspectives on two central issues – society and culture. That is, the ways that human groups organize themselves, and the ways that they view the world that they inhabit.

## MEDICAL ANTHROPOLOGY

Medical anthropology has emerged over the past 30 years as one of the most important subfields of anthropology, and the one most directly relevant to cultural psychiatry. It can be defined as:

> *The study of how people in different cultures and social groups explain the causes of ill-health, the types of treatment they believe in, and to whom they turn if they do get ill. It is also the study of how these beliefs and behaviours relate to biological, psychological and social changes in the human organism – in both health and disease. It is the study of human suffering, and the steps that people take to explain and relieve that suffering.*
>
> (Helman, 2007)

Medical anthropology therefore focuses on how cultural and social realities can shape the clinical presentation, recognition and treatment of different forms of illness – both mental and physical (Kleinman, 1980; Johnson and Sargent, 1991; Hahn, 1995; Swartz, 1998). In doing so, it tries to answer the 'Why?' questions, such as: 'Why are types of behaviour regarded as "bad" in one society, regarded as "mad" in another?' 'Why are behaviours regarded as "mental illness" in one group, seen as "normal" in another?' 'Why do definitions of "normality" and "abnormality" differ so widely between human populations?' 'Why do some religious (or ethnic) groups have higher levels of alcohol (or drug) use, than others?' 'Why are some forms of mental illness brought to doctors, but others to priests or traditional healers?' 'Why do some psychiatric conditions seem to be more "culture-bound", while others seem relatively "culture-free"?'

Cross-cultural psychiatry can be regarded as one of the most important components of medical anthropology. In its early years it owed its main conceptual and comparative approach to anthropology (two of the founders of British anthropology, WH Rivers and CG Seligman, were both psychiatrists), and particularly to its notions of the role of culture and social context in understanding human behaviour. As Kleinman (1988) puts it:

> *Of all the medical specialities, I contend, psychiatry has the most pervasive relationship to culture. Psychiatry is, to begin with, a window on a culture's sources of distress and on the human consequences of such distress. . . . The psychiatrist experiences, moreover, in his own professional identity, the fears and stigma that attach to serious mental illness. His diagnostic criteria are infiltrated with cultural norms and biases. His treatment is founded on the very apparatus of culture – words, symbols, meanings, not least of all his own social persona and charisma.*

This suggests that psychiatry itself is not 'culture-free'. Like other forms of medicine, it is the product of a particular time, place and social context. Furthermore, it is shaped by – and expresses – many of the underlying concepts, values and prejudices of that context, such as social, economic, gender or ethnic inequalities – including racism (Littlewood and Lipsedge, 1989). In many cases, psychiatric diagnoses are not purely objective and scientific, but can be influenced by the cultural, social and political context in which they take place (Wing, 1978; Pichot, 1982; Merskey and Shafran, 1986).

## THE CONCEPT OF 'CULTURE'

As well as its comparative approach, anthropology has contributed the useful concept of culture, though anthropologists have defined it in different ways. For cultural psychiatry, Keesing and Strathern's (1998) definition is particularly useful. It stresses the ideational aspect of culture, whereby cultures comprise: 'systems of shared ideas, systems of concepts and rules and meanings that underlie and are expressed in the ways that human beings live'. Without such a shared perception of the world, therefore, both the cohesion and continuity of any human group would be impossible.

Culture can thus be seen as a set of guidelines – both explicit and implicit – that individuals inherit as members of a particular human group, and which tell them how to view the world, how to experience it emotionally, and how to behave in it in relation to other people, to supernatural forces or gods and to the natural environment. It also provides them with a way of transmitting these guidelines to the next generation, by the use of language, symbols, art and ritual. To some extent, culture thus can be seen as an inherited 'lens' through which individuals perceive and understand the world that they inhabit and learn how to live within it (Helman, 2001).

Growing up within any society is a form of enculturation, whereby the individual slowly acquires the cultural 'lens' of that society. Immigrants or newcomers to a society may undergo a process of acculturation, whereby they gradually acquire some or all of the cultural beliefs and behaviours of their new environment. In an increasingly diverse and mobile world, therefore, many individuals may perceive themselves as having more than one cultural identity – depending on the context in which they find themselves.

Although useful, the concept of culture has often been misunderstood, or even misused. It has been used to stereotype groups and individuals as notional 'cultural types', and also used as a form of 'victim-blaming' – providing a false explanation for inequalities in health status, which are really due to ethnic or religious discrimination. Culture must always be seen in a particular context of time, place and local circumstances – for it is never the only determinant of human beliefs, behaviours and social organizations. Other important determinants are: individual factors – such as personal idiosyncrasy, personality or experience; social and economic factors – such as poverty, racism, unemployment, bad housing, social isolation or immigrant status; educational factors – both formal and informal, including education into a religious or ethnic tradition; and environmental factors – both physical and social – such as weather, population density, rural or urban habitat, and natural disasters, as well the types of health care facilities available. In recent years, the focus has shifted towards an understanding that 'pure' culture cannot exist apart from a particular context. Increasing emphasis has thus been placed on the role of structural factors – such as economic inequality, poverty, gender and power relationships, racism and other forms of discrimination – in shaping health-related beliefs and behaviours.

## RESEARCH METHODOLOGIES

The most unique research method of anthropology is fieldwork or ethnography. This usually involves highly detailed studies of a particular group or community, usually carried out over several months or years. Usually the researcher lives full-time within that group, taking part in their daily activities, and closely observing them, in order to understand how they see the world, and how and why they organize their lives in particular ways. An example of this type of ethnography is Goffman's detailed ethnography of a British psychiatric hospital (1961). In each case the ethnographer should approach the research with an open mind, and with as few preconceptions as possible (Peacock, 1986). Peacock concedes, therefore, that the very presence of the ethnographer may have some influence on the actual phenomena under study.

Such in-depth local studies can reveal differences between what people say they believe or do, and what they actually do in practice – and explain the reasons for these discrepancies. They can also illustrate how health policy formulated at the national (or international) level – for example, a national AIDS prevention programme – may have its efficacy reduced at the local level by the political, economic and gender realities in that village or community (Lyttleton, 1994).

As ethnography was developed mainly among non-literate people, instead of relying on written replies to questionnaires, anthropologists have 'fallen back on human powers, to learn, understand and communicate. . . [and] avoided many of the devices that spuriously objectify human encounters' (Keesing and Strathern, 1998). Anthropology has recognized, therefore, that not everything can be measured, or converted into numbers – and this insight is especially important in understanding and describing phenomena that cannot easily be quantified: such as myths, rituals, religious practices, belief systems, body image and the meanings that people give to human suffering and disease: particularly how they answer questions such as 'Why has it happened to *me*?', 'Why *now*?', or even: 'Who has done this to me?' Despite this, anthropologists do not only collect qualitative data.

Many also collect more quantitative data such as population censuses, genealogies, infant mortality rates, crop output or levels of caloric intake.

More recently, medical anthropology has utilized a whole new set of research methodologies, many of them borrowed from psychology, sociology, cultural studies or even literary criticism. They include the use of focus groups, narrative analysis, pile sorting and rank ordering methods, videotapes, open-ended questionnaires, rapid ethnographic assessment techniques and computer analyses of the data generated by these methods (Helman, 2007).

## ANTHROPOLOGY AND CULTURAL PSYCHIATRY

For cultural psychiatry, anthropology has the advantage of being a comparative discipline. It offers a detailed database of in-depth studies of a wide range of local communities, in many parts of the world, which can then be compared and contrasted in order to understand what patterns of human behaviour are universal, and what patterns are unique and shaped by local social or cultural conditions. This comparative approach can illustrate, for example, how (and why) definitions of 'normality' and 'abnormality' vary so widely cross-culturally. They can also show how variations in the definition of mental illness vary considerably, but how there is often wide cross-cultural agreement on the major psychoses, and on what types of behaviours are universally seen as 'mad' (Edgerton, 1977) – though often less agreement on the significance of more moderate conditions, such as neuroses or personality disorders (Littlewood, 1990).

Anthropology also sheds light on the role of social and cultural factors in the aetiology of certain mental illnesses; on clinical presentations such as somatization (Kirmayer and Young, 1998); and on the ways that these illnesses are recognized, labelled, explained and treated by members of a particular society (Swartz, 1998). The concept of culture-bound psychiatric disorders is especially useful (Simons and Hughes, 1985). These are a group of psycho-social syndromes, each of which

is unique to a particular group of people, geographical area or culture. However, as cultures are rarely homogeneous, and local contexts often play a greater role in producing and shaping these conditions, they should more accurately be described as context-bound psychiatric disorders. Each of them is a specific cluster of symptoms, signs or behavioural changes recognized by members of a particular group and responded to in a standardized way. They usually have a range of symbolic meanings, moral, social or psychological, for both the victims and those around them, and can link that victim's case to wider social concerns, including their relationships with other people, with supernatural forces, or with the natural environment. In some cases they play an important role in expressing and resolving both antisocial emotions and social conflicts in a culturally patterned way. However, some anthropologists have criticized this model of culture-bound disorders. Hahn (1995), for example, does not see them as a unique class of syndromes because, to some extent, all syndromes are 'culture-bound'. Furthermore, the term overemphasizes the role of 'culture' (while ignoring social, economic and biological factors), and has also mostly been applied to syndromes from 'exotic', non-Western communities, rather than to those from the industrialized world. Despite these reservations, most medical anthropologists would see a value of this diagnostic category, provided that the roles of social and economic context are also taken into account.

## LIMITATIONS OF ANTHROPOLOGY

Although it has many useful applications for cultural psychiatry, anthropology also has certain limitations. These include:

- Anthropological knowledge may be too local, and too focused on a particular small community – especially in the non-industrialized world – to provide a basis for valid generalizations.
- Traditional anthropological studies have mostly been carried out in small, rural communities in poorer countries – leaving more urban or

industrial societies in the West to be studied by sociology, social psychology and cultural studies (though this is now changing) – and this may make them less relevant to some cultural psychiatrists.

* Many anthropologists studying mental illness may not be *au fait* with recent developments in genetics, physiology, psychopharmacology, psychology and epidemiology – and their relevance to modern psychiatry.
* The long duration of traditional ethnography (often up to 2–3 years), followed by a lengthy analysis of the data, can make changes to mental health policy based on this ethnographic data impractical.
* Many traditional ethnographies still lack a historical perspective, and present the societies they study as essentially static, unchanging and bound to 'traditions' – especially if those societies are illiterate, and without any written history of their own. (Increasingly, though, modern anthropology now focuses on social change, the effects of globalization on local communities and phenomena such as migration and urbanization.)
* Like other social sciences, anthropology is essentially the study of groups, rather than of individuals – and its conclusions may therefore not be applicable to individual patients.
* Among some anthropologists there is a rather low tolerance of any 'applied' offshoots of their discipline, such as cultural psychiatry, and they prefer to focus on more theoretical debates within their own subject, rather than on its practical applications.

## REFERENCES

Edgerton, R.B. 1977: Conceptions of psychosis in four East African societies. In Landy, D. (ed.) *Culture, Disease and Healing: Studies in Medical Anthropology*. New York: Macmillan, 358–67.

Editorial 1980: More anthropology and less sleep for medical students. *British Medical Journal* 281, 1662.

Goffman, E. 1961: *Asylums*. Harmondsworth: Penguin.

Hahn, R.A. 1995: *Sickness and Healing: An Anthropological Perspective*. New Haven, CT: Yale University Press, 40–56.

Helman, C.G. 2007: *Culture, Health and Illness* (5th edn). London: Hodder Arnold, 1–18, 456–66.

Johnson, T.M. and Sargent, C.F. (eds) 1991: *Medical Anthropology*. New York: Praeger.

Keesing, R.M. and Strathern, A.J. 1998: *Cultural Anthropology: A Contemporary Perspective* (3rd edn). Fort Worth, TX: Harcourt Brace, 2–25.

Kleinman, A. 1980: *Patients and Healers in the Context of Culture*. Berkeley, CA: University of California Press.

Kleinman, A. 1988: *Rethinking Psychiatry*. New York: Free Press, 182–83.

Kirmayer, L.J. and Young, A. 1998: Culture and somatization: clinical, epidemiological, and ethnographic perspectives. *Psychosomatic Medicine* 60, 420–30.

Littlewood, R. 1990: From categories to contexts: a decade of the new cross-cultural psychiatry. *British Journal of Psychiatry* 156, 308–27.

Littlewood, R. and Lipsedge, M. 1989: *Aliens and Alienists* (2nd edn). London: Unwin Hyman.

Lyttleton, C. 1994: Knowledge and meaning: the AIDS education campaign in rural northeast Thailand. *Social Science and Medicine* 38, 135–46.

Merskey, H. and Shafran, B. 1986: Political hazards in the diagnosis of 'sluggish schizophrenia'. *British Journal of Psychiatry* 148, 247–56.

Peacock, J.L. 1986: *The Anthropological Lens*. Cambridge: Cambridge University Press.

Pichot, P. 1982: The diagnosis and classification of mental disorders in French-speaking countries: background, current views and comparison with other nomenclatures. *Psychological Medicine* 12, 475–92.

Simons, R.C. and Hughes, C.C. 1985: *The Culture-Bound Syndromes*. Dordrecht: Reidel.

Swartz, L. 1998: *Culture and Mental Health: A Southern African View*. Cape Town: Oxford University Press.

Wing, J.K. 1978: *Reasoning about Madness*, Oxford: Oxford University Press, 167–93.

# 3

# Sociology of health and illness

Karen Iley and James Nazroo

## INTRODUCTION

This chapter will consider how sociology has influenced and contributed to the critical debates in the study of mental health and illness. A number of sociological perspectives will be explored and considered in relation to aspects of mental health, including work developed from social interactionist perspectives, the critique of medicalization and social constructionism. Sociology has also made a major contribution to our understanding of ethnicity and culture (Modood *et al.*, 1997; Bulmer and Solomos, 1999) and ethnicity and mental health (Nazroo, 1997; Iley and Nazroo, 2001).

Mental health is an area of medicine that has long been associated with a number of controversies, such as the system of treatment and care within asylums and, more recently, the impact of community care (Pilgrim and Rogers, 1999). Issues such as how society views mental illness and the role of health professionals in defining and managing mental illness remain topical. Sociologists' interest in mental health was triggered and framed by the rise of the anti-psychiatry movement in the 1950s, which challenged the beliefs and methods of treatment used by psychiatrists.

The sociological perspectives presented in this chapter have their origins in this era, but nevertheless continue to influence health care professionals who come into contact with those with mental health problems.

## INTERACTIONIST APPROACHES: DEVIANCE, LABELLING AND STIGMA

Symbolic interactionism is a sociological perspective that considers how individuals use, and reproduce, socially created symbols as a resource to manage their interactions with each other. The main strands in this perspective are how individuals use symbols of what they mean to convey in communication with one another and the effects these symbols have on the behaviour of people during a social interaction (Jones, 2003). In the context of mental health and psychiatry, the concepts of deviance, labelling and stigma are examples of where this sociological perspective has been particularly productive.

Deviance can be described as 'non conformity to a norm, or set of norms, which is accepted by a significant proportion of local citizens or inhabitants' (Scambler, 2003). Therefore defining deviant behaviour can be problematic as it depends on what a particular society considers to be unacceptable; what is deviant behaviour will vary across context and time. In his classic work Lemert (1967) proposed that deviance consisted of two elements: primary deviance and secondary deviance. Primary deviance concerns the attribute or behaviour that is deemed within a particular context to be deviant. Secondary deviance is concerned with how assignment into a deviant status has consequences for subsequent social interactions, behaviour and attitudes; consequences that follow from the symbolic meanings associated with the primary deviant status. Take, for example, how the assignment of a behaviour as deviant and being schizophrenic impacts on the social interactions of those with that behaviour as a consequence of the symbolic meanings it carries.

Secondary deviance typically flows from the application of a symbolically laden label to primary deviance. Labelling theory is concerned with this process: how society labels individuals on the basis of the behaviour they exhibit and the consequences of such labelling. According to Becker (1963), a label defines an individual as a particular kind of person. The label is not neutral; it contains an evaluation of the person it is applied to. And if sufficiently powerful, the label can become a 'master-status' for the individual, who in most situations is viewed and responded to in terms of the label rather than anything else, including the assumption that the individual has all of the negative characteristics normally associated with such labels. For example, the assignment of a label might mean that an individual's behaviour is judged first as a consequence of mental illness, and he or she is considered as mentally ill, rather than considering other factors. This may produce what Becker (1963) describes as a 'self-fulfilling prophecy', which is where the deviant identification becomes the controlling one. Becker describes this process as occurring in a number of possible stages, including the definition of the individual and predictions or prophecies being made about the individual's behaviour. Interactions with the individual are then made on the basis of these prophecies and the individual's actions are interpreted within the context of what others expect of him or her and, in this way, the prophecy is fulfilled. Becker suggests that this leads to the deviant person developing 'deviant routines' out of necessity and that the deviant career is complete when the individual joins an organized deviant group.

Scheff (1966) claimed that labelling was the most important cause of mental illness. He argued that there exists a residue of odd, eccentric and unusual behaviour that does not fit into the norms of a society. Scheff suggested that most psychiatric symptoms can be categorized as instances of residual deviance. By this he meant that some types of behaviour are viewed as deviant, because they are labelled or categorized by society. There also exists a cultural stereotype of mental illness in that when such deviant or unacceptable behaviour is exhibited in a public place, the cultural stereotype of insanity becomes the guiding imagery for action. Therefore the person is taken or sent to a psychiatric unit by either a doctor or the police for diagnosis, treatment and management. Secondary deviance inevitably follows. Scheff clearly saw psychiatrists as those who labelled individuals as mentally ill. Another example of the impact of the labels allocated by psychiatrists was given by Rosenhan (1973), who undertook a study where a number of health care professionals gained admission to a psychiatric unit by displaying behaviours such as hearing voices. Once admitted, they ceased to complain of any symptoms and asked to go home, but they were all diagnosed with either schizophrenia or manic depression and were treated for up to seven weeks as inpatients before being discharged back into the community.

Closely related to the concept of deviance is that of stigma. The notion of stigma also introduces a role for the public and lay perceptions of normality and deviance as a major driver for labelling. This is particularly important in cross-cultural settings where the norms of one social group may be imposed on another, and mismatches will then attract a deviance label. Stigma is identified by Goffman (1963) as consisting of three different types: stigmas of the body, such as deformities or blemishes; stigmas of character, such as mental illness or being a criminal; and stigmas attached to social collectivities, such as tribal or racial. Goffman (1963) stressed that all of these types of stigma were socially, culturally and historically variable. Stigmatizing conditions vary in terms of their visibility and obtrusiveness and thereby in the extent to which they are recognized by others. Where stigma is immediately apparent, Goffman described the individual as being 'discredited'. Those with a discredited stigma, such as blindness or visible scarring, often find that they have to cope with situations made awkward by their stigma, something Goffman refers to as 'managing tension'. In contrast, Goffman describes those who have a stigma that may be apparent only occasionally as the 'discreditable'. For example, a person with schizophrenia may have infrequent episodes of changes in their behaviour, a fact that is known to only a few people. The 'discreditable' group usually find they have to 'manage information' to pass as 'normal' or to censor what others know about them. Here, of course, the process of labelling is significant and, in relation to mental illness, Goffman believed that the family, psychiatrists and the 'total institution' (meaning the hospital and systems of care) were responsible for applying the label.

Similarly, research by Scambler and Hopkins (1986) extended this theory further. They found in their study of epilepsy that individuals tended to conceal their epilepsy whenever possible because of their fear of discrimination. In relation to this, Scambler and Hopkins (1986) were able to make a distinction between felt stigma and enacted stigma. Felt stigma refers to the shame associated with being epileptic, for example, and the fear of being discriminated against solely on the grounds of an implied cultural inferiority or unacceptability. Enacted stigma is the actual discrimination shown to individuals. Scambler (1989) developed this theory further to include a 'hidden distress model' in which those with epilepsy do their utmost to conceal their felt stigma. He concluded that this process was actually more disruptive to the individual's wellbeing and life than enacted stigma, which was rarely experienced.

Although it has been suggested that the concepts of labelling and stigma are dated (Pilgrim and Rogers, 1999), the body of work around deviance, labelling and stigma remains of great relevance. The media continue to portray individuals in a particular way (Coppock and Hopton, 2000), which both affects and reflects the way they are viewed by health professionals as well as society. Indeed, in their study of the use of medication by mentally ill patients in the community, Rogers et al. (1998) found that patients chose not to disclose their illness to others in case they were seen as dangerous or violent and to avoid discrimination. An understanding of stigma, deviance and labelling should extend our understanding of the impact of a diagnosis of mental illness and how individuals with mental health problems are viewed. People from minority ethnic, racial and religious groups already fear ill treatment or discredited treatment within institutionally racist public services. Their skin colour, religious practices and beliefs, and any visible markers of their minority status can compound the stigma associated with having a mental illness. The cumulative effect is that they have to manage more tension and this can have health consequences.

## MEDICALIZATION

Whereas labelling and stigma consider how society views the individual, medicalization is concerned with how doctors use the diagnosis of an illness as a method of social control. Medicalization has been explored in a number of clinical specialisms, including mental illness. Zola (1972) and others, such as Freidson (1970), argued that social life had increasingly been viewed as within the remit of medicine, and social problems as diseases, and therefore had become medicalized. The process occurs once a disease category covering certain social problems is developed, thereby allowing doctors to diagnose those exhibiting these problems as suffering from an illness or disease. From this point, individuals are viewed in terms of their illness and are regarded as (having) a problem to be dealt with by medical treatments (Szasz, 1961). There are many examples of how social problems have been defined in terms of mental illness, both historically, such as homosexuality, and in contemporary medical practice, such as post-traumatic stress disorder. A dimension that has been omitted from these classic papers is the cultural dimension, whereby certain societies and religious and cultural beliefs associated with those societies may label certain behaviours as deviant or as pathology; for example, homosexuality and gender, which vary between Muslim and non-Muslim countries. Owing to the authority and power ascribed to the medical profession by the state, medicalization has the potential to be used in the service of sustaining cultural beliefs and values, and ensuring conformity.

Ivan Illich (1975) took medicalization a step further and described doctors as being a 'major threat to health', creating 'iatrogenesis'. He believed that doctors created a dependency which removed a lot of the individual's control over life and reduced the autonomy that people had in managing their own health. Illich also suggested that iatrogenesis caused harm instead of improving people's health because of the side-effects of medical treatments prescribed by doctors. An example of this in mental health is the ever increasing reliance on medication to control mental health problems, instead of using alternatives such as psychotherapy, even though many drugs have unpleasant long-term side-effects (Pilgrim and Rogers, 1999).

Although this description of medicalization is helpful in considering the role of medicine in controlling individuals and maintaining social order in society, it contains an assumption that society continues to have an uncritical acceptance of medical knowledge. In contrast, Williams and Calnan (1996) have suggested that the general public are more critical and more aware of the risks, as well as the benefits, of medical interventions. They show how patients are less accepting of medical expertise than they have been and that doctors must prove themselves to maintain their position as experts of medicine. Within the field of mental health, this can be seen in the actions of mental health charities and patient groups.

## SOCIAL CONSTRUCTIONISM

Closely related to discussions of medicalization is the understanding offered by the social constructionist critique of the power of medical knowledge and practitioners. This sociological perspective is influenced by a relativist view of the world, one which considers knowledge to not be universal and that there is more than one truth, with knowledge only capable of being assessed against criteria set in specific cultures, periods and social conditions. From this perspective, assumptions about truth and knowledge should be challenged. Social constructionism thus provides an opportunity to examine the creation of biomedical knowledge and to challenge the assumptions made by doctors, especially psychiatrists. It has also enabled a shift towards acknowledging that the creation of medical knowledge is a political rather than technically neutral enterprise. Wright and Treacher (1982) describe social constructionists as those who:

> begin by taking as problematic the very issues which appeared to be self-evident and uninteresting to the earlier writers. They, therefore, insist on enquiring how it should be that certain areas of human life come or cease to be regarded as medical in particular historical circumstances.

In other words, medical knowledge is problematic and its creation and the form it takes becomes the central issue to be investigated. Scambler (2003) describes the social constructionist view as being: 'marked by an interest in how health and illness are created and understood by society and social processes, rather than seeking to find a biological basis for them'. This is in contrast to a common belief within society that medical knowledge is the only true and valid knowledge about health, illness and disease.

Within the social constructionist perspective there are a number of themes identified (Bury, 1986). However, three relevant themes will be considered here: the problematization of reality; the social creation of medical 'facts'; and the mediation of social relations through medical knowledge (Bury, 1986). The first theme is concerned with how it is that objects of medical science are not what they appear to be. The human body and disease are seen as inventions, rather than discoveries, and this means that they exist only because of medical tests proposed by doctors, as these tests simply prove what doctors already believe is true.

The second theme considers the social creation of medical 'facts', which are demonstrated to medical students who are trained to see and interpret what they are looking at. This theme is based upon the ideas of Foucault (1976). He considered the development of the clinic as a base for medical training by doctors in the eighteenth century. The clinic allowed them to study and develop their expertise of the body and illnesses using large numbers of people who could be observed and studied in one place. As a result of this, Foucault suggested that a catalogue of clearly defined diseases replaced the 'sick man' approach to medicine during this period of time and, importantly, argued that this knowledge was a product of this (historically located) process, rather than a reflection of some more universal truth.

The third theme is also based upon the ideas of Foucault (1976) and was further developed by Armstrong (1987), who considers how medical knowledge is used to mediate social relations. Armstrong discussed how medical techniques were important expressions of medical power and claimed that procedures such as using a stethoscope served a purpose to de-humanize patients, so to render them quiet, passive and co-operative in their relationship with the doctor. Through this process the patient became an object of study, which enabled a very personal encounter to become depersonalized. Armstrong suggested that the physical examination of the patient enabled this process further as the patient is reduced to being a body that can be manipulated and its clinical signs and symptoms compared with what the 'expert' knows about normal anatomy and physiology. This process is reinforced by the growth of medical technology which supports the doctor's decision-making, reinforcing the scientific status of medicine, and maintains the powerful position of the doctor.

Although social constructionism provides a useful perspective on how individuals are affected by their interactions with doctors and health care, a number of criticisms of this perspective have been made (Bury, 1986). These include that it does not fully acknowledge the real impact and experience of illness. Bury suggests that how knowledge of the diseased body is gained or developed does not matter, because sickness, pain and disability remain real for those who suffer them. Bury also claims that the social constructionist view sidesteps the recognition of medical advances and does not acknowledge how medical knowledge and interventions have impacted (positively) on the quality of modern life. A final, more fundamental criticism (from a number made by Bury) concerns the relativist perspective of social constructionism. However, as the relativist viewpoint holds that there is no one truth and that knowledge is only capable of being assessed against measures set in specific cultures, times and social conditions, it may be useful when considering how those from ethnic groups or cultural locations that are different from Western psychiatry may experience mental illness in ways that are in conflict with modern psychiatric knowledge and practice. This is a theme that has been developed by a number of cross-cultural psychiatrists (Kleinman, 1987; Littlewood, 1992; Jadhav, 1996).

## SOCIOLOGY OF ETHNICITY AND CULTURE

Sociological approaches to ethnicity have been concerned with understanding how ethnicity relates both to social structures and to social relationships and identities. In this, sociology has attempted to provide a sensitive and contextual understanding of ethnicity, rather than resort to explanations based on stereotypes. Much of this work has demonstrated the social and economic inequalities faced by ethnic minority people (Modood et al., 1997; Mason, 2003) and how economic inequalities and racism relate to ethnic inequalities in physical and mental health (Nazroo, 2001, 2003; Karlsen and Nazroo, 2002). In addition, within the sociological literature many writers place importance on the notion of ethnicity as an identity that reflects self-identification with cultural traditions that provide both meaning and boundaries between groups. So, although there is strong evidence to show that socioeconomic disadvantage contributes to ethnic inequalities in health, it is suggested that there remains a cultural comonent to ethnicity that could play a major defining role

(Smaje, 1996), and explain ethnic inequalities that are not socio-economically determined.

When considering the relationship between culture, ethnicity and mental health, however, it is vital to avoid reducing ethnic differences in mental health down to stereotyped notions of fixed cultural or biological difference (Iley and Nazroo, 2001). Not surprisingly, the sociological focus on ethnicity as identity has mirrored the anti-essentialism found in work on identity more generally (Modood, 1998). So, although ethnicity is considered to reflect identification with sets of shared values, beliefs, customs and lifestyles, it has to be understood dynamically, as an active social process (Smaje, 1996). In particular, the influence of an ethnic identity on individuals and their health depends on the wider context in which that identity is lived.

It is informative to see how decontextualized, stereotyped notions of South Asian communities have been mobilized in markedly different ways to explain both low and high rates of different and sometimes the same illness. It has been suggested that the overall lower rates of mental illness among South Asian people could be a consequence of a strong and protective Asian culture, which provides extended and strong communities with protective social support networks (Cochrane and Bal, 1989). In contrast, in the attempt to explain the high mortality rates of suicide among young women born in South Asia and living in the UK, South Asian communities are portrayed as constraining, demanding and conflictual, rather than supportive and cohesive, and so contributing to the high suicide rates (Merrill and Owens, 1986; Soni Raleigh and Balarajan, 1992).

Of course, these stereotypes will not hold when closely examined. Culture is seized upon to explain such findings rather than more plausible explanations such as a lack of access to appropriate care and different illness expressions being perceived as a lower rate of mental illness; similarly, among those with suicidal ideas, interpersonal conflicts are inevitable and perhaps a cause of self-harming behaviours rather than 'culture' being a central and unique determinant of self-harm behaviour and suicidal ideas. For example, despite the focus on patriarchal South Asian families, there

are, in fact, great similarities between the motives of white and South Asian patients for their suicidal actions (Handy et al., 1991). Indeed, a study of coroners' reports on actual suicides in London found that only one-third of the 12 South Asian women who had committed suicide had 'family conflict' cited among the reasons for the suicide, and only by stretching the imagination could these be considered as specific to South Asian cultures (Karmi et al., 1994). So, although it is worth considering how culture informs our understanding of ethnic minority people and their experiences of illness, it is necessary to question the stereotypes we use and to understand ethnic identities as dynamic and dependent on context.

## CONCLUSION

In this chapter we have summarized the main sociological perspectives that have been applied to the study of ethnicity and of mental health and illness. This has included: the contribution of symbolic interactionism to our understanding of deviance, labelling and stigma; the critique offered by medicalization; how social constructionism has contributed to our understanding of the historical and contextual nature of medical knowledge and the forces that have shaped its creation; and how considering the structural and cultural dimensions of ethnicity can add to our understanding of mental illness. These issues remain pertinent, as shown by contemporary discussions of the impact of being labelled with a mental illness (Department of Health, 1999) and of the potential impact of the proposed revisions in mental health legislation in the UK (Department of Health, 2004). The proposed legislation is now not going to be implemented in its full form. It had extended the scope of medical surveillance to enable the detainment of people who had no clearly identified treatable mental illness. A race impact assessment of the proposed legislation (a legal requirement) had not taken place, and it is highly likely that had the legislation been introduced it would have risked an even greater overrepresentation of black and minority ethnic people within mental health care.

Therefore, sociology, alongside other basic sciences such as anthropology and epidemiology, will continue to contribute a critical and relevant perspective from which the impact of mental health and illness upon individuals and society, and ethnic variations in this, can be explored and explained.

# REFERENCES

Armstrong, D. 1987: Bodies of knowledge: Foucault and the problem of human anatomy. In Scambler G. (ed) *Sociological Theory and Medical Sociology*. London: Tavistock, 59–76.

Becker, H. 1963: *Outsiders: Studies in the Sociology of Deviance*. New York. Free Press.

Bulmer, M. and Solomos, J. 1999: *Racism*. Oxford: Oxford University Press.

Bury, M. 1986: Social constructionism and the development of medical sociology. *Sociology of Health and Illness* 8, 137–69.

Cochrane, R. and Bal, S.S. 1989: Mental hospital admission rates of immigrants to England: a comparison of 1971 and 1981. *Social Psychiatry and Psychiatric Epidemiology* 24, 2–11.

Coppock, V. and Hopton, J. 2000: *Critical Perspectives on Mental Health*. London: Routledge.

Department of Health 1999: *National Service Framework for Mental Health – Modern Standards and Service Models*. London: The Stationery Office.

Department of Health 2004: *Draft Mental Health Bill*. London. The Stationery Office.

Foucault, M. 1976: *Birth of the Clinic: An Archaeology of Medical Perception*. London: Tavistock.

Freidson, E. 1970: *Professional Dominance: The Social Structure of Medical Care*. Chicago: Aldine.

Goffman, E. 1963: *Stigma: Notes on the Management of Spoiled Identity*. Harmondsworth: Penguin.

Handy, S., Chithiramohan, R.N., Ballard, C.G. and Silveira, W.R. 1991: Ethnic differences in adolescent self-poisoning: a comparison of Asian and Caucasian groups. *Journal of Adolescence* 14, 157–62.

Iley, K. and Nazroo, J.Y. 2001: Ethnic inequalities in mental health: a critical examination of the evidence. In Culley L. and Dyson, S. (eds) *Sociology, Ethnicity and Nursing Practice*. Basingstoke: Palgrave, 67–89.

Illich, I. 1975: *Limits to Medicine*. Harmondsworth: Penguin.

Jadhav, S. 1996: The cultural origins of Western depression. *International Journal of Social Psychiatry* 42, 269–86.

Jones, P. 2003: *Introducing Social Theory*. Oxford: Polity Press.

Karlsen, S. and Nazroo, J.Y. 2002: The relationship between racial discrimination, social class and health among ethnic minority groups. *American Journal of Public Health* 92, 624–31.

Karmi, G., Abdulrahim, D., Pierpoint, T. and McKeigue, P. 1994: *Suicide among Ethnic Minorities and Refugees in the United Kingdom*. London: NE & NW Thames RHA.

Kleinman, A. 1987: Anthropology and psychiatry: the role of culture in cross-cultural research on illness. *British Journal of Psychiatry* 151, 447–54.

Lemert, E. 1967: *Human Deviance, Social Problems and Social Control*. Englewood Cliffs: Prentice-Hall.

Littlewood, R. 1992: Psychiatric diagnosis and racial bias: empirical and interpretative approaches. *Social Science and Medicine* 34, 141–49.

Mason, D. 2003: *Explaining Ethnic Differences: Changing Patterns of Disadvantage in Britain*. Bristol: The Policy Press.

Merrill, J. and Owens, J. 1986: Ethnic differences in self-poisoning: a comparison of Asian and white groups. *British Journal of Psychiatry* 148: 708–12.

Modood, T. 1998: Anti-essentialism, multiculturalism and the 'recognition' of religious groups. *Journal of Political Philosophy* 6, 378–99.

Modood, T., Berthoud, R., Lakey, J., Nazroo, J., Smith, P., Virdee, S. and Beishon, S. 1997: *Ethnic Minorities in Britain: Diversity and Disadvantage*. London: Policy Studies Institute.

Nazroo, J.Y. 1997: *Ethnicity and Mental Health: Findings from a National Community Survey*. London: Policy Studies Institute.

Nazroo, J.Y. 2001: *Ethnicity, Class and Health*. London: Policy Studies Institute.

Nazroo, J. 2003: The structuring of ethnic inequalities in health: economic position, racial discrimination and racism. *American Journal of Public Health* 93, 277–84.

Pilgrim, D. and Rogers, A. 1999: *A Sociology of Mental Health and Illness* (2nd edn). Buckingham: Open University Press.

Rogers, A., Day, J.C., Williams, B., Randall, F., Wood, P., Healy, D. and Bentall, R.P. 1998: The meaning and management of neuroleptic medication: a study of patients with a diagnosis of schizophrenia. *Social Science and Medicine* 47, 1313–23.

Rosenhan, D.L. 1973: On being sane in insane places. *Science* 179, 250–58.

Scambler, G. 1989: *Epilepsy*. London: Routledge.

Scambler, G. 2003: *Sociology as Applied to Medicine* (5th edn). London: W.B. Saunders.

Scambler, G. and Hopkins, A. 1986: Being epileptic: coming to terms with stigma. *Sociology of Health and Illness* 8, 26–43.

Scheff, T. 1966: *Being Mentally Ill: A Sociological Theory*. Chicago: Aldine.

Smaje, C. 1996: The ethnic patterning of health: new directions for theory and research. *Sociology of Health and Illness* 18, 139–71.

Soni Raleigh, V. and Balarajan, R. 1992: Suicide and self-burning among Indians and West Indians in England and Wales. *British Journal of Psychiatry* 161, 365–68.

Szasz, T.S. 1961: The uses of naming and the origin of the myth of mental illness. *American Psychologist* 16, 59–65.

Williams, S. and Calnan, M. 1996: The 'limits' of medicalisation? Modern medicine and the lay populace. *Social Science and Medicine* 42, 1609–20.

Wright, P. and Treacher, A. 1982: *The Problem of Medical Knowledge: Examing the Social Construction of Medicine.* Edinburgh: Edinburgh University Press.

Zola, I. 1972: Medicine as an institution of social control. *Sociological Review* 20, 487–503.

## KEY REFERENCES/FURTHER READING

Pilgrim, D. and Rodgers, A. 1999: *A Sociology of Mental Health and Illness* (2nd edn).Buckingham: Open University Press.

# 4

# The epidemiological method and its contribution to international and cross-cultural comparative mental health research

## Martin Prince

## INTRODUCTION

This chapter sets out the purpose, nature and process of epidemiological research, and its contribution to 'comparative mental health research', which, by design, includes populations of different cultures or ethnicities with the explicit aim of learning from any intergroup heterogeneity that is observed. Some epidemiological study designs are presented along with their application to cross-cultural or international research, with a particular focus on the inferences that can be drawn from such studies. Finally, there is a presentation of some innovative quantitative approaches for the confirmation of construct validity of outcome measures used in culturally diverse populations.

## WHAT IS EPIDEMIOLOGY?

Epidemiology has been defined as 'The study of the distribution and determinants of health-related states or events in specified populations, and the application of this study to the control of health problems' (Last, 2001). Epidemiological studies may be used to describe the distribution of health states (extent, type, severity) within a population (descriptive epidemiology). Alternatively epidemiologists may try to explain the distribution of health states (analytical epidemiology). The basic strategy is to compare the distribution of disease between groups or between populations, looking for associations between hypothesized risk factors (genes, behaviours, lifestyles and environmental exposures) and health states.

**Table 4.1** *Epidemiological study designs*

| Observational | | | | | Experimental |
|---|---|---|---|---|---|
| 1. Population prevalence/ incidence a. Geographic variation b. Temporal ('secular') variation | 2. Ecological correlation | 3. Cross-sectional survey | 4. Case–control study | 5. Cohort study a. prospective b. retrospective 'historical' | 6. Randomized controlled trial |
| Descriptive | | | Analytic | | |

**Table 4.2** *Five of the nine criteria favouring causality as developed by Austin Bradford Hill (1897–1991)*

| | |
|---|---|
| 1. Strong associations | |
| 2. Temporality | The exposure should precede the onset of the disease |
| 3. Dose–response relationships | |
| 4. Consistency | With findings from other studies |
| 5. Plausibility/coherence | Given our understanding of possible underlying biological, psychological or sociological mechanisms |

| | Cases | Controls |
|---|---|---|
| Exposure$^+$ | a | b |
| Exposure$^-$ | c | d |
| Odds of being exposed if a case | = a/c | |
| Odds of being exposed if a control | = b/d | |
| Odds ratio | $= \dfrac{a/c}{b/d}$ | $= \dfrac{ad}{bc}$ |

Figure 4.1  *Case–control studies.*

Epidemiological studies are generally not controlled experiments (see Table 4.1 for types of studies). Observations are made on individuals living freely in the 'real world'; these non-experimental studies are referred to as 'observational'. Observed associations between risk factors and diseases may represent the effects of chance (random sampling error), or bias (non-random error) or confounding. Occasionally the apparent risk factor may be a consequence rather than a cause of the disease. This is called 'reverse causality'. Two key functions for epidemiologists are therefore to design and analyse studies in order to maximise the precision and validity of their findings. Even then great care must be taken with the inferences drawn from the

research findings. Inference is the 'process of passing from observations to generalisations'. This is a key activity in epidemiological investigation. An association need not signify that the risk factor causes the outcome with which it is associated. The role of chance, bias, confounding and reverse causality must first be considered. Only if these competing explanations can be confidently excluded may a causal attribution be entertained. Even then there are criteria for assessing whether causality can be inferred (see Table 4.2 for some Bradford Hill criteria). Different study designs (see Table 4.1) have distinct advantages and disadvantages over others. Figures 4.1 and 4.2 show the analytic strategy used in case–control studies and cohort studies, where

|  | Cases | Non-cases | Total |
|---|---|---|---|
| Exposed⁺ | a | b | a + b |
| Exposed⁻ | c | d | c + d |

Incidence risk in exposed $= a/a + b$

Incidence risk in non-exposed $= c/c + d$

Risk ratio $= \dfrac{a/(a + b)}{c/(c + d)}$

Figure 4.2 *Cohort studies.*

**Table 4.3** *Case–control and cohort studies. Characteristics, advantages and disadvantages*

|  | Case–control | Cohort |
|---|---|---|
| Subjects selected according to: |  |  |
|  | Caseness | Exposure |
| Perspective: | Retrospective | Prospective (usually) |
|  | (Subjects recall exposure) | (Observers attend outcome) |
| Sources of bias: | Selection bias | Information (outcome only) |
|  | Information bias | Non-response bias |
|  | (recall and observer) | (loss to follow-up) |
| Resources: | Quick | Lengthy |
|  | Relatively cheap | Relatively expensive |
| Useful for: | Rare outcomes | Rare exposures |
|  | Single outcomes | Single exposures |
|  | Multiple exposures | Multiple outcomes |
| Measure of effect | Odds ratio | Relative risk |

those exposed to a risk factor are compared with those not exposed, in terms of the disease outcome. Table 4.3 compares some of the strengths and weaknesses of case–control and cohort studies.

# COMPARATIVE AND CORRELATIONAL RESEARCH

## Comparative studies of disease frequency

The simplest studies are those of single populations, identifying clusters of low or high prevalence for a disorder. These are of great interest to epidemiologists, and may give important clues about aetiology. For example, there is a high prevalence of motor neuritides in Guam (Zhang *et al.*, 1995), and a rarity of multiple sclerosis in Southern Africa

(Dean *et al.*, 1994). These are examples of ecological variations which have led to the formulation of aetiological hypotheses (Hoffman *et al.*, 1983; Alter *et al.*, 1987; Spencer, 1987). Early studies of schizophrenia have reported clusters of strikingly low prevalence, for example, among the Hutterite Anabaptist sect in the USA (Nimgaonkar *et al.*, 2000), and an unusually high prevalence in Croatia (Cooper and Eagles, 1994).

Several research collaborations have been established with the explicit aim of making much broader comparisons of the frequency of mental disorders between countries and cultures. The main conclusion from the World Health Organization (WHO) Collaborative Study on Determinants of Outcome of Severe Mental Disorders (Sartorius *et al.*, 1986) was that when both clinical interview techniques and case criteria were standardized, there was little variability in prevalence and incidence rates between different centres, in North and South America, Europe, Africa, South Asia and

East Asia. That said, there was a twofold variation in the annual incidence of schizophrenia using narrow criteria from 7/100 000 in Denmark and 8/100 000 in urban India, to 15/100 000 in the UK centre. Prognosis also seemed to be better in some of the developing country centres (Sartorius *et al.*, 1986; Leff *et al.*, 1992).

In the 15-site WHO International Study of Psychological Problems in General Health Care (PPGHC), there was a 15-fold variation in the prevalence of major depression. Depression was assessed using the lay administered Composite International Diagnostic Instrument (CIDI-PC), with the lowest prevalence in Asia, the highest prevalence in Latin America and intermediate prevalence in Europe and North America (Simon *et al.*, 2002). In the ongoing World Mental Health Survey (Kessler, 1999) a new version of the CIDI (WMH-CIDI) is being administered to samples of those aged 18 and over in 28 centres worldwide. Preliminary findings have been published from 15 surveys in 14 countries in the Americas (Colombia, Mexico and USA), Europe (Belgium, France, Germany, Italy, Netherlands, Spain and Ukraine), the Middle East and Africa (Lebanon and Nigeria), and Asia (Japan, separate surveys in Beijing and Shanghai in the People's Republic of China; see Demyttenaere *et al.*, 2004). Sample sizes ranged from 1663 (Japan) to 9282 (USA), with a total of 60 463 participating adults. This study indicates considerable between-centre heterogeneity in the prevalence of all common mental disorders. The prevalence of any mental disorder, as defined in the *Diagnostic and Statistical Manual of Mental Disorders* (DSM-IV), varies from 4.3 to 26.4 per cent (interquartile range 9.1–16.9 per cent), with strikingly low prevalence in Shanghai (4.3 per cent) and Nigeria (4.9 per cent), and strikingly high prevalence in the USA (26.4 per cent). Even within Europe there was a more than twofold variation in prevalence between Italy (8.2 per cent), Germany (9.1 per cent), Spain (9.2 per cent), Belgium (12.0 per cent), the Netherlands (14.0 per cent), France (18.4 per cent) and Ukraine (20.5 per cent).

If genuine (an important proviso – see below), differences in disease frequency between populations may be explained by the main effect of genetic factors or environmental exposures, or by interactions between genes and environment, genes and other genes, or between different environmental factors (Cooper and Kaufman, 1998).

Quite apart from the difficulty of attributing differences to individual risk factors, it is not generally possible to adduce direct evidence to support genetic or environmental explanations. Genetic explanations have fallen into relative disfavour, given that as little as 10 per cent of genetic variation is found across as opposed to within continents (Barbujani *et al.*, 1997). Cooper asserts that 'race, at the continental level, has not been shown to provide a useful categorization of genetic information about the response to drugs, diagnosis, or causes of disease' (Cooper *et al.*, 2003). However, recent evidence suggests that the 10 per cent among-population genetic variability seems to include relatively recent population-specific adaptations to environmental changes and cultural innovations (Voight *et al.*, 2006); the genes most strongly affected by recent population-specific selection appear to be those associated with skin colour, bone structure and the metabolism of different foods. Several of these genes have already been identified as implicated in disease processes (Voight *et al.*, 2006). Both genetic and environmental explanations for regional differences in disease frequency are, therefore, tenable in most cases.

A variant on the single population study is the migration study, in which the health outcomes of migrants from a high-prevalence setting to a low-prevalence setting (or vice versa) are compared with those of the population at origin. Such studies can offer insights into the likely genetic or environmental contribution to the observed differences. Sustained high or low prevalence despite dietary acculturation, as is seen with type 2 diabetes among South Asian migrants to the UK, for example (Dhawan *et al.*, 1994), suggests that one or more genetic factors may be relevant. Convergence of disease frequency with that of the host population, as has been noted for cardiovascular disease among Japanese Americans (Worth *et al.*, 1975), suggests that environmental (lifestyle) risk factors were involved. Hendrie *et al.* (1995) sought to match for population genetics in comparing the prevalence of dementia and Alzheimer's disease among Africans in Ibadan, Nigeria and African Americans in Indianapolis. While racial admixture in the USA after the abduction of Africans for the purpose of slavery will have undermined this aim somewhat, the much lower prevalence (Hendrie *et al.*, 1995) and incidence (Hendrie *et al.*, 2001) of both outcomes in the Nigerian centre is most consistent with an environmental explanation for the observed difference.

Studies of ethnic minority groups in the UK consistently report a particularly high incidence of schizophrenia and bipolar disorder among those of African and African Caribbean ancestry. The recent Aetiology and Ethnicity in Schizophrenia and Other Psychoses (AESOP) studies of first-onset psychosis indicate that high incidence rates are relatively specific to these diagnoses and these ethnic groups although more modest elevations of risk for psychosis are also seen in white and Asian migrants (Kirkbride *et al.*, 2006; Morgan *et al.*, 2006). Risk in second-generation migrants seems if anything to be higher than for first generation. These are effectively migration studies without an adequate comparison group in the country of origin. While investigators have focused upon the interaction between the process of migration and the experience of racism and disadvantage as a plausible explanation for these findings, genetic differences remain a parsimonious but unlikely alternative (Sharpley *et al.*, 2001). Clearly more work is needed on the prevalence and incidence of psychosis in the countries of origin of African and Caribbean migrants to the UK.

Any observed differences in disease frequency between regions, countries, cultures and ethnicities need to be interpreted with due care, for the following reasons: first, the history of psychiatric epidemiology has demonstrated that much of the heterogeneity in reported disease frequency between studies may be attributable to methodological differences in the studies rather than true findings of difference. Relevant factors include selection bias in sampling methods, and the influence of inclusion and exclusion criteria, biased or invalid measures of mental disorder (scale-based versus diagnostic interview, lay versus clinician administered) and, particularly, diagnostic criteria. As operationalized criteria are established,

diagnostic interview technologies are developed, and study methodologies increasingly standardized, the heterogeneity between estimates is minimized (Sartorius *et al.*, 1986; Beekman *et al.*, 1999; Lobo *et al.*, 2000).

Second, diagnostic procedures for psychiatric disorders that have been standardized and validated in a specific cultural setting may not be applied indiscriminately to another. They may turn out to be culturally biased, giving a misleadingly high or low estimate of the prevalence of the disease. This might arise if, for example, use of identical diagnostic methods identifies different levels of disease severity in different language or cultural groups (Simon *et al.*, 2002). Attempts to validate standard assessments across a range of countries and cultures are relatively few and far between (Goldberg *et al.*, 1997; Prince *et al.*, 2003, 2004; Kessler *et al.*, 2004; Bhui *et al.*, 2006). Even where they have been carried out they may be limited by the underlying universalist assumption that it is appropriate to apply a common external criterion across countries and cultures, whether that be local clinician-diagnosed DSM-IV dementia (Prince *et al.*, 2003), local clinician SCID (structured clinical interview for DSM-IV) interviews (Kessler *et al.*, 2004) or DSM-IV diagnoses using the primary care version of the Composite International Diagnostic Instrument (CIDI-PC) (Goldberg *et al.*, 1997). Some have argued that mental disorders as defined in the Eurocentric DSM-IV may not exist, or may exist in different forms in other cultural settings (Mezzich *et al.*, 1999). The fact that they are consistently identified does not mitigate the risk of a category fallacy (Kleinman, 1987) as the associated disabilities and prognoses and wider web of meanings and therefore illness behaviour may vary across cultures even for the same diagnosis.

Third, in unstable populations low prevalence may be accounted for either by selective out-migration of susceptible persons, or by in-migration of those unlikely to develop the disorder, and vice versa for high prevalence. Such an effect has been noted upon the recorded admission risk rates for schizophrenia in Croatia (Cooper and Eagles, 1994). There is little available information on the effects of either mental disorder or susceptibility for mental disorder on migration behaviour.

Fourth, differing response rates between studies make it very difficult to make valid comparisons of disease frequency. In the World Mental Health Survey the proportions of non-responders varied from 45.9 per cent (France) to 87.7 per cent (Colombia), with a weighted average of just 69.9 per cent (Demyttenaere *et al.*, 2004).

Fifth, as prevalence is the product of incidence and duration, low prevalence rates may indicate a high recovery rate or a low survival rate for those with the disorder, rather than a true difference in incidence. Longitudinal studies measuring disease incidence and duration are needed if valid comparisons are to be made between settings (Hendrie *et al.*, 2001; Perkins *et al.*, 2002).

Sixth, the make-up of the population under study will influence disease frequency. For mental health outcomes these will include such attributes as age, gender, socio-economic status and physical health status. Technically, these can be controlled for (essentially treated as potential confounders of the association between the population and the mental health outcome) by standardization or other statistical procedures. However, in many cases we are more likely to be interested in compositional effects as mediators of the association between population and mental health outcome; that is, factors which have the potential to explain the observed variation in disease frequency.

## Ecological correlational studies

Ecological studies provide a crude quantitative framework for analysing factors that might contribute to variation in disease frequency. An aggregate measure of the hypothesized exposure at population level (the proportion exposed, or the mean level of the exposure in the population) is correlated with an aggregate measure of the outcome (population prevalence or incidence) across centres. For example, the relationship between sun exposure and melanoma was established following the observation of an association between latitude and incidence (Elwood and Koh, 1994). In sub-Saharan African societies there is a general inverse association at the societal level between the prevalence of male circumcision and

the seroprevalence of human immunodeficiency virus (HIV), leading to the suggestion that male circumcision may reduce the risk of sexual transmission (Moses *et al.*, 1990). Hare (1956) noted a correlation at the ecological level, in electoral districts in Bristol, between the proportion of single households (as an indicator of anomie) and the prevalence of schizophrenia.

This last example can be used to illustrate the main problems specific to ecological correlational studies. Both exposure and outcome are aggregate measures at the level of community districts. We do not know if the people with schizophrenia are necessarily those living in single person households. Thus, an ecological correlation need not imply a correlation at the level of individuals within populations. This problem is referred to as the 'ecological fallacy'. The exposure may be considered to be a property of the locale and/or the population, rather than of the individuals living within the district. These are referred to as contextual factors. Thus, the effect of living in an anomic neighbourhood, as indicated by a high proportion of single-person households, may apply to all individuals living in the area regardless of their individual living circumstances. Other ecological correlational studies have demonstrated the salience of the contextual effects of income inequality on risk for schizophrenia (Boydell *et al.*, 2004) and common mental disorder (Weich *et al.*, 2001), and for the effect of ethnic density (living in an area with few non-white migrants) upon risk for schizophrenia among ethnic minorities in London (Boydell *et al.*, 2001).

Second, adjusting for confounding effects is tricky in ecological studies. If a factor is operating at the contextual level, other contextual factors may be associated with it and confound the association. Hence areas with a high proportion of single person residences may also be of lower socio-economic status, and it may be living in a low socio-economic status area (regardless of personal socio-economic status) that is the real causal contextual factor. We could adjust for this at the ecological level (if we have a suitable aggregate measure, which is often not the case). However, it is never possible to adjust for confounding at the individual level.

A further problem is that as with any cross-sectional study, we do not know if the anomic nature of the neighbourhoods has caused the schizophrenia, or whether people developing schizophrenia move into such areas. This would be an example of reverse causality – the disease causing the 'exposure' rather than vice versa.

For all of these reasons it is difficult to make causal inferences from ecological correlational studies. They may be used, however, to develop hypotheses for further investigation. For exposures that can be meaningfully considered to apply to individuals rather than populations, these are best carried out on individuals within a single population, where there is a reasonable variance in the exposure – this work has now been carried out on the association between male circumcision and HIV risk (Bailey *et al.*, 2001), largely confirming that the ecological correlation is also reflected in an inverse association at the level of individuals.

## Multilevel modelling

For contextual factors, multilevel study designs offer a more sophisticated approach, allowing the simultaneous study of compositional and contextual effects. Multiple communities are selected to ensure variance in the contextual factors under study (for example social capital); individuals are then selected within each community cluster so that information can be collected on compositional individual level risk factors, and mental health outcomes. The independent effects of compositional and contextual variables can then be assessed in a statistically and methodologically robust fashion (Veenstra, 2005). For international and/or cross-cultural research, 'culture' can be considered to be a contextual variable. In multilevel analyses, any centre-level variation that remains unaccounted for after controlling for compositional and other measurable contextual factors may be considered to represent the effect of culture (as well as other unmeasured contextual effects, and error). Therefore, if minimal we may conclude that the effect of culture on the outcome is limited.

## Analytical studies

The defining characteristics of case–control and cohort studies are described and compared in Figures 4.1 and 4.2. Where analytical studies have been conducted across a range of different countries and cultures, it may be possible to compare findings regarding aetiological associations. This can be useful to demonstrate the wider generalizability of findings from individual studies. For example, the INTERHEART cross-national (52 country) case–control study suggests that risk factors for myocardial infarction (abnormal lipids, smoking, hypertension, diabetes, abdominal obesity, psycho-social factors, consumption of fruits, vegetables and alcohol, and regular physical activity) account for 90 per cent of the risk of myocardial infarction worldwide in both sexes and at all ages in all regions; thus approaches to prevention can be based on similar principles worldwide (Yusuf *et al.*, 2004). The EURODEM consortium carried out meta-analyses of case–control studies for risk factors for dementia and Alzheimer's disease (Brayne, 1991), and later demonstrated in a concerted series of European incidence studies that cigarette smoking was an internationally consistent and robust risk factor for cognitive decline (Ott *et al.*, 2004). Such exercises are just as valuable when they demonstrate heterogeneity in risk factor profiles; for example, the US–Nigeria dementia study has shown that the Apo-E genotype is not associated with risk for dementia and Alzheimer's disease in Nigerians in Ibadan but is associated with both of these outcomes among African Americans in Indianapolis (Gureje *et al.*, 2006), as well as in most other studies worldwide, suggesting a gene–environment interaction.

The potential for comparative studies of aetiology is currently underdeveloped in psychiatric epidemiology. One reason for this may be the ongoing concerns regarding the universal applicability of case definitions and cross-cultural validity of diagnostic assessments. This omission will soon be partly corrected by the World Mental Health study (Demyttenaere *et al.*, 2004), the AESOP studies on incident psychosis (Morgan *et al.*, 2006), and for older people the 10/66 studies of risk for dementia and other mental disorders (Prince and Acosta, 2006).

## Experimental studies – randomized controlled trials

The evidence base for psychological and psychopharmacological interventions needs to be extended to countries and cultures beyond Europe and North America, where the vast majority of trials have been carried out (Patel and Sumathipala, 2001). Patel identifies four reasons for potential non-generalizability for trial evidence from developed countries (Patel, 2000).

* The explanatory models of common mental disorders in many developing countries are unlikely to acknowledge a role for biomedical interventions, influencing the acceptability of psychiatric interventions.
* While it may be assumed that cultural factors are unlikely to influence treatment response for physical treatments such as antidepressants, there may be genetically mediated effects on the pharmacokinetics and pharmacodynamics of drug therapies, affecting dosage and therapeutic windows. There may also be cultural effects on the acceptability and tolerance of side-effects.
* Widely varying and rapidly changing health system-related factors can profoundly influence the applicability of treatment research.
* While effectiveness may vary relatively little, the cost of drugs is strongly influenced by regional economic factors such as the differing interpretations of drug patent rules, the production of generic drugs and the variable dose strengths of pharmaceutical preparations. The relative cost-effectiveness and cost–benefit ratios associated with treatments are therefore likely to vary between settings.

Most importantly, the prioritization of mental health care will be much more heavily influenced by locally conducted research. The drug policies in many countries require at least phase IV trials before new medications are licensed for use, even if they are being widely used elsewhere. Trials in developing countries might usefully focus also on the interface between mental health and established health priorities, such as, for example, the management of common mental disorders in those presenting for treatment of HIV/AIDS. Good-quality trials already indicate effectiveness for selective serotonin reuptake inhibitor (SSRI) antidepressants in India (Patel et al., 2003), stepped care psychological/pharmacological interventions in Chile (Araya et al., 2003) and group interpersonal therapy in Uganda (Bolton et al., 2003).

In summary, comparative mental health research has identified significant variation in the prevalence and incidence of mental disorders worldwide. The interpretation of such differences, and in particular their attribution to underlying aetiological factors, is much more problematic, particularly given the difficulty of excluding the role of methodological factors, chief among these being measurement. Is the same outcome being measured in the same way and with comparable validity between the different groups or populations under study?

## QUANTITATIVE INSIGHTS ON MEASUREMENT VALIDITY IN COMPARATIVE RESEARCH

Much of the literature on the cross-cultural application of assessments of mental health and psycho-social phenomena has concentrated on the application of measures developed in one cultural setting (usually the UK or the USA) to another: typically a non-English-speaking low- or middle-income country in Latin America, Africa or Asia. The need to establish the relevance of the construct to the new setting, to make the necessary cultural adaptations, and to use bicultural and bilingual translators to arrive at a local language version aiming for conceptual equivalence is well established; the methods and procedures are well rehearsed in this volume and elsewhere (Patel, 2003; Bhui et al., 2006).

Construct validity is highly relevant to the establishment of a case for the validity assessments across populations and cultures. The term was proposed by the American Psychiatric Association Committee on Psychological Tests in 1954 (Cronbach and Meehl, 1955). Pre-existent concepts of validity had focused on content validity (essentially referring to the considerations in the previous paragraph) and criterion-related validity (concurrent and predictive validity), where a gold standard for the construct was already established. Construct validity referred to a situation in which 'the tester has no definite criterion measure of the quality with which he is concerned, and must use indirect measures. Here the (elucidation of the) trait or quality underlying the test is of central importance'. Cronbach and Meehl (1955) considered that expert ratings of these matters would be of limited value. Construct validity would be involved in answering questions such as: To what extent is this test culture-free? Does this test measure reading ability, quantitative reasoning, or response sets? How does a person with a high score on trait 'A' differ from a person with a low score? The answers to these questions would be derived from quantitative research, essentially through a series of hypothesis-driven investigations aimed at identifying the 'nomological net' or theoretical framework consisting of more or less proximate identifiers for the construct, at least some of which would need to be observable. The quantitative procedures advocated for establishing construct validity included inter-item correlations and internal consistency, factor analysis, test–retest reliability, and test–'criterion' correlations. While some observables may be regarded as 'criteria', the construct validity of the criteria themselves is also under investigation. The investigation of a test's construct validity is compared to that for developing and confirming theories.

## EXPLORATORY FACTOR ANALYSIS

Principal component analysis (PCA) is an exploratory technique (Olsson, 1979). Qadir *et al.* (2005) used this approach to study the applicability of the Parental Bonding Interview (PBI) to young women in Pakistan. In the PBI (Parker and Tupling,

1979), adults provide retrospective descriptions of their perceptions of parenting from their father and mother, when they were children; it has two subscales referring to traits of 'care' and 'overprotection'. Local Pakistani experts identified items from the overprotection scale, which they felt could evoke a culture-specific response from the Pakistani women because they might interpret them as signifying care as opposed to 'control' or 'overprotection'. However, a quantitative pilot investigation provided no empirical evidence to support their concerns. First, during the interview, it was clear that most young women regarded 'liberal' responses to the following items as reflecting favourably upon their mothers: item 21: 'Gave me as much freedom as I wanted'; item 22: 'Let me go out as much as I wanted'; item 25: 'Let me dress in any way I pleased'. Second, in the factor analysis all of the items concerned loaded heavily on the overprotection dimension. Third, consistent with previous findings (Parker, 1989), there was a strong negative correlation between the PBI 'care' and 'overprotection' subscales, suggesting that women who scored high on the care scale perceived their mothers as more autonomy granting, and women with low scores on the care dimension felt more overprotected by their mothers. This pattern of findings supported the construct validity of the overprotection items and that of the overprotection scale as a whole. It also underlined that, in this instance, neither lay nor expert opinions on content validity were correct and that these should not be accepted uncritically. The factor analysis replicated the previously reported two- and three-factor solutions for the PBI.

The clear delineation of the two subscales with their high factor loadings, high internal consistencies and negative total score correlations, supported the notion that young Pakistani women perceived and responded to these items as addressing parental 'control' or 'overprotection' in a similar way to respondents from Western Anglophone cultures. This provided further support for the essential construct validity of PBI, and indicated a perhaps surprising degree of sensitivity to the cultural nuances of parenting. The construct validity of the PBI in Pakistan was further supported by the observation of the hypothesized associations between common mental disorder and low care and high overprotection. Consistent with previous research, maternal overprotection was also associated with reports of marital dissatisfaction.

## NOVEL HYPOTHESIS-DRIVEN APPROACHES TO TESTING CONSTRUCT VALIDITY ACROSS CULTURES

Confirmatory factor analysis (CFA) and Rasch models can be used to assess whether a scale measures the same trait dimension in the same way when applied in qualitatively distinct groups; this is referred to as 'measurement invariance'. In a worked example, Reise *et al.* (1993) demonstrate these approaches with respect to mood symptoms assessed in Minnesota and China. The demonstration of measurement invariance across countries, cultures and/or ethnic groups provides strong evidence to support the construct validity of an assessment for the purposes of comparative research.

### Confirmatory factor analysis

In CFA a model is tested that specifies in advance the relations between observed variables and latent factors. Testing for measurement invariance (Sorbom, 1974) involves an assessment of whether the best factor solution relates to the latent trait or traits in the same way in each of several populations. Two models can be compared in which all item loadings are (1) constrained and (2) not constrained to be identical between countries. The absolute fit of a CFA model can be evaluated by means of a $\chi^2$ statistic (Bentler and Bonett, 1980). Several other absolute and relative indices of fit are recommended (Tucker & Lewis, 1973; Akaike, 1987; Browne, 1990; Dunn *et al.*, 1993; Marsh *et al.*, 1996; Burnham and Anderson, 1998).

This approach has been used to validate the PBI across European centres participating in the World Mental Health Survey (Heider *et al.*, 2005), providing strong evidence for the invariance of a three-factor solution suggested by exploratory factor analysis, across six countries, both genders and all age groups. Despite its evident applicability

to cross-cultural validity of assessments of mental health status, there are few if any examples of the use of CFA in this area to date.

## Rasch models

Rasch analysis belongs to a family of statistical models developed from Item Response Theory (IRT) (Reise *et al.*, 1993; Nunnally and Bernstein, 1994). Whereas CFA models account for the covariance between test items, IRT models account for patterns of item responses. The Rasch model (Rasch, 1993) suggests that the responses to a set of items can be justified by a person's position on the underlying trait that is being measured and by the item severity (also referred to as item calibration). It is measured on the same scale as the severity of the underlying trait. Participants with severity scores below the calibration for the given item are more likely to deny than endorse the item, while those with severity scores above the calibration for the item are more likely to endorse it. It follows that the items with higher calibrations are less frequently endorsed. Also, a participant who endorses an item of middling severity is likely to have endorsed all items with lower calibrations. While there can be no single satisfactory test of model adequacy, techniques can be used to assess different aspects of goodness-of-fit of Rasch models.

This approach was used in the WHO international study of mental disorder in general health care settings (PPGHC). Strong evidence was provided to support a common hierarchy for CIDI symptoms (in order of item severity: sleep, mood, concentration, fatigue, loss of interest, suicidality, guilt, agitation/retardation, appetite change) across three groups of countries categorized by level of prevalence of major depression (low/intermediate/high). This impression was confirmed by a formal test for differential item functioning; the goodness-of-fit for a model allowing different symptom thresholds for the three prevalence groups was not significantly better than that for a simpler model assuming identical symptom thresholds ($P = 0.38$). The authors concluded from these findings that there was no evidence that prevalence differences were explained by cross-cultural differences in the form or validity of the depressive syndrome, and that therefore the apparent differences in depression prevalence could not be attributed to 'category fallacy'.

## CONCLUSIONS

This chapter sets out some basic epidemiological issues, and how epidemiology has contributed to international and cultural psychiatry. Many of the basic assumptions of epidemiology may challenge and be challenged by alternative research methods (see Chapters 2, 3, 5 and 9). Nonetheless, epidemiological methods do focus on what can be concluded if all sources of bias and confounding are removed, and in this endeavour innovations in research methods and mixed methods are emerging as part of the new cultural epidemiology.

## REFERENCES

Akaike, H. 1987: Factor analysis and AIC. *Psychometrika* 52, 317–32.

Alter, M., Zhen-xin, Z., Davanipour, Z., Sobel, E. and Min Lai, S. 1987: Does delay in acquiring childhood infection increase risk of multiple sclerosis? *Italian Journal of Neurological Science* 8, 23–28.

Araya, R., Rojas, G., Fritsch, R., Gaete, J., Rajas, M., Simon, G. and Peters, T.J. 2003: Treating depression in primary care in low-income women in Santiago, Chile: a randomised controlled trial. *The Lancet* 361, 995–1000.

Bailey, R.C., Plummer, F.A. and Moses, S. 2001: Male circumcision and HIV prevention: current knowledge and future research directions. *Lancet Infectious Diseases* 1, 223–31.

Barbujani, G., Magagni, A., Minch, E. and Cavalli-Sforza, L.L. 1997: An apportionment of human DNA diversity. *Proceedings of the National Academy of Sciences of the USA* 94, 4516–19.

Beekman, A.T.F., Copeland, J.R.M. and Prince, M.J. 1999: Review of community prevalence of depression in later life. *British Journal of Psychiatry* 174, 307–11.

Bentler, P.M. and Bonett, D.G. 1980: Significance tests and goodness of fit in the analysis of covariance structures. *Psychological Bulletin* 88, 588–606.

Bhui, K., Craig, T., Mohamud, S., Warfa, N., Stansfeld, S.A., Thornicroft, G., Curtis, S. and McCrone, P. 2006: Mental disorders among Somali refugees: developing culturally appropriate measures and assessing socio-cultural risk factors. *Social Psychiatry and Psychiatric Epidemiology* 41: 400–408.

Bolton, P., Bass, J., Neugebauer, R., Verdeli, H., Clougherty, K.F., Wickramaratne, P., Speelman, L., Ndogoni, L. and Weissman, M. 2003: Group interpersonal psychotherapy for depression in rural Uganda: a randomized controlled trial. *Journal of the American Medical Association* 289, 3117–3124.

Boydell, J., van Os, J., McKenzie, K., Goel, R., McCreadie, R.G. and Murray, R.M. 2001: Incidence of schizophrenia in ethnic minorities in London: ecological study into interactions with environment. *British Medical Journal* 323, 1336–38.

Boydell, J., van Os, J., McKenzie, K. and Murray, R.M. 2004: The association of inequality with the incidence of schizophrenia – an ecological study. *Social Psychiatry and Psychiatric Epidemiology* 39, 597–99.

Brayne, C. 1991: The EURODEM collaborative re-analysis of case-control studies of Alzheimer's disease: implications for public health. *International Journal of Epidemiology* 20(Suppl 2), S68–S71.

Browne, M.W. 1990: *MUTMUM PC: User's Guide*. Columbus: Ohio State University.

Burnham, K.P. and Anderson, D.R. 1998: *Model Selection and Inference: A Practical Information-Theoretic Approach*. New York: Springer-Verlag.

Cooper, B. and Eagles, J.M. 1994: Folnegovic & Folnegovic-Smalc's 'Schizophrenia in Croatia: inter-regional differences in prevalence and a comment on constant incidence'. *British Journal of Psychiatry* 164, 97–100.

Cooper, R.S. and Kaufman, J.S. 1998: Race and hypertension: science and nescience. *Hypertension* 32, 813–16.

Cooper, R.S., Kaufman, J.S. and Ward, R. 2003: Race and genomics. *New England Journal of Medicine* 348, 1166–70.

Cronbach, L.E. and Meehl, P.E. 1955: Construct validity in psychological tests. *Psychological Bulletin* 52, 281–302.

Dean, G., Bhigjee, A.I., Bill, P.L., Fritz, V., Chikanza, I.C., Thomas, J.E., Levy, L.F. and Saffer, D. 1994: Multiple sclerosis in black South Africans and Zimbabweans. *Journal of Neurology, Neurosurgery and Psychiatry* 57, 1064–1069.

Demyttenaere, K., Bruffaerts, R., Posada-Villa, J. and the WHO World Mental Health Survey Consortium. 2004: Prevalence, severity, and unmet need for treatment of mental disorders in the World Health Organization World Mental Health Surveys. *Journal of the American Medical Association* 291, 2581–90.

Dhawan, J., Bray, C.L., Warburton, R., Ghambhir, D.S. and Morris, J. 1994: Insulin resistance, high prevalence of diabetes, and cardiovascular risk in immigrant Asians. Genetic or environmental effect? *British Heart Journal* 72, 413–21.

Dunn, G., Everitt, B. and Pickles, A. 1993: *Modelling Covariances and Latent Variables using EQS*. London: Chapman & Hall.

Elwood, J.M. and Koh, H.K. 1994: Etiology, epidemiology, risk factors, and public health issues of melanoma. *Current Opinion in Oncology* 6, 179–87.

Goldberg, D.P., Gater, R., Sartorius, N., Ustun, T.B., Piccinelli, M., Gureje, O. and Rutter, C. 1997: The validity of two versions of the GHQ in the WHO study of mental illness in general health care. *Psychological Medicine* 27, 191–97.

Gureje, O., Ogunniyi, A., Baiyewu, O., Price, B., Unverzagt, F.W., Evans, R.M., Smith-Gamble, V., Lane, K.A., Gao, S., Hall, K.S., Hendrie, H.C. and Murrell, J.R. 2006: APOE epsilon4 is not associated with Alzheimer's disease in elderly Nigerians. *Annals of Neurology* 59, 182–85.

Hare, E.H. 1956: Mental illness and social conditions in Bristol. *Journal of Mental Science* 102, 349–57.

Heider, D., Matschinger, H., Bernert, S., Vilagut, G., Martinez-Alonso, M., Dietrich, S., Angermeyer, M.C.; ESEMeD/MHEDEA investigators 2005: Empirical evidence for an invariant three-factor structure of the Parental Bonding Instrument in six European countries. *Psychiatry Research* 135, 237–47.

Hendrie, H.C., Osuntokun, B.O., Hall, K.S., Ogunniyi, A.O., Hui, S.L., Unverzagt, F.W., Gureje, O., Rodenberg, C.A., Baiyewu, O., Musick, B.S. 1995: Prevalence of Alzheimer's disease and dementia in two communities: Nigerian Africans and African Americans. *American Journal of Psychiatry* 152, 1485–92.

Hendrie, H.C., Ogunniyi, A., Hall, K.S., Baiyewu, O., Unverzagt, F.W., Gureje, O., Gao, S., Evans, R.M., Ogunseyinde, A.O., Adeyinka, A.O., Musick, B. and Hui, S.L. 2001: Incidence of dementia and Alzheimer disease in 2 communities: Yoruba residing in Ibadan, Nigeria, and African Americans residing in Indianapolis, Indiana. *Journal of the American Medical Association* 285, 739–47.

Hoffman, P.M., Robbins, D.S., Gibbs, C.J., Jr. and Gajdusek, D.C. 1983: Immune function among normal Guamanians of different age. *Journal of Gerontology* 38, 414–19.

Kessler, R.C. 1999: The World Health Organization International Consortium in Psychiatric Epidemiology (ICPE): initial work and future directions – the NAPE Lecture 1998. Nordic Association for Psychiatric Epidemiology. *Acta Psychiatrica Scandinavica* 99, 2–9.

Kessler, R.C., Abelson, J., Demler, O., Escobar, J.I., Gibbon, M., Guyer, M.E., Howes, M.J., Jin, R., Vega, W.A., Walters, E.E., Wang, P., Zaslavsky, A. and Zheng, H. 2004: Clinical calibration of DSM-IV diagnoses in the World Mental Health (WMH) version of the World Health Organization (WHO) Composite International Diagnostic Interview (WMHCIDI). *International Journal of Methods in Psychiatric Research* 13, 122–39.

Kirkbride, J.B., Fearon, P., Morgan, C., Dazzan, P., Morgan, K., Tarrant, J., Lloyd, T., Holloway, J., Hutchinson, G., Leff, J.P., Mallett, R.M., Harrison, G.L., Murray, R.M. and Jones, P.B. 2006: Heterogeneity in incidence rates of schizophrenia and other psychotic syndromes: findings from the 3-center AeSOP study. *Archives of General Psychiatry* 63, 250–58.

Kleinman, A. 1987: Anthropology and psychiatry. The role of culture in cross-cultural research on illness. *British Journal of Psychiatry* 151, 447–54.

Last, J.M. 2001: *A Dictionary of Epidemiology* (4th edn). New York: Oxford University Press.

Leff, J., Sartorius, N., Jablensky, A., Korten, A. and Ernberg, G. 1992: The International Pilot Study of Schizophrenia: five-year follow-up findings. *Psychological Medicine* 22, 131–45.

Lobo, A., Launer, L.J., Fratiglioni, L., Andersen, K., Di Carlo, A., Breteler, M.M., Copeland, J.R., Dartigues, J.F., Jagger, C., Martinez-Lage, J., Soininen, H. and Hofman, A. 2000: Prevalence of dementia and major subtypes in Europe: a collaborative study of population-based cohorts. Neurologic Diseases in the Elderly Research Group. *Neurology* 54, S4–S9.

Marsh, H.W., Balla, J.R. and Hau, K.T. 1996: An evaluation of incremental fit indices: a clarification of mathematical and empirical properties. In Marcoulides, G.A. and Schumacker, R.E. (eds) *Advanced Structural Equation Modelling: Issues and Techniques*. Mahwah: Lawrence Erlbaum Associates, 315–55.

Mezzich, J.E., Kirmayer, L.J., Kleinman, A., Fabrega, H. Jr, Parron, D.L., Good, B.J., Lin, K.M. and Manson, S.M. 1999: The place of culture in DSM-IV. *Journal of Nervous and Mental Disease* 187, 457–64.

Morgan, C., Dazzan, P., Morgan, K., Jones, P., Harrison, G., Leff, J., Murray, R., Fearon, P. and the AESOP study group. 2006: First episode psychosis and ethnicity: initial findings from the AESOP study. *World Psychiatry* 5, 40–46.

Moses, S., Bradley, J.E., Nagelkerke, N.J., Ronald, A.R., Ndinya-Achola, J.O. and Plummer, F.A. 1990: Geographical patterns of male circumcision practices in Africa: association with HIV seroprevalence. *International Journal of Epidemiology* 19, 693–97.

Nimgaonkar, V.L., Fujiwara, T.M., Dutta, M., Wood, J., Gentry, K., Maendel, S., Morgan, K. and Eaton, J. 2000: Low prevalence of psychoses among the Hutterites, an isolated religious community. *American Journal of Psychiatry* 157, 1065–70.

Nunnally, J.C. and Bernstein, I.H. 1994: *Psychometric Theory* (3rd edn). New York: McGraw-Hill.

Olsson, U. 1979: Maximum likelihood estimation of the polychoric correlation coefficient. *Psychometrika* 44, 443–60.

Ott, A., Andersen, K., Dewey, M.E., Letenneur, L., Brayne, C., Copeland, J.R., Dartigues, J.F., Kragh-Sorensen, P., Lobo, A., Martinez-Lage, J.M., Stijnen, T., Hofman, A., Launer, L.J. and the EURODEM Incidence Research Group. 2004: Effect of smoking on global cognitive function in nondemented elderly. *Neurology* 62, 920–24.

Parker, G. 1989: The Parental Bonding Instrument: psychometric properties reviewed. *Psychiatric Developments* 7(4), 317–35.

Parker, G. and Tupling, H. 1979: A parental bonding instrument. *British Journal of Medical Psychology* 52, 1–10.

Patel, V. 2000: The need for treatment evidence for common mental disorders in developing countries. *Psychological Medicine* 30, 743–46.

Patel, V. 2003: Cultural issues in measurement and research. In Prince, M., Stewart, R., Ford, T. and Hotopf, M. (eds) *Practical Psychiatric Epidemiology*. Oxford: Oxford University Press, 434–655.

Patel, V., Chisholm, D., Rabe-Hesketh, S., Dias-Saxena, F., Andrew, G. and Mann, A. 2003: Efficacy and cost-effectiveness of drug and psychological treatments for common mental disorders in general health care in Goa, India: a randomised, controlled trial. *Lancet* 361, 33–39.

Patel, V. and Sumathipala, A. 2001: International representation in psychiatric literature: survey of six leading journals. *British Journal of Psychiatry* 178, 406–409.

Perkins, A.J., Hui, S.L., Ogunniyi, A., Gureje, O., Baiyewu, O., Unverzagt, F.W., Gao, S., Hall, K.S., Musick, B.S. and Hendrie, H.C. 2002: Risk of mortality for dementia in a developing country: the Yoruba in Nigeria. *International Journal of Geriatric Psychiatry* 17, 566–73.

Prince, M. and Acosta, D. 2006: Ageing and dementia in low- and middle-income countries – the work of the 10/66 Dementia Research Group. *International Psychiatry* 3(4), 3–6.

Prince, M., Acosta, D., Chiu, H., Scazufca, M., Varghese, M. and the 10/66 Dementia Research Group. 2003: Dementia diagnosis in developing countries: a cross-cultural validation study. *The Lancet* 361, 909–17.

Prince, M., Acosta, D., Chiu, H., Copeland, J., Dewey, M., Scazufca, M., Varghese, M. and the 10/66 Dementia Research Group. 2004: Effects of education and culture on the validity of the Geriatric Mental State and its AGECAT algorithm. *British Journal of Psychiatry* 185, 429–36.

Qadir, F., Stewart, R., Khan, M. and Prince, M. 2005: The validity of the Parental Bonding Instrument as a measure of maternal bonding among young Pakistani women. *Social Psychiatry and Psychiatric Epidemiology* 40, 276–82.

Rasch, G. 1993: *Probabilistic Models for Some Intelligence and Attainment Tests*. Chicago, IL: Mesa Press.

Reise, S.P., Widaman, K.F. and Pugh, R.H. 1993: Confirmatory factor analysis and item response theory: two approaches for exploring measurement invariance. *Psychological Bulletin* 114, 552–66.

Sartorius, N., Jablensky, A., Korten, A., Ernberg, G., Anker, M., Cooper, J.E. and Day, R. 1986: Early manifestations and first-contact incidence of schizophrenia in different cultures. *Psychological Medicine* 16, 909–28.

Sharpley, M., Hutchinson, G., McKenzie, K. and Murray, R.M. 2001: Understanding the excess of psychosis among the African-Caribbean population in England. Review of current hypotheses. *British Journal of Psychiatry* Suppl. 40, S60–68.

Simon, G.E., Goldberg, D.P., Von Korff, M. and Ustun, T.B. 2002: Understanding cross-national differences in depression prevalence. *Psychology and Medicine* 32, 585–94.

Sorbom, D. 1974: A general method for studying differences in factor means and factor structure between groups. *British Journal of Mathematical and Statistical Psychology* 27, 229–39.

Spencer, P.S. 1987: Guam ALS/parkinsonism-dementia: a long-latency neurotoxic disorder caused by 'slow toxin(s)' in food? *Canadian Journal of Neurological Sciences* 14, 347–57.

Tucker, L. and Lewis, C. 1973: A reliability coefficient for maximum likelihood factor analysis. *Psychometrika* 38, 1–10.

Veenstra, G. 2005: Location, location, location: contextual and compositional health effects of social capital in British Columbia, Canada. *Social Science and Medicine* 60, 2059–71.

Voight, B.F., Kudaravalli, S., Wen, X. and Pritchard, J.K. 2006: A map of recent positive selection in the human genome. *PLoS Biology* 4, e72.

Weich, S., Lewis, G. and Jenkins, S.P. 2001: Income inequality and the prevalence of common mental disorders in Britain. *British Journal of Psychiatry* 178, 222–27.

Worth, R.M., Kato, H., Rhoads, G.G., Kagan, K. and Syme, S.L. 1975: Epidemiologic studies of coronary heart disease and stroke in Japanese men living in Japan, Hawaii and California: mortality. *American Journal of Epidemiology* 102, 481–90.

Yusuf, S., Hawken, S., Ounpuu, S., Dans, T., Avezum, A., Lanas, F., McQueen, M., Budaj, A., Pais, P., Varigos, J. and Lisheng, L. and the INTERHEART Study Investigators. 2004: Effect of potentially modifiable risk factors associated with myocardial infarction in 52 countries (the INTERHEART study): case-control study. *The Lancet* 364, 937–52.

Zhang, Z.X., Anderson, D.W., Mantel, N. and Roman, G.C. 1995: Motor neuron disease on Guam: temporal occurrence, 1941–85. *Acta Neurologica Scandinavica* 92, 299–307.

# 5

# Philosophical tools for cultural psychiatry

KWM Fulford, David Sallah and Kim Woodbridge

## INTRODUCTION

Recent years have witnessed an unprecedented expansion of cross-disciplinary work between philosophy and psychiatry. In this chapter we outline developments in the new philosophy of psychiatry and illustrate the relevance of these developments to service development and delivery in cultural psychiatry.

## THE NEW PHILOSOPHY OF PSYCHIATRY

The new philosophy of psychiatry took off in the 1990s, the so-called 'decade of the brain' (Fulford *et al.*, 2003). There had been cross-disciplinary contact throughout the twentieth century, some of which, notably in the foundational work of the German philosopher-psychiatrist Karl Jaspers, on descriptive psychopathology, had a decisive impact on practice (Meares, 2003). But the 1990s witnessed a rapid expansion of new groups in many parts of the world and the establishment of a support network, the International Network for Philosophy and Psychiatry, the launch of a new international journal, *PPP – Philosophy, Psychiatry, and Psychology*, new book series from the USA, UK, France, Germany and the Netherlands, a series of annual international conferences, and the establishment of new research and teaching programmes, including new 'Chairs' for the discipline.

It was no coincidence that the emergence of a vigorous discipline of philosophy of psychiatry should coincide with the decade of the brain. As no less a neuroscientist than the American functional imaging researcher Nancy Andreasen has pointed out, the new neurosciences have pushed some of the deepest questions of general philosophy – such as freedom of the will, determinism, and the relationship between mind and brain – to the top of our practical research agenda in psychiatry (Andreasen, 2001).

Equally important, though, have been two fundamental shifts in practical service delivery: (1) from professional-centred to patient-centred decision-making; (2) from doctor-led to multidisciplinary service provision (Department of Health, 2005a, 2005b). These shifts, which were anticipated and to some extent provoked by the anti-psychiatry movement of the 1960s and 1970s, have required a radical re-thinking of the values and concepts, or models of disorder, guiding service development and delivery, and hence of the skills required for effective practical work in mental health and social care (Fulford, 2003). It is here, in the conceptual and values challenges of the new services, as much as in the neurosciences, that the practical impact of the new philosophy of psychiatry has been felt (Fulford *et al.*, 2006a). It is here, too, that the new philosophy of psychiatry has most to contribute in the way of practical tools for cultural psychiatry.

In the remainder of this chapter we illustrate the practical tools for service development and delivery in mental health and social care from four areas of the new philosophy of psychiatry: phenomenology (and related disciplines), the philosophy of science, philosophical value theory and conceptual analysis.

## PHENOMENOLOGY

Phenomenology is perhaps the area of philosophy that is most familiar to mental health practitioners. As the basis of Karl Jaspers' *General Psychopathology* (Jaspers, 1913), phenomenology in the early years of the twentieth century was a foundational discipline for modern descriptive psychopathology. Although somewhat neglected by British and American psychiatry, a strong tradition of phenomenology continued throughout the twentieth century in Continental Europe and in many other parts of the world (Fulford *et al.*, 2003). In recent years, with phenomenology becoming a key driver of the new philosophy of psychiatry, there has been a renewal of interest in the role of phenomenology as a partner to empirical methods in providing new insights into the structure of consciousness and of disturbances of consciousness (e.g. Varela *et al.*, 1992; Stanghellini, 2004).

In relation to service development and delivery, phenomenology is important to effective patient-centred practice because it provides insights into, and ways of characterizing, individual differences of experience. Matthew Philpott, for example, at the time a philosophy PhD student at Warwick University, used the work of the French phenomenologist

Maurice Merleau-Ponty to analyse the experience of dyslexia (Philpott, 1998). Merleau-Ponty's phenomenology, which was clinically grounded in the disturbances of consciousness following damage to the brain, for example by strokes, was concerned with the ways in which we come to make sense of the world, in particular in its temporal and spatial aspects. Philpott showed that the 'surface changes' of dyslexia (for example, reversing letters) reflected deeper underlying changes in the way that experiences are organized temporally by people with dyslexia.

Philpott's phenomenological insights were found to be directly helpful in the interpretation of brain imaging studies of dyslexia (Rippon, 1998). In relation to patient-centred practice, they were significant in shifting the way in which dyslexic experience is understood from 'defect' to 'difference'. Philpott's work suggests that children with dyslexia have different ways of learning to make sense of the spatial and temporal aspects of their experience and that much of their difficulty arises from well-intentioned attempts to train them in non-dyslexic ways of experiencing the world – somewhat like the correspondingly well-intentioned ways in which people used to try to turn natural left-handers into right-handers. Moreover, once dyslexic experience is recognized to be different rather than necessarily defective, different approaches to education and training that build on the particular strengths of the dyslexic become possible.

Other examples of the practical contributions to service development and delivery of phenomenology and related disciplines include an Irish psychiatrist and philosopher's use of Heideggerian phenomenology as the basis of new approaches to managing trauma in developing countries (Bracken, 2002), an approach that has been influential in policy and practice through the work of Amnesty International; the development by a Dutch philosopher of a hermeneutic approach to improved communication and conflict resolution with people with Alzheimer's disease (Widdershoven and Widdershoven-Heerding, 2003); and a powerful set of interpretive tools again for working with people with Alzheimer's disease, based on discursive methods (Sabat, 2001; Sabat and Harré, 1997).

Work in each of these areas illustrates the way in which phenomenology and related disciplines, as rigorous approaches to analysing experience supported by detailed theoretical frameworks, provide tools for more effective and inclusive ways of understanding differences not only between individuals but also between cultures in the way they experience the world. Much individual testimony, for example by an ex-service user researcher and writer, suggests that the (again well-intentioned but) profound mismatches between cultures in mutual understanding is one important source of the failure of conventional mental health and social care services to deliver race equality (King, 2007). Here, as in the better-recognized abuses of psychiatry (Fulford *et al.*, 1993), differences from the norm are misinterpreted as deficiencies, and culturally normal expressions of distress are misinterpreted as pathology. There are other tools for remedying this of course, notably from cultural anthropology, but phenomenology and related disciplines bring a new and potentially powerful set of theories and skills.

## PHILOSOPHY OF SCIENCE

Developments in the philosophy of science as applied to psychiatry provide the basis for a more culturally appropriate approach to psychiatric classification and diagnosis. The strongly empiricist orientation of current psychiatric classifications such as the *International Classification of Diseases* (ICD) (World Health Organization, 1992) and *Diagnostic and Statistical Manual of Mental Disorders* (DSM-IV) (American Psychiatric Association, 1994) reflects a model of science, called logical empiricism, that was dominant through the middle decades of the twentieth century. Indeed we owe these classifications, and the descriptive psychopathologies on which they are based, to the work of one of the great exemplars of logical empiricism, the American philosopher Carl Hempel. It was Hempel's intervention at a key meeting of the World Health Organization in the late 1950s (Hempel, 1961), interpreted and developed by the British psychiatrist Aubrey Lewis (Fulford *et al.*,

2006b), that led to the first exclusively symptom-based classification, the *Manual of the International Statistical Classification of Diseases, Injuries, and Causes of Death* (ICD-8) (World Health Organization, 1967), and hence to our current classifications in both the ICD series from the World Health Organization and the DSM series from the American Psychiatric Association.

As a model of science, logical empiricism has had many benefits for psychiatry: clearer definitions of diagnostic terms and improved reliability have been fundamental to advances in fields as diverse as epidemiology and functional imaging. There is a growing recognition, however, that these gains have been made at the expense of validity (Kupfer *et al.*, 2002), not only in relation to the neurosciences but also, and crucially, in cultural psychiatry (Alarcón *et al.*, 2002). There are many possible explanations for the failure of validity but from the perspective of the new philosophy of psychiatry this can be understood as reflecting the limitations of logical empiricism. The essential point here is that, just as logical empiricism, although a powerful model of science, has proved to be insufficient for psychiatry (as reflected in the failure of validity), so logical empiricism itself has proved to be an insufficient model of the way that science actually works – Hempel was indeed perhaps the last advocate of this model (Fulford *et al.*, 2006b).

The up-side to this interpretation is that, if logical empiricism is too limited a model, it turns out that what might now be called post-logical empiricist philosophy of science offers many resources for strengthening the scientific basis of psychiatry and, thereby, for improving the extent to which psychiatric classification and diagnosis are culturally appropriate. In the first place, a post-logical empiricist model opens up the conceptual space for there to be more than one way of understanding mental disorder (Fulford *et al.*, 2006b). Logical empiricism implies that there is ultimately one correct way of seeing the world that can be established through observations that are perspective-free. Post-logical empiricist philosophy of science shows, to the contrary, that observation, even in a 'hard' science like physics, is necessarily a matter of perspective. A failure to recognize this, combined with the 'one right view' of logical empiricism, tends inevitably to lead to one perspective becoming dominant. Post-logical empiricism, by contrast, provides a richer model of science that is capable of encompassing coherently a family of different views. Steps towards such a family have already been taken in the form of a 'comprehensive' model of psychiatric diagnosis (Mezzich *et al.*, 2003) incorporating personal idiographic as well as generalized descriptive criteria (Mezzich, 2002), as the basis of what one of us has called elsewhere a culturally competent psychiatry (Fulford, 1999).

The second way in which the post-logical empiricist philosophy of science opens up the conceptual space for more culturally appropriate models of psychiatric classification and diagnosis is that it shows the extent to which values are important in the way in which science actually proceeds. Values are important in psychiatric diagnosis because of their critical place, for example in relation to diagnostic judgements of clinical significance (Fulford, 2002), and the relevance of such judgements to culturally problematic differential diagnoses such as that between delusion and spiritual experience (Jackson and Fulford, 1997).

The traditional view, as in the logical empiricist model, is that science and values, like oil and water, are immiscible. In post-logical empiricist philosophy of science, modelled remember on the hard sciences such as physics, values are recognized as being woven into the scientific process at all stages, from the selection of research topics, through the definition of criteria of significance, to the interpretation of results and their applications in practice. It is small wonder then, that as the American psychiatrist and philosopher John Sadler has shown (Sadler, 2004), values are woven right through the most self-consciously scientific of psychiatry's classifications, the DSM. From the perspective of a traditional understanding of science, the value-ladenness of DSM is at best an embarrassment. But once it is recognized to be a reflection of the nature of science itself, this opens up the resources of philosophical value theory alongside those of the philosophy of science for the development of more culturally appropriate approaches to psychiatric classification.

## PHILOSOPHICAL VALUE THEORY

The importance of values even in the traditional heartland of scientific psychiatry, that is, in the art of classification, has traditionally been interpreted, for example in the 'psychiatry/anti-psychiatry' debate of the 1960s and 1970s, as a mark of scientific deficiency (Kendell, 1975). Work in philosophical value theory, by contrast, as developed in the new philosophy of psychiatry, shows that it is a mark rather of psychiatry being an area in which the values by which we define disorder itself are highly diverse (Fulford, 1989): values are present in all diagnostic concepts, bodily as well as mental, but we notice them in psychiatry because psychiatry is concerned with areas such as emotion, desire, motivation and sexuality, in which human values are inherently diverse, between individuals and between cultures, and hence may be problematic in practice.

The insights of philosophical value theory have been translated into practical tools for mental health and social care through a new approach to working with complex and conflicting values, called values-based practice. Briefly, values-based practice is a clinical skills-based approach to working with complex and conflicting values in health care (Fulford, 2004). Where traditional regulative ethics identifies and promotes particular values, values-based practice starts from respect for differences of values and relies on 'good process' for balanced decision-making in individual cases (Woodbridge and Fulford, 2003, 2004a).

It is the particularly wide diversity of values between cultures that makes the tools of values-based practice important in cultural psychiatry. In relation to ethics, for example, as the Egyptian psychiatrist Ahmed Okasha has pointed out, the dominant bioethical model, in reflecting particularly 'Western' values such as individual autonomy, may be inappropriate in cultures where families and relationships are of greater significance (Okasha, 2000). But the diversity of values between cultures also has a much wider significance, for psychiatric classification for example, as we described in the last section, and also at the cutting edge of cultural psychiatry, in the challenge of delivering race

---

**Box 5.1  Values in the vision for delivering race equality**

**Values in 'The Vision'**
**defined in policy (see text)**
bold = explicit values
italic = implicit values

1. *less fear* of mental health services among BME communities and service users;
2. **increased satisfaction** with services;
3. a reduction in the *disproportionate rate of admission* of people from BME communities to psychiatric inpatient units;
4. a reduction in the **disproportionate** *rates of compulsory detention* of BME users in inpatient units;
5. fewer violent incidents that are secondary to *inadequate treatment* of mental illness;
6. a reduction in the *use of seclusion* in BME groups;
7. *the prevention of deaths* in mental health services following physical intervention;
8. an increase in the population of BME service users who **feel they have recovered** from the *illness*;
9. a *reduction* in the proportion of prisoners from BME communities;
10. a *more balanced* range of **effective** therapies such as peer support services, psychotherapeutic and counselling treatments, as well as pharmacological interventions that are *culturally appropriate* and **effective**;
11. *a more active role* for BME communities and BME service users in the training of professionals, in the development of mental health policy, and in the planning and provision of services; and
12. a workforce and organization *capable* of delivering *appropriate* and *responsive* mental health services to BME communities.

---

equality in mental health services. In the UK, for example, the importance of values in this respect is reflected in the fact that a majority of the components of the current policy agenda for delivering race equality are deeply embedded in values, some of which, as Box 5.1 shows, are explicit, while others, although no less important, are implicit.

Values-based practice offers two specific and well-developed tools for responding to this agenda. First, it provides a strong policy framework (National Institute for Mental Health in England, 2005). This framework, which is reproduced in Box 5.2, emphasizes that values-based practice, in starting from respect for differences of values, explicitly excludes racism and other discriminatory attitudes. Second, the tools of values-based practice include a well-developed set of training materials covering four key areas of clinical skills: awareness, reasoning, knowledge and communication skills (Woodbridge and Fulford, 2004b, 2005). This training manual, which was launched by the British Minister for Health at a conference in London in 2004, is now the basis of a national generic skills training programme (Department of Health, 2004), and of a number of other national policies, covering such areas as multidisciplinary teamwork (Department of Health, 2005b) and the auditing and commissioning of services (Welsh Assembly Government, 2005).

Again, the tools of values-based practice are generic to psychiatry, and indeed to any area of health care decision-making where complex and conflicting values are involved, but they bear particularly on cultural psychiatry because of the extent of the differences of values between cultures.

## CONCEPTUAL ANALYSIS

The value-ladenness of psychiatric diagnostic concepts, and hence of the overall concept of mental disorder, compared with their counterparts in bodily medicine was at the heart of the 'psychiatry/anti-psychiatry' debate in the 1960s and 1970s. Much of this debate, indeed, has a 'values-in versus values-out' structure that has been carried through to the present day in relation to concepts of dysfunction and clinical significance (Fulford, 2000).

These debates, to the extent that they are concerned with the meanings of the very concepts by which psychiatry as a medical discipline is defined,

**Box 5.2   The National Institute for Mental Health in England (NIMHE) values framework**

The work of the National Institute for Mental Health in England (NIMHE) on values in mental health care is guided by three principles of values-based practice:

1. Recognition – NIMHE recognizes the role of values alongside evidence in all areas of mental health policy and practice.
2. Raising awareness – NIMHE is committed to raising awareness of the values involved in different contexts, the role(s) they play and their impact on practice in mental health.
3. Respect – NIMHE respects diversity of values and will support ways of working with such diversity that makes the principle of service-user centrality a unifying focus for practice. This means that the values of each individual service user/client and their communities must be the starting point and key determinant for all actions by professionals.

Respect for diversity of values encompasses a number of specific policies and principles concerned with equality of citizenship. In particular, it is anti-discriminatory because discrimination in all its forms is intolerant of diversity. Thus respect for diversity of values has the consequence that it is unacceptable (and unlawful in some instances) to discriminate on grounds such as gender, sexual orientation, class, age, abilities, religion, race, culture or language.

Respect for diversity within mental health is also:

- *user-centred* – it puts respect for the values of individual users at the centre of policy and practice;

- *recovery oriented* – it recognizes that by building on the personal strengths and resiliencies of individual users, and on their cultural and racial characteristics, there are many diverse routes to recovery;
- *multidisciplinary* – it requires that respect be reciprocal, at a personal level (between service users, their family members, friends, communities and providers), between different provider disciplines (such as nursing, psychology, psychiatry, medicine, social work), and between different organizations (including health, social care, local authority housing, voluntary organizations, community groups, faith communities and other social support services);
- *dynamic* – it is open and responsive to change;
- *reflective* – it combines self-monitoring and self-management with positive self-regard;
- *balanced* – it emphasizes positive as well as negative values;
- *relational* – it puts positive working relationships supported by good communication skills at the heart of practice.

NIMHE will encourage educational and research initiatives aimed at developing the capabilities (the awareness, attitudes, knowledge and skills) needed to deliver mental health services that will give effect to the principles of values-based practice.

are essentially philosophical in nature: one way of understanding the distinctive remit of philosophy is that it is, as the great twentieth-century philosopher-psychologist William James put it, 'an unusually stubborn effort to think clearly' about the meanings of concepts of this higher level or general kind (James, 1987, p. 296).

There are many ways of thinking clearly about meanings (Fulford *et al.*, 2006c, 2006d). Within the new philosophy of psychiatry, effective use has been made of a method of conceptual analysis called

'linguistic analysis'. Particularly associated with Oxford philosophy in the middle decades of the twentieth century, linguistic analysis, although only one way of proceeding philosophically, is a particularly powerful tool for philosophical work in an applied discipline like psychiatry (Fulford, 1990). First, linguistic analysis is a natural ally of empirical research in that its distinctive feature is that it focuses on language use as a guide to meaning rather than simply reflecting on definitions: the Oxford philosopher J.L. Austin called this, by direct

| ELEMENTS | MODELS | | | | | |
|---|---|---|---|---|---|---|
| | Medical (Organic) | Social (Stress) | Cognitive behavioural | Psycho-therapeutic | Family (interaction) | Conspiratorial |
| 1  Diagnosis/ Description | P | | | S | | |
| 2  Interpretation of behaviour | P | | | S | | |
| 3  Labels | P | | | S | | |
| 4  Aetiology | P | | | S | | |
| 5  Treatment | P | S | | | S | |
| 6  Function of the hospital | S  P | S | P | | | S  P |
| 7  Hospital & Community | P | S | | S | | |
| 8  Prognosis | P | | | S | | |
| 9  Rights of the Patient | S  P | S | | | | S |
| 10  Rights of Society | S  P | | | | | |
| 11  Duties of the Patient | P | | S  P | | | |
| 12  Duties of Society | P | S | | | | |

Figure 5.1  *Graphical representation of a models grid.*

analogy with empirical methods, 'philosophical field work' (quoted in Warnock, 1989, p. 25). Second, the philosophical field work approach is, like a medical discipline, most effectively employed in relation to case studies: this makes the approach naturally inclusive of diverse views rather than focusing on a currently dominant received view. Third, the inclusiveness of linguistic analysis is further reinforced by the nature of its characteristic outputs: linguistic analysis gives us a more complete or comprehensive view of the complex meanings of higher level concepts, a view that another Oxford philosopher, Gilbert Ryle, characterized as a more complete view of the 'logical geography' (Ryle, [1949] 1963, p. 9).

The potential of linguistic analysis as a practical tool in psychiatry is illustrated by a study carried out by the British social scientist, Anthony Colombo and colleagues, at Warwick University into the models of disorder held by different stakeholders – psychiatrists, social workers, psychiatric nurses, users and carers – involved in the community care of people with long-term schizophrenia (Colombo *et al.*, 2003).

The main findings from the study are illustrated by Figure 5.1. This 'models grid' as it is called, can be thought of as a Rylean logical geography that compares the implicit model of disorder held by the group of psychiatrists with that held by the group of psychiatric social workers. As can be seen, these two groups did indeed show significantly different implicit models of disorder: they coincided on only six out of a total of 72 elements of the overall grid. Equally important though, was the finding (not shown) of a similar split of models within the group of users of services: this group divided up naturally into one subgroup whose models looked very like those of psychiatrists, and a second subgroup whose models looked very like those of social workers. This was a surprise finding because the service user group had been recruited through the local branch of a mental health advocacy group Mind (National Association for Mental Health), and the expectation was that their models would be broadly anti-psychiatric.

Findings of this kind might suggest the need for one model to become dominant or perhaps for a 'super model' in which all the variety of different models are merged. The inclusive approach of linguistic analysis, however, provides a coherent framework within which these different models, once they are made explicit as part of professional training programmes, provide a balanced approach in which different professional perspectives from within a well-functioning multidisciplinary team can be tailored appropriately to the different perspectives of individual users and carers.

The findings and the methods developed in the course of the 'models project' have now been incorporated into the training materials in values-based practice described in the last section, as developed and piloted with front-line staff (Woodbridge and Fulford, 2004b). Colin King, the British researcher noted earlier, working with the Mental Health Foundation (a London-based mental health nongovernmental organization), is currently running an extension of the models project adapted to the particular challenges of developing race equality in mental health services (http://www.mentalhealth.org.uk/ck-project-survey).

## CONCLUSIONS

Philosophy is sometimes thought to be too abstract to be relevant in a practical discipline like psychiatry. The new cross-disciplinary field of philosophy of psychiatry, by contrast, as we have shown in this chapter, is already producing practical tools from within four areas: phenomenology, the philosophy of science, philosophical value theory and conceptual analysis. As we noted at the start of the chapter, there are also significant cross-disciplinary developments with the neurosciences but we have concentrated here on the practical tools from philosophy that directly support policy and service development in mental health and social care.

These practical tools from philosophy, as we have also indicated, are complementary to the tools derived from other disciplines. What is added by philosophy is, in effect, depth and breadth: a particular power of penetration of deeply embedded meanings (William James's 'stubborn effort' to think clearly); and a widening of understanding (Gilbert Ryle's 'more complete' view). The depth and breadth added by philosophy is particularly important in cultural psychiatry, and particularly in relation to race equality in mental health and social care, as a basis for inclusiveness in service development and delivery, an inclusiveness that arises not from ethical or political considerations

(important as these are), but from the very meanings of the concepts by which our discipline is defined.

If, however, the new philosophy of psychiatry has particular 'added value' for cultural psychiatry, it is cultural psychiatry, too, that shows the limits of the discipline as it has developed to date. The four areas of philosophy outlined in this chapter are all broadly 'Western' in origin. Powerful as these have been in the early development of the field, there are of course many other philosophies in other parts of the world with quite different but equally powerful resources for psychiatry: African philosophy (Coetzee and Roux, 2002), for example, and the more praxis-oriented Asian philosophies (Depraz, 2003, drawing on Yuasa, 1987 and Yamaguchi, 1997), could both be important in this respect. Cultural psychiatry is thus the natural conduit for the further development of philosophy and psychiatry as a discipline that is fully representative of the rich diversity of both philosophical and practice traditions around the world.

## REFERENCES

Alarcón, R.D., Bell, C.C., Kirmayer, L.J., Lin, K-M., Üstün, B. and Wisner, K.L. 2002: Beyond the funhouse mirrors: research agenda on culture and psychiatric diagnosis. In Kupfer, D.J., First, M.B. and Regier, D.E. (eds) *A Research Agenda for DSM-V.* Washington, DC: American Psychiatric Association, 219–82.

American Psychiatric Association 1994: *Diagnostic and Statistical Manual of Mental Disorders* (4th edn) (DSM-IV). Washington, DC: American Psychiatric Association.

Andreasen, N.C. 2001: *Brave New Brain: Conquering Mental Illness in the Era of the Genome.* Oxford: Oxford University Press.

Bracken, P. 2002: *Trauma: Culture, Meaning and Philosophy.* London: Whurr Publishers.

Coetzee, P.H. and Roux, A.P.J. (eds) 2002: *Philosophy from Africa* (2nd edn). Cape Town: Oxford University Press.

Colombo, A., Bendelow, G., Fulford, K.W.M. and Williams, S. 2003: Evaluating the influence of implicit models of mental disorder on processes of shared decision making within community-based multi-disciplinary teams. *Social Science and Medicine* 56, 1557–70.

Department of Health 2004: *The Ten Essential Shared Capabilities: A Framework for the Whole of the Mental Health Workforce.* London: The Sainsbury Centre for Mental Health, the NHSU (National Health Service University), and the NIMHE (National Institute for Mental Health England).

Department of Health 2005a: *Creating a Patient-led NHS: Delivering the NHS Improvement Plan*. London: Department of Health; Available at: http://www.dh.gov.uk/assetRoot/04/10/65/07/04106507.pdf.

Department of Health 2005b: *New Ways of Working for Psychiatrists: Enhancing effective, person-centred services through new ways of working in multidisciplinary and multi-agency contexts (Final report 'but not the end of the story')*. London: Department of Health. Available at: http://www.dh.gov.uk/assetRoot/04/12/23/43/04122343.pdf.

Depraz, N. 2003: Putting the *époché* into practice: schizophrenic experience as illustrating the phenomenological exploration of consciousness. In Fulford, K.W.M., Morris, K.J., Sadler, J.Z. and Stanghellini, G. (eds) *Nature and Narrative: An Introduction to the New Philosophy of Psychiatry*. Oxford: Oxford University Press, chapter 12.

Fulford, K.W.M. 1989 reprinted 1995 and 1999: *Moral Theory and Medical Practice*. Cambridge: Cambridge University Press.

Fulford, K.W.M. 1990: Philosophy and medicine: the Oxford connection. *British Journal of Psychiatry* 157, 111–15.

Fulford, K. W. M. 1999: From culturally sensitive to culturally competent: a seminar in philosophy and practice skills. In Bhui, K. and Olajide, D. (eds) *Mental Health Service Provision for a Multi-cultural Society*. London: W.B. Saunders Company, 21–42.

Fulford, K.W.M. 2000: Teleology without tears: naturalism, neo-naturalism, and evaluationism in the analysis of function statements in biology (and a bet on the twenty-first century). *Philosophy, Psychiatry, and Psychology* 7, 77–94.

Fulford, K.W.M. 2002: Values in psychiatric diagnosis: executive summary of a report to the chair of the ICD-12/DSM-VI Coordination Task Force (Dateline 2010). *Psychopathology* 35, 132–38.

Fulford, K.W.M. 2003: Mental illness: definition, use and meaning. In Post, S.G. (ed.) *Encyclopedia of Bioethics* (3rd edn). New York: Macmillan, 1789–1800.

Fulford, K.W.M. 2004: Ten principles of values-based medicine. In Radden, J. (ed.) *The Philosophy of Psychiatry: A Companion*. New York: Oxford University Press, 205–34.

Fulford, K.W.M., Smirnov, A.Y.U. and Snow, E. 1993: Concepts of disease and the abuse of psychiatry in the USSR. *British Journal of Psychiatry* 162, 801–10.

Fulford, K.W.M., Morris, K.J., Sadler, J.Z. and Stanghellini, G. 2003: Past improbable, future possible: the renaissance in philosophy and psychiatry. In Fulford, K.W.M., Morris, K.J., Sadler, J.Z. and Stanghellini, G. (eds) *Nature and Narrative: an Introduction to the New Philosophy of Psychiatry*. Oxford: Oxford University Press, pp. 1–41.

Fulford, K.W.M., Thornton, T. and Graham, G. 2006a: Progress in five parts. In Fulford, K.W.M., Thornton, T. and Graham, G. (eds) *The Oxford Textbook of Philosophy and Psychiatry*. Oxford: Oxford University Press, chapter 1.

Fulford, K.W.M., Thornton, T. and Graham, G. 2006b: Natural classifications, realism and psychiatric science. In: Fulford, K.W.M., Thornton, T. and Graham, G. (eds) *The Oxford Textbook of Philosophy and Psychiatry*. Oxford: Oxford University Press, chapter 13.

Fulford, K.W.M., Thornton, T. and Graham, G. 2006c: Philosophical methods in mental health research and practice. In Fulford, K.W.M., Thornton, T. and Graham, G. (eds) *The Oxford Textbook of Philosophy and Psychiatry*. Oxford: Oxford University Press, chapter 4.

Fulford, K.W.M., Thornton, T., Graham, G. and Sturdee, P. 2006d: Arguments good and bad: an introduction to philosophical logic for practitioners. In Fulford, K.W.M., Thornton, T. and Graham, G. (eds) *The Oxford Textbook of Philosophy and Psychiatry*. Oxford: Oxford University Press, chapter 5.

Hempel, C.G. 1961: Introduction to problems of taxonomy. In Zubin, J. (ed.) *Field Studies in the Mental Disorders*. New York: Grune and Stratton, 3–22. Reproduced in Sadler, J.Z., Wiggins, O.P. and Schwartz, M.A. (1994) *Philosophical Perspectives on Psychiatric Diagnostic Classification*. Baltimore, The Johns Hopkins University Press, 315–31.

Jackson, M. and Fulford, K.W.M. 1997: Spiritual experience and psychopathology. *Philosophy, Psychiatry, and Psychology* 4, 41–66.

James, W. 1987: Review of Grunzuge der Physiologischen Psychologie, by Wilhelm Wundt 1975. In *Essays, Comments and Reviews*. Cambridge, MA: Harvard University Press.

Jaspers, K. 1913: *Allgemeine Psychopathologie*. Berlin, Springer-Verlag. trans. J. Hoenig and M.W. Hamilton (1963) *General Psychopathology*. Chicago: University of Chicago Press. New edition (two volumes, paperback), with a Foreword by Paul R. McHugh (1997). Baltimore: The Johns Hopkins University Press.

Kendell, R.E. 1975: The concept of disease and its implications for psychiatry. *British Journal of Psychiatry* 127, 305–15.

King, C. 2007: They diagnosed me a schizophrenic when I was just a gemini: the other side of madness. In Chung, M., Fulford, K.W.M. and Graham, G. (eds) *Reconceiving Schizophrenia*. Oxford: Oxford University Press, chapter 2.

Kupfer, D.J., First, M.B. and Regier, D.E. 2002: Introduction. In Kupfer, D.J., First, M.B. and Regier, D.E. (eds) *A Research Agenda for DSM-V*. Washington, DC: American Psychiatric Association, xv.

Meares, R. 2003: Towards a psyche for psychiatry. In Fulford, K.W.M., Morris, K.J., Sadler, J.Z. and Stanghellini, G. (eds) *Nature and Narrative: An Introduction to the New Philosophy of Psychiatry*. Oxford: Oxford University Press, chapter 2.

Mezzich, J.E. 2002: Comprehensive diagnosis: a conceptual basis for future diagnostic systems. *Psychopathology* 35, 162–65.

Mezzich, J.E., Berganza, C.E., Von Cranach, M., Jorge, M.R., Kastrup, M.C., Murthy, R.S., Okasha, A., Pull, C., Sartorius,

N., Skodol, A. and Zaudig, M. 2003: IGDA. 8: Idiographic (personalised) diagnostic formulation. In Essentials of the World Psychiatric Association's International Guidelines for Diagnostic Assessment (IGD). *British Journal of Psychiatry* 182 (Suppl. 45), 5–57.

National Institute for Mental Health in England 2005: *Values Framework*. Available at: http://nimhe.csip.org.uk/ValuesBasedPractise.

Okasha, A. 2000: Ethics of psychiatric practice: consent, compulsion and confidentiality. *Current Opinion in Psychiatry* 13, 693–98.

Philpott, M.J. 1998: A phenomenology of dyslexia: the lived-body, ambiguity, and the breakdown of expression. *Philosophy, Psychiatry, and Psychology* 5, 1–20.

Rippon, G. 1998: Commentary on 'A phenomenology of dyslexia'. *Philosophy, Psychiatry, and Psychology* 5, 25–28.

Ryle, G. [1949] 1963: *The Concept of Mind*. London: Penguin Books.

Sabat, S.R. 2001: *The Experience of Alzheimer's Disease: Life Through a Tangled Veil*. Oxford: Blackwell Publishers.

Sabat, S.R. and Harré, R. 1997: The Alzheimer's disease sufferer as semiotic subject. *Philosophy, Psychiatry, and Psychology* 1, 145–60.

Sadler, J.Z. 2004: *Values and Psychiatric Diagnosis*. Oxford: Oxford University Press.

Stanghellini, G. 2004: *Deanimated Bodies and Disembodied Spirits. Essays on the Psychopathology of Common Sense*. Oxford: Oxford University Press.

Varela, F.J., Thompson, E.T. and Rosch, E. 1992: *The Embodied Mind: Cognitive Science and Human Experience*. Cambridge, MA: The MIT Press.

Warnock, G.J. 1989: *J.L. Austin*. London: Routledge.

Welsh Assembly Government 2005: *Healthcare Standards for Wales: Making the Connections Designed for Life*.

Widdershoven, G. and Widdershoven-Heerding, I. 2003: Understanding dementia: a hermeneutic perspective. In Fulford, K.W.M., Morris, K.J., Sadler, J.Z. and Stanghellini, G. (eds) *Nature and Narrative: An Introduction to the New Philosophy of Psychiatry*. Oxford: Oxford University Press, 103–12.

Woodbridge, K. and Fulford, K.W.M. 2003: Good practice? Values-based practice in mental health. *Mental Health Practice* 7, 30–34.

Woodbridge, K. and Fulford, K.W.M. 2004a: Right, wrong and respect. *Mental Health Today* September, 28–30.

Woodbridge, K. and Fulford, K.W.M. 2004b: *Whose Values? A Workbook for Values-based Practice in Mental Health Care*. London: Sainsbury Centre for Mental Health.

Woodbridge, K. and Fulford, K.W.M. 2005: Values-based practice. In Basset, T. and Lindley, L. (eds) *The Ten Essential Shared Capabilities Learning Pack for Mental Health Practice*. For the National Health Service University (NHSU) and the National Institute for Mental Health in England (NIMHE), module 4. London: The National Health Service University.

World Health Organization 1967: *Manual of the International Statistical Classification of Diseases, Injuries and Causes of Death (ICD-8)*. Geneva: World Health Organization.

World Health Organization 1992: *The ICD-10 Classification of Mental and Behavioural Disorders: Clinical Descriptions and Diagnostic Guidelines*. Geneva: World Health Organization.

Yuasa, Y. 1987: *The Body. Toward an Eastern Mind-Body Theory*. New York: State University of New York Press.

Yamaguchi, I. 1997: *Ki also leibhaftige Vernunft, Beitrag zur interkulturellen Phànomenologie de Leiblichkeit*. München: Fink Verlag.

# 6

# Religion and mental health

Goffredo Bartocci and Simon Dein

## INTRODUCTION

The past ten years have seen increasing interest amongst academics in the topic of religion and mental health (Bhugra, 1996; Bartocci, 2000; Koenig *et al.*, 2001; Dein, 2004). This chapter presents an overview of the area and is divided into several themes. First, the problems defining religion and spirituality and their relation to mental health are outlined. Second, religion and differential diagnosis are discussed. Third the 'healing effect' of religious experience is explored.

## THE DIVORCE OF RELIGION AND PSYCHIATRY

The study of the role played by religious beliefs and experiences in mental health care is becoming one of the priority epistemological targets of postmodern psychiatry (Wulff, 1991; Schumaker, 1992; Littlewood, 1993; Bartocci *et al.*, 1998; Boehnlein,

2000). Due to the recent phenomena of globalization, creolization and colonization of people and religions, both the secular and the spiritual movements in medicine are moving towards a converging path. There is a tendency of religious institutions to encompass domains that up to now fell under the competence of psychiatric disciplines; at the same time, in the anthropological, psychological and neurological fields of scholarship, there is now a general inclination to undertake the task of analysing the influence, either positive or negative, of religious factors on human behaviour and sometimes even brain functioning.

Until the early nineteenth century religion and psychiatry were closely connected. Much of the 'healing' of mental illness was conducted within the church context. Highly influenced by the processes of modernization, professionalization and secularization, medicine, with its emphasis on technical procedures and legitimated by scientific 'authority', became increasingly divorced from the subjective experience of illness; and consequently religion was relegated to the sphere of subjectivity rather than science (Glas, 2001). Hence psychiatry with its objective, morally neutral application of scientific knowledge became separated from religion.

However there is evidence for a recent rapprochement of the two disciplines, as suggested by the burgeoning literature on religion and psychiatry (for example, Bhugra, 1996; Koenig *et al.*, 2001) and the increasing involvement of religious professionals in mental health care. Although the roots of this reunion are unclear, it is likely that several factors might play a mediating role: the increasing influx to the industrialized world of people from developing countries who hold strong religious convictions, disillusionment with materialism, a search for more spiritual ways of being, the inability of psychiatry to address existential questions of ultimate concern and an internal underlying tension among psychiatrists relating to a perception that their current practice is too limited (Glas, 2001). There is increasing recognition that psychopathology is intimately connected to and influenced by spiritual and religious issues.

The importance of taking into account patients' spiritual and religious views has become increasingly recognized, as exemplified by the American Psychiatric Association's call for a 'respectful clinical assessment' of patients including areas related to religion and spirituality. Similarly Sims (1994), a past president of the Royal College of Psychiatrists, noted:

> For too long psychiatry has avoided the spiritual realm . . . but psychiatrists have neglected it at their patients' peril. We need to evaluate the religious and spiritual experience of our clients in aetiology, diagnosis, prognosis and treatment.

These thoughts are echoed by the World Health Organization position paper on Quality of Life (World Health Organization, 1995) which emphasizes the importance of recognizing religion/spirituality and personal beliefs.

## RELIGION AND SPIRITUALITY

The term 'religion' has generally been used to refer to some institutionalized set of beliefs and practices relating to a community. The word religion derives from the Latin term *religare* (to hold together, bind) which refers to the binding together of a conglomerate of persons (Cicero, second century AD). This has taken on the meaning of a state of dependence on a superior entity (in Tertullian's usage, third century AD). Surrender to God, and the transcendental thrust that oneness with the Absolute is the human ultimate wish, opened the way for a new religious era in Western civilization: 'the characteristic of the new faith, compared to pagan cults, was represented by the bondage of pity and of dependence seen as a duty of faith paid to God. Thus the old concept of the Roman *religio* disappears making way for its modern meaning' (Frighi, 1996).

The term religion is to be differentiated from the term spirituality, which refers to a connectedness with a higher power and the sense of meaning deriving from this connectedness (King *et al.*, 2001; Dein, 2005). One can be spiritual but not religious. The two terms are often used synonymously in the literature. The distinction between religion and spirituality is largely a Western (Christian) phenomenon with less distinction being made in Judaism and Islam. This increasing division between religion and spirituality is rooted in a number of cultural trends: the emphasis on individualization, the Western preoccupation with the pursuit of meaning and discontentment with materialism. Dein (2005) has written an overview of this area. The dependence on God still remains today in the definition of spirituality. For example Hughes and Wintrob (2000), quoting Miller and Martin (1988), state: 'As a working definition, we propose that spirituality entails the acknowledgement of a transcendent being, power, or reality greater than ourselves. . . . Furthermore spirituality involves an attempt to align and conform one's life (both covert and overt behaviour) toward this higher power.'

## CONCEPTS OF THE SELF AND RELIGION

Cultural variations in concepts of the self and person, and the perceived boundaries between the self and other, might predispose some groups to transcend the 'mundane' world and commune with spiritual entities. It appears that some devotees, once their world has been split in two parts (the mundane and the spiritual), learned to enjoy mastering the experience of travelling between the two domains. This includes an experience of risk and associated pleasure, and experience of vanishing from daily perceptions, then making contact with the Absolute as the turning buoy from which to return back to the abandoned world which momentarily disappeared. Such pervasive experiences may be reflected in the biblical condemnation of having lost forever the garden of Eden.

In Western culture, particularly in the Judaeo-Christian tradition, where the split of the mundane and extramundane world is particularly evident, a definition of a separate self is widely accepted. This individual self is associated with the capacity for self-direction and responsibility. Evidence from other cultures suggests that our conception of the individual self is constituted by a set of cultural rules and practices and that autonomous individuality which we presume to be universal is, in fact, culturally specific (Geertz, 1975). Heelas and Lock (1981) point out that all cultures make some distinction between self and non-self but radically differ both in regard to their boundaries and the existence of improper relations between the varying parts. For instance, among the Balinese there is only a minimal role for the unique individual self in everyday life. For the Ilongot there is no recognition of an autonomous self apart from outward behaviour (Rosaldo, 1984) and the Ifaulk who are collectivists find any reference to unique autonomous individuality to be excessively egocentric. Traditional Hindu culture defines the self fluidly in and through others rather than sharply differentiating between them (Schweder and Miller, 1985).

In a similar way the Western conceptualization of the self is historically recent. Lyons (1978) argues it was not until the late eighteenth century that people reinforced the view of their individual selves as central. Before this they saw themselves in terms of group membership categories. This change may have been exaggerated by the religious choice introduced by the reformation and the distinction between the public and private self made possible by capitalization and the cultivation of the inner spiritual self during the romantic era. These conceptualizations of the self are seminal in understanding religious experience and the relationship with non-human worlds.

## RESEARCH ON RELIGION AND MENTAL HEALTH: PSYCHOLOGY OF RELIGION PERSPECTIVES

A significant problem in examining the relation of religion and mental health relates to the measurement of religiosity. We suggest that religion is best seen as a multidimensional phenomenon. The term can be divided up into a number of components: church attendance, beliefs about God, the use of ritual, the importance of religion in everyday life, religion as coping with life events, intrinsic and extrinsic religiosity. The latter two terms refer to being religious for its own sake (intrinsic religion) or for what religion can do for a person (extrinsic religion). Each of these components may relate to mental health outcomes in different ways. Each dimension has its own problems when researchers try to provide operational details and definitions. Until recently, studies that have included a religious variable had largely focused on church or synagogue attendance. This is problematic as those who are mentally ill may not be able to attend church. This would provide a biased view in any research that assessed the relationship between religion and mental health. Recently there has been a move to examine the ways that religion is used for coping with everyday life stresses (Pargament *et al.*, 1990). In terms of mental health, Pargament *et al.* (1990) found that beliefs in a just benevolent God and the experience of God as a supportive partner in coping are positively related to various indices of mental health. Studies on the relation between religion and mental health have deployed a wide range of definitions of 'mental health'. Some studies have stopped at measuring general sense of wellbeing or optimism. Other studies have looked at more specific types of mental illness, such as depression, schizophrenia, alcoholism, suicide, marital stability or delinquency.

Koenig *et al.* (2001) have reviewed over 1200 published research studies providing data on the positive and negative relationships between religion/spirituality and physical, mental and social health. Overall, the literature suggests that on average, being religious is related to better indices of mental health (Koenig *et al.*, 2001; Koenig and Larson, 2001). Specifically, several studies have found religious/spiritual factors to be linked with lower rates of depression (McCullough and Larson, 1999) and suicide (Koenig and Larson, 2001). Being religious might also speed up recovery from depression (Koenig *et al.*, 1998a,b). The findings in relation to schizophrenia appear to be more contradictory.

## BY WHAT MECHANISMS MIGHT RELIGIOSITY ENHANCE MENTAL HEALTH?

There are a number of ways religion might enhance mental health throughout the life cycle. The major religious groups provide positive models of parenting which are conducive to the development of positive self-esteem in children. Specifically, those who have a history of mental illness are supported by the religious community, which may act to minimize any genetic effects on children. Although not formally empirically demonstrated, it is likely that community support will reduce rates of puerperal illness.

Religion often protects against abuses that occur in the secular world, for instance drug or alcohol abuse, and against stressful life events. For instance, divorce is less common in some religious groups than in the secular world. It may provide a number of cognitions that can enhance wellbeing. Experiencing a severe life event but knowing that God is taking responsibility and that He is supporting you, may offer transcendent salvation so avoiding the risk of a mundane acute psychogenic reaction and thus enhancing mental health. Religion may provide a meaningful perspective into which adverse experiences can be put. For example, when a person

experiences an adverse life event it may be given extra meaning by the religious context. For instance, severe illness may not be readily understandable but in the wider scope of things can be seen as a learning experience. Ultimately religions argue that we do not understand God's ways and even this may be comforting for some people.

## THE ADVERSE EFFECTS OF RELIGION

Not all religious practices lead to positive mental health benefits. It is well recognized that some religious groups such as Catholicism and Judaism emphasize guilt. This may adversely affect mental health. Some religious groups may be antipsychiatry, and therefore, may prevent their practitioners from obtaining treatment and worsen their prognosis when they do become mentally ill. Rarely, some groups advocate suicide. For instance, some cult groups may advocate that the end of the world is coming and there will be an apocalypse. To avoid suffering people may commit suicide (Dein and Littlewood, 2000). Beyond this, there is emerging evidence that 'negative religious coping', seeing illness as a punishment from God or questioning God's power (Pargament, 1998), can be detrimental to mental health.

## RELIGION AND DIFFERENTIAL DIAGNOSIS

The recent V code in the *Diagnostic and Statistical Manual of Mental Disorders* (DSM-IV) illustrates the increasing acknowledgement by mental health professionals of the overpathologization of religious states. The code discusses a number of experiences that are not necessarily pathological but may be misdiagnosed as symptoms of psychiatric disorder: becoming over-religious, religious conversion and losing religious faith. Although these may result in formal mental illness, they are not in themselves symptoms of mental disorder and may result in issues which might be dealt with by religious professionals. One contentious area involves the close links between mystical experiences and schizophrenia. It cannot be denied, however, that there are some similarities between the two types of experience (Clarke, 2001). For instance, both often share a religious or paranormal content, or association with a divine calling. Both involve a sense of presence or experience of discarnate entities and a sense of being guarded by external power. Visions and voices may occur in both. There are also some phenomenological parallels between the two types of experience (Jackson and Fulford, 1997).

The central characteristics of mystical states include 'noesis'. This can be experienced at the onset of psychosis (Buckley, 1981). Both mystical states and psychoses share a sense of disruption of time. The mystic may claim to be in the presence of God for what seems like hours whereas the psychotic may experience trance-like lapses of time. Generally mystical experiences are short-term phenomena, which are associated with insight. They are usually positive experiences, whereas psychoses are usually negative experiences (Clarke, 2001).

Another problematic differential diagnosis is in terms of obsessional illness. Sometimes it can be difficult to differentiate between hyper religiosity and obsessional illness. However, in obsessional religiosity, a person's religious practice, for instance prayer, is carried out in accord with accepted religious practice in the congregation but perhaps at the expense of being part of the religious group. There is an excessive focus on a single practice rather than the full range of practices. Also the themes exemplified in religious practices, cleanliness for example, may also be found in obsessive-compulsive disorders.

## RELIGIOUS EXPERIENCE AND HEALING

In 1979 Prince argued that both psychosis and religious experience could be seen as endogenous attempts to heal the psyche and argued that a spontaneous healing mechanism is also apparent in a good proportion of extrovertive mystical experiences. He provides as evidence the experiences of a number of people such as Arthur Koestler, Claire

Myers Owen and Malcolm Muggeridge who experienced these mystical states during periods of privation or depression. Prince viewed religious experience as a homeostatic self-healing mechanism which the brain has evolved to resolve acute stress; the notion that religious and spiritual experiences are adaptive psychological processes is shared by many expert authors (James, 1902; Jung, 1960; Batson and Ventis, 1982; Grof and Grof, 1986; Storr, 1996). Persinger (1983) argues that the capacity for such experiences has evolved as a species-specific buffer against death anxiety. For Batson and Ventis (1982) spiritual experience is a problem-solving process that is triggered by existential crises involving both emotional and cognitive tension. In the case of benign spiritual experience, the problem-solving process is homeostatic and reduces their level of tension. From a statistical point of view we witness that religious-based or religious-interwoven healing procedures are seen as successful up to the point that pain-killing transcendence techniques are widely recommended even by good housekeeping magazines.

So it is not true that scientific civilization has obscured the light emanating from the heavens, as was once believed by religious leaders. As biomedicine increasingly succeeded in treating the body, it was believed that alternative healers would disappear. Despite biomedicine's extraordinary achievements, a multitude of alternative healing forms have continued to flourish; indeed we can even now add the flourishing of holy thaumaturgists (Bartocci and Littlewood, 2004).

## CONCLUSION

Before us lies a clinical path laden with responsibility: 'In order to meet the demands of patients of diverse cultures, it is essential to add the dimensions of religion and spirituality to the training of future psychiatrists' (Tseng, 2003). In order to provide future psychiatrists with adequate training that might be both politically correct, in the sense of respecting different cultural backgrounds, but also scientifically correct, that is to say endorsed by the scientific paradigms that are consistent with the motivations that led us to choose the medical profession, it is necessary to be able to assess clinically all cultural and dynamic factors producing peak experiences. This is essential in order to prevent a patient presenting an irruption of the supernatural from being treated 'for a biogenetic (incurable) brain disease rather than a curable spiritual illness' (Castillo, 2003).

## REFERENCES

Bartocci, G. 2000: WPA 2000 Forum on Culture Psychiatry Spirituality. *Current Opinion in Psychiatry* 13, 525–43.

Bartocci, G. and Littlewood, R. 2004: Modern techniques of the supernatural: a synchretism between healing and the mass media. *Social Theory and Health* 2, 18–28.

Bartocci, G., Frighi, L., Rovera. G.G., Lalli, N. and Di Fonzo, T. 1998: Cohabiting with magic and religion in Italy: cultural and clinical results. In Okpaku, S. (ed.) *Clinical Methods in Transcultural Psychiatry.* Washington: American Psychiatric Press, 321–35.

Batson, C. and Ventis, L. 1982: *The Religious Experience.* Oxford: Oxford University Press.

Bhugra, D. (ed.) 1996: *Psychiatry and Religion. Context, Consensus and Controversies.* London: Routledge.

Boehnlein, J. 2000: *Psychiatry and Religion.* Washington, DC: American Psychiatric Press.

Buckley, P. 1981: Mystical experience and schizophrenia. *Schizophrenia Bulletin* 7, 516–21.

Castillo, R. 2003: Trance, functional psychosis and culture. *Psychiatry* 66, 9–21.

Clarke, I. 2001: *Psychosis and Spirituality: Exploring the New Frontier.* London: Whurr.

Dein, S. 2004: Working with patients with religious beliefs. *Advances in Psychiatric Treatment* 10, 287–94.

Dein, S. 2005: Spirituality, psychiatry and participation: a cultural analysis. *Transcultural Psychiatry* 42(4), 526–44.

Dein, S. and Littlewood, R. 2000: Apocalyptic suicide. *Mental Health, Religion and Culture* 3, 109–14.

Frighi, L. 1996: Qualità della vita e dimensione spirituale. *Attualità in Psicologia* XI, 465–70.

Geertz, C. 1975: *The Interpretation of Cultures.* New York: Basic Books.

Glas, G. 2001: Angst. *Beleving, Structuur, Macht.* Amsterdam: Boom.

Grof, S. and Grof, C. 1986: Spiritual emergency: the understanding and treatment of transpersonal crises. *Revision* 8, 7–20.

Heelas, P. and Lock, A. 1981: *Indigenous Psychologies: Anthropology of the Self.* London: Academic Press.

Hughes, C. and Wintrob, R. 2000: Psychiatry and religion in cross-cultural context. In Boehnlein, J. (ed.) *Psychiatry and Religion.* Washington, DC: American Psychiatric Press, 27–52.

Jackson, M. and Fulford, K. 1997: Spiritual experience and psychopathology. *Philosophy, Psychiatry and Psychology* 1, 41–65.

James, W. 1902: *The Varieties of Religious Experience.* New York: Longman.

Jung, C. 1960: On the psychogenesis of schizophrenia. *Collected Work,* Vol. 3. London: Routledge & Kegan Paul.

King, M., Speck, P. and Thomas, A. 2001: The Royal Free interview for spiritual and religious beliefs: development and validation of the self report version. *Psychological Medicine* 31: 1015–23.

Koenig, H. and Larson, D. 2001: Religion and mental health: evidence of an association. *International Review of Psychiatry* 13, 67–78.

Koenig, H., Larson, D. and Weaver, A. 1998a: Research on religion and serious mental illness. In Fallott, R.D. (ed.) *Spirituality and Religion in Recovery from Mental Illness.* San Francisco: Jossey-Bass, 80, 81–95.

Koenig, H., George, L. and Peterson, B. 1998b: Religiosity and remission from depression in medically ill older patients. *American Journal of Psychiatry* 155, 536–42.

Koenig, H., McCullough, M. and Larson, D. 2001: *Handbook of Religion and Health.* Oxford: Oxford University Press.

Littlewood, R. 1993: *Pathology and Identity.* Cambridge: Cambridge University Press.

Lyons, J. 1978: *The Invention of the Self.* Carbondale, IL: Southern Illinois University Press.

McCullough, M. and Larson, D. 1999: Religion and depression: a review of the literature. *Twin Research* 2, 126–136.

Miller, W.R. and Martin, J.E. 1988: Spirituality and behavioral psychology: toward integration. In Miller, W.R. and Martin, J.E. (eds) *Behavior Therapy and Religion: Integrating Spiritual and Behavioral Approaches to Change.* Newbury Park, CA: Sage, 13–23.

Pargament, K. 1998: Patterns of positive and negative religious coping with major life stressors. *Journal for the Scientific Study of Religion* 37, 710–24.

Pargament, K., Ensing, D., Falgout, K. *et al.* 1990: God help me: religious coping efforts as predictors of outcome to significant life events. *American Journal of Community Psychology* 18(6), 793–834.

Persinger, M. 1983: Religious and mystical experience as artefacts of temporal lobe function: a general hypothesis. *Perception and Motor Skills* 57, 1255–62.

Prince, R. 1979: Religious experience and psychosis. *Journal of Altered States of Consciousness* 5, 1979–80.

Rosaldo, R. 1984: Towards an anthropology of the self and feeling. In Schweder, R. and Le Vine, R. (eds) *Culture*

*Theory: Essays on Mind, Self and Emotion.* Cambridge: Cambridge University Press.

Schumaker, J. (ed.) 1992: *Religion and Mental Health.* New York: Oxford University Press.

Schweder, R.A. and Miller, J.G. 1985: The social construction of the person: how is it possible? In Gergen, K.J. and Davis, K.J. (eds) *The Social Construction of the Person.* New York: Springer-Verlag.

Sims, A. 1994: Psyche-spirit as well as mind. *British Journal of Psychiatry* 165, 441–46.

Storr, A. 1996: *Feet of Clay – Saints, Sinners, and Madmen: A Study of Gurus.* New York: The Free Press.

Tseng, W.S. 2003: *Clinician's Guide to Cultural Psychiatry.* San Diego, CA: Academic Press.

World Health Organization 1995: The World Health Organization quality of life assessment (WHOQAL): position paper from the World Health Organization. Geneva: WHO.

Wulff, D. 1991: *Psychology of Religion.* New York: Wiley & Sons.

# 7

# Mental health law and clinical practice: An international and cultural perspective

Albert Persaud, Anand Satyanand, Nemu Lallu, Charles Pace and Li Zhanjiang

## INTRODUCTION

As civilization evolved so have laws and attitudes to the treatment of the mentally ill. Attitudes to mental health care and legislation can be traced back to Hippocrates – Patriarch of Greek medicine. More recently, governments across the world have had to respond to an ever-expanding evidence base, and rapid political and policy changes, and most importantly more emphasis on the rights of the individual to free choice. This chapter describes the evolution of four models of mental health legislation in England, Malta, New Zealand and China. It also captures the policy context which sets the tone for the use of mental health legislation (see Chapter 9).

## THE ENGLAND EXPERIENCE

Mental health legislation has always been a major cornerstone of England's mental health policy and practice. Following the publication in 1998 of a government White Paper called *Modernising Mental Health Services – safe, sound and secure* (Department of Health, 1998) and the *National Service Framework (NSF) for Mental Health* (Department of Health, 1999), clear priorities were set for the development and funding of mental health services. The emphasis was on standards of care and service models that provide effective treatment in primary care, in community settings as well as in hospitals. *The National Health Service (NHS) Plan* (Department of Health, 2000) reinforced these initiatives in 2000 by making mental health one of the top three clinical priorities for the NHS. It also gave assurances of resources to support the development of services.

*The NHS Plan* states that 'The Mental Health Act 1983 will be reformed to create a new legislative framework reflecting modern patterns of care and treatment for severe mental illness'. English mental health legislation is relatively young when compared with other countries in the world, yet the government wishes to introduce new mental health legislation as a priority for the improvement of mental health care. This does raise a question of what should come first – standards of care and a philosophy of care that enables new legislation to be enacted in practice, or does new legislation itself create a process for improved standards of care?

## History of mental health law in England

Early legislation associated with mental health dates back to the sixteenth century. The 1890 Lunacy Act's principal aim was to ensure that sane people were not committed to hospital. The 1930 Mental Treatment Act introduced the first notion of voluntary admission. The most significant piece of legislation that transformed the way policy-makers and practitioners think in the twentieth century was the 1959 Mental Health Act. This was seen as more liberal than all previous legislation, and was influenced by patients, legal activists and others interested in reform. It was developed and implemented at the time of the great American civil rights movement, which in turn influenced a global trend towards more liberal attitudes. The 1959 Act aimed to bring mental health care into greater congruency with other health care, to remove the emphasis on a certification process with a legal review of continuing detention after admission. Furthermore, it broadened admission criteria and the role of professional discretion.

## The current 1983 Mental Health Act in the UK

The 1983 Mental Health Act preserved the essential principles of the 1959 Act but also introduced external audits and monitoring. This included several safeguards:

- The creation of the Mental Health Act Commission. The principal function of the Commission is to monitor the treatment and care of detained patients; it appoints Commissioners who visit and interview detained patients about the quality and safety of care. The Mental Health Act Commission publishes a bi-annual report which is considered by Parliament.

- The Mental Health Act Commission appoints Second Opinion Appointed Doctors, whose principal duty is to assess and give consent to patients receiving specific forms of treatment, after they have already been detained (Section 58 of the Act). This is a form of medical peer review to ensure that enforced treatment is still necessary at a time after three months of detention when voluntary treatment might be expected due to some recovery.
- The Mental Health Review Tribunal has a range of powers that include discharge from detention.
- The Approved Social Worker is appointed by the local Social Services Authority having achieved the approved and appropriate competence in dealing with people suffering from mental disorder.
- The Nurses Holding Powers Section 5(4) authorizes a nurse of a prescribed class to detain an informal patient who is already being treated for a mental disorder as an inpatient in a psychiatric hospital for up to six hours if it appears to them that:
  (a) The patient is suffering from mental disorder to such a degree that it is necessary for his or her health and safety, or for the protection of others for him or her to be immediately restrained from leaving the hospital and
  (b) it is not practicable to secure the immediate attendance of a medical practitioner for applying the doctor's holding power Section 5(2).
- A Code of Practice provides practical guidance on the application of the Act.

The 1983 Act has worked; reforms are proposed to modernize the current legislation in response to growing community-based treatment and care, the expanding range of effective interventions that make this possible, the European Convention on Human Rights and the development of user-led services. However, there remain concerns with regard to the over-representation of some ethnic minority groups amongst the detained population (Department of Health, 2003), and the costs of running the proposed new and intensive tribunal system. The full proposed Act is not now going to be enacted, but modifications of the existing Act are proposed to update legislation and make it suitable for community-based care where patients' preferences and choices are maximized.

## Future legislation

The proposed changes introduce a new range of safeguards, such that all patients should have a written treatment plan, rights to advocacy and an automatic right to a tribunal hearing. In addition five conditions have been proposed for compulsion, all of which must be met before a patient can be treated compulsorily:

- The patient must have a mental disorder (defined as a disorder or disability of the mind).
- The mental disorder must be of a nature or degree that requires the provision of medical treatment (defined as treatment that includes nursing, care, therapy, habilitation and rehabilitation).
- The treatment is necessary to protect the patient from suicide or serious self-harm or from serious neglect by them of their health or safety, or for the protection of others.
- Compulsory treatment is necessary either because the patient has not consented to treatment or because of the degree of risk associated with proceeding based on a patient consent.
- Treatment is available that is appropriate in the patient's case, taking into account the nature and degree of the mental disorder and all other circumstances.

The challenge facing the English systems is how to adapt a law developed for specific cultural groups and values to meet the needs of culturally diverse groups.

## THE MALTA EXPERIENCE

In contrast, Maltese mental health law makes for an interesting case study of adapting mental health legislation from pluri-cultural sources. This poses special challenges of adaptation to the local context and local philosophies of care and treatment of the mentally ill. The Maltese Mental Health Act (Ministry for Justice and Home Affairs, 1981) is a simplified version of the 1959 English Mental Health Act. Malta's Mediterranean island population of 400 000, crowded on 315 km$^2$, is compact, but largely stable for many generations. Family, community and acquaintance ties are deep and close-knit. While competitiveness is evident, in many areas an atmosphere of community feeling and protectiveness tends to be strong.

Malta's population has been classified as the second densest in Europe, with the fifth best health system in the world. In the World Health Organization 2000 World Report, Malta scored very highly in health status, very high in equity of distribution, and second highest in the world for value for money. Malta has a very strong hospital system, available free of charge, and very high levels of doctors' services and medicines. Specialists outside hospital are mostly privately paid.

Maltese law is based on Roman law, Napoleonic code, Italian criminal codes, British commercial law, and other European models including a strong influence from British rule (1814–1964) and membership of the European Union (EU). Anglo-Saxon statutes reflect a greater penchant for detail while Latin laws leave more room for discretion, consideration for context and the operation of complementary laws. Malta's five-page Children's Care Order Act has long been considered as over-simple, but it has not yet been widened in scope, whereas the Mental Health Act runs into 28 pages, retaining a substantial part of the English Act's complexity and practices (Ministry of Education, 1980).

While allowing for voluntary admission to hospital, the Maltese Mental Health Act regulates a person's compulsory admission to mental hospitals. Normally this needs 'medical recommendation' of two doctors, one being a listed specialist, but also an application by the 'nearest relative' or a 'mental welfare officer', certifying:

*(a) that he is suffering from mental disorder of a nature or degree, which warrants the detention of the patient in a hospital and*

*(b) that it is necessary that he be so detained in the interests of his own health or safety or with a view to the protection of other persons.*

The authority expires after one year but can be extended for one year in the first instance and then two years at a time for admission for treatment. It allows an admission for 28 days for observation (not precluding treatment), and this can be converted to a formal admission for treatment. A 72-hour emergency admission can be resorted to on the basis of one medical recommendation, if getting two is seen to involve too much delay.

Admission for treatment is open to appeal to a Mental Health Review Tribunal, or objection by the nearest relative. The latter may also order discharge, restricted only by a medical declaration of the patient's danger to self or others, which would in turn lead to immediate review by the Tribunal. However, a nearest relative can be divested of powers if judged by the Family Court (a non-adversarial civil High Court), after a valid request, not to be acting in the interest of the patient.

Persons accused of criminal offences, if suspected or considered by the Court to be 'insane' during proceedings or at the time of the offence, may be detained by Court order, either for observation prior to sentencing or for detention and treatment following sentencing. Only the Home Minister may agree release, or refer them to Tribunal, consulting the latter and the doctor responsible.

Transfer between hospitals in different countries, as well as ministerial regulatory and inspection powers, are also regulated. A mental welfare officer is also empowered to 'enter and inspect any premises (not being a hospital) in which a mentally disordered person is living, if he has reasonable cause to believe that the patient is not receiving care'. Apart from the reference to 'insanity during the offence', there is nothing in the above that is not in the parent English law. However, four types of adaptations can be found, in the law and its implementation; these can be attributed to attempts to achieve greater congruence (Pace, 2003) within the Maltese context.

## Adaptations in the law as formulated

The following English 1959 provisions are notably excluded in current Maltese law:

* Decisions for long-term compulsory admission of psychopaths are restricted to the courts.
* Disallowing the certifying doctors from being partners or employed in the same hospital (there are provisions in the code of practice to prevent two doctors from the same employing authority authorizing admission; and professional regulations prevent doctors from being involved in the treatment of relatives including partners).
* Special punishments for staff who abuse patients.
* Providing for Guardianship (though discharge 'in the custody' of a third person is authorized).
* Enforce the power for police to remove a person to a place of safety, if that person appears to be 'in immediate need of care and control' due to mental disorder (Section 136).
* Moves to reduce the time a patient on leave can be kept under compulsory 'admission' (and treatment) status.

## 'On the ground' adaptations

The vast majority of compulsory admissions are emergency admissions that are transferred to longer-term admissions once in hospital. In Malta, free home visits and community interventions by state-employed specialists are not provided. However, it is considered good practice to involve a specialist whenever a case is insufficiently clear, especially if there is no previous episode of illness.

Police use their protective powers to take people needing treatment to a general hospital emergency department. Long-term 'leave' from the detention order during an extended admission for treatment order has served to give compulsory long-term treatment in the community where this has seemed appropriate. This approach in England was considered unlawful and in part motivated the new amendments in English law. Compulsory admission for psychopaths and substance abusers was in fact only resorted to for clear danger to self or others, otherwise this was a court prerogative.

## Differences in practice resulting from other laws

The Care Order Act was used to order minors to reside at the hospital's Young People's Unit. Recourse to advocacy and defence at the tribunal was widely seen as not being necessary, as the perception was of a benevolent tribunal.

## Envisaging reforms

The 1959 parent Act was made obsolete in England only two years after it was adopted in Malta. The EU Green Paper on Mental Health offers Malta an opportunity to seek considered legislative reforms. This will enable Malta to develop capacity and design modern mental health services. In addition, the Public Curator Act, enacted in 1982, can be put into force, to protect the property of persons admitted to hospital, and of other vulnerable persons, from the abuse, neglect or inattention of relatives, procurators or curators (Ministry for Justice and Home Affairs, 1982).

## THE NEW ZEALAND EXPERIENCE

## Policy development

New Zealand first developed a national mental health strategy in 1994; this was called *Looking Forward*. The strategy proposes developments of mental health services similar to those of many other countries. Mental health was a priority for the Government and the policy emphasized the need for more services and a commitment to develop community-based services. The five strategic directions announced in 1994 were to:

* develop comprehensive community-based mental health services,
* develop specific and appropriate mental health services for Māori,
* focus on increasing the quality of service delivery,

* maintain a balance between individual rights and public protection, and
* develop a national drug and alcohol policy, and in so doing integrate drug and alcohol services with mental health services.

Three years later in 1997, the New Zealand Ministry of Health published *Moving Forward* (Ministry of Health, 1997). This emphasized the need for better services and included two more strategic directions:

* To develop the systems infrastructure to enable the further development of mental health services such as information systems and workforce development.
* To strengthen promotion and prevention approaches, and address the discrimination and stigma associated with mental illness.

The Mental Health Commission is an independent agency established under legislation to monitor the Ministry of Health and the mental health sector on progress with funding mental health services. In 1998 the Mental Health Commission proposed a blueprint that gave details of a costed service and developments needed to implement *Moving Forward* (Mental Health Commission, 1998).

In June 2005, *Te Tāhuhu Improving Mental Health 2005–2015, The Second New Zealand Mental Health and Addiction Plan 2005* was launched by the Government. The plan takes account of health sector developments that have impacted on the way mental health services are delivered such as the establishment of 21 District Health Boards and over 70 Primary Health Organizations. The plan sets out the Government's priorities that must be tackled if the outcomes are to be met. Some of the key priorities for *Te Tāhuhu* are:

* to move from 'mental illness' to 'mental health',
* to move from inputs and outputs to 'outcomes' to be more encompassing, for example, a shift to public health, primary health, specialist mental health services,
* to shift from 'community care' to 'community liaison', and
* to give new opportunities for new ideas.

## Mental health legislation

Mental health legislation in New Zealand has provided the parameters for the treatment and detention of people with mental illness since the first mental health legislation was passed in 1882 (Department of Health, 2003). The most comprehensive reform for this area occurred in 1992 with a new Mental Health (Compulsory Assessment and Treatment) Act. The new Mental Health Act redefined the circumstances and conditions a person may be subject to during compulsory psychiatric assessment and treatment. It also made explicit the rights of such persons and provided a system for the better protection of these rights. In addition, the Act reformed and consolidated law relating to assessment and treatment of persons suffering from a mental disorder, and created congruence with the shift from the provision of treatment in psychiatric hospitals to compulsory community care. The 1992 Act was amended in 1999 to include better involvement of families (*whanau*) in legal and clinical processes, and to improve the rights of victims of violent acts committed by certain persons with mental illness (New Zealand Statutes, 1999a,b). These provisions are compatible with the Nations Declaration of the Rights of Disabled Persons and the United Nations Principles for the Protection of Persons with Mental Illness.

There are a number of other statutes of direct relevance. Criminal justice legislation concerns the disposition of mentally disordered offenders and has recently been updated in New Zealand. The Criminal Procedure (Mentally Impaired Persons) Act (2003) (Ministry of Health, 1994; New Zealand Statutes, 2003b) replaced Part VII of the Criminal Justice Act 1985 (New Zealand Statutes, 1985; Ministry of Health, 1997). The new Act introduces a new and undefined concept of mental impairment and changes certain procedures for people found by the courts to be unfit to plead to criminal offences. Other recent legislative changes include forensic mental health services, the Victims Rights Act 2002 (Mental Health Commission, 1998; New Zealand Statutes, 2002) and the Intellectual Disability (Compulsory Care and Rehabilitation) Act 2003 (New Zealand Statutes, 2003a; Ministry of Health, 2005).

The Protection of Personal and Property Rights Act 1988 (New Zealand Statutes, 1882) reworked the law concerning disabled people's property administration and gave the Family Court new powers over the personal lives of disabled adults, including the power to appoint welfare guardians. Additional legislation in New Zealand provides a broader platform for protecting privacy (Privacy Act 1994) (New Zealand Statutes, 1994) and emphasizing health consumer rights (Code of Consumer Rights under the Health and Disability Commissioner Act 1995). This gives the Health and Disability Commissioner the right to investigate all complaints of breach of this Code. This includes all people who are assessed and treated for mental illness by any health service.

## Mental health services

Most of the mental health services in New Zealand are community-based, with mobile 24-hour crisis services and general hospital acute wards. There are some hospital-based rehabilitation services and a range of supported accommodation and vocational training options, as well as day programmes and drop-in centres that are often run by consumers. Supported accommodation services have been reviewed and District Health Boards need to help people make the transition to supported accommodation and to other appropriate community-based services by 2006. There is a range of specialty services that are regionally based; for example, early intervention services for psychotic disorders, alcohol and other drug treatment services including residential services, child and youth services, eating disorder services, and forensic services including inpatient facilities that are locked and appropriately secure for mentally disordered offenders.

## Māori mental health

The 1997 strategy included a strong policy encouraging Māori development, where Māori own and run their own services. This fostered a bicultural approach to health care in mainstream services to ensure culturally competent treatment. In 2002,

*Te Puawaitanga: Mäori Mental Health National Strategic Framework* was developed to provide District Health Boards with a nationally consistent framework for planning and delivery of services for *tangata whaiora*. The *Te Tähuhu* challenge continues to broaden the range, quality and choice of mental health and addiction services for Mäori. The emphasis includes:

* enabling Mäori to present earlier to mental health and addiction services
* promoting choice by supporting the implementation of Kaupapa Mäori models of practice
* increasing Mäori participation in planning and delivery of mental health and addiction services for Mäori.

## A confidential forum to address grievances of mental health service users

In early 2005, the New Zealand Government established a confidential forum for people who were inpatients of psychiatric hospitals before November 1992, their families and staff of that era. The cut-off date of November 1992 arises because since then better legislative protections for mental health patients have been introduced. A new mental health act (the Mental Health Compulsory Assessment and Treatment Act 1992) came into force on 1 November 1992. This Act redefined the (limited) circumstances in which, and the conditions under which, people in New Zealand may be subjected to compulsory psychiatric assessment and treatment. The Act defines the rights of such people, including the right to respect for a person's cultural and ethnic identity, language and religious or ethical beliefs and protection for those rights.

The Act provides for district inspectors who are lawyers and are appointed to safeguard the rights of people under the Mental Health Act. Their responsibilities include arranging legal representation for patients at hearings before a judge to decide if a compulsory treatment order should be made, investigating complaints about breaches of patients' rights and visiting and inspecting hospitals and other services.

In 1994 the Health and Disability Commissioner Act was established and following that a Code of Health and Disability Consumers' Rights was established in 1996. The Health and Disability Commissioner Act asks a Commissioner to promote and protect the rights of health and disability consumers and facilitates the fair, simple and speedy resolution of complaints about health and disability services. This Act also paved the way for the establishment of a national network of independent advocates, whose role is to advise patients of their rights, ensure the rights of patients are respected and to assist patients to resolve concerns about the quality of the service they are receiving.

### Why a confidential forum?

A number of people who received treatment as inpatients in psychiatric hospitals prior to 1992 have raised concerns about their treatment – with many claiming to have suffered abuse while in hospital. Some have been able to obtain assistance in kind, such as counselling, or financial payment through New Zealand's no-fault Accident Compensation Scheme, in cases where assault or sexual assault had occurred. Some have commenced litigation against hospital authorities for compensation or damages because they allege the treatment they received while in hospital was a breach of the law, particularly about the administration of electroconvulsive treatment (ECT) and some medications. There have also been allegations of physical and sexual assault. There is a further category of people who are not able to litigate, or not willing to do so, for reasons such as disclosure of identity in open court, or for whom the strain of cross-examination would be undesirable or who might not be able to establish cases to the standard required in civil litigation.

For these people the Government decided that a different approach might be useful, namely that of setting up a Confidential Forum which people could attend and tell of their experiences of inpatient care and to speak of the unresolved issues. A panel was chosen comprising a former judge and ombudsman, a senior health official and a former consumer group member. Publicity was generated through newspapers, consumer networks and community organizations. To date some 350 people have made contact via a free telephone number or website, with a view to making arrangements to meet the panel. At the time of writing, meetings have been held with 80 people.

Participants are encouraged to relate to the panel what happened in their own words, and to indicate the issues they might have with that. In the first grouping of those seen, people retain resentment at:

* the lack of communication about diagnosis or treatment with either patient or family,
* the administration of treatment or medication without consent being sought and obtained, and
* the rigorous discipline of hospitals, albeit this was in a former era.

Regrettably there have been examples of misbehaviour and the misuse of authority, including assault and sexual violation. These may take the form of staff condoning patients' activity or staff themselves perpetrating the assault. A recurring theme in the first bracket of cases has been a desire to 'tell the story' and 'let the government know what happened'.

The powers of the Forum are restricted to listening and reporting to the Government in a regular quarterly cycle but without any remit to make judgments or order compensation. It has the ability to assist people to access current means of assistance such as obtaining their clinical records, correcting errors on files, making advance directives, accessing counselling and seeking out or encouraging current means of treatment that may be available. The Forum has adopted a kind of 'truth and reconciliation' approach. Its final report will be furnished in mid 2006 and its views may establish a new kind of alternative dispute reso-lution methodology that fits into a restorative justice framework without the need for court proceedings and without damages being the central goal.

## THE CHINA EXPERIENCE

In ancient China, mentally ill patients were cared for using principles and treatment within the framework of Traditional Chinese Medicine. This holistic approach is much valued as it makes no distinction between mind and body, and emphasizes healing and recovery rather than pathology. The Traditional Chinese Medicine approach, however, has not stopped some instances of ill treatment of the mentally ill due to misunderstanding or ignorance. Indeed, such instances are documented in most mental health systems, particularly the asylums, before the advent of effective treatments. At the beginning of the twentieth century, Western medical psychiatry enabled a much better understanding of mental illness. Consequently, the mentally ill are now better cared for than before. Whilst the science of effective mental health treatment and cure were still in their infancy, many patients were locked up, banded together, tied down, or simply taken into custody in hospital settings. In the 1950s, the rapid advancement of psychopharmacology enabled the development of better treatment methods for psychoses. The benefits for those seen as 'madmen' become better than before, although we have more to do.

In China, the Government and academics began to pay greater attention to the issues surrounding mental health services, rehabilitation and legal rights protection. Guidance for medical care at psychiatric hospitals was established. This led to enhanced regulations governing mental hospitals, better public mental health promotion, improved awareness of mental health issues and discussion around the better protection of the legal rights of mentally ill people through legislation. In particular, in 1991, after the United Nations Convention passed resolution 46/119 'Principles for the protection of persons with mental illness and the improvement of mental health care', the Chinese Government became even more active in their work in the area of mental health law. The more economically developed regions in China took on a leading role in devising local laws to regulate mental health services, strengthening the responsibility of the Government, protecting mentally ill citizens' rights in areas of study and work.

The Hong Kong Special Administrative Region was the first region in China to implement mental health legislation. In the 1970s, Hong Kong was governed by the British Government and at that time there were some laws relating to mental health care. It was not a comprehensive and systematic legal framework. Mental health care and legal protection were provided by a number of legislations. The Mental Health Act 1983 was first introduced in Hong Kong in 1983. This was followed by the Hong Kong Mental Health (Amendment) Ordinance, which was officially enacted on 1 February 1999. The said Ordinance consists of four parts and 74 sections. The first part mainly defines the terminology of mental health care, service provisions, staff duties and delegation. The second part included management of property and affairs of patients for those lacking the mental capacity to deal with these matters. The third part covers hospital admissions, compulsory detention and treatment, and sets out specific powers for the detention, monitoring and treatment of patients involved in criminal proceedings or under sentence. The fourth part deals with transfer, detention and rehabilitation regulations and reviews of prisoners under sentence.

The Mental Health Law 1990 in Taiwan came into force on 7 December 1990. The Act is divided into six parts and 52 sections. Its primary aim is to prevent and treat mental illness, protect patients' legal rights, promote their welfare, improve citizens' mental wellbeing as well as safeguarding social peace and harmony. It also sets out explicit requirements for establishing and implementing effective mental health services as well as proposing a medical guardian of the mentally ill patient. This includes clear procedures for diagnoses, treatment and admission; respect and protection for patients' personal and legal rights; and forbidding of discrimination, abuse, and exploitation of the mentally ill. Twenty-three implementation guidelines were introduced the year after in order to ensure the Act was carried out comprehensively.

In Mainland China, the development of mental health legislation has been inconsistently applied across different regions. Most regions have yet to have an integrated local mental health law. At present, the legal protection for the mentally ill and the legal responsibilities of mental health services are mainly addressed in various related laws and statutes. For instance, the National Constitution stipulates the protection of citizen rights such as personal freedom, human dignity, communication, confidentiality, employment and study. The law on the Protection of Disabled Persons sets out the rights to work, to have employment, to study and provides for medical care for the disabled including the mentally ill. Matters relating to marital, civil or criminal laws are dealt with through invoking the Marriage Law, the Civil Law, the Civil Procedure Law, and the 'Criminal Law'. In Mainland China, Shanghai was the first region that formally adopted the Shanghai Municipality Regulations on Mental Health on 1 April 2002. It contains seven parts and 49 sections. These regulations are comprehensive and systematic and help to strengthen the quality of mental health care in Shanghai by protecting the legal rights of the mentally ill. It sets out the guidelines for a range of mental health services including counselling, prevention, treatment and rehabilitation. This legal framework also sets out the responsibilities of services and staff, including how to deal with failure of duty, malpractice or illegal activities.

Currently, a national Mental Health Law of China is being developed and has so far gone through numerous drafts. Such development is being guided by groups of mental health professionals and related departments. In the meantime, a draft of the 'Beijing Mental Health Regulations' are under consultation with experts; comments will be incorporated into the Government legislative procedure. It is likely that this will be announced and implemented next year. It looks hopeful that a comprehensive and authoritative Mental Health Law will be enacted in Mainland China before 2008.

## CONCLUSIONS

This chapter explored mental health legislation in different countries, and traced how the English legislation in some of them is being revised, as it is in England. Different forms of legislation and variations in readiness for legislation reflect, in part, the differing cultural contexts and values, and attitudes to treatment of the mentally ill in each country.

Practitioners in each country strive to improve the care of mentally ill people, but there are challenges with existing legislation in each country, and whether this reflects national and international values about how care might best be provided for the wellbeing of patients. Furthermore, even though there are international agreements on what should constitute mental health care, there is less expectation that all countries will have the same legislative framework, in part, as this requires similar cultural contexts and values to produce similar benefit. Differing histories of care, different use of legislation, and different populations within each country also require adaptation of imported legislation to the specific environments in which it is to be applied. Nonetheless, there are standards of practice that can be introduced to all countries, supported by service users and the non-governmental organization sector, in order to raise the quality of care and the effectiveness of interventions. Differing levels of spend on mental health care, and the diverse economies of the countries discussed will also limit some shared actions. Legislation to improve the quality of mental health care can introduce new value systems, but it also reflects a readiness to move into a particular culture of care. The negotiation of these influences is the challenge facing all countries, governments, policy-makers and practitioners.

## REFERENCES

Department of Health 1998: *Modernising Mental Health Services: Safe, Sound and Secure*. London: Department of Health.

Department of Health 1999: *National Service Framework for Mental Health: Modern Standards and Service Models*. London: The Stationery Office.

Department of Health 2000: *The National Health Service (NHS Plan – Creating a 21st Century Health Service*. London: Department of Health.

Department of Health 2003: *Inside Outside: Improving Mental Health Services for Black and Minority Ethnic Communities in England*. London: Department of Health.

Ministry of Education 1980: Laws of Malta: http://www.education.gov.mt/ministry/doc/pdf/children_and_young_persons_care%20Orders_act.pdf (accessed May 2006).

Ministry for Justice and Home Affairs 1981: Laws of Malta: http://docs.justice.gov.mt/lom/legislation/english/leg/vol_6/chapt262.pdf (accessed May 2006).

Ministry for Justice and Home Affairs 1982: Laws of Malta: http://docs.justice.gov.mt/lom/legislation/english/leg/vol_6/chapt299.pdf (accessed May 2006).

Mental Health Commission 1998: *Blueprint for Mental Health Services in New Zealand: How Things Need to Be*. Wellington: Mental Health Commission.

Ministry of Health 1994: *Looking Forward: Strategic Directions for the Mental Health Services*. Wellington: Ministry of Health.

Ministry of Health 1997: *Moving Forward: The National Mental Health Plan for More and Better Services*. Wellington: Ministry of Health.

Ministry of Health 2005: *Te Tahuhu: Improving Mental Health 2005–2015. The Second New Zealand Mental Health and Addiction Plan 2005*. Wellington: Ministry of Health.

New Zealand Statutes 1882: *Lunatics Act 1882*. Wellington: Brookers Ltd.

New Zealand Statutes 1985: *Criminal Justice Act 1985*. Wellington: Brookers Ltd.

New Zealand Statutes 1994: *Privacy Act 1994*. Wellington: Brookers Ltd.

New Zealand Statutes 1999a: *(Compulsory Assessment and Treatment) Amendment Act 1999*. Wellington: Brookers Ltd.

New Zealand Statutes 1999b: *Mental Health (Compulsory Assessment and Treatment) Act 1999*. Wellington: Brookers Ltd.

New Zealand Statutes 2002: *Victims Rights Act 2002*. Wellington: Brookers Ltd.

New Zealand Statutes 2003a: *Intellectual Disability (Compulsory Care and Rehabilitation) Act 2003*. Wellington: Brookers Ltd.

New Zealand Statutes 2003b: *Criminal Procedure (Mentally Impaired Persons) Act 2003*. Wellington: Brookers Ltd.

Pace, C. 2003: Adapting services to culture, capability and need: can a cumulative methodology be achieved? In Bartocci, G., Wintrob, R. and Pace, C. (ed.) *Psychiatric Care Across Cultures: World Psychiatric Association Transcultural Psychiatry Section Symposium 2003, November 9–10: Proceedings*. Malta: Malta University Services. CD-ROM, 261–75.

Trapski, P.J. 2006: *Trapski's Family Law*. Wellington: Brookers Ltd.

# 8

# Management studies and organizational development

## Zoë K Reed

## INTRODUCTION

This chapter addresses the fundamental issue of
how to deliver effective mental health services in
a multicultural context. It proposes that providing
quality and equality in mental health services
requires skilful managers as well as skilful clinicians.
It is about recognizing management as an essential
skill and discipline in the delivery of quality health
care. The theoretical study of management and
managers has a long history. As Drucker says, the
functions of management include planning, organizing, motivating, performance measurement and
the development of people (Drucker, in Stewart,
1963). A working definition of management is given
to us by Brech as: 'planning and regulating (or guiding) the activities of an enterprise in relation to its
procedures, and to the duties or tasks of its personnel' (Brech, in Stewart, 1963).

Tackling inequalities and addressing cultural
issues in care, as captured in policy documents,
encompasses more than policies and processes
to address 'race or ethnicity'. Management and
organizational development programmes need to

be seen to be tackling all forms of discrimination,
including prejudicial responses to gender, sexuality, age and physical and mental disabilities.
However, there is a risk that by focusing on a large
number of significantly different issues, attention
to race and ethnicity can become ephemeral, or
simply inadequate to reach a critical mass of
actions to effect change in the way services are
organized and delivered.

For mental health services, a significant issue is
the impact of racism on service users. However,
the impact of racism on staff has been given less
attention (Coker, 2001). Staff and service users can
experience racism both within public institutions
and within the wider society. Similarly the management agenda is larger than quality and equality,
with the efficient, economic and effective use of
resources as centrally important. The management
task is to deliver such policies in a way that ensures
quality and equality.

This chapter takes the UK's National Health
Service (NHS) as an example of a health care system
and offers a 'kitbag' (Clarkson, 1995) of management and organizational theories that help with

surviving and thriving in turbulent times. It is hoped that this brief introduction to some really useful perspectives and approaches will encourage the reader to follow up the references listed at the end of the chapter.

An important cultural consideration is to what extent the findings in the UK are transferable to other world contexts. Indeed do all service management initiatives have to be grounded in the local experiences and health care economies? Clearly, this has to be true to some extent, but in a global society the use of knowledge sharing is on the increase, and barriers to sharing knowledge are diminishing. I hope in this chapter to offer some ways of thinking about organizational management that can be applied to other health care economies, in order to deliver culturally appropriate care at a cost that can be supported locally.

## WHICH MANAGEMENT THEORIES HELP PROVIDERS OF MENTAL HEALTH SERVICES IN A MULTICULTURAL SOCIETY?

When mental health provider organizations are in a stable context and do not have plans to change their practices, then little attention need be paid to organizational development theories. However, this 'stability' scenario is rare. It has not been the circumstance in the UK or USA for some while and will not be so for the foreseeable future in most of the developed or developing world. In Western countries the relentless shift towards individualization means that in the NHS health care system, as in all other aspects of life, providers are required to deliver a flexible service, responsive to each individual's needs and wishes. In order to survive a multitude of requests, health care systems need to have the capacity and capability to co-evolve with the changes around them. These demands come from the public, from politicians, and from neighbouring countries and from global organizations such as the World Health Organization. For example the European Union has influenced the UK health economy, the health and social workforce, and it has led to the implementation of the Human Rights Act. A more recent phenomenon is campaigning

by non-governmental organizations in the voluntary or charitable sector. These often have the support of service users and the public and are now a powerful voice for change, and often deliver services also.

Technological advances as well as individual needs and wishes will mean that agile health care teams need to be created and sustained (Fraser *et al.*, 2003). Therefore a growing number of theories are being adopted within the NHS to help shape and guide the ongoing process of change. Alongside these are a number of tools and techniques that help design and measure the impact of change programmes. The theories can be grouped into categories where they are most helpfully applied.

- Organizations and systems
- Individuals in groups – the leadership task
- Individuals.

## THEORIES ABOUT ORGANIZATIONS AND SYSTEMS

Complexity sciences (Battram, 1998) contain a number of principles and ideas that help designers to shape change and survival programmes. Central to these are the idea that organizations are complex adaptive systems. Complex adaptive systems are defined as: 'A collection of individual agents who have the freedom to act in ways that are not entirely predictable and whose actions are interconnected such that one agent's action changes the context for other agents' (Wheatley, 1999). This definition can be applied at every level of nested systems. For example, each team member within the team, each team within the organization, each organization within the health services community, each health service community within the broader public sector.

Thinking about organizations and individuals in this way leads to the design of change programmes profoundly different from those used in a more traditional view of health services and professionals. Most conventional management theories view organizations as machines, and staff within them as component parts. From this worldview, designers assume that people can be told what to do and that they will do it in a consistent manner. They assume that learning from one area will be automatically replicated in another area. They believe that a 'plan for change' can be worked out in advance in detail and that it must be and can be executed as planned.

Complexity perspectives provide a more organic and holistic view. Biological metaphors are frequently used to deepen understanding of successful approaches. Two of these are birds flocking and termites building. Both these describe the idea that central command and control is neither necessary nor helpful in orchestrating action. Birds and termites achieve amazing results through the individual agents following a few simple rules. Some modern organizational development work is focused around seeking to identify the few simple rules – often characterized as values or guiding principles – which will enable every individual to shape their behaviour in accordance with organizational goals.

The termite hill emerges from the patterns of behaviour of the termites following their simple rules – there was no grand plan, the hills simply emerged from the behaviour. The intrinsic motivation of the termites coupled with the simple rules ensures that the termites self-organize to achieve the desired result. Emergence, intrinsic motivation and self-organization are key concepts in the complexity sciences. They are the underpinning theory to techniques such as whole-group brainstorming and Post-it note exercises. The aim of such exercises is to involve everybody and create a possibility space into which solutions will emerge (Battram, 1998). This contrasts with more conventional management methods where top management creates a plan and then seeks to involve staff through consultation exercises.

Birds are also used to illustrate the need for attractors within the system. As a way of getting people to understand that organizations are living entities not machines, the contrast is given between a rock and a bird. If you want to get a rock into the corner of a room, with a bit of practice on your aim you will be able to achieve it by throwing it. By contrast if you want to get a bird into the corner of a room you certainly will not achieve it by throwing the bird; instead your only chance is by placing the attractor (for birds) of birdseed in the corner.

Using words like systems and drawing on biological metaphors has another important message for organizations. It is that the life continues, evolves and proceeds; things are never static, and flow and movement are an intrinsic part of organizations and systems. This contrasts with more conventional approaches where there is an assumption that once the change has occurred and the problem has been fixed it will remain so.

## THEORIES ABOUT INDIVIDUALS IN GROUPS – THE LEADERSHIP TASK

Understanding that the management task is about enabling a living system rather than controlling a machine brings a different set of tasks. A metaphor that is frequently used to describe the organization is a garden, and this can help managers understand that their role is to create the most favourable conditions for emergence and self-organization. They must tend their gardens with care and continually work on improving the conditions to maximize the chance of development, but what they cannot do is make the plants grow! This helps managers and leaders let go of thinking their role is to figure it all out and then create a plan and then force the system to implement it. Instead a much more nurturing role becomes apparent. A key role for managers and leaders in this worldview is to manage the context and the relationships around their work area to enable it to thrive and grow. Leaders start something, see what happens and give feedback in a continuous cycle; they watch to see when the required patterns of behaviour emerge and then manage the conditions so that those patterns are reinforced and sustained. As Battram says, 'possibility spaces' are a very important component in this way of working. Leaders need to become skilled at designing them and in observing the whole system to spot the 'tipping point' when the whole system starts to move in the required direction (Gladwell, 2000).

Helpful guidance for managers comes from the idea of learning organizations, with the leader's new work being to act as designers, stewards and teachers (Senge, 1993). In learning organizations leaders design the processes and systems within which the vision can be generated and articulated; they are stewards of that vision with a special sense of responsibility without possessiveness towards it; as a teacher they help people achieve more accurate views of reality and hold the creative tension which is generated. This vision of leadership contrasts with the more conventional theories of leader as hero, leading from the front, leader as most knowledgeable expert on the subject area they are leading. It calls for knowledge, skills and attention to process to get the best out of everyone – leadership as guardian of process rather than expert on content.

Complexity sciences help managers and leaders look for order rather than control; they provide a conceptual framework for inviting participation – every voice is valid – rather than curtailing contribution (for fear that someone will speak out against the plan). They foster a real belief in the intrinsic motivation of people. Even in chaotic circumstances, individuals can make congruent decisions when there are a few simple principles that everyone is accountable for but where the condition within which everyone is operating is one of individual freedom.

In this mindset much management time is spent on developing and sustaining a shared vision which will guide and shape the behaviour of the individuals in the team. Creating the conditions for team learning becomes an essential leadership task since 'do something and see what happens – then repeat' is the way in which the organization will move forward and adapt to its shifting context. The incremental effect of small changes to achieve big service improvements is a core feature of the NHS Improvement Leaders Guides. 'Plan, do, study, act' (PDSA) cycles are the bedrock of modernization programmes in the NHS.

## THEORIES THAT HELP INDIVIDUALS THRIVE IN THIS CONTEXT

To be effective in complex adaptive systems people need to have highly developed emotional intelligence (Goleman, 1996). This is defined as 'The capacity for recognising our own feelings and those of others, for motivating ourselves, and for managing emotions well in ourselves and in our relationships.' The research evidence is that competent leaders who also exhibit high levels of emotional intelligence lead teams who have the competitive edge. Crucially, if managers are to lead from the perspective that all staff have intrinsic motivation then it follows that high levels of emotional intelligence need to be developed in all individuals.

The concepts of personal mastery and mental models are crucial skill areas for continuous development (Senge, 1993). They complement the development of emotional intelligence and enable individuals to understand what motivates them and to work at clarifying and articulating how they are thinking about people and issues and understanding that their response is based on their mental models not objective reality. Crucial to progress in learning organizations is the development of the ability for each individual in the group to articulate their mental models and suspend them before everyone else so others can understand and respond. Individuals in learning organizations need to become skilled in dialogue rather than discussion (Battram, 1998). This approach starts with listening, it encourages reflection, suboptimal solutions are preferred with a focus on generating many ideas and synthesizing the way forward.

## THE UK'S NATIONAL HEALTH SERVICE – A TURBULENT HEALTH CARE SYSTEM

The UK's National Health Service is the largest health services organization in the world. Until recently (August 2005) it viewed itself as a single organization comprising 1.3 million workers commissioning and providing the full range of health care services to all residents of the UK. Care is free at the point of delivery. The quality of care and treatment is maintained at an internationally high standard by the close symbiotic working relationship with UK's world-renowned academic institutions.

The NHS was created in 1948 and has a high political profile. This means it has been subject to many short-term (within the life of one government approximately five years) 'solutions' to perceived problems. These have included:

- Structural changes – to professions and institutions.
- Process changes – incremental locally determined and unilateral system-wide.
- Cultural patterns analysis and interventions – locally and nationally.
- Philosophical changes coupled with promotional campaigns to raise awareness and expectation.

Since the election of the Labour Government in 1997 (in its third term in August 2005) the NHS has undergone unprecedented change on a scale unknown anywhere else in the world. The pace of change has accelerated and the radical nature of the reforms has deepened. A number of policy thrusts are being pursued with the intention of destabilizing the context and achieving the stated ambition of a truly patient-centred service. Amongst the most significant are 'payment by results' and 'practice-based commissioning' – both of which are about the money following the patient. 'Contestability in provision' (the public sector no longer being sacrosanct for the provision of NHS health care) and patient 'choice of provider' are intended to drive up quality. Foundation Hospital Trusts are a new form of NHS organization that are independent and must function as financially robust institutions. 'Patient and public involvement' legislation aims to ensure local ownership and connection of services as well as driving efficiency, effectiveness and economy.

Mental health services are provided by the NHS, the independent (for profit) sector and the voluntary (non-profit distributing) sector. They are commissioned by the NHS and social care (within local government) institutions. A typical portfolio for an area might comprise:

- All primary mental health care and treatment – by the NHS via GP practices and the primary care trusts.
- All secondary mental health and addictions services – both for inpatient care and treatment and those provided whilst patients remain in the community (in people's own homes or from outpatient and other trust premises) – by the NHS in a single mental health trust.
- Tertiary services – highly specialized services available nationwide on referral from secondary care (with associated primary care trust funding) – by some NHS mental health trusts usually where linked to an academic institution.
- Specialist high-cost inpatient provision (e.g. forensic or for patients with complex needs requiring long-term residential care) – by the independent (for profit) sector.
- Specialist community-based services for particular groups of patients (e.g. assertive outreach for African Caribbean people) – by the voluntary (non-profit distributing) sector.

This is a complex terrain of provision for clinicians to operate within and it is also constantly changing. It is clear that to survive and create the capacity to deliver increasingly efficient and effective treatments and care, all mental health provider organizations need to be flexible and responsive. For staff to thrive in such times they need to be emotionally intelligent as people and to be able to cope with high levels of uncertainty. Traditional thinking – for example managers who think that it is their responsibility to control (Stewart, 1963) as opposed to designing and managing the context (Senge, 1993) are likely to suffer high levels of personal stress in a health care system which is inherently unstable and uncontrollable. Having a complexity worldview makes for a mentally healthier workplace and a more confident workforce.

## SO HOW DOES ALL THIS LINK TO PROVIDING MENTAL HEALTH SERVICES IN A MULTICULTURAL SOCIETY?

The point about a multicultural society is that it is just that. Staff and service users are likely to come from cultural backgrounds that are different from one another. In one London mental health trust, the South London and Maudsley NHS Trust, for example, 58 different languages are regularly used for interpretation and the majority of nurses in training are from a black or minority ethnic group (mainly African). In this context it is not about a 'host' culture learning about the needs and preferences of a couple of newer migrant communities. Running effective mental health services in these circumstances is about alerting staff to the expectation that they are likely not to have any prior knowledge or understanding of the culture of the patient before them or of their other staff colleagues. They need therefore to be exceptionally skilled communicators, particularly good at listening and enquiring to aid understanding and promote dialogue (Battram, 1998) with high levels of emotional intelligence which enable them to build rapport across cultures.

The added dimension of multiculturalism makes it harder to respond to patients' needs and wishes in a way that ensures they feel respected and heard. It is therefore vital that all staff feel they have sufficient autonomy to adapt and adjust the provision of their service as is required. Entrepreneurial approaches and creativity will become paramount. Traditional management theories take a command and control approach and this can stultify the necessary creativity which is essential if each patient is to feel they have a personalized service. Many traditional approaches assume that the thinking is done by senior staff, this is then written down in protocols and policies and all staff are required to follow them exactly. Complexity approaches, by contrast, will recognize that whilst guidelines in the form of protocols and policies are clearly essential, they must be operated in a way that fosters a sense of personal responsibility in staff to respond to each patient's needs and wishes.

These theories and ways of thinking are helpful for people in organizations and they are also helpful for practitioners in relation to their patients. Key components are (a) that we need to believe in people and their abilities – an asset-based approach, and (b) that the leadership task is to set the context and nurture the conditions for the preferred behaviour to emerge. Developing dialogue skills with patients is particularly helpful in a multicultural context where prior knowledge cannot be assumed on any dimension of the patient and their life experience. Skills in inclusive working and an understanding that your task is to value every voice and contribution also support cross-cultural working. Seeing systems and understanding the value of networks makes more relevant to the practitioner the fact that in a multicultural context with a policy driver on pluralism of provision, connecting with communities is a key part of the day job. Flexing and flowing as the living system moves forward on the wave of many policy drivers is essential for organizational survival and for individuals to thrive in the modernizing NHS.

It is frequently said that ensuring equal opportunities and valuing diversity is simply good management. The point is that the management theories that guide the management behaviour need to be good too. Complexity sciences, organizational and personal development and learning and emotional intelligence provide the key to good management. In circumstances where these skill sets and frameworks for understanding are continually developed and practised, providing mental health services in a multicultural society is no more or less difficult than in a monocultural one.

## REFERENCES

Battram, A. 1998: *Navigating Complexity.* London: The Industrial Society.

Clarkson, P. 1995: *Change in Organisations.* London: Whurr Publishers.

Coker, N. (ed.) 2001: *Racism in Medicine: An Agenda for Change.* London: King's Fund Publishing.

Fraser, W., Conner, M. and Yarrow, D. (eds) 2003: *Thriving in Unpredictable Times.* Chichester: Kingsham Press.

Gladwell, M. 2000: *The Tipping Point – How Little Things can Make a Big Difference.* London: Little, Brown and Company.

Goleman, D. 1996: *Emotional Intelligence.* London: Bloomsbury Publishing.

Senge, P. 1993: *The Fifth Discipline – the Art and Practice of the Learning Organisation.* London: Century Business.

Stewart, R. 1963: *The Reality of Management.* London: William Heinemann.

Wheatley, M. 1999: *Leadership and the New Science – Discovering Order in a Chaotic World.* San Francisco: Berrett-Koehler Publishers.

# 9

# Health services research and policy

## Rachel Jenkins

## INTRODUCTION

This chapter addresses the interface between culture, health systems and health services research, with particular reference to mental health. Culture may broadly be defined as social structures, systems, ideas and assumptions, which together form human societies. These influential social structures include nuclear and extended families, kinship networks, community and neighbourhood. Factors that nurture social capital and social networks are embedded in cultures and generate cultures. Other factors found within cultures include leadership patterns, professional status of health care professionals, and social stratifying systems such as religion, caste and class. In every culture there are prevalent and popular ideas, and assumptions that reflect expectations of how and why things should be done. For example, cultures include attitudes about the meaning and significance of life, and prescribe rules of behaviour for different groups of people within a society. Culture also determines which behaviours or rituals are confined to or cross the public and private realms or the religious and secular realms.

It is shared cultural rules and principles that keep cultures and subcultures together to form societies and social collectives that act as a cohesive unit because its members share a common view of the world. Other senses in which the term culture is often used include the material objects of past civilizations, and the high culture or arts, music and literature of present society (Dunbar, 2004). Culture is omnipresent and can contribute as well as influence protective and risk factors for mental illness. Culture is thus a pervading influence on all of us (see Chapter 2). There are cultural differences across ethnic groups, across countries, but also within occupational groups and political persuasions. Culture therefore necessarily impacts on key aspects of both health systems and health services research due to the various cultural contexts within which we live, to the cultural orientations of professionals, and to the diverse range of cultural, religious, racial and ethnic backgrounds of the people who use health services. There are also markedly diverse political climates across the world's countries which may support or challenge specific health care practices.

## CULTURE, HEALTH POLICY AND HEALTH SYSTEMS

### What is a mental health policy?

A mental health policy is a written statement of intent by the government on mental health issues and mental health services. Health policy at national level will identify the range of health, morbidity, disability and mortality issues it intends to tackle, the relevant settings covered by the policy, the overall framework for implementing policy in the relevant settings including, for example, health services, social services, the education sector, the workplace and the criminal justice sector. The policy may set our desired goals and will set a framework for planning at local level. The policy document addresses the issues in mental health which require multidisciplinary and intersectoral collaboration at all levels of human development as well as socio-economic development.

### Why is it important to have a mental health policy?

A written national mental health policy is important because it can inform all other general health sector policies as well as the policies of other sectors such as social care, employment, housing and welfare. A policy brings into sharp focus all mental health issues that affect individuals, families, communities and the nation at large, and may act as an advocacy tool for equitable resource allocation at individual, family, community, national and international levels.

The effect of a policy, if fully supported by government(s), is to place mental health issues on the mainstream agenda at all levels, and to bring mental health priorities to the same level as physical health and social wellbeing. Thus the policy itself, if fully supported and properly integrated with other health and social policies, can be a good starting point to address issues of stigma. Stigma is not just found in the general public but also in professionals and government officials.

Economic forecasting of a policy and its implications can assist in the national allocation of both human and non-human resources such as mental health personnel, financing and supplies and equipment. National mental health policy helps government include mental health in the health and social sector plans so it is not marginalized. Mental health policy can inform the process of reviewing mental health legislation which should reflect the nature of the service and its operation, values and resources to ensure legal care (see Chapter 7). It is a key pillar for the development of a national mental health programme of action and mental health service delivery in an integrated decentralized manner. Some aspects of mental health care can be included in co-programming with health programmes for HIV, malaria, other infectious diseases, reproductive and child health. This helps raise awareness in other government departments, whilst addressing co-morbid conditions.

Thus an integrated national mental health policy will be integrated with the overall national health policy (including the general health sector reform strategy, the package of essential health interventions, the essential medicine kit, health information systems, curriculum for all health workers, and country level work on global burden of disease); with overall government policy and budgetary and public expenditure processes, involving ministries of finance, education, social welfare, home affairs/criminal justice and employment; and with the poverty reduction strategy.

## CULTURE AND THE NEED FOR LOCALLY TAILORED SOLUTIONS

Each country is unique, with a different context, culture, resource base and types of existing services. Each will require its own mental health strategy to reflect the needs of the population, and their preferred solutions for managing distress and mental disorder. Locally tailored solutions must address both the general and specific challenges and issues (Jenkins *et al.*, 2002). Within these major contextual and cultural differences and influences, there are some common aims for mental health policy which include:

- the promotion of mental health,
- the reduction of the incidence and prevalence of mental disorder through prevention and treatment,
- the reduction of the extent and severity of associated disability (rehabilitation),
- the development of services for people with mental illness,
- reduction of stigma,
- the promotion of human rights and dignity of people with mental illness,
- the promotion of psychological aspects of general health care,
- the reduction of mortality associated with mental illness from suicide and from premature physical mortality (Harris and Barraclough, 1998; Jenkins *et al.*, 2002; Jenkins, 2003).

Some of the components within mental health policy need to be addressed in both rich and poor countries. First, the national components must be addressed, including the construction of a national strategy to promote mental health, reduce morbidity and reduce mortality, as well as the establishment of policy links with other government departments including home affairs, criminal justice, education, housing, finance, etc. The enactment of specific mental health legislation will include an overall philosophy of approach to the care of people with mental disorders. It will also offer safeguards for precise assessment and effective and humane treatment without consent, for those meeting predefined criteria set in each country.

Under these conditions the interests of the individual and the public must be balanced with regard to safeguarding human rights. There must be adequate financing to remove perverse incentives that undermine effective humane treatment, or which promise services that are not sustainable.

There should be funding for disseminating good practice models, including an overall system of accountability and governance.

Second, the supportive infrastructure components should include a human resources strategy, a consumer involvement strategy, a research and development strategy, and a mental health information strategy (which should include context, needs, inputs, processes and outcomes). Information systems provide an essential resource for clinicians, managers, planners and policy-makers. They allow the audit cycle to proceed. Service users and carers also require relevant information, and the general public requires information for public accountability.

Third, the service components should be addressed. The necessary service components include primary care, specialist care, the links between the two, good practice guidelines, liaison with non-governmental organizations, police, prisons, social sector, dialogue with traditional healers, mental health promotion in schools, workplaces and the community (Jenkins *et al.*, 2002).

In all countries, especially poor ones, finance is a major limiting factor and prioritization of services will be necessary. However, a basic minimum package will probably include:

- the provision of medicines for patients at primary care level with psychosis, epilepsy and severe depression,
- the ability to refer very ill patients for hospital admission,
- primary care workers supported by mental health specialist workers (for liaison, education and supervision) in the community,
- mental health promotion in the community,
- intersectoral linkages.

## DEFINITION OF HEALTH SYSTEM

A health system includes all actors, organizations, institutions and resources whose primary purpose is to improve health (Pang *et al.*, 2003). Health systems are varied within and between countries, but often broadly consist of health interventions delivered to people in their own homes, interventions delivered by traditional health practitioners, interventions delivered by primary care and interventions delivered by specialist care either in outpatient or inpatient settings. Health care is also delivered in a variety of non-health settings such as schools, prisons, other institutions and social services. Health care may be publicly or privately funded, or charitably provided. Many factors influence access to and provision of care within each of these levels and sectors.

## THE PURPOSE OF HEALTH SYSTEMS AND THE NEED FOR RESEARCH

The main purpose of a health system is to improve health outcomes (Jenkins, 1990; Jenkins and Singh, 2000; World Health Organization, 2004). A secondary aim is to be responsive to the local population which it serves. Therefore it is important to gather information about population needs, and to evaluate how resources (human, physical, financial) are deployed to provide care to meet those needs. How far does such deployment achieve improved health and social outcomes, altered service designs, interventions, human resource development and configurations? These changes can only be judged on the basis of improved effectiveness and efficiency (Jenkins et al., 2003). Such evaluations linking change to outcomes, a complex process (see Chapter 8), comprise the body of health services research.

## INFLUENCE OF CULTURE ON HEALTH SYSTEMS

Culture and history influence the way in which health systems – including public, private, traditional and informal health services within a country – have been shaped, and the types of professionals, organizations and institutions that have been developed. Through the priority given to mental health issues and the mentally ill, culture and history also shape health policies and strategic action plans to reflect this priority, which is again reflected in actual service implementation.

## EPIDEMIOLOGY AND RESEARCH ON HEALTH SYSTEMS AND ASSESSMENT OF POPULATION NEEDS

### The value of epidemiology

Assessment of population needs is a basic prerequisite for the assessment of whether health systems meet population needs and contribute to the development and refinement of mental health policy. Mental health policy will not only need to take account of contextual factors, but also the epidemiology (range, severity, frequency and duration) of disorders, their accompanying social disability, their mortality and relationship to sociodemographic, including geographic, variations of the epidemiology of disorders.

Thus, epidemiology is fundamental to the overall goals of mental health policy (Jenkins, 2001). A few countries are embarking on a rolling programme of detailed national surveys of mental health problems in the community (Jenkins and Meltzer, 2002). The World Health Organization is coordinating a world mental health survey programme in a variety of participating countries (Demyttenaere et al., 2004), and a number of epidemiological surveys have been carried out in low income countries (Institute of Medicine, 2001).

Epidemiological information about incidence, prevalence and risk factors for illness are valuable indicators of population health, and can be obtained either for specific localities from local studies or for countries as a whole from nationally representative studies. Surveys can reveal:

- the prevalence of psychiatric morbidity either as individual symptoms, specific disorders, or for above-threshold disorders combined;
- associations between psychiatric disorders and substance use and abuse;
- the nature and extent of social disabilities associated with mental illness;
- the use of health and social services;
- the association between psychiatric morbidity and recent life events;

- the experience of social support and socio-economic circumstances;
- the links to other potential risk factors such as measures of deprivation, living conditions, employment, housing;
- the links to physical illness and physiological measures;
- the cost effectiveness of interventions; and
- the costs for people and their families.

Surveys can also:

- compare findings between populations or within populations;
- compare health trends over time;
- estimate the likely impact of potentially preventable health problems; and
- describe the impact of health problems.

## The development of hypotheses and research design

Cultural differences in life experiences include variations of particular types of event, for example political turmoil, armed conflict, natural disasters as well as the cultural processes and systems in place to manage those events and the impacts. These can lead to chronic social stresses as well as make use of social supports to influence the range and gravity of specific health needs. There are also cultural variations of the recognition of emotional distress and mental health needs. Therefore, culture and its impact need to be taken into account when assessing population needs. Culture also needs to be taken into account in the design of research instruments, the choice of such instruments, the way in which questions about symptoms are phrased and whether they should use local idioms, and the way in which screening instruments are calibrated (see Chapters 2 and 4).

## HEALTH SYSTEMS AND SERVICES RESEARCH

Health services research may be broadly defined as the generation of knowledge about health services which can be used to promote health, treat and rehabilitate illness and prevent mortality. Health services research therefore needs to mirror the complexity of the health system which it seeks to examine. This requires a multilevel and multisectoral approach. Each of these sectors and levels will have its own perspective on the impact of culture on health care delivery, and these subcultural differences between professionals and disciplines and other stakeholders will need reconciliation. Culture is a key issue to be taken into account at all stages and levels of health services research, irrespective of which country, population or service is being studied. The possibilities are limitless but a few examples will be given here.

## Social capital

Culture is a major influence on social capital (Putnam, 1993). For example, culture influences the nature and degree of community social support, mutual trust and practical help, and the extent to which people are prepared to give towards unfunded community activities. For example, spending time with people who are mentally ill can be very valuable to the person living with mental illness but may not be perceived to be valuable by a busy working professional working in a society where individual success is more greatly valued and promoted.

## Stigma

Similarly, stigma can lead to shame, a sense of disgrace, or disapproval from authority figures and loved ones, or the public. This can result in an individual being shunned or rejected by others and discriminated against by services (World Health Organization, 1999). Although forms of stigma are ubiquitous, its particular manifestations are influenced by culture within communities and, regrettably, within professional, managerial and policy groups.

## Pathways to care within public service provision

There are cultural variations in pathways to and through these levels of care provision (Goldberg and Huxley, 1992). Culture can influence the value placed by society on mental health, wellbeing and individual versus collective success. Culture also influences the expression of distress, and its presentation as symptoms, and the forms of illness behaviour that follow, including access to services, the way individuals and families manage illness, the way the community responds to illness, the degree of acceptance and support, and the degree of stigma and discrimination. These culturally influenced factors will in turn influence for example the likelihood of detection of illness by the health professional, the interventions offered and the likelihood of referral to specialist services, and the likelihood of admission to hospital.

## Traditional health service provision

Traditional and alternative health practitioners are important service providers in many countries, either because of their wide availability relative to public or private health services, or because they are perceived as effective, or because they are experienced as more user friendly. Many people consult both. In sub-Saharan Africa, where traditional health practitioners are very common (1 per 50 population compared with 1 health professional per 10 000 population), they will remain a key provider of health care for large proportions of the population for many decades, if not centuries. Their practice is variable, and there is no doubt that some traditional practice is very harmful; but it is also likely that some of the herbal medicines used have helpful psychoactive properties and that some of the interventions give important psycho-social support to individuals, families and communities. Rather than seek to destroy all traditional healing, it would be more productive to research their provision and outcomes (Bodeker *et al.*, 2001), to seek dialogue with the aim of eliminating frankly harmful practices, and to engage in joint training using diagnostic algorithms to encourage referral and shared systems of support and supervision of difficult or chronic cases, including psychosis (Saeed *et al.*, 2002).

It is therefore important to research them in all cultures, whether in low, middle or high income countries. There may be culturally unique variants of who might be called a traditional healer in a developing country or an alternative or complementary practitioner in the West. A useful function of health providers is to establish the different kinds of traditional health practice that exist in each country, what the role of each of these is in mental health care, and whether they are organized into formal associations that operate some kind of professional accountability and regulation. It is useful to know what interventions are used, for whom, and with what efficacy. It is also helpful to study how traditional healers can interface with modern health systems and collaborate to improve health and social outcomes.

## Frequently unresearched mental health policy issues in most cultures

Some of the generic social policy issues that impact on mental health are policies on education, employment, housing, prisons, police, social welfare, environment and urban regeneration, rural issues, and transport. Effective inter-agency working at national, local and individual level is fundamental to the delivery of good mental health care, and needs to be firmly addressed at policy level. There may need to be a pan-government working group on mental health, as well as regional and local groups to monitor and facilitate joint working. There may need to be policy action to address co-terminosity of geographic boundaries, synchronization and communication of planning cycles, lines of accountability for joint working, joint financial and information systems, shared good practice guidelines and removal of perverse incentives against cooperation between agencies.

## Schools

Children are a nation's most precious resource, and yet receive too little policy attention: specific learning difficulties, including dyslexia in schools, educational failure, school drop-out, trajectories to unemployment and over-representation in prisons.

## Looked after children

Large numbers of children across the world are looked after in orphanages and children's homes which often contain children who have been abused and neglected, children whose home life has broken down, and children with developmental delay and retardation, speech delay, fits, severe overactivity and aggression, chronic physical illness, disability and handicap. It should be an important policy imperative to ensure adequate mental and physical health promotion and care to 'looked after' children and to prevent their subsequent over-representation in the prisons.

## Prisons

Prisons are another key setting of concern for policy-relevant mental health research. Mental illness is very common in prisons, and in some countries suicide is very high in prisoners. Guidelines for health care staff in prisons may be useful (Paton and Jenkins, 2002). We need systems to prevent and treat anxiety and depression in prison, to ensure that people with psychosis are treated in hospital rather than prison, to prevent suicide and suicidal attempts, and to tackle dyslexia and educational failure in prisoners.

## Preparedness for disasters

No country can afford to ignore the possibility of disasters, whether man-made or natural. More than 50 countries have experienced conflict in the last 20 years. Conflicts are much more common in poor countries, and 15 of the 20 poorest countries of the world have had a major conflict in the last 15 years. Nearly all low-income countries are next to a country that has experienced war and are therefore frequently caring for refugees. Women and children are particularly vulnerable to war and are frequently witnesses to or forced participants in

murder and rape; they may also be at high risk of infection with AIDS and suffer rejection by local society. There is also a separate issue to do with the abduction of child soldiers and the subsequent difficulty rehabilitating them back to childhood and adolescence and a less disabled and more fruitful life away from conflict zones.

Psycho-social issues are often neglected in post-conflict situations, despite the knowledge that the presence of psycho-social disorders contributes to low compliance with vaccination, nutrition, oral rehydration, antibiotics and also contributes to high-risk sexual behaviour. Psycho-social disorders are therefore linked to high morbidity and mortality from preventable and treatable infectious disease. Sometimes the sheer volume of refugees and their movements make practical arrangements very difficult. For example, in Macedonia during the Kosovo crisis, there were over 250 000 refugees and large transfers at short notice between camps as new refugees arrived, making psycho-social work very difficult during the initial phase (World Health Organization, 2000). In Georgia, with a population of around 5 million, and an economic crisis which has reduced government health expenditure from US$200 to $7 per head per year, there are over 250 000 internally displaced people with largely unmet needs for psychological support, and a further 7000 refugees from Chechnya for whom the government does not accept responsibility so they have no access to medical care other than that supplied by the Red Cross (Jenkins et al., 2001). The central importance of involving primary care teams in the management of the medium- and long-term psychological consequences of a disaster has long been argued (Lima et al., 1988).

# CULTURE AND HEALTH RESEARCH SYSTEMS

## What is a health research system?

A health research system can be defined as the people, institutions and activities whose primary purpose is to generate, disseminate and apply high-quality knowledge that can be used to promote health, treat and rehabilitate illness and disability, and prevent mortality. Health systems and health research systems should ideally be mutually dependent (World Health Organization, 2004). The range of research that it is possible to do is infinite and all countries will need to prioritize relatively scarce resources, but this is especially true of low-income countries, where the priority is likely to be collecting the basic information that is required for planning, financing and implementing health and related other sector services. Collecting information can detract from service provision in low-income and developing countries.

## Relative resource allocations to mental and physical health research

Mental health research is poorly funded relative to physical health research, and mental health services research is the poor relation of biological research on mental disorders. This disparity is a reflection of the present health culture which values physical health over mental health, places a higher priority on communicable than non-communicable disease, and which places more value on physical aspects of mental health and mental illness (e.g. genes and hormones) rather than on the socio-cultural aspects of health and illness. The strength of these cultural issues is exemplified in *The Global Burden of Disease* (Murray and Lopez, 1996), which analysed global patterns of death and disability over the last decade. Despite mental health being centre stage in the relative burden of disease, nonetheless this has not translated into greatly increased research funding, relative to other subject areas.

## Relative resource allocations to research on biological and social causes of mental illness

The pace of research on mental and neurological disorders in rich countries is high. There has been considerable investment, particularly in biological research, on aetiological factors including genes and biochemical factors, but also in social research on epidemiology, disability and outcome, and on social risk factors including life events and social networks.

## Resource allocation to health services research on effective interventions

There is also a growing body of investment in assessment of interventions and in health services and health systems research, although this investment remains inadequate given the pre-eminent role of this type of research to improve health systems. There has been far less investment in such research in developing countries, but nonetheless a significant amount is now known about prevalence, risk factors and effectiveness of treatments in low-income countries. Cost-effectiveness studies in relation to both specific interventions and to health service delivery have been relatively well researched in richer countries for many of these conditions, but there is little cost-effectiveness research or health services research or service systems research in low-income countries (Shah and Jenkins, 2000); and large numbers of individuals living in low-income countries do not receive needed treatment.

## Research on generic medicines

Research about new medicines is a constant preoccupation in relatively rich countries, but in middle and low-income countries, which can barely afford the cheaper generic medicines, the main priority research issues to do with medicines are around evaluating the effectiveness of the cheaper generic medicines, optimum dosage levels and side-effects in different ethnic populations, and evaluating basic training and continuing education in their use, management of side-effects and reduction of relapse. Equitable access to new medicines is a luxury which most countries cannot afford, and where expenditure is still required simply to support the basic service infrastructure. However, it is extremely difficult to obtain funding for research about the older generic medicines. Research donors rarely if ever fund such work on generic medicines in low-income countries, which are then left to develop best practice on clinical experience alone rather than on the information which could be obtained from randomized controlled trials within their populations.

A crucial randomized controlled trial that needs to be done is the optimum dosage of amitriptyline in sub-Saharan Africa, where clinical experience suggests that 50 mg as opposed to 75–150 mg is a normal therapeutic dose. Despite the clear economic constraints, pharmaceutical companies are nonetheless heavily lobbying low-income countries to use the expensive new psychotropics within their public service. Such lobbying is counterproductive when it causes policy-makers to then consider that effective interventions for mental illness are so expensive that nothing can be used in the foreseeable future.

Research is urgently needed on the cost-effectiveness of the expensive, newer medicines in achieving improved health and social outcomes in low-income countries, compared with using cheaper alternatives and with the impact of using other crucial investments in health and social care such as strengthening primary care systems. All countries should make available some generic psychotropics and the psycho-social skills necessary to provide all forms of treatment.

## Research on practical difficulties in primary care service delivery

In low-income countries, specialist care is usually extremely scarce. For example, there is one psychiatrist per million population in low-income countries as opposed to one per 10 000 in the USA and in Eastern Europe. Most mental health care is delivered through primary care services. However low-income countries experience many practical difficulties in the delivery of basic primary health care (all the more crucial because of the relative paucity of specialist services), including lack of access to good practice guidelines, continuing professional development, means of transport for liaison, outreach and supervision, and lack of

access to regular means of communication (post, telephone or email). This communication is important not only in terms of social networks and economic development of countries, but is also important when taking place between levels in the health system and with other sectors. It is probably impossible to secure research funding to evaluate the cost-effectiveness, in terms of improved health and social outcomes achieved by ensuring that primary care centres in low-income countries have access to phone, email and suitable means of transport, and yet these are key limiting factors in the practical delivery of care.

## CULTURE AND RESEARCH PRIORITIES

### Methods of research prioritization

There is all too often a large cognitive dissonance between the research priorities of governments, funding institutions and academics. There is a need to develop needs-based criteria for research prioritization by donors, including the magnitude and urgency of the problem, as suggested from quantitative and qualitative data in the requisite situation analysis; the extent of previous research in discovering, developing or evaluating new interventions; feasibility of carrying out the research in terms of the technical, economic, political, socio-cultural and ethical aspects; expected impact of the research, considering both direct and indirect effects, short- and long-term benefits, as well as its implications on issues of affordability, efficacy, equity and coverage. Such needs-based criteria need to draw on the views of relevant stakeholders.

### Undue influence of donor agencies

Existing research is often the result of collaborative partnerships between rich and poor countries, and the donor agency usually has more power in deciding the research agenda, which can skew both research activities and qualified staff on to research areas that are not actually priorities for the local population. This is especially problematic for low-income countries, but is also a major problem in richer countries. The World Health Organization's Ad Hoc Committee on Health Research Relating to Future Intervention Options (1996) outlined a five-step priority-setting approach to decide how health research funds should be allocated in developing countries. These were subsequently refined by the Council for Health Research and Development and the Global Forum for Health Research (COHRED, 2000; Ghaffer *et al.*, 2004; World Health Organization, 2004).

The Global Forum for Health Research has recently funded a project to support the development of grassroots mental health research prioritization in the different regions of the world, and this will report next year (Khandelwal *et al.*, 2007 in preparation).

## Gender bias in research systems and hence in research content

Women's representation in senior research positions, on research committees and on editorial boards has not kept pace with women's expansion into medicine and science (Keiser *et al.*, 2003). There is cultural bias in the determination of journal content, so studies from developing countries receive less attention in the major peer review journals which are based in the rich countries. This is likely to have influenced the extensive gender bias in research. Whereas in physical health research female subjects are often excluded because of fears that the menstrual cycle will introduce potentially confounding effects or that an intervention will harm the foetus, paradoxically women are researched much more frequently than men in mental health research. This has arisen because of presumptions in the research culture that mental disorder is more of an issue for women than for men, and that men are more difficult to locate for research. Whatever the cause, it has resulted in a major gap in studies of mental disorder in men. In addition, studies of women have tended to focus on women's frequent higher rates of depression, while still ignoring women's greater exposure to many key risk factors, including rape and sexual violence, sexually transmitted diseases, prostitution, female genital mutilation, forced sterilization, involuntary abortion and partners who demand unprotected sex.

Rates of depression are high in caregivers for AIDS and other disorders and these caregivers are usually women. The impact of HIV/AIDS on women's mental health is likely to be enormous in countries such as Zimbabwe, where 30 per cent of pregnant women attending antenatal health clinics were found to be HIV-positive. In such situations, women must cope not only with illness in their male partners, but also with their own failing health and that of their children.

Although domestic violence is widespread in all countries, culture plays a role in how socially unacceptable it is, and how possible it is for the victim and indeed the perpetrator to seek help. For example, domestic violence resulting in death occurs through dowry deaths of brides in India and female infanticide in India and China. The perceived burden of female infants and the role of women in society influence attitudes to these practices. Domestic violence is frequently alcohol-related and women are overwhelmingly the targets. This is a largely hidden problem but routine battering is estimated to affect 25 per cent of women across diverse cultures, and this rate is often much higher in certain groups and certain countries.

## CULTURE AND RESEARCH CAPACITY

Two recent reports on neuropsychiatric disorders in developing countries summarize the existing state of knowledge, and highlight their importance and the urgent need to develop an international framework that will assist low-income countries to undertake the long-term research (Institute of Medicine, 2001; World Health Organization, 2001). Interdisciplinary research combined with partnership with implementing agencies is needed to overcome the barriers to care for persons with mental and neurological disorders in poor countries and to effectively change unhealthy behaviours in high-risk groups in these countries. There is a critical lack of research capacity in low-income countries in these fields and barriers to the translation of research results into action.

## Stigma and lack of advocacy

The substantial funding gap on mental health research between rich, middle- and low-income countries arises partly because of stigma about these conditions, and partly because neurologists and psychiatrists lack access to funders and decision-makers allocating resources.

## Brain drain

Human resource constraints are also critical. There is a substantial movement of psychiatrists, neurologists and specialist nurses to the West, some of whom might otherwise engage in operational research helpful to their local health systems (Ndetei *et al.*, 2004; Patel, 2003).

There is also a lack of identified career pathways for researchers in low-income countries, which makes them highly vulnerable to recruitment from institutions in rich countries. Some Western donors now do make research fellowships available to people from low-income countries, but scrutiny of the criteria reveals that they are directed at people who already have a serious research track record, and there is a need to develop mechanisms to support people at an earlier stage in their careers if research potential is to be fully developed, so that when project funding opportunities are available there will be expertise ready to make use of it. There is a need to fund posts as well as projects.

## Inequity in research partnerships

There are a growing number of research centres focusing on mental health in low- and middle-income countries, and growing number of partnerships between centres in richer and poorer countries. Publications from poorer countries are still very much in the minority of the journals.

Authors frequently find publication assisted if they have a Western partner. A further serious issue is ease of publication. Often those studies from poor countries which Western journals will publish are, for example, studies of effectiveness rather than of efficacy, and cannot for practical and logistical reasons be widely implemented.

Often research funding organizations for low-income countries do not have specific initiatives or programmes to fund research on mental health. Some funding is available from rich-country donors, and medical research councils in some middle-income countries now have some dedicated funding for mental health research, although little is yet available for the type of practice-based research that assists real implementation in the field. Few low-income countries, however, have indigenous mental health research funding as yet. This means that it is crucial to develop partnerships between countries, particularly South–South, as well as North–South, and to develop mechanisms for maximizing the research potential of all health professionals in training. It is also crucial to maximize the potential of newly developing and existing health information systems in primary and secondary care to gather useful data, and to ensure that sentinel surveillance sites and other generic health research projects address mental health issues.

## Lack of utilization of research skills acquired within clinical training

Many basic training courses for psychiatric nurses, psychiatrists and neurologists do include a research component and production of a research thesis, but this early exposure to research methodology and skills is then not utilized in the person's subsequent clinical career. For example, the nurses trained by the College of Health Sciences in Zanzibar receive a four-year training, of which the fourth year is devoted to psychiatry, and as part of this year, a research study is conducted. Similarly, the trainee psychiatrists in Kenya complete a research project for their MMed degree, and trainee diploma nurses at the Kenya Medical College Training Centre are expected to complete a research project. These research projects are rarely published and are relatively inaccessible to the wider research, health services and policy community, although scrutiny shows that they frequently address important local issues. Such students also form a willing and useful labour force for more complex studies which can thereby be conducted relatively cheaply, as well as providing an excellent educational opportunity for the students who will have the potential to carry such principles forwards into their working lives (Bondestan *et al.*, 1990).

Unfortunately there is a lack of attention to mechanisms whereby people can pursue research as an integral part of their clinical careers so that research activity does not inadvertently cause damage to fragile health care systems by further reducing the availability of well-informed clinical leadership. When developing research programmes there is a need to consider the existing specialist and primary care capacity in a country, and the way in which services can be developed and deployed to enable professionals to undertake operational research as well as their service commitments in a way that is mutually beneficial.

## Culture and reasons for lack of use of research findings

All too frequently research results are not applied in practice. Sometimes this is because the research was not designed to succeed within the logistical constraints of the country or the overall framework and direction of the health and social sector reform. There is then a need for further practice-based health services research to demonstrate how the findings can be used within the local context. It is of course often very difficult to obtain funding for such practically orientated research. Sometimes it is because researchers are not effective advocates and so have no regular dialogue with policy-makers. Researchers often feel that governments should read their research and implement it, without the researchers either making adequate efforts to disseminate the research results and their implications in ways that are tailored for policy-makers or, more fundamentally, without consulting governments from the

onset of the research so that the research design can be tailored to meet local needs, rather than simply informing governments later.

## VALUE OF RESEARCH–POLICY PARTNERSHIPS

There is clearly a need for closer developmental partnerships between policy-makers and researchers if researchers want their studies to contribute to the policy process. It is also true that mental health is often stigmatized by national policy-makers, and regional and district health management teams so that, even when the research is highly relevant, no action is taken. A helpful mechanism is to have a person with a broad mental health services research track record take up a post within a country's ministry of health to develop policy on mental health, so that there is a closer integration between policy-making and use of research. However, a number of countries are taking the retrograde step of removing specialist health advisers from their ministries of health, which is likely to aggravate the above problems. A further helpful mechanism is to organize appropriate mental health contributions to the annual meetings of public health officials, general medical and nursing conferences, and provincial/regional and district health management teams, etc.

## MAKING RESEARCH RELEVANT TO NATIONAL POLICY

### Need for overall health systems research

National policy development, implementation and evaluation are informed by research on overall systems as well as on individual services and interventions. National policy, by definition, has to take a broad overview and digestive role. It has to ensure that connections are made, that all the elements of the jigsaw puzzle are in place, that the system will work as an integrated and coherent whole, and that the policy can be implemented. Thus, there is a need for evidence about the health system as a whole rather than simply a summation of the bits. However, this is extremely difficult to get, and mental health services research is usually about small segments of the system rather than about the system as a whole. There is substantial expertise in the development of generic models for the design and reform of health systems (e.g. Roemer, 1991; Frenk, 1994; Cassels, 1995; Murray and Frenk, 2000) but rather less interest, until recently, in mental health-specific systems and the ways in which mental health systems interact with general health systems, broader social policy and other contexts within countries, and the way in which they are influenced by cultural issues.

Such policy-relevant mental health services research needs to cover the multiple sectors involved (not only public and private health sectors, but also the traditional health sector, and social welfare, housing, education, criminal justice, non-governmental organizations, media, etc.), and the linkages between them.

## Broad and narrow research questions

Broad information helps to inform decisions such as how much money should be spent overall and how it should be divided up between promotion, prevention, treatment and rehabilitation services. It also helps to decide the balances that should be sought between public and private health care, generalist and specialist health care and mental health care and social care. Finally, it helps to determine the importance of public policy on mental health. In contrast, narrow information helps to inform decisions on specific treatment options and interventions.

However, there are few studies available on which to base 'broad information' decision-making and useful information that can be shared between countries is urgently needed. The systematic review is the 'narrow information' instrument of choice to guide decision-making and has proved very useful. However, the quality of the systematic review is entirely dependent on the quality and quantity of the existing investigations on which it is based and

high-quality investigations aimed at issues relevant to policy are not always available, especially in middle- and low-income countries. Only a very restricted set of policy questions have been addressed by systematic review and as soon as one looks beyond the specific to broader health care and the interplay of health care, welfare, criminal justice, education and environmental policies, experimental trials become difficult or impossible. Given these circumstances, there are a number of steps we can take to improve evidence-based mental health policy-making.

## Evaluation of existing research

Knowledge depends as much on evaluation of existing research as it does on the generation of new research, but the research culture favours acquisition of new knowledge over evaluation of existing research. There is a need to ensure that policy-makers have ready access to the information and evidence that already exists but which they may find difficult to access. They may not even know that it exists. This means that there is insufficient use of limited resources and missed opportunities for health gain. Systematic review has become the gold standard for evaluating research. The Cochrane Collaborations and the National Institute for Health and Clinical Excellence (NICE) are very helpful in increasing access to the evidence base around specific medicines and psychological interventions. They contain as yet little information on the broader questions beyond specific medicines, psychological interventions or a specific service structure such as 24-hour nursed care.

Even where helpful information on cost-effective interventions does exist, it frequently seems to be given far less weight in practice than long-standing political and public imperatives, for example to reduce waiting lists in the UK. In addition, cost-containment rather than cost-effectiveness may be seen as an underlying imperative rather than the broader goal of maximizing health and social outcomes for a given level of expenditure. There are few systematic reviews of mental health questions in low-income countries and few such reviews are carried out by developing country personnel. Much of the research in developing countries is unfunded, and is conducted as research theses by trainee nurses or doctors, and is therefore difficult for reviewers and policy-makers to access.

## Stakeholder views

Policy-makers also have to take into account, or are well advised to take into account, the views of multiple stakeholders whose views would not necessarily be counted as admissible evidence in a systematic review. In particular, policy-makers need to consult and listen to users of primary care, specialist care and non-governmental organization services, of users of the education and criminal justice systems, as well as to managers, professionals and the public. These views are required, not just on the content of policy, but also on the practicalities of implementation. Health services research can provide a systematic methodology for such consultations, and culture is a key variable to be taken into account in such assessments.

## Country profile tools to integrate information and research

For policies and their implementation strategies to be credible and evidence based, they need to be highly tailored to the local situation to which they are intended to be applied, and should take into account the local context, needs, existing resources, structures, processes and outcomes, with particular attention to problems, challenges, strengths and opportunities (Cassels, 1995; Jenkins, 2001). The process of reform and the difficulty of implementing policy and institutional change have been relatively neglected (Walt and Gilson, 1994) compared with the debate about the content of reform, and both require a detailed prior situation appraisal.

It is important for policy-makers to have ready access to both qualitative and quantitative information about mental health (the context, needs, resources, provision and outcomes) in any country, and in a form that is accessible, organized, accurate, triangulated (Jick, 1979), usable, and

owned by key stakeholders (Smith, 1989; Kelle, 2001). There is a need for information about systemic as well as programmatic issues (Hafner and Heiden, 1991), and a need to analyse carefully the political, economic and institutional context in order to assess both the need and the potential for reform (Cassels, 1995).

However, this is rarely if ever available. Information is patchy, disorganized, inaccurate, not triangulated, and not discussed with key stakeholders. Information is not always accessible or available outside the narrow confines of government, and one part of government may not have data from another part of government. For example the prison service may not release data.

Information is often narrowly focused on the processes of specialist services and does not cover either the broader aspects of mental health within the health care system or the wider contextual factors that impinge on mental health. Furthermore, the information is not integrated in a coherent way that might facilitate broad understanding of the way in which the system articulates a whole as opposed to only understanding a small segment of the overall system. Much that goes wrong within health services is often to do with those interfaces, which are frequently neglected both in policy-thinking and in practice (Department of Health, 1996).

The fields of quantitative information that currently exist or which are thought about include household surveys, surveys of patients at various levels in the service, routine data on patients within the service, routine data on service inputs and processes. The data are often collected and published years later, too late to be of use in health planning and decision-making (Smith, 1989) and too little synthesized with qualitative information to be easily interpreted by the decision-makers.

Conceptual tools are therefore needed which help planners and policy-makers design and reform strategies, predict and subsequently trace the effects of policy, institutional and systems change (Cassels, 1995). It is also important that such tools respond to the charge that attention on the content of health sector reform has neglected the actors involved in the policy reform as well as the processes contingent on developing and implementing change and the context within which the policy is developed (Walt and Gilson, 1994; Koivusalo and Ollila, 1996).

The mental health country profile (Jenkins *et al.*, 2004) was designed to be such a conceptual and practical tool for low- and middle-income countries. It is both theory-driven and practice-based and extends the application of the some of the methodology of rapid situation appraisal to mental health at national level.

The country profile is designed to be used by local policy-makers, planners, professionals, users, and other key stakeholders. It allows the speedy synthesis of qualitative and quantitative information from multiple sources and is immediately useful for key stakeholders to improve policy and programmes. The multidisciplinarity inherent within the country profile brings different perspectives into the appraisal and planning process, acknowledges the complexities of the mental health situation and the need to pool disciplinary expertise. The development of the country profile had capacity building at its core, via networking, linking, visits, workshops, conferences and participation (Eade, 1997).

## CONCLUSIONS

Culture and stigma pervade attitudes towards most mental and neurological disorders, impact on the research attention to the disease burden, and need to be taken into account in health systems and services research. The whole spectrum of health services research needs to take culture into account, whether it be research instrumentation, research design, resource allocation, training of researchers and dissemination of research findings or implementation of the researched intervention. Good governance of both health systems and health research systems (stewardship, public accountability, good public health practice) is particularly important to address. Careful studies of cost-effectiveness and financing mechanisms within varying cultural contexts will improve service delivery and outcomes. A better understanding of cultural risk factors and culture-specific health care

delivery issues is crucial to tailor interventions to local conditions. All countries are a mixture of developed and developing, and we can learn from each other. Large-scale applications are dangerous and we need locally tailored solutions.

An important component of the way forward includes building cultural capacity for policy development, health monitoring and research architecture, for innovation, development and empowering leadership. This means creative use of attachments and secondments during training and career development. We also need to know much more about national and local epidemiology, and so need to build capacity in local epidemiology.

The Commission on Health Research for Development drew attention to the importance of health research as the essential link to equity in development. The research funding agencies have a key role to play in adopting a multi-country approach, investing in young researchers, in research centres, and in acknowledging the complexity of health services research and evaluating preventive interventions. Long-term commitment from governments, international bodies, donors and ourselves is needed. It is important to monitor research funding (Global Forum for Health Research, 2004). Access to the Internet, the Cochrane Collaboration, and international journals are all essential if countries are to avail themselves of the international evidence base. There is also a pressing need for cost-effectiveness studies in low-income countries (Shah and Jenkins, 2000).

## REFERENCES

Bodeker, G., Jenkins, R., Burford, G. 2001: International Conference on Health Research for Development (COHRED), Bangkok, Thailand, October 9–13, 2000: Report on the Symposium on Traditional Medicine, October 9, 2000. *Journal of Alternative and Complementary Medicine* 7, 101–108.

Bondestan, S., Garssen, J., Abdulwakil, A.I. 1990: Prevalence and treatment of mental disorders and epilepsy in Zanzibar. *Acta Psychiatrica Scandinavica* 81, 327–31.

Cassels, A. 1995: Health sector reform: key issues in less developed countries. *Journal of International Development* 7, 329–47.

COHRED (Commission on Health Research for Development) Working Group on Priority Setting 2000: Priority setting for health research: lessons from developing countries. *Health Policy and Planning* 15(2), 130–36.

Department of Health 1996: *Building Bridges*. London: HMSO.

Demyttenaere, K., Bruffaerts, R., Posada-Villa, J., Gasquet, I., Kovess, V., Lepine, J.P., Angermeyer, M.C., Bernert, S., De Girolamo, G., Morosini, P., Polidori, G., Kikkawa, T., Kawakami, N., Ono, Y., Takeshima, T., Uda, H., Karam, E.G., Fayyad, J.A., Karam, A.N., Mneimneh, Z.N., Medina-Mora, M.E., Borges, G., Lara, C., De Graaf, R., Ormel, J., Gureje, O., Shen, Y., Huang, Y., Zhang, M., Alonso, J., Haro, J.M., Vilagut, G., Bromet, E.J., Gluzman, S., Webb, C., Kessler, R.C., Merikangas, K.R., Anthony, J.C., Von Korff, M.R., Wang, P.S., Brugha, T.S., Aguilar-Gaxiola, S., Lee, S., Heeringa, S., Pennell, B.E., Zaslavsky, A.M., Ustun, T.B. and Chatterji, S. 2004: Prevalence, severity, and unmet need for treatment of mental disorders in the World Health Organization World Mental Health Surveys. *Journal of the American Medical Association* 291, 2581–2590.

Dunbar, R.I.M. 2004: *Grooming, Gossip and the Evolution of Language*. London: Faber and Faber.

Eade, D. 1997: *Capacity Building – An Approach to People Centered Development*. Oxford: Oxfam.

Frenk, J. 1994: Dimensions of health system reform. *Health Policy* 27, 119–34.

Ghaffer, A., de Francisco, A. and Matlin, S. (eds) 2004: *The Combined Matrix Approach: A Priority-setting Tool for Health Research*. Geneva: Global Forum for Health Research.

Global Forum for Health Research 2004: *The 10/90 Report on Health Research 2003–4*. Geneva: Global Forum for Health Research.

Goldberg, D. and Huxley, P. 1992: *Common Mental Disorders – A Biopsychosocial Model*. London: Routledge and Kegan Paul.

Hafner, H. and Heiden, W. 1991: Methodology of evaluative studies in the mental health field. In Freeman, H. and Henderson, J. (eds) *Evaluation of Comprehensive Care of the Mentally Ill*. London: Gaskell, 1–23.

Harris, E.C. and Barraclough, B. 1998: Excess mortality of mental disorder. *British Journal of Psychiatry* 173, 11–53.

Institute of Medicine 2001: *Neurological, Psychiatric and Developmental Disorders. Meeting the Challenge in the Developing World*. Washington, DC: National Academy Press.

Jenkins, R. 1990: Towards a system of outcome indicators for mental health care. *British Journal of Psychiatry* 157, 500–14.

Jenkins, R. 2001: Making psychiatric epidemiology useful: The contribution of epidemiology to mental health policy. *Acta Psychiatrica Scandinavica* 103, 2–14.

Jenkins, R. 2003: Supporting governments to adopt mental health policies. *World Psychiatry* 2, 14–19.

Jenkins, R. and Meltzer, H. 2002: A decade of national surveys of psychiatric epidemiology in Great Britain: 1990–2000. *International Review of Psychiatry* 15, 5–200.

Jenkins, R. and Singh, B. 2000: General population strategies of suicide prevention. In Hawton, K. and van Heeringen, K. (eds) *The International Handbook of Suicide and Attempted Suicide*. Chichester: Wiley, 597–615.

Jenkins, R., Tomov, T., Puras, D., Nanishvili, G., Kornetov, N., Sherardze, M., Surguladze, S. and Rutz, W. 2001: Mental health reform in Eastern Europe. *Eurohealth* 7, 15–21.

Jenkins, R., McCulloch, A., Friedli, L. and Parker, C. 2002: *Developing a National Mental Health Policy*. Maudsley Monograph. Andover: Psychology Press.

Jenkins, R., Baingana, F., Gulbinat, W., Khandelwval, S., Manderscheid, R., Mayeya, J., Minoletti, A., Mubbashar, M., Murthy, S., Parmeshvara, D., Schilder, K., Tomov, T. and Whiteford, H. 2003: International Project on Mental Health Policy and Services. Phase 1: Instruments and country profiles. *International Review of Psychiatry* 16(1–2).

Jenkins, R., Gulbinat, W., Manderscheid, R., Baingana, F., Whiteford, H., Khandelwal, S., Deva, M., Lieh Mak, F., Baba, A., Townsend, C., Harris, M. and Mohit, A. 2004: The mental health country profile: background, design and use of a systematic method of appraisal. The International Consortium on Mental Health Policy and Services – objectives, design and project implementation. *International Review of Psychiatry* 16, 31–47.

Jick, T.D. 1979: Mixing qualitative and quantitative methods: triangulation in action. *Administrative Science Quarterly* 24, 602–11.

Keiser, J., Utzinger, J. and Singer, B.H. 2003: Gender composition of editorial boards of general medical journals. *Lancet* 362, 1336.

Kelle, U. 2001: Sociological explanations between micro and macro and the integration of qualitative and quantitative methods. Forum Qualitative Sozial Forschung/Forum. *Quantitative Social Research* (online journal) 2, 1. Available at http://qualitative-research.net/fqs-eng.htm

Kessler 2004: The world Mental Health Survey Programme

Khandelwal, S., Mayeya, J., Cruz, M., Puras, D., Lopez, C., Gulbinat, W., Silberberg, D. and Jenkins, R. 2007 (in preparation): Mental and neurological research priorities in low- and middle-income countries.

Koivusalo, M. and Ollila, E. 1996: *International Organisations and Health Policies*. Helsinki: Stakes.

Lima, R.R., Santaonz, H., Lazano, J. and Lima, J. 1988: Planning for health: mental health integration in emergencies. In Lystad, M. (ed.) *Mental Health Response to Mass Emergencies – Theory and Practice*. Psychosocial Stress series No. 12. New York: Brunner Mazel, 371–92.

Murray, C.J.L. and Frenk, J. 2000: A framework for assessing the performance of health systems. *Bulletin of the World Health Organization* 78, 717–39.

Murray, C. and Lopez, A.D. 1996: *The Global Burden of Disease – A Comprehensive Assessment of Mortality and Disability from Diseases, Injuries and Risk Factors in 1990 and Projected to 2020*. Boston, MA: Harvard University Press.

Ndetei, D., Karim, S. and Mubbashar, M. 2004: Recruitment of consultant psychiatrists from low and middle income countries. *International Psychiatry* 6, 15–18.

Pang, T., Sadana, R., Hanney, S., Bhutta, Z.A., Hyder, A.A. and Simon, J. 2003: Knowledge for better health – a conceptual framework and foundation for health research systems. *Bulletin of the World Health Organization* 81, 815–20.

Patel, V. 2003: Recruiting doctors from poor countries: the great brain robbery. *British Medical Journal* 327, 926–28.

Paton, J. and Jenkins, R. 2002: *Mental Health Primary Care in Prisons*. London: Royal Society of Medicine.

Putnam, R.D. 1993: *Making Democracy Work*. Princeton, NJ: Princeton University Press.

Roemer, M. 1991: *National Health Systems of the World*, Vol. 1. Oxford: Oxford University Press.

Saeed, K., Gater, R. and Mubbashar, M.H. 2002: The prevalence, classification and treatment of mental disorders among attenders of native healers in rural Pakistan. *Social Psychiatry and Psychiatric Epidemiology* 35: 480–85.

Shah, A. and Jenkins, R. 2000: Mental health economic studies from developing countries reviewed in the context of those from developed countries. *Acta Psychiatrica Scandinavica* 101, 87–103.

Smith, G.S. 1989: Development of rapid epidemiologic assessment methods to evaluate health status and delivery of health services. *International Journal of Epidemiology* 18, S2–S15.

Walt, G. and Gilson, L. 1994: Reforming the health sector in developing countries: the central role of policy analysis. *Health Policy and Planning* 9, 353–70.

World Health Organization 1999: *Fact Sheet on Stigma*. Geneva: World Health Organization.

World Health Organization 2000: *Health in Emergencies: The Experience in the Former Yugoslav Republic of Macedonia in 1999*. Report from the workshop, Skopje, May 2000 WHO regional office for Europe, Humanitarian Assistance Office, Skopje, FYR Macedonia.

World Health Organization 2001: *The World Health Report 2001. Mental Health: New Understanding, New Hope*. Geneva: World Health Organization.

World Health Organization 2004: *World Report on Knowledge for Better Health: Strengthening Health Systems*. Geneva: World Health Organization.

World Health Organization Ad Hoc Committee on Health Research Relating to Future Intervention Options 1996: *Investing in Health Research and Development* (document TDR/Gen.96.1). Geneva: World Health Organization.

# 10

# Psychopathology and culture: disorders of possession and dissociation in intercultural clinical practice

Michael Odenwald, Marjolein van Duijl and Tobias Schmitt

## INTRODUCTION

Trance and possession phenomena exist in most cultures (Sar, 2006). Consequently, clinicians can come across phenomena in their daily practice and are confronted with challenging issues concerning the diagnostic and management process. [Note: Most experts dealing with the topic use the term 'possession' as an emic experiential term, not necessarily requiring that they themselves also believe in the existence of entities like spirits (Cardena, 1992).] For example, they will need to be able to distinguish normal from pathological phenomena, differentiate from other disorders, recognize the relationship with stress and trauma, deal with conflicting explanatory systems and ideas on treatment, and negotiate a path of management with the client and his or her relatives in accordance with their own ethical values. Here we want to briefly address some basic issues for clinical practice without further elaborating on the distinction between trance and possession phenomena (Tseng, 2001).

## EPIDEMIOLOGY, PHENOMENOLOGY, AETIOLOGY AND CLASSIFICATION

Trance and possession phenomena range from indigenous cultural presentations such as shamanism, trance dance, *amok* and *latah* (American Psychiatric Association, 2000), to modern Christian exorcism practice in the USA (Fountain, 2000) and further include the involvement of spirit mediums in African political issues (Behrend, 2000). While some claim that their prevalence seems to decrease with increasing industrialization of the culture (American Psychiatric Association, 2000), others describe how presentations of trance and possession phenomena seem to adapt to cultural, political and social change and disturbance (Ong, 1987; Igreja, 2003; Halliburton, 2005). Bourguignon demonstrated that from 488 societies reviewed, 74 per cent believe that spiritual forces can influence the individual and 52 per cent that an individual's personality can be replaced by that of another being (Bourguignon, 1976).

## Cultural perspectives

Lewis-Fernandes (1992, pp. 304–305) points out that decades of transcultural research suggest:

> the overwhelming majority of trance states across cultures are normal, and probably represent the voluntary use of non-distressing dissociative ability for the purposes of culturally-accepted healing rituals, religious and philosophical practices, and secular rituals of various kind.

Possession phenomena are also part of the normal range of human experience, and besides being typical expressions of stress, they belong as well to therapy, healing and shamanism (Tseng, 1999; Somer, 2006).

In anthropological studies, spirit possession is often described as occurring among marginal, subordinate and underprivileged people (O'Connel, 1982) and has been regarded as a response to intrapsychic tension, difficulties with relatives, and situations associated with low expectations for aid and support (Ward, 1980) or socio-economic change (De Jong, 1987). It is generally believed that possession states have a function within traditional societies, for example, to enable the expression of desires and wishes of underprivileged members (Somer, 2006).

For instance, Zar possession in northeastern Africa is common among Muslim women who live isolated, oppressed lives and is traditionally not seen as a pathological state. They can become possessed by a male spirit who argues with the husband about the wife's material needs. For treatment she is taken to a Zar specialist (often a female) where she is shown how to manage her spirit while in a group of women (Boddy, 1992). The spirits seem to help this woman survive by expressing her needs and relieving her from her isolated, exploited position (Grisaru et al., 1997; Al-Adawi et al., 2001).

It is important to acknowledge, though, that besides the non-pathological forms of trance and possession phenomena, pathological forms do exist (Wijesinghe et al., 1976; Saxena and Prasad, 1989) and produce significant impairment. For example, in southern India, possession per se is not considered pathological (Castillo, 1994a) and being possessed by a god or a benevolent spirit is generally seen as a gift. It is only when the possession agent is considered a bad spirit that traditional healing is sought. When the possessing agent is the soul of a deceased human being, the condition is seen as pathological and medical help is frequently preferred. In Box 10.1 we briefly

### Box 10.1 Example from Uganda

Martin was a 19-year-old boy who had been referred to the psychiatric ward, suffering from attacks of aggressive and threatening behaviour followed by amnesia. He had been to medical clinics before, where tests for malaria and typhoid fever had been positive. He had received treatment for these, but the attacks had continued and he wondered if it could be cerebral malaria. It was only after it was asked whether other causes, such as spirits, had been considered in the family that he admitted that according to his family he was bewitched by an aunt because she had not received her part of the dowry when his sister married. During some attacks he was reported to have actually spoken in her voice, so the family believed that he was possessed by her spirit. He had been taken to traditional healers by his family, where rituals were performed, including a reconciliation ritual, and his aunt had received her part. The attacks still continued, however.

By taking an extensive psycho-social history, further multiple problems were revealed. He wanted to study law but due to financial constraints in his family he was not allowed to attend the (more expensive and better quality) school of his choice. He felt enormous pressure to perform well at school as his older brothers and sisters were university graduates, but at the same time he feared that, being the youngest at home, he would have to take care of his mother who was mentally ill and needed intensive care. He also felt bad about having deserted the (poor) girl he loved under pressure of a dominating rich girlfriend.

present a case of pathological possession in Uganda who was seen by the second author.

Typical cases of pathological possession might involve more than one possessing agent at a time or consecutive agents (Castillo, 1994b). In general, spirit possession is a social phenomenon, which implies that others recognize the possessing agent(s) (Tseng, 2001).

## Psychological perspective

Anthropological and medical research on pathological trance and possession phenomena in non-Western cultures nowadays relies on the theory of dissociation (van der Kolk and van der Hart, 1989; Spiegel and Cardena, 1991), as well as the culture-centred descriptive anthropological perspective, which – in contrast to the former – postulates that states of altered consciousness are only to be explained by culture-specific theories (Lambek, 1992). Dissociation is defined as a disruption in the usually integrated functions of consciousness, memory, identity or perception (American Psychiatric Association, 2000). An amalgamation of both approaches is increasingly applied to the study of possession phenomena in non-Western cultures. Castillo (1994a) postulated on these grounds that it is a universal psychological mechanism that human beings might enter into spontaneous trance states when faced with extreme and overwhelming stress, and that this leads to phenomena of symptom quality according to the specific cultural background. In Western cultures, trauma-related dissociation can be conceived as a continuum from single somatoform and anxiety symptoms to dissociative identity disorder at the extreme poles (van der Kolk and van der Hart, 1989). Some researchers postulate that in non-Western cultures, pathological forms of spirit possession might be at the extreme end of this continuum, being explained by the same underlying mechanism as dissociative identity disorder (Suryani and Jensen, 1993; Castillo, 1994a; Butler *et al.*, 1996). Today, most researchers agree that from a cultural perspective, possession is a common way of experiencing and describing dissociative phenomena (Lewis-Fernandes, 1988; Cardena, 1996; Kirmayer, 1998).

This position is strengthened by the research on the effects of trauma on dissociation, trance and possession. Retrospective research has not only shown the association between trauma exposure and dissociative symptoms in the Western world (Van der Kolk *et al.*, 1996; Chu *et al.*, 1999) but also in countries such as Turkey (Sar *et al.*, 2000). Many authors concluded that potentially traumatizing events can be antecedents of dissociative symptomatology, particularly when the events are severe and recurrent, when they involve threat to physical integrity, and when the individual is young or was previously traumatized (Freyd, 1996; Van der Kolk *et al.*, 1996; Nijenhuis *et al.*, 1998; Chu *et al.*, 1999).

The few studies on the relationship between spirit possession and potentially traumatizing events go the same line: in a Buthanese refugee camp, Van Ommeren *et al.* (2001) identified trauma, early loss and recent loss as predictors of attacks of medically unexplained illness, involving alterations of consciousness, fear of spirit possession and hallucinations of supernatural beings. Van Duijl *et al.* (2006) showed that Ugandan patients consulting traditional healers because of spirit possession had experienced more traumatic events than a randomly selected control group from the same communities. In northern Uganda, our work with former child soldiers revealed that, shortly after having been liberated, many report that the spirits of the people they were ordered to kill come to haunt them, for example, in their dreams. After the return to their communities of origin they are often treated with suspicion and find it difficult to be accepted. Some develop severe dissociative attacks during which they might lose control over behaviour and commit violent acts or scream or shout aloud; afterwards they are amnesic for it. The local explanation is that the spirits of the victims have taken control over the former child soldier (Thomas Harlacher and Elisabeth Schauer, personal communications 2006). This is in line with the findings of Castillo (1994a,b) who suggested, based on the re-analysis of previously published case reports, that trauma was a risk factor for spirit possession in South Asia. It is also in agreement with studies on increased rates of non-traumatic stressful life experiences in persons suffering from possession (Gaw *et al.*, 1998; Trangkasombat *et al.*, 1998).

In all these settings, symptoms of possession and trance were culturally attributed to possession by spirits, rather than to traumatic experiences.

## DIAGNOSTIC CLASSIFICATION

In their latest editions, the *Diagnostic and Statistical Manual of Mental Disorders* (DSM-IV) and the *International Classification of Diseases* (ICD) have included a set of criteria to define abnormal trance and possession phenomena in non-Western cultures, relying on the combined theoretical approach described above in order to 'set out a Western nosological niche for a whole class of dissociative illness experiences previously unaccounted by the DSM system' (Lewis-Fernandes, 1992).

In DSM-IV the section on dissociative disorders covers amnesia, fugue, dissociative identity disorder, depersonalization, and dissociative disorders not otherwise specified (DDNOS). Pathological trance and possession states can be classified under the residual category DDNOS as dissociative trance disorder or possessive trance disorder. The ICD-10 (World Health Organization, 1992) includes trance and possession disorders (F44.3) under the section Dissociative Disorders.

According to the DSM, dissociative trance disorder is defined by an involuntary state of trance that is not accepted as a normal part of a collective or cultural ritual. This state is accompanied by narrowing of awareness of immediate surroundings and stereotyped behaviour or movement which one experiences as beyond one's control. In possession trance disorder a single or episodic alteration in the state of consciousness is accompanied by the replacement of the customary sense of personal identity by a new identity that is attributed to the influence of a spirit, power, deity or other person (American Psychiatric Association, 2000). The stereotyped and culturally determined behaviours are experienced as being controlled by the possessing agent and there is full or partial amnesia for the event.

The DSM-IV emphasizes that it is only when the trance or possession state is not accepted as a normal part of a collective cultural or religious practice that it can be considered as a disorder.

The inclusion of these categories has been discussed extensively because this diagnosis requires that manifested symptoms are considered as culturally not sanctioned and abnormal (Antze, 1992; Boddy, 1992; Leavitt, 1993); consequently this criterion differs between cultures and from the Western diagnostic categories (Bourguignon, 1992; Lewis-Fernandes, 1992; Kirmayer, 1998). Furthermore, syndromes attributed to spirit possession can overlap several diagnoses (Kirmayer, 1996; American Psychiatric Association, 2000). Many researchers agree that the established dissociation disorders section in the DSM and ICD systems need to be further revised in order to achieve validity in non-Western cultures (Alexander *et al.*, 1997; Van Duijl *et al.*, 2005; Sar, 2006), implying the need for further transcultural research in this field. Using the experimental criteria for possessive and dissociative trance disorder in clinical practice and research, further evaluation of dissociative and possessive trance symptoms is necessary in order to gain experience of how useful these categories might be.

The group of patients who are, in emic terms, possessed by a spirit, is made up of a heterogeneous group of etic disorders. For example, among an Indian sample of possessed patients, schizophrenia, mania and hysteria were diagnosed (Teja *et al.*, 1970), but there were also people without any disorder. Therefore, a clinician working with this group needs to be equipped with knowledge about the patient's culture (Tseng, 1999).

In the clinical diagnostic process, the clinician has to be aware of 'category fallacy', that is, 'the reification of a nosological category developed for a particular cultural group that is then applied to members of another culture for whom it lacks coherence and its validity has not been established' (Kleinman, 1987, p. 452). Applying a Western nosological category like dissociative disorders or psychotic disorders to an emic phenomenon loses the connection to its meaning in the original culture concerning ideas on causes and management.

There is also a risk that trance and possession phenomena, which are not considered pathological within the respective culture, are taken as disorders based on the Western diagnostic criteria (Lewis-Fernandes, 1992; Leavitt, 1993). But the necessary evaluation of the respective phenomena might not be easy as the distinction between normal and abnormal may not be beyond dispute within one culture. For example, in northern Sudan, because of the increased influence of Islamic thinking official opinion now might judge Zar possession as a psychiatric disorder (Boddy, 1992).

## Assessment of social context

For the diagnosis of possession trance disorder, DSM-IV and ICD-10 require the social and cultural context to be assessed in order to evaluate whether the phenomenon is culturally sanctioned or abnormal by local indigenous criteria of normality (Lewis-Fernandes, 1992). Thus, the decision on diagnosis should rely not just on the clinical examination and personal history but should necessarily include information from other areas, including family members and cultural informants. In non-Western cultures, health and disease, falling ill and healing, are not understood as related to an individual, but merely as depending on the family and the problems within the community, as our above-mentioned example shows. The information needed will encompass description and interpretation of symptoms and the disease concept by the patient's culture in general, by the family and the patient, social relationships, recent and past stressors or social conflicts and their interpretation, previous attempts to seek assistance (for example, from traditional healers and churches), previous confrontation with spirit possession and exorcism, etc.

Furthermore, relevant information, especially traditional explanatory models such as spirit possession, might not be easily revealed to a doctor because they might be considered irrelevant in the context of Western medicine; or shame, mistrust or 'cultural transference and countertransference' prevent their expression (Tseng, 1999; Halliburton, 2005). In this context, thorough and respectful enquiry, being non-judgemental towards cultural and religious meanings and giving them a place in the treatment process are of utmost importance.

Presented symptoms should, therefore, be held in the light of locally known explanatory models.

## Differential diagnosis

The typical case requires a multilevel diagnostic process, as a patient typically presents with multiple co-morbidities and unmet basic needs. The following steps of assessment and evaluation of clinical signs can be followed by the clinician in the diagnostic process:

- *Physical illness and substances*: infectious diseases, brain injury and substance abuse, intoxications, epilepsy, etc.
- *Psychiatric disorders*: psychotic disorders, bipolar disorders, depression; dissociative disorders including DDNOS (possession trance disorder), dissociative fugue, or other diagnoses involving dissociative symptoms.
- *Psychological problems* such as loss experiences, conflicts between individual needs and social expectations, potentially traumatic events.
- *Family problems* (including with the deceased) and social problems such as financial problems, jealousy and conflicts concerning land issues, inheritance, power, religion, unapproved marriages.
- *Cultural and religious conflicts*, such as unpaid dowries, unperformed (burial) rituals, mixed religious marriages.

The distinction between possessive and dissociative trance disorder and other psychiatric disorders can be challenging, because of the symptomatic overlap. Here we briefly present some aspects relevant to differential diagnosis.

### Psychotic disorders

It is known that psychotic disorders can present with delusions of being possessed (Goff *et al.*, 1991). Cross-cultural research has shown that especially in non-Western societies the delusions of psychotic patients are shaped by beliefs in witchcraft and religion (Ndetei, 1988). Furthermore, states of absorption by hallucinatory phenomena might be confused with trance states and a decision on the presence of formal thought disorder might not be easy, as incoherent thoughts, inadequate emotional expressions and thematic jumping might be related to possession. However, the duration and course of the two disorders can help to separate them; one dissociative shift in the course of a possession or trance phenomenon usually lasts minutes to hours, and only certain syndromes like the possession syndrome in southern India can include several subsequent shifts with a total duration of days to weeks (Lewis-Fernandes, 1992). Cardena labels possession delusions as 'attribution of illness to possession' in the absence of altered states of consciousness and possession trance (Cardena, 1992).

### Dissociative identity disorder, dissociative fugue and other syndromes involving dissociative symptoms

The diagnosis of dissociative identity disorder might not be relevant in the case of a clear-cut culture-bound possession syndrome, but most symptom criteria would match both disorders (Antze, 1992). Some authors try to make a distinction through the locality of possessing agent as external (possession trance) versus internal (dissociative identity disorder; Cardena, 1992). The course and duration of dissociative identity disorder and dissociative fugue might be different compared with possession syndromes, with temporarily clearer circumscribed dissociative shifts and better prognosis in the latter (Kua et al., 1986; Castillo, 1992; Lewis-Fernandes, 1992). Somatization and conversion-like symptoms are frequently found in persons with culture-bound possession syndromes. A clear understanding of the emic explanation and meaning of somatic symptoms is required.

### Trauma spectrum disorders

In Western countries, post-traumatic stress disorder and dissociative identity disorder are very frequently co-morbid conditions (Ross et al., 1989). Assuming a similar aetiology related to trauma, we can expect that possessed patients also might suffer from post-traumatic symptoms, such as nightmares which are interpreted as being haunted by spirits or avoidance symptoms explained by fear of spirit possession. The clinical exploration of trance-like symptoms provides the information needed to distinguish flashbacks from possession states.

## MANAGEMENT AND TREATMENT

Research in low-income countries and among immigrant groups in Western countries showed that people afflicted by mental distress search for help in different places/entities. These institutions have different explanations for mental distress, which sometimes contradict each other; for example, traditional or religious healers as well as medical doctors may be consulted (Alem et al., 1999; Assion et al., 1999; Odenwald et al., 2004). There is a wide range of different actors in the provision of services to people afflicted with pathological forms of possession and trance phenomena: traditional healers (shamans working with spirits, or others with herbal medicine), religious instances (sheikhs, shrines, temples or Christian churches), traditional medicine (Ayurvedic or Traditional Chinese Medicine), pharmacies, counselling services and Western-trained health professionals.

## Effectiveness of traditional and religious approaches

The traditional practices used to treat spirit possession generally try to involve the whole social environment of the patient, based on the model that the reasons why somebody became possessed are within the family, often involving already deceased members. These principles are close to Western concepts of systemic or family therapy.

In the experience of many authors, traditional and religious healers in the local communities are often effective in dealing with emotional problems and dissociative states in resource-poor countries (Somasundaram et al., 2000; De Jong, 2002), however, quantitative studies to evaluate traditional healing practices are widely lacking. The research of the second author in Uganda showed that most possessed patients felt the treatment by the traditional healers had helped them well (45 per cent felt better and 54 per cent completely healed after treatment). Other authors also acknowledged that traditional healing practices can bring subjective relief in the case of emotional problems (Eyber and Ager, 2002) or even severe psychiatric illnesses (Raguram et al., 2002). In Sri Lanka, Catani et al.

(2005) reported that four weeks' post-treatment chanting mantras and meditation and Narrative Exposure Therapy (Schauer *et al.*, 2005) were equally effective in the treatment of war-related post-traumatic stress disorder in schoolchildren – both treatments being delivered by teacher counsellors at school. On the other hand, it is also known that certain local or traditional practices are noxious; for example, severe beatings in order to drive out a spirit or prescription of Western drugs by untrained healers (Somasundaram *et al.*, 2000).

## Cooperation between Western medicine and traditional healers

Some experts have recommended the involvement of traditional healers in the official health service system or encouraged collaboration between Western-trained experts and local healers (Alem *et al.*, 1999). The second author's experience as head of a psychiatric unit in Uganda confirms that a mutually fruitful work relationship with traditional healers can be established with frequent referrals from the one to the other for diagnostic and treatment purposes (see Chapters 2 and 18). However, one has to be aware that in the field of traditional healing, as in Western medicine, there is a wide range of services on offer, from downright quacks charging exorbitant fees, to wise and insightful healers (Thomas Harlacher, personal communication). In order to identify a trustworthy counterpart, the clinician will need the assistance of cultural experts and probably needs to establish a personal contact.

## Providing Western-style treatment

In some cases, a patient, although holding a clear emic explanation of possession, wants or needs to get treatment by a Western-trained physician or psychotherapist (Somer, 1997); for example, in the case of severe medical conditions or psychiatric disorders involving immediate threat to the patient's wellbeing or that of others. In this case, careful preparation of the treatment is required to secure the compliance of the patient and his or her family, which focuses on treatment motivation and on

explanatory models for the problem and its treatment. The general aim is to find a viable compromise between all sides involved. In doing so, the use of the patient's or family's own terminology, combining it with Western medical thinking is advised (Suryani and Jensen, 1993; Somer, 1997). In Western Cognitive Behavioural Therapy this is conceptualized as System Adoption Strategies (Tuschen and Fiegenbaum, 1997; Fiegenbaum and Tuschen-Caffier, 2000) and has been applied in cases when the patient's disease model strongly diverged from the psychological model – making psychotherapy impossible at first.

In recent years, various efforts have been made to develop culture-sensitive approaches to counselling and psychotherapy (Bolton *et al.*, 2003; Van Duijl, 2003). Making use of the fact that most non-Western cultures have strong oral traditions, narrative methods for the treatment of the consequences of severe trauma have been developed in which the survivor assumes not the role of a patient but the one of a testimony (Cienfuegos and Monelli, 1983; Igreja *et al.*, 2004; Onyut *et al.*, 2005). Regardless of the explanatory model, facilitating verbal expression of past traumatic experiences enables emotional expression and subjective relief, helps the individual to restore peace with the past by developing new solutions and interpretations, to build up trust to others, and enables the resumption of social interactions in the community (Straker, 1994; Weine and Laub, 1995; Agger and Jensen, 1996).

The experience of the first author's department with the treatment of traumatized individuals in Uganda shows that the patient might automatically frame the narrative approach within emic explanatory systems. In particular, the belief that the spirits of the deceased blame the patient for their actions (killing them or not performing funeral rituals) leads to the patient's strong wish to explain in detail the problems and obstacles that led to this behaviour. For example, in the treatment of formerly abducted child soldiers one frequently found problem is that they believed that the ghosts of the people they had killed were haunting them because they had not heard that the commander had ordered them to do it. During the development of a detailed narration they felt that they made the spirit understand the reasons why they had killed them and, finally, felt relief and that they had forgiven them (Elisabeth Schauer, personal communication 2006). However, as the above-mentioned study in Sri Lanka shows, not all spirit-possessed patients need their traumatic experiences to be extensively explored or addressed in order to feel better (see Chapters 2 and 4 on the limitations of emic perspectives).

Here we come back to the case presented in Box 10.1. From a psychological viewpoint we could identify the conflict between Martin's individual needs and ambitions and the interests and expectations of the family as core problems; his identification with another disadvantaged family member, his aunt, was important for the symptomatic arrangement. The traditional explanation, however, was a conflict between family members on bridal price, witchcraft and possession. The solution to his problem was sought in reconciliation rituals involving the whole family and material compensation. However, this approach did not result in a solution of his individual stress as he kept on having attacks. He approached the Western medical system by presenting with physical symptoms, which were treated without success on the core complaint. Finally, he was presented to the psychiatric service, maybe in an act of despair. He finally participated in couselling sessions in an outpatient setting. During the counselling he expressed his grief concerning the fact that since his sister's marriage, her new husband did not allow her to support Martin any more financially, for example with school fees and maintenance costs. Here there appeared to be a parallel with the possessing agent, the spirit of his aunt who was financially disadvantaged by the wedding. During the course of the therapy, he started to become aware of his anger about others deciding for him. He became more assertive and identified some friends in his environment with whom he could share his feelings. After some months his attacks disappeared.

## CONCLUSIONS

Trance and spirit possession are frequent phenomena all around the world, being more common in non-Western cultures. Most of these phenomena have to be considered as normal, perhaps as part of religious rituals. In some cases, trance and spirit possession are expressions of distress and can be understood as pathological dissociative processes, often related to traumatic or stressful experiences. DSM-IV and ICD-10 have made attempts to include culture-bound syndromes and pathological trance and possession states. Although experts agree that in both classification systems these sections need further revision, it is helpful to use the experimental criteria to evaluate possessive and trance symptoms, and to explore and integrate different concurring explanatory models in their assessment and management. For a clinician, it is a good idea to explore the specific cultural context of the complaints. Many traditional and religious healing practices can be beneficial for the emotional relief of patients, but Western medical, psychiatric and counselling approaches are also applicable, in combination with traditonal approaches or alone. Psychiatric research in this field is just beginning, providing challenging opportunities for developing and evaluating culturally appropriate and accessible clinical practice and further research.

## REFERENCES

Agger, I. and Jensen, S.B. 1996: *Trauma and Healing under State Terrorism.* London, New Jersey: Zed Books.

Al-Adawi, S.H., Martin, R.G., Al-Salmi, A. and Ghassani, H. 2001: Zar: Group distress and healing. *Mental Health, Religion and Culture* 4, 47–61.

Alem, A., Jacobsson, L., Araya, M., Kebede, D. and Kullgren, G. 1999: How are mental disorders seen and where is help sought in a rural Ethiopian community? A key informant study in Butajira, Ethiopia. *Acta Psychiatrica Scandinavica* 397, S40–S47.

Alexander, P.J., Joseph, S. and Das, A. 1997: Limited utility of ICD-10 and DSM-IV classification of dissociative and conversion disorders in India. *Acta Psychiatrica Scandinavica* 95, 177–82.

American Psychiatric Association 2000: *Diagnostic Criteria from DSM-IV-TR.* Washington, DC: American Psychiatric Association.

Antze, P. 1992: Possession trance and multiple personality: psychiatric disorders or idioms of distress? *Transcultural Psychiatric Research Review* 29, 319–23.

Assion, H.J., Dana, I. and Heinemann, F. 1999: [Folk medical practices in psychiatric patients of Turkish origin in Germany]. *Fortschritte in Neurologie und Psychiatrie* 67, 12–20.

Behrend, H. 2000: Power to heal, power to kill: spirit possession and war in northern Uganda (1986–1994). In H. Behrend and U. Luig (eds) *Spirit Possession: Modernity and Power in Africa.* Oxford: James Currey, 20–31.

Boddy, J. 1992: Comment on the proposed DSM-IV criteria for trance and possession disorder. *Transcultural Psychiatric Research Review* 29, 323–30.

Bolton, P., Bass, J., Neugebauer, R., Verdeli, H., Clougherty, K.F., Wickramaratne, P., Speelman, L., Ndogoni, L. and Weissman, M. 2003: Group interpersonal psychotherapy for depression in rural Uganda: A randomized controlled trial. *Journal of the American Medical Association* 289, 3117–24.

Bourguignon, E. 1976: *Possession.* San Francisco, CA: Chandler.

Bourguignon, E. 1992: The DSM-IV and cultural diversity. *Transcultural Psychiatric Research Review* 29, 330–32.

Butler, L.D., Duran, R.E., Jasiukaitis, P., Koopman, C. and Spiegel, D. 1996: Hypnotizability and traumatic experience: a diathesis-stress model of dissociative symptomatology. *American Journal of Psychiatry* 153, S42–S63.

Cardena, E. 1992: Trance and possession as dissociative disorders. *Transcultural Psychiatric Research Review* 29, 287–300.

Cardena, E. 1996: Dissociative disorders: Phantoms of the self. In Turner, S.M. and Hersen, M. (eds) *Adult Psychopathology and Diagnosis.* New York: John Wiley, 384–403.

Castillo, R.J. 1992: Cultural considerations for trance and possession disorder in DSM-IV. *Transcultural Psychiatric Research Review* 29, 333–37.

Castillo, R.J. 1994a: Spirit possession in south Asia, dissociation or hysteria? Part 1: Theoretical background. *Culture, Medicine and Psychiatry* 18, 1–21.

Castillo, R.J. 1994b: Spirit possession in south Asia, dissociation or hysteria? Part 2: Case histories. *Culture, Medicine and Psychiatry* 18, 141–62.

Catani, C., Kohiladevy, M., Neuner, F., Ruf, M. and Schauer, M. 2005: Treating children shattered by war and disaster: a controlled clinical trial in Sri Lanka's north-eastern coastal region affected by the tsunami. *9th European Conference on Traumatic Stress (ECOTS).* Stockholm: European Society for Traumatic Stress Studies (ETSS).

Chu, J.A., Frey, L.M., Ganzel, B.L. and Matthews, J.A. 1999: Memories of childhood abuse: dissociation, amnesia, and corroboration. *American Journal of Psychiatry* 156, 749–55.

Cienfuegos, A.J. and Monelli, C. 1983: The testimony of political repression as a therapeutic instrument. *American Journal of Orthopsychiatry* 53, 43–51.

De Jong, J.T. 1987: *A Descent into African Psychiatry.* Amsterdam: Royal Tropical Institute.

De Jong, J.T. 2002: Public mental health, traumatic stress and human rights violations in low-income countries. In De Jong, J.T. (ed.) *Trauma, War and Violence: Public Mental Health in Socio-cultural Context.* New York: Kluwer Academic/Plenum Publishers.

Eyber, C. and Ager, A. 2002: Conselho: Psychological healing in displaced communities in Angola. *Lancet* 360, 871.

Fiegenbaum, W. and Tuschen-Caffier, B. 2000: [Systemimmanent communication and exposure as treatments of sexual disorders]. *Verhaltenstherapie* 10, 32–39.

Fountain, J.W. 2000: Exorcists and exorcism proliferate across U.S. *The New York Times,* Tuesday 28 November, 16.

Freyd, J.J. 1996: *Betrayal Trauma: The Logic of Forgetting Childhood Trauma.* Cambridge, MA: Harvard University Press.

Gaw, A.C., Ding, Q., Levine, R.E. and Gaw, H. 1998: The clinical characteristics of possession disorder among 20 Chinese patients in the Hebei province of China. *Psychiatric Services* 49, 360–65.

Goff, D.C., Brotman, A.W., Kindlon, D., Waites, M. and Amico, E. 1991: The delusion of possession in chronically psychotic patients. *Journal of Nervous and Mental Disease* 179, 567–71.

Grisaru, N., Budowski, D. and Witztum, E. 1997: Possession by the 'Zar' among Ethiopian immigrants to Israel: Psychopathology or culture-bound syndrome? *Psychopathology* 30, 223–33.

Halliburton, M. 2005: 'Just some spirits': The erosion of spirit possession and the rise of 'tension' in south India. *Medical Anthropology* 24, 111–44.

Igreja, V. 2003: 'Why are there so many drums playing until dawn?': Exploring the role of gamba spirits and healers in the post-war recovery period in Gorgongosa, central Mozambique. *Transcultural Psychiatry* 40, 459–87.

Igreja, V., Kleijn, W.C., Schreuder, B.J., Van Dijk, J.A. and Verschuur, M. 2004: Testimony method to ameliorate post-traumatic stress symptoms. Community-based intervention study with Mozambican civil war survivors. *British Journal of Psychiatry* 184, 251–57.

Kirmayer, L.J. 1996: Confusion of the senses: implications of ethnocultural variations in somatoform and dissociative disorders for PTSD. In Marsella, A.J., Friedman, M.J., Gerrity, E.T. and Scurfield, R.M. (eds) *Ethnocultural Aspects of Posttraumatic Stress Disorder.* Washington DC: American Psychological Association, 131–63.

Kirmayer, L.J. 1998: The fate of culture in DSM-IV. *Transcultural Psychiatry* 35, 339–42.

Kleinman, A. 1987: Anthropology and psychiatry. The role of culture in cross-cultural research on illness. *British Journal of Psychiatry* 151, 447–454.

Kleinman, A. 1988: *Rethinking Psychiatry, from Cultural Category to Personal Experience.* New York: Free Press.

Kua, E.H., Sim, L.P. and Chee, K.T. 1986: A cross-cultural study of the possession-trance in Singapore. *Australian and New Zealand Journal of Psychiatry* 20, 361–64.

Lambek, M. 1992: Discreteness or discretion? *Transcultural Psychiatric Research Review* 29, 345–47.

Leavitt, J. 1993: Are trance and possession disorders? *Transcultural Psychiatric Research Review* 30, 51–57.

Lewis-Fernandes, R. 1988: A cultural critique of the DSM-IV dissociative disorders section. *Transcultural Psychiatry* 35, 387–400.

Lewis-Fernandes, R. 1992: The proposed DSM-IV trance and possessions disorder category: potential benefits and risks. *Transcultural Psychiatric Research Review* 29, 301–17.

Ndetei, D.M. 1988: Psychiatric phenomenology across countries: constitutional, cultural, or environmental? *Acta Psychiatrica Scandinavica* 344, S33–S44.

Nijenhuis, E.R.S., Spinhoven, P., Van Dyck, R., Van der Hart, O. and Vanderlinden, J. 1998: Degree of somatoform and psychological dissociation in dissociative disorders is correlated with reported trauma. *Journal of Traumatic Stress* 11, 711–30.

O'Connel, M.C. 1982: Spirit possession and role stress among the Xesibe of eastern Transkei. *Ethnology* 21, 21–37.

Odenwald, M., Catani, C. and Lingenfelder, B. 2004: [Where do people in Somaliland seek assistance for mental disorders]. *Neurologie and Psychiatrie* 13, 23.

Ong, A. 1987: *Spirits of Resistance and Capitalist Discipline: Factory Women in Malaysia*. Albany: State University of New York Press.

Onyut, L.P., Neuner, F., Schauer, E., Ertl, V., Odenwald, M., Schauer, M. *et al.* 2005: Narrative Exposure Therapy as a treatment for child war survivors with posttraumatic stress disorder: Two case reports and a pilot study in an African refugee settlement. *BMC Psychiatry* 5, 7.

Raguram, R., Venkateswaran, A., Ramakrishna, J. and Weiss, M.G. 2002: Traditional community resources for mental health: A report of temple healing from India. *British Medical Journal* 325, 38–40.

Ross, C.A., Norton, G.R. and Wozney, K. 1989: Multiple personality disorder: an analysis of 236 cases. *Canadian Journal of Psychiatry* 34, 413–18.

Sar, V. 2006: The scope of dissociative disorders: an international perspective. *Psychiatric Clinics of North America* 29, 227–44.

Sar, V., Kundakci, T., Kiziltan, E., Bakim, B. and Bozkurt, O. 2000: Differentiating dissociative disorders from other diagnostic groups through somatoform dissociation. *Journal of Trauma and Dissociation* 1, 67–80.

Saxena, S. and Prasad, K.V. 1989: DSM-III subclassification of dissociative disorders applied to psychiatric outpatients in India. *American Journal of Psychiatry* 146, 261–62.

Schauer, M., Elbert, T. and Neuner, F. 2005: *Narrative Exposure Therapy: a Short-Term Intervention for Traumatic Stress Disorders after War, Terror, or Torture*. Toronto: Hogrefe and Huber.

Somasundaram, D., Sivayokan, S. and Jongh, J.D. 2000: *Mental Health in the Tamil Community*. Jaffna: Transcultural Psychosocial Organization (TPO).

Somer, E. 1997: Paranormal and dissociative experiences in middle-eastern Jews in Israel: diagnostic and treatment dilemmas. *Dissociation* 10, 174–81.

Somer, E. 2006: Culture-bound dissociation: a comparative analysis. *Psychiatric Clinics of North America* 29, 213–26.

Spiegel, D. and Cardena, E. 1991: Disintegrated experience: the dissociative disorders revisited. *Journal of Abnormal Psychology* 100, 366–78.

Straker, G. 1994: Integrating African and western healing practices in South Africa. *American Journal of Psychotherapy* 48, 455–67.

Suryani, L.K. and Jensen, G.D. 1993: *Trance and Possession in Bali: a Window on Western Multiple Personality, Possession Disorder, and Suicide*. Kuala Lumpur, New York: Oxford University Press.

Teja, J.S., Khanna, B.S. and Subrahmanyam, T.B. 1970: Possession states in Indian patients. *Indian Journal of Psychiatry* 12, 71–81.

Trangkasombat, U., Su-Umpan, U., Churujiporn, V., Nukhew, O. and Haruhanpong, V. 1998: Risk factors for spirit possession among school girls in southern Thailand. *Journal of the Medical Association of Thailand* 81, 541–46.

Tseng, W.S. 1999: Culture and psychotherapy: review and practical guidelines. *Transcultural Psychiatry* 36, 131–79.

Tseng, W.S. 2001: *Handbook of Cultural Psychiatry*. New York: Academic Press.

Tuschen, B. and Fiegenbaum, W. 1997: Techniques of exposure. In Roth, W.T. and Yalom, I.D. (eds) *Treating Anxiety Disorders*. San Francisco: Jossey-Bass, 31–55.

Van der Kolk, B.A. and van der Hart, O. 1989: Pierre Janet and the breakdown of adaptation in psychological trauma. *American Journal of Psychiatry* 146, 1530–40.

Van der Kolk, B.A., Pelcovitz, D., Roth, S., Mandel, F.S., McFarlane, A. and Herman, J. 1996: Dissociation, somatization, and affect dyregulation: the complexity of adaption to trauma. *American Journal of Psychiatry* 153, S83–S93.

Van Duijl, E.M. 2003: Culturally sensitive counselling in Uganda. *Memisa Medisch* 69, 18–27.

Van Duijl, E.M., Cardena, E. and De Jong, J.T. 2005: The validity of DSM-IV dissociative disorders categories in south-west Uganda. *Transcultural Psychiatry* 42, 219–41.

Van Duijl, E.M., Nijenhuis, E., Komproe, I., Gernaat, H. and De Jong, J.T. 2006: Dissociative symptoms and reported trauma among patients with spirit possession and matched healthy controls in Uganda. Paper presented at the First World Congress of Cultural Psychiatry of the

World Association of Cultural Psychiatry, Beijing, China (S-IV-38).

Van Ommeren, M., Sharma, B., Komproe, Poudyal, B.N., Sharma, G.K., Cardena, E. *et al.* 2001: Trauma and loss as determinants of medically unexplained epidemic illness in a Bhutanese refugee camp. *Psychological Medicine* 31, 1259–67.

Ward, C. 1980: Spirit possession and mental health: a psycho-anthropological perspective. *Human Relations* 33, 149–63.

Weine, S. and Laub, D. 1995: Narrative constructions of historical realities in testimony with Bosnian survivors of 'ethnic cleansing'. *Psychiatry* 58, 246–60.

Wijesinghe, C.P., Dissanayake, S.A. and Mendis, N. 1976: Possession trance in a semi-urban community in Sri Lanka. *Australian and New Zealand Journal of Psychiatry* 10, 135–39.

World Health Organization 1992: *International Classification of Diseases, 10th Revision (ICD-10)*. Geneva: World Health Organization.

# 11

# The history and relevance of culture-bound syndromes

Keith Lloyd

## INTRODUCTION

In Chapter 2, Helman sets out the role of anthropology in mental health care, and draws some attention to culture-bound syndromes as part of the history of cultural understanding of mental distress. This chapter, however, explores some specific phenomena in order to ensure that researchers and practitioners who encounter such diagnoses and associated symptoms are prepared to challenge such concepts, and to ensure there is critical application of these diagnoses. It could be argued that, like the working steam train, culture-bound syndromes are becoming confined to fewer and fewer parts of the world, largely swept aside by the diesel locomotive of globalization and DSM-IV, and consigned to museums where they are lovingly tended by a small group of enthusiasts. Others see things differently. Guarnaccia and Rogler (1999) applauded the inclusion of culture-bound syndromes in DSM-IV as an overdue acknowledgement of both the cultural diversity of many modern societies, as well as acknowledging the global reach of DSM-IV. The way was now open, they suggested, to investigate these syndromes within their cultural context and to analyse the relationship between these syndromes and psychiatric disorders. A third view is that the very concept of a culture-bound syndrome is a tautology because there can be no such thing as a culture-free syndrome – all disease classifications have to exist in a cultural context (Lee, 1996). And that it is only by becoming aware of the cultural context of all consultations and research, by becoming reflexive, that we can truly practise cultural psychiatry.

It is by examining the development of the concept in a historical context that we can see how successive waves of anthropologists and psychiatrists have each created culture-bound syndromes in their own image. By and large, the anthropologists have emphasized the cultural specificity and relativist aspects of culture-bound syndromes whilst the psychiatrists have emphasized the universalist and biological aspects (Prince, 2000). This chapter does not attempt an exhaustive categorization of culture-bound syndromes but rather attempts to look at some of the cultural and historical assumptions behind the concept.

Current concerns have been elegantly summarized by Kirmayer (2006) who proposes that the future of cultural psychiatry lies in advancing a broad perspective that: (a) is inherently multidisciplinary; (b) recognizes psychological processes as fundamentally social as well as individual; and (c) critically examines local and global systems of power. As he notes, globalization has brought with it many ironies for cultural psychiatry. Transcultural migrations have resulted in cultural hybridization at the same time as ethnicity has become more salient. Evidence-based medicine can seem to limit the scope for and impact of cultural research which is lacking in methodologies, capacity and the foundations or inheritance of previous research. Furthermore, some suggest that cultural psychiatry has itself been co-opted by the pharmaceutical industry to inform marketing campaigns to promote conventional treatments for new populations, rather than adapt existing interventions or inform their development to better suit the needs of the culturally diverse populations.

## HISTORY OF THE CONCEPT

Kraepelin is widely credited with being the first, from a psychiatric perspective at least, to propose integrating cultural concerns into clinical psychiatric practice (Kraepelin, 1904). He identified the potential value of a comparative psychiatry focused on ethnic and cultural aspects in mental health and disease and was interested in the role of sociocultural factors in psychopathology.

It was Yap, half a century later, who coined the term 'culture-bound syndrome' in a number of early articles in the field (Yap, 1951, 1965). In a posthumously published article (Yap, 1974), Yap nailed several of the difficulties with the concept of culture-bound syndromes. He noted that,

*Whether or not there are new psychiatric illnesses to be found in folk cultures or non-metropolitan populations is a question that requires semantic resolution. Undoubtedly there are, in certain cultures, some clinical manifestations quite unlike those described in standard psychiatric textbooks which historically are based on the experiences of western psychiatrists. In these senses illnesses presenting so strangely can be regarded as new. However, each of the same textbooks also espouses a system of disease classification*

*that by its own logic is meant to be final and exhaustive. From this point of view, no more new illnesses are to be discovered, and any straight clinical condition can only be a variation of something already recognized and described. Two problems then arise: firstly how much do we know about the culture-bound syndromes for us to be able to fit them into a standard classification and secondly whether such a standard and exhaustive classification in fact exists.*

He then continues,

*It has long been known that there are, in certain groups, particular aberrations of behaviour which are regarded as abnormal. Over the years a number of terms taken from indigenous languages have crept into the psychiatric literature to denote these conditions but many of them do not point to novel and distinct forms of disorder unknown elsewhere. Some are simply generic terms for mental disorder, without definitive meaning, others refer to healing rituals, and still others to supernatural notions of disease causation. From a psychiatrist's point of view the field has, with notable recent exceptions, remained confused and barren. Interest has tended to wither after the syndromes have been disdainfully labelled exotic and the colourful names are then surrendered to the belletrist. To avoid stagnation in the field, it is essential to apply the concepts of clinical psychopathology to the analysis of these disorders, to integrate them into recognised classifications of disease if possible or to broaden the classification if necessary.*

After Yap, much of the research into culture-bound syndromes appears to have had the goal of attempting to fit these syndromes into the standard classificatory systems without fully investigating them on their own terms (Guarnaccia and Rogler, 1999). Nonetheless, their inclusion in both the *Diagnostic and Statistical Manual of Mental Disorders* (DSM-IV) and the *International Classification of Diseases* (ICD-10) was an important move. In this chapter, culture-bound syndromes are presented as a historical classification phenomenon that warrants some revision, in the face of increasing information about culturally determined patterns of behaviour and expressions of distress.

## DEFINITIONS OF CULTURE-BOUND SYNDROMES

Ritenbaugh (1982) suggested four criteria for a culture-bound syndrome: (1) it cannot be understood apart from its specific cultural or subcultural context; (2) the aetiology summarizes and symbolizes core meanings and behavioural norms of that culture; (3) diagnosis relies on culture specific technology as well as ideology; (4) successful treatment is accomplished only by participants in that culture. This definition ties culture-bound syndromes to folk or emic models of illness and locates them outside etic, global biomedical models. This perspective is at odds with subsequent attempts to include them within mainstream psychiatric classificatory systems.

More prosaically, DSM-IV defines a culture-bound syndrome as denoting:

*Recurrent, locality-specific patterns of aberrant behaviour and troubling experience that may or may not be linked to a particular DSM-IV diagnostic category. Many of these patterns are indigenously considered to be illnesses, or at least afflictions and most have local names. Although presentations conforming to the major DSM-IV categories can be found throughout the world, the particular symptoms, course, and social response are very often influenced by local cultural factors. In contrast, culture-bound syndromes are generally limited to specific societies or culture areas and are localized, folk, diagnostic categories that frame coherent meanings for certain repetitive, patterned, and troubling sets of experiences and observations.*
(**American Psychiatric Association, 1994**)

In ICD-10 the culture-bound syndromes are included as an annex outside the main classificatory system and the terminology used differs from that in DSM-IV. ICD-10 refers to culture-specific disorders which are described as:

*having diverse characteristics but sharing two principal features: 1) they are not easily accommodated by the categories in established and internationally used psychiatric classifications; 2) they were first described in, and subsequently closely or exclusively associated with, a particular population or cultural area.*

The authors then go on to comment that these

*syndromes have also been referred to as culture-bound or culture-reactive, and as ethnic or exotic psychoses. Some are rare and some may be comparatively common; many are acute and transient, which makes their systematic study particularly difficult. The status of these disorders is controversial: many researchers argue that they differ only in degree from disorders already included in existing psychiatric classifications, such as anxiety disorders and reactions to stress, and that they are therefore best regarded as local variations of disorders that have long been recognized. Their exclusive occurrence in specific population or cultural areas has also been questioned.*

Like Guarnaccia and Rogler (1999) the authors of ICD-10 note that there is a clear need for research that will help to establish reliable clinical descriptions of these disorders and clarify their distribution, frequency and course. In the hope of stimulating and facilitating such research, the best-described culture-bound syndromes are described, and then critiqued. Some of these might better be described as local illness categories (for example, *nervios*, *susto*) rather than culture-bound syndromes as initially conceived, where these were alien syndromes not found in part or whole in Euro-American societies.

## SOME CULTURE-BOUND DISORDERS IN ICD-10

Twelve frequently described culture-bound syndromes are included in ICD-10 (World Health

Organization, 1993). These are *amok, dhat, koro, latah, nerfizo* or *nervios, pa-leng* or frigophobia, *pibloktoq* or Arctic hysteria, *susto, taijin kyofusho* or anthropophobia, *ufufuyane, uqamairineq* and *windigo*.

## Amok

*Amok* is described mainly in Malaysia and Indonesia. It is

> *an indiscriminate, seemingly unprovoked episode of homicidal or highly destructive behaviour, followed by amnesia or fatigue. Many episodes culminate in suicide. Most events occur without warning, although some are precipitated by a period of intense anxiety or hostility. Some studies suggest that cases may derive traditional values placed on extreme aggression and suicidal attacks in warfare.*

ICD-10 classifies it under 'F68.8 Other specified disorders of adult personality and behaviour' and identifies a number of potentially related syndromes: *ahade idzi be* (the island of New Guinea), *benzi mazurazura* (southern Africa (among Shona and affiliated groups)), *berserkergang* (Scandinavia), *cafard* (Polynesia), *colerina* (the Andes of Bolivia, Colombia, Ecuador, and Peru), *hwa-byung* (Korean peninsula), *iich'aa* (indigenous peoples of south-western America) (Yap, 1951; Simons and Hughes, 1985).

An earlier description is provided by the 1911 *Encyclopaedia Britannica*, which describes *amok* or 'running amuk' as:

> *the native term for the homicidal mania which attacks Malays. A Malay will suddenly and apparently without reason rush into the street armed with a kris or other weapon, and slash and cut at every-body he meets till he is killed. These frenzies were formerly regarded as due to sudden insanity. It is now, however, certain that the typical* amok *is the result of circumstances, such as domestic jealousy or gambling losses, which render a Malay desperate and weary of his life. It is, in fact, the Malay equivalent of suicide. The act of running amuck is probably due to causes*

> *over which the culprit has some amount of control, as the custom has now died out in the British possessions in the peninsula, the offenders probably objecting to being caught and tried in cold blood.*

> **(Britannica, 1911)**

Little information is available on incidence. Both the above descriptions are of interest in terms of how they are so firmly rooted in their own historical time and place. For the universalist, syndromes such as *amok* are to be understood as a local variant of epidemic hysteria. For the cultural relativist, there is little value in comparing it with other geographical locations.

## Dhat

Also known as *dhatu, jiryan* and *shen-k'uei, dhat* is described mainly in India and Taiwan. ICD-10 gives the core features as:

> *Acute anxiety and somatic complaints such as fatigue and muscle pain, related to a fear of semen loss in men or women (also thought to secrete semen). Precursors are said to include excess coitus, urinary disorders, imbalances in body humours, and diet. The main symptom is a whitish discharge in urine, interpreted as semen loss. Traditional remedies focus on herbal tonics to restore semen or humoral balance.*

Suggested ICD-10 codes are 'F48.8 Other specified neurotic disorders' or 'F45.34 Somatoform autonomic dysfunction of the genitourinary system'. It is seen as potentially related to *koro* in China and *rabt* in Egypt.

In a subtle analysis of culture-bound syndromes, Sumathipala *et al.* (2004) argue that the symptoms of *dhat* are, or have been, much more widely distributed in the world than might at first appear, again raising doubts about whether the 'culturally bound' perception is a reality at a particular time and place, or indeed simply a product of explorers and researchers looking for the 'alien' in the other and finding inexplicable phenomena where these are understandable and not culturally bound.

## Koro

*Koro* is described mainly in South-East Asia, China and India and involves an acute panic or anxiety reaction involving fear of genital retraction. In severe cases, men become convinced that the penis will suddenly withdraw into the abdomen; women sense that their breasts, labia, or vulva will retract. Victims expect the consequences to be fatal. Studies cite factors such as illness, exposure to cold or excess coitus as precursors, but interpersonal conflict and sociocultural demands reportedly exert greater influence on the condition. Onset is rapid, intense and unexpected. Responses vary, but include grasping of the genitals by the victim or a family member, application of splints or devices to prevent retraction, herbal remedies, massage or fellatio (Simons and Hughes, 1985). It is classified under ICD-10 as 'F48.8 Other specified neurotic disorders' or 'F45.34 Somatoform autonomic dysfunction of the genitourinary system' (World Health Organization, 1993).

## Latah

*Latah* involves highly exaggerated responses to a fright or trauma, followed by involuntary echolalia, echopraxia or trance-like states. Studies variously interpret cases as a neurophysiological response that is possessed by all, but that is enhanced in particular societies through culturally determined value being placed on the state; it also includes a hypersuggestible state, or a mechanism for expressing low self-image. Onlookers usually find such imitative episodes amusing, while victims feel humiliated. It occurs mainly in Indonesia and Malaysia (Murphy, 1976). Suggested ICD-10 codes are 'F48.8 Other specified neurotic disorders' and 'F44.88 Other specified dissociative [conversion] disorders'.

## Nervios

Also described as *nerfiza*, nerves, *nevra* or *nervios* in, respectively, Egypt, northern Europe, Greece and Mexico, Central and South America, this condition is depicted by common, often chronic, episodes of extreme sorrow or anxiety, inducing a complex of somatic complaints such as head and muscle pain,

diminished reactivity, nausea, appetite loss, insomnia, fatigue, and agitation. The syndrome is more common in women than in men. Research links the condition to stress, anger, emotional distress and low self-esteem. Cases are traditionally treated with herbal teas, 'nerve pills', rest, isolation and family support. The suggested ICD-10 codes are 'F32.11 Moderate depressive episode with somatic syndrome' (this is the most likely code); 'F48.0 Neurasthenia, F45.1 Undifferentiated somatoform disorder'.

## Susto, espanto

This is highly diverse, chronic complaints attributed to 'soul loss' induced by a severe, often supernatural, fright (Mexico, Central and South America). In some cases, traumatic events are not personally experienced; individuals may be stricken when others (usually relatives) suffer a fright. Symptoms often include agitation, anorexia, insomnia, fever, diarrhoea, mental confusion and apathy, depression and introversion. Studies variously attribute cases to hypoglycaemia, non-specific organic disease, generalized anxiety, and stress resulting from social conflict and low self-esteem (Good and Good, 1982). Suggested ICD-10 codes: F45.1 Undifferentiated somatoform disorder; F48.8 Other specified neurotic disorders.

## Windigo

ICD-10 lists *windigo* as a culture-bound syndrome among indigenous people of north-east America and then concedes that it is based solely on 'rare, historic accounts of cannibalistic obsession'. Traditionally, cases were ascribed to possession, with victims (usually male) turning into cannibal monsters. Symptoms included depression, homicidal or suicidal thoughts, and a delusional, compulsive wish to eat human flesh. Most victims were socially ostracized or put to death. Early research described episodes as hysterical psychosis, precipitated by chronic food shortages and cultural myths about starvation and *windigo* monsters. Some studies question the syndrome's legitimacy, claiming cases were actually a product of hostile accusations invented to justify the victim's ostracism or execution (Simons and Hughes, 1985). The existence of the syndrome has largely been discredited.

## Western culture-bound syndromes and limitations of the concept

Despite the progress in ICD-10 and DSM-IV, it is ethnocentric to list as culture-bound syndromes only those conditions that do not occur in the culture that permeates the disease classification and is the cultural context of the authors that determine what is understandable and what is not. As far as ICD-10 and DSM-IV are concerned, culture-bound syndromes almost all arise in 'exotic other' cultures and are not found in Western society. From an anthropological perspective classificatory systems cannot exist outside of culture so all disease classificatory systems are culture bound. The issue then becomes which one has the greatest utility in terms of relieving distress.

Perhaps the best examples of Western culture-bound syndromes are the eating disorders anorexia nervosa, bulimia nervosa and obesity. Once confined to North America and Western Europe, these disorders are now found across wide swaths of the world, like Coca-Cola, markers of globalization or the spread of modernity (Lee, 2002).

Other examples of Western culture-bound syndromes are type A behaviour (Simons and Hughes, 1985) and deliberate self-harm (Littlewood and Lipsedge, 1987). That these conditions might not appear to meet Ritenbaugh's (1982) criteria for a culture-bound syndrome is indicative of the extent to which we have difficulty seeing the cultural context within which we work, and it highlights the limitations of a construct of culture-bound syndromes.

## WHAT DO CULTURE-BOUND SYNDROMES SHARE?

A number of overlapping categories can be differentiated among phenomena often described as culture-bound syndromes:

- An apparent psychiatric illness, not attributable to an identifiable organic cause, which is locally recognized as an illness and which does not correspond to a recognized Western disease category (*e.g. amok*).
- An apparent psychiatric illness, not attributable to an identifiable organic cause, which is locally recognized as an illness and which resembles a Western disease category, but which has locally salient features different from the Western disease, and which may be lacking some symptoms seen as salient in the West. One example is *shenjing shaijo* or neurasthenia in China, which resembles major depressive disorder but has more salient somatic features and often lacks the depressed mood which defines depression in the West. Another is *taijin kyufusho*, which is widely regarded as being a peculiarly Japanese form of social phobia.
- A discrete disease entity not yet recognized by Western medicine. The most famous example of this is *kuru*, a progressive psychosis and dementia indigenous to cannibalistic tribes in New Guinea. *Kuru* was eventually classified as a slow-virus disease, and is now believed to result from an aberrant protein or prion which is capable of replicating itself by deforming other proteins in the brain (a 1997 Nobel prize was awarded for the elucidation of prions). *Kuru* has been identified with a form of Creutzfeldt–Jakob disease, and may be equivalent or related to scrapie, a disease of sheep, and bovine spongiform encephalopathy (BSE) or mad cow disease.
- An illness which may or may not have an organic cause, and may correspond to a subset of a Western disease category or may elaborate symptoms not recognized as constituting a Western disease into an illness category. In other words, this is a phenomenon which occurs in many cultural settings, but which is only elaborated as an illness in one or a few. A possible example is *koro*, the fear of retracting genitalia, which may sometimes have a physiological–anatomical reality, and which appears to occur independently in a non-culturally elaborated way as a delusion or phobia in numerous cultural settings.

- Culturally accepted explanatory mechanisms or idioms of illness which do not match allopathic mechanisms or Western idioms, and which, in a Western setting, might indicate culturally inappropriate thinking and perhaps delusions or hallucinations. Examples of this include witchcraft, rootwork (Caribbean) and the evil eye (Mediterranean and Latin America).
- A state or set of behaviours, often including trance or possession states; hearing, seeing and/or communicating with the dead or spirits; or feeling that one has 'lost one's soul' from grief or fright; which may or may not be seen as pathological within their native cultural framework, but which if not recognized as culturally appropriate could indicate psychosis, delusions or hallucinations in a Western setting.
- A syndrome allegedly occurring in a given cultural setting which does not in fact exist, but which may be reported to the anthropologist or psychiatrist. A possible example is *windigo* (Algonquian Indians), a syndrome of cannibal obsessions whose reality has been challenged (Marano, in Simons and Hughes, 1985) but may in fact be used to justify the expulsion or execution of an outcast in a manner similar to witchcraft allegations.

Debates over culture-bound syndromes often revolve around confusions or conflations among these different categories. Many so-called culture-bound syndromes actually occur in many unrelated cultures, or appear to be merely locally flavoured varieties of illnesses found elsewhere. Some are not so much actual illnesses as explanatory mechanisms, like witchcraft or humoral imbalances. Beliefs in witchcraft and humoral imbalances can lead to behaviours which would seem to indicate disordered thought processes outside their cultural context, such as avoidance of cold and drafts in Chinese *pa-feng* and *pa-leng*, but which actually make sense in context (Hall, 1998; Jilek, 2000).

## REFLEXIVE PSYCHIATRY

Guarnaccia and Rogler (1999) are optimistic about the inclusion of culture-bound syndromes in DSM-IV; they see this as providing the opportunity for highlighting the need to study such syndromes and the occasion for developing a research agenda to study them. Perhaps it is more that their inclusion might prompt us to be more sceptical about our own cultural baggage and create a truly reflexive context in which to practise culturally informed psychiatry that can both recognize the utility and effectiveness of biomedicine but also practise it with an awareness of history and context as shaping our disease classifications and treatment approaches. As Prince (1985) noted, the culture-bound syndrome concept is useful for medical anthropologists or transcultural psychiatrists who are concerned about relationships between symptom patterns and cultural processes. It is also useful to epidemiologists who, for example, may be interested in estimating the prevalence of depression; it is important to know that they must count some cases of culture-bound syndromes along with cases of depression with more typically Western symptoms. The concept may seem redundant to doctors who can treat many culture-bound syndromes with the same drugs. But the rise of individualized drug therapy may again highlight the importance of context. On the other hand, we should not uncritically assign local folk illnesses the same nosological status as ICD-10 or DSM-IV (themselves folk categories but fairly successful ones).

The concept of culture-bound syndromes is therefore useful insofar as it brings culture to the attention of psychiatrists trained in a different cultural tradition. Awareness of culture-bound syndromes allows psychiatrists and physicians to make culturally appropriate diagnoses. The concept is also interesting to medical and psychiatric anthropologists; in that culture-bound syndromes provide examples of how culturally salient symptoms can be elaborated into illness experiences. The concept is problematic, however, in that it is not a homogeneous category, and the designation of culture bound can imply that the illness is somehow not real, or that a patient's experience can be dismissed as merely exotic (Hall, 1998).

Psychiatric diagnosis and classification reflect the social and political context of an era and are embedded in it. In the last few decades, culture-bound syndromes reported in non-Western societies constituted the major focus of contention over the validity and universality of psychiatric diagnosis. In contemporary times, social, economic and political factors, such as the hegemony of the DSM discourse, the managed care culture, pharmaceutical forces and studies of the global burden of disease, have virtually made culture-bound syndromes 'disappear'. Once widely believed to be rare outside of the developed West, depression has rapidly become the master narrative of mental health worldwide. In the context of global mental health, the field of psychiatric classification must go beyond routine debates over categories. In order to address the growing discrepancy between needs and services, international cultural psychiatry must engage key social forces, such as psychiatric epidemiology, primary care psychiatry, integration of diagnostic systems, stigma and advocacy (Lee, 2002; Bhugra and Mastrogianni, 2004). Collecting culture-bound syndromes as psychiatric train spotting is to be avoided; bringing a proper cultural focus to clinical practice is to be applauded.

## REFERENCES

American Psychiatric Association 1994: *Diagnostic and Statistical Manual of Mental Disorders*, DSM-IV (4th edn). Washington, DC: American Psychiatric Association.

Bhugra, D. and Mastrogianni, A. 2004: Globalisation and mental disorders. Overview with relation to depression. *British Journal of Psychiatry* 184, 10–20.

Britannica 1911: *Encyclopaedia Britannica*. London: Britannica.

Good, B. and Good, M.J.D. 1982: Toward a meaning-centered analysis of popular illness categories: fright illness and heart distress in Iran. In Marsella, A.J.W.G.M. (ed.) *Cultural Conceptions of Mental Health and Therapy*. Dordrecht: Kluwer, 150–58.

Guarnaccia, P.J. and Rogler, L.H. 1999: Research on culture-bound syndromes: new directions. *American Journal of Psychiatry* 156, 1322–27.

Hall, T.M. 1998: Culture bound syndromes. http://homepage.mac.com/mccajor/cbs.html (accessed 15 December 2006).

Jilek, W.D. 2000: Culturally related psychoses. In Gelder, M.G., Lopez-Ibor, J.J. and Andreason, N. (eds) *New Oxford Textbook of Psychiatry*. Oxford: Oxford University Press, 1061–66.

Kirmayer, L.J. 2006: Beyond the 'new cross-cultural psychiatry': cultural biology, discursive psychology and the ironies of globalization. *Transcultural Psychiatry* 43, 126–44.

Kraepelin, E. 1904: Vergleichende Psychiatrie. *Centralblatt fur Nervenheilkunde und Psychiatrie* 27, 433–37.

Lee, S. 1996: Reconsidering the status of anorexia nervosa as a western culture-bound syndrome. *Social Science and Medicine* 42, 21–34.

Lee, S. 2002: Socio-cultural and global health perspectives for the development of future psychiatric diagnostic systems. *Psychopathology* 35, 152–57.

Littlewood, R. and Lipsedge, M. 1987: The butterfly and the serpent: culture, psychopathology and biomedicine. *Culture, Medicine and Psychiatry* 11, 289–335.

Murphy, H.P.M. 1976: Notes for a theory on latah. In Lebra, W.P. (ed.) *Culture Bound Syndromes, Ethnopsychiatry and Alternate Therapies*. Honolulu: University Press of Hawaii, 3–21.

Prince, R. 1985: The concept of culture-bound syndromes: anorexia nervosa and brain-fag. *Social Science and Medicine* 21, 197–203.

Prince, R. 2000: Transcultural psychiatry: personal experiences and Canadian perspectives. *Canadian Journal of Psychiatry* 45, 431–37.

Ritenbaugh, C. 1982: Obesity as a culture bound syndrome. *Culture, Medicine and Psychiatry* 6, 347–50.

Simons, R.C. and Hughes, C. 1985: *The Culture-Bound Syndromes: Folk Illnesses of Psychiatric and Anthropological Interest*. Dordrecht: Reidel Publishing Company.

Sumathipala, A., Siribaddana, S.H. and Bhugra, D. 2004: Culture-bound syndromes: the story of dhat syndrome. *British Journal of Psychiatry* 184, 200–209.

World Health Organization 1993: *The ICD-10 Classification of Mental and Behavioural Disorders Diagnostic Criteria for Research*. Geneva: World Health Organization.

Yap, P.M. 1951: Mental diseases peculiar to certain cultures: a survey of comparative psychiatry. *Journal of Mental Science* 97, 313–27.

Yap, P.M. 1965: Koro – a culture-bound depersonalization syndrome. *British Journal of Psychiatry* 111, 43–50.

Yap, P.M. 1974: *Comparative Psychiatry: A Theoretical Framework*. Toronto: University of Toronto.

# 12

# Russian culture and psychiatry

Valery N Krasnov and Isaak Ya Gurovich

## HISTORICAL OVERVIEW

### Buildings and hospitals

In Kiev Rus' (ninth to tenth centuries AD), mental patients were under the patronage of the church authorities and could easily find asylum in the monasteries. Even at that time, the written sources (chronicles) mention two principal groups of mental patients: first, the so-called 'devilish' who were disturbed and agitated; second, the 'odd and feeble-minded'. These distinctions are not dissimilar to ancient Roman classifications of people into either *furiosi* or *dementes*. On the whole, people practising witchcraft and *klikushestvo* (translated as: 'drawing attention to oneself by means of demonstrative behaviour') were condemned and sometimes even prosecuted. However, in the majority of cases such behaviours were understood as symptoms of disease. Another group comprised 'God's fools' or 'holy fools'. These were wandering beggars, probably with some mental deficit and residual symptoms of schizophrenia and paranoia; they were allowed to make heretical statements and criticize the authorities.

As for psychiatric care, until the eighteenth century it was confined to care in the monasteries, and less commonly in big community asylums, which also housed the old, the sick and physically handicapped people. The early prototype of a psychiatric institution was first created in 1706 as the specialist department of the general hospital for disabled people in Novgorod region (now known as the Kolmovskaya Psychiatric Hospital). Several special asylums – so-called 'dullhauses' – were opened during the reign of the Russian Empress Catherine (Ekaterina) the Great. One of them was opened in 1779 at Obuchovskaya Hospital in St Petersburg. During her travel from St Petersburg to Moscow in 1785, Catherine the Great ordered the building of the first psychiatric hospital in Moscow. This still exists today, as the Preobrajenskaya Hospital.

### Leaders in psychiatry and psychology

In 1847, the first original Russian manual on psychiatry was published by P.P. Malinovsky. He divided all mental disorders (in tune with his epoch) into monomania, mania, dementia and idiotism. The first faculty of psychiatry in Russia was opened in 1857 at the St Petersburg Medicosurgical Academy, with I.M. Balinsky (1827–1902) as its first director. He worked to develop teaching and learning in the new discipline, and trained many future teachers and directors of more structured and well-run psychiatry departments. One of the best European clinical departments of psychiatry, with a theatre, greenhouse and separate occupation therapy premises, was built by Balinsky in 1867 in the St Petersburg Medicosurgical Academy. He was also interested in psychopathology, and became famous for understanding the 'crystallization of delusions'.

The close connection between theory and practice was a feature of the best Russian psychiatry at that time. Victor Kandinsky (1849–1889), chief psychiatrist at a psychiatric hospital in St Petersburg, developed a classification of psychoses that was later adopted by the first Congress of Russian Psychiatrists in 1887. His work on general psychopathology called *About Pseudohallucinations* received worldwide recognition, and the Kandinsky–Klerambo syndrome is named after him: the syndrome comprises pseudo-hallucinations, delusions of persecution and influence, feelings of mastery and connectedness with the world.

In 1893 V. Bekhterev (1857–1927) took up a place at the faculty of psychiatry in the Medical Surgical Academy in St Petersburg. His particular interest was brain structure and his name is now associated with a number of brain structures, including a vestibular nucleus in the 4th cerebral ventricle, and the myelin zone of tangential cortex fibres. He also described a number of new neurological symptoms, new reflexes and developed various pieces of research apparatus. In the field of psychiatry, he mainly aspired to find anatomical–physiological correlates of abnormal phenomena. Bekhterev spoke at a 1893 congress at St Petersburg about the necessity of 'objective' study of the human being. From these insights he considered the idea of a complex of sciences about human behaviour – in his terminology psychoneurology – embracing anatomy and nervous system, physiology, neurology, psychiatry, psychohygiene, psychology and pedology (pedagogics). He spoke about psychoneurology as a certain synthesis of the sciences, providing a comprehensive study of the behaviour of a person (healthy person and the patient) at all stages of development.

Bekhterev was also interested in hypnosis and other phenomena associated with suggestion, such as cases of 'mental infection' and epidemics of mental disorders (Bekhterev, 1908). At the end of the nineteenth and the beginning of the twentieth century, along with Tokarsky, Krainsky and other Russian psychiatrists, he described hysterical psychoses in ethnic minorities in the north of Russia and in Siberia. These were associated with experiences of witchcraft, sorcery and possession by evil spirits. These mass and group (e.g. in a family or village) disorders were characterized by speech and motor stereotypical phenomena and partial or temporary withdrawal. In eastern Siberia they were known as *meryachenie* ('enchantment'), while in European northern Russia they were referred to as *ikotka* ('hiccup-like'). Disorders resembling *ikotka*, though predominantly single cases, were also described in the rural Slavonic population of Russia. Bekhterev pointed out that group suggestibility and the risk of 'mental infection' increased at times of social crisis, change and revolutions.

After 1903 Bekhterev began to develop a psychoneurological institute:

*a higher educational institution for scientific development and distribution of knowledge in the field of psychology and neurology, allied disciplines dealing with general and experimental psychology, psychiatry, pedagogical and social psychology, criminal anthropology with psychology of criminals, and also philosophical sciences.*

With his extraordinary energy, Bekhterev was able to attract large private donations and also to obtain funds from the Ministry of Finance and was given land for the institute from the Government. The institute opened on 3 February 1908 and is known today as the Bekhterev Research Psychoneurological Institute.

In Moscow the study of psychiatry as an independent subject started in 1887 in the psychiatric department of Moscow University. Professor S. Korsakov (1854–1900) founded the classification approach, as opposed to a symptom-based approach. His name is associated, for example, with Korsakov syndrome (organic amnesic syndrome as a result of chronic alcoholism with the main symptom being loss of memory for immediate events). Korsakov was a brilliant clinician, and taught tenacity in the search for symptoms and disease states, but he also emphasized that the personality required detailed individual description.

He understood that the professional's duty in the psychiatrist–patient relationship was not only to provide treatment for symptoms and the mental illness, but also to try to improve the social life and occupations of people. A large number of followers developed his heritage further. The Moscow Psychiatric School was mainly represented by Korsakov's pupils and coworkers, for example, Bazhenov, Gannushkin and Rybakov.

What about the organization of psychiatric care? The period from the 1860s to the revolution of 1917 is known as the 'Zemstvo' period in Russian medicine and psychiatry. Zemstvo medicine focused on local services under both administrative and community supervision. It was provided by district doctors in cooperation with regional medical institutions, including general and specialized hospitals. The advantages of such medical services were that they provided:

- treatment and preventive orientation,
- education and health promotion,
- free medical help,
- reduction of the area that any one service had to cover,
- outpatient care,
- public health approaches that included improvements of conditions of living,
- interventions to reduce the incidence and changing prevalence of illness, and
- improved communications on all medical topics.

In the last quarter of the nineteenth century a network of comfortable psychiatric hospitals was constructed, in which humane patient care was realized. However, new psychiatric hospitals were filled quickly by patients with chronic diseases. It became apparent that hospitals mainly housed patients from nearby districts, but patients from more distant districts continued to stay at home and received less care. It became necessary to reconsider how to make psychiatric care accessible to all the population. After intense discussion, the solution proposed was further decentralization. It implied building smaller hospitals which could admit all patients, instead of one large hospital in the region. In many ways this emphasis on public health and locally based care was well ahead of the West, where community focus and public health approaches came to the fore only in the late 1900s.

The total number of patients treated in all Zemstvo psychiatric hospitals in 1911 numbered 49 789; by 1 January 1912, 29 781 patients were discharged, 4699 had died; 25 309 stayed in hospital, 1837 were under supervision; 808 stayed in district hospitals with a payment from Zemstvo, while 1062 were with their own families. The personnel noted on 1 January 1912 were: 214 doctors, 177 medical assistants (trained nurses), 431 observers, 309 assistants of observers, and 4477 hospital attendants. On 1 January 1912, the population of St Petersburg included more than 5300 inpatients from a total population of 1 686 000. There were 3.1 psychiatric beds per 1000 inhabitants located in 18 psychiatric hospitals, including five private clinics. Other facilities included urban and rural psychiatric control, urban asylums, and shelter for children with epilepsy and mental retardation. In 1912 Moscow had a population of 1 399 000, with 2890 patients with mental disorders with slightly fewer beds per head of population than St Petersburg (two patients for 1000 inhabitants). Historical records show that in 1910 the Moscow municipal government spent 819 179 rubles on psychiatric care; this was 16 per cent of all charges for medical health promotional purposes and amounted to 2.1 per cent of the total city budget. For comparison, in the Arkhangelsk region, in 1912 there were only 62 patients (Yudin, 1951).

Practical attempts to improve the delivery of psychiatric care to the population were postponed because of revolutions and wars that unexpectedly followed this initial foundation work. However, during this period the number of psychiatrists and neurologists in the country increased. At the first psychiatry congress in the year 1887, 93 experts attended, whilst at the second held in Kiev in 1905, there were 276 neurologists and psychiatrists. In 1912 the number of doctors with at least three years' experience and who were members of the Society of Psychiatry and Neurology reached 538 (Yudin, 1951).

The discoveries of the great Russian physiologists I. Sechenov (1829–1905) and I. Pavlov (1849–1936) exerted a substantial influence on Russian psychiatry, especially on the theory of the pathogenesis of mental disorders. In his outstanding work *Reflexes of the Head Brain*, published in 1863, Sechenov established experimentally the presence of the braking phenomenon in the nervous system. He proved that thinking is a constrained reflex, and that the initial reason for any act lies in external sensual excitation, without which any idea is impossible. He began experimental methods to investigate the physiological bases of mental activity. He considered the mental phenomena sensations, representations and thinking as integrated parts of all processes.

The scientific activity of Pavlov deserves more detailed illumination. Although he was primarily a scientist (physiologist), his research had a strong influence not only on Russian but also universally on psychiatry, psychology and psychotherapy. He was initially interested in the finding that there were regularities of formation in the most elementary and initial conditional reflexes.

In the Soviet period (the 1920s and 1930s) Pavlov became interested in the psychopathology of the person, the mechanism of hypnosis and especially in the origin of psychology. Unfortunately, soon after his death, Pavlov's work began to be used in the Soviet Union for the prohibition of other approaches that diverged from physiological, psychological or psychiatric sciences. This situation persisted for decades and harmed the development of Russian science.

The psychiatry of the Soviet period in Russia was constructed on the principles of preventive medicine, the rights of the patients to free and qualified psychiatric help, an integrated approach and planning of that help, alongside the introduction of innovations in practice. Frequently these principles remained declarative. In August 1919 a first all-Russian neuropsychiatric congress was held, with 70 delegates. They decided to restore the psychiatric services that were destroyed during the civil war. In 1919 in Moscow a new section of psychiatric care called out-hospital psychiatry was introduced. In this form of help a method was found to bring psychiatric help closer to the population, as originally sought by Zemstvo psychiatry. Out-hospital psychiatric help was organized into neuropsychiatric (later psychoneurological) dispensaries, which were opened in all large cities of the Soviet Union. The first of these was opened in 1924 in Moscow. By the end of 1924 in the Russian Federation there were 80 psychiatric institutions with 14 000 regular beds. At 1 January 1925, there were 16 608 patients (8574 men and 8034 women). The new research institutes were gradually organized, and the number of faculties of psychiatry increased with greater scientific and practice-based developments.

In 1920, Rybakov founded the Moscow Institute of Psychiatry, the second research institute of psychiatry in Russia. This institute played an important role in the development of a system of territorial psychiatric care facilities, which was organized around city and regional dispensaries and district psychiatric units with day-hospitals. The hospitals were, in the majority of cases, subordinate to dispensaries and they provided care in accordance with territorial principles. Psychiatric care was free. Hospitals and dispensaries set up rehabilitation workshops and some of these provided workplaces for mental patients.

At the beginning of the twentieth century, psychoanalysis, and specifically psychodynamically oriented therapy, had been developing fast in Russia, primarily due to the efforts of I. Ermakov. In contrast, in the early 1930s it was virtually forbidden, and in the period from the 1930s to the 1950s it was considered to be an anti-scientific direction. One must also discuss here the obstacles to the scientific development of psychiatry in the USSR: the persecution of geneticists, and the belief that the genetics of mental disorders was not scientific or acceptable, and there were dramatic restrictions in the numbers of clinical psychologists; for example, the famous psychologist Vygotsky was attacked 'for being critical and following the fashionable bourgeois theories'.

Despite an emphasis on genetics, psychology remained influential in Russian psychiatry. Professor Melekhov played a major role in the development of the theoretical grounds for labour rehabilitation. He used the achievements of the Russian psychological school and especially Vygotsky and Leontyev and their 'psychology of activity' and 'psychology of values'. In St Petersburg, Professor Myasischev, being a psychologist, developed psychotherapy and rehabilitation approaches in psychiatry. On the basis of the 'psychology of attitudes', he proposed that it was the understanding of the person as a system of relationships with social environments that was important.

The history of Soviet psychiatry is closely intertwined with the development of world psychiatry, contributing to the theory and science and practice. Indeed, the problem of finding an effective treatment for psychoses before modern medication (neuroleptics and antidepressants) and improving the effectiveness of psychotherapy for mental disorders received worldwide attention in the field of psychiatry during this period.

## CRITICAL PERIOD IN RUSSIAN PSYCHIATRY: THE DEVELOPMENT OF MODERN LEGISLATION AND BIOMEDICAL ETHICS

The development and practical applications of modern ethical principles in Russian psychiatry are interesting from a moral, professional and historic perspective. From an ethical and legal point of view, a serious disadvantage was the lack of a special law on psychiatric care in soviet psychiatry. Professional instructions which regulated the rights of physicians and patients have always existed. At the same time the rights of psychiatrists in the examination and hospitalization of a patient were exaggerated while patients' rights were limited.

This system was based on the principle of paternalism, in which the physician was completely responsible for the patient, the treatment, the protection of the patient's social rights, including providing access to social benefits or restricting activities due to severity of illness. The physician took care of the patient's living conditions if his or her lodgings were unfit or taken away. The physician also addressed the patient's psycho-social problems and sometimes the problems of the family as well. It was very far from a partnership: the physician had a dominant position in all aspects of psychiatric care. Clinical psychologists never took part in therapeutic work and only solved diagnostic problems. The number of clinical psychologists in psychiatric facilities was very low, as was the number of social workers. In addition, from the end of the 1950s a system of obligatory registration was introduced for everyone seeking help, even if the patient needed just a consultation with a psychiatrist or insignificant psychiatric treatment. For example, people with transient, short neurotic-like disorders and behavioural disturbances were required to register.

Registration in a psychiatric dispensary could become a barrier to enter some educational institutions or to find a job in some companies if their administration had the right to make requests about the presence or the absence of a person's registration in a psychiatric dispensary. It could be said that a psychiatrist protected the interests of the state and society, sometimes to the detriment of the patient's interests (Gurovich *et al.*, 1994).

## Misuse of psychiatry

In the 1970s and 1980s the psychiatric system in the Soviet Union was used for political purposes. Psychiatric facilities and separate psychiatrists were involved in using their psychiatric expertise, leading to involuntary hospitalization and treatment of so-called dissidents; dissidents were those who criticized and opposed the Soviet political system. The political authorities imposed methods for the conduct of forensic psychiatric evaluations of people who made anti-Soviet statements or had anti-Soviet publications, and psychiatrists were compelled to follow these instructions. Thus political persecution was replaced with psychiatric examination and hospitalization in psychiatric clinics. From the point of view of modern diagnostics in some cases experts' conclusions were connected with excessive diagnostic patterns for schizophrenia, psychopathy or other mental disorders. Some of these cases were made public and fairly criticized by the whole world.

This course of action within the psychiatric services led to a greater stigmatization of psychiatric services and mental illness, with more fear of psychiatric centres. There were also other less widely publicized violations of patients' rights. For example, there were mass 'prophylactic' hospitalizations of registered patients before major international actions such as international youth festivals, Olympic Games and others. Many patients with the capacity to make decisions were even deprived of voting rights during elections.

In the early 1980s the All-Union Society of Neurologists and Psychiatrists was threatened with expulsion from the World Psychiatric Association because of opposition from international human rights organizations. To avoid expulsion the Society suspended its membership of the World Psychiatric Association. Unfortunately, official representatives of psychiatry who took part in the political abuse of psychiatry never acknowledged the lack of evidence for their actions and diagnostics. Such an acknowledgement of psychiatric abuse for political purposes would have been understood and appreciated by all psychiatrists both inside the country and abroad (see Chapter 7, specifically the discussion on the Truth and Reconciliation Council in New Zealand, as a method of dealing with complaints about psychiatric abuses in New Zealand). Although there had in fact been few cases of wrong diagnoses, the absence of such an acknowledgement and the absence of an analysis of errors committed cast a shadow upon all psychiatrists in the Soviet Union, but specifically in Russia.

At best, the response was aimed at saving dissidents from political persecution (Polubinskaya, 2000; Krasnov, 2002; Krasnov and Mosolov, 2002, Gurovich, 2005). At the same time this painful process had its positive side and led to criticism from abroad and growing discontent among the majority of psychiatrists in Russia. In the mid 1980s there was a more dramatic period of change driven by 'Perestroika', and so further work on improving the legal status of psychiatric patients began. Discussions in the media and in professional spheres stimulated law-making activities involving psychiatrists and lawyers.

## Mental health legislation

In 1991 the Soviet Union fell apart and several other countries were formed (the former Union republics). Russia was the first country where a Law on Psychiatric Care was passed. In 1992 this Law was confirmed by the Parliament and took effect in January 1993, 10 years after the current legislation in the UK (see Chapter 7). The provisions of the Russian Law on Psychiatric Care and its guarantees of citizens' rights were constructed from the principles in the USA, the UK, the Netherlands, Germany and other countries. It was accepted and commended by international experts. The law considerably widened patients' rights and restricted the possibility of unlawful actions in the course of psychiatric treatment.

The obligatory registration of the mentally ill in psychiatric centres was cancelled. All assistance is now given confidentially. Some patients with the most serious forms of disorder can now receive treatment in dispensaries either at their own request or, if necessary, after the decision of the court. By 1993 membership of the Russian Society of Psychiatrists in the World Psychiatric Association was completely restored. The Russian Society of Psychiatrists now cooperates with the World Psychiatric Association and other international organizations and is more open to discussions about the human rights of the mentally ill.

## Ethical principles

Nevertheless, the introduction of basic laws in psychiatry did not solve the problems in the Russian approach to scientific and practical psychiatry. The necessity of solving different questions at the level of biomedical ethics arises more and more frequently. In 1994 the Russian Society of Psychiatrists adopted its code of professional ethics (Russian Society of Psychiatrists, 1994). The ethical committee, including members of the Board of the Russian Society of Psychiatrists, was formed in 1995 at the Society's Congress and over the next years ethical committees were created in regional psychiatric associations. In 1996, after the World Congress on Psychiatry in Madrid, the Russian Society of Psychiatrists adopted the Madrid Declaration. Even today psychiatry (not only in Russia) is the scene of ethical collisions: between paternalism and autonomy, between the danger of non-medical abuse of psychiatry and the danger of not helping due to formal legal criteria, between confidentiality and openness, between informed consent and the difficulty of explaining the mechanisms of therapeutic actions of some treatment methods, between keeping medical secrecy and informing patients and their relatives about illness, between the responsibility of a psychiatrist and of a patient, between the good for patients and for their relatives and close social environment (see Chapters 5, 7 and 9).

## MODERNIZATION OF PRACTICE AND SERVICES

Of course, these ethics policies cannot control each step of mental health professionals' practice or scientific knowledge, but they do define some moral guidelines for modern mental health services in a democratic society. These documents reflect modern notions of rights and the freedom of citizens, at the same time they contain rules for special situations and relationships. The rudiments of excessive centralization of inpatient mental health care still exist – 20 per cent of hospitals in Russia still have 1000 or more beds; another 35 per cent have from 600 to 1000 beds. The huge task of rebuilding large hospitals remains, but economic difficulties hinder this aspiration. The number of mentally ill who are disadvantaged in the public health system is growing due to the difficulties of providing employment and adaptation in the settings of a market economy. There are also fewer sheltered jobs for mentally ill people. Moreover,

the Mental Health Law, in force since 1993, prevents and minimizes the institutionalization of mentally ill people if their behaviour does not pose a threat to others. Many mentally ill people appear to live on the streets, though most either live in specialized institutions ('internats') for the chronically mentally ill (without active therapy) or at home under the care of their relatives.

The unfavourable living conditions in many psychiatric clinics (rooms with too many beds, lack of space and equipment) pose serious ethical and legal problems. Costly but effective remedies remain unavailable to many patients, especially outpatients. The economic difficulties of this transition period of Russia's social development make it unlikely that these difficulties will be overcome in the short term. Until recently, psychiatry was not a priority in the state's health care strategy, unlike paediatrics and cardiosurgery. There are difficulties in the quality of collaboration between psychiatric and general medical institutions when helping people with somatoform disorders, somatized depressions and anxiety disorders. These problems are being actively discussed and some of them are gradually being solved (Krasnov, 1999a, 2000). For example, the rules of informed consent have become the norm when new medicines are tested and they have gradually spread to all forms of therapeutic activity.

## CURRENT STATE OF RUSSIAN PSYCHIATRY

In the past 20 years radical and, for some population groups, dramatic changes have taken place in the politics, economy, social infrastructure, ideology and legal relationships within society in Russia. These have had an impact on many aspects of public consciousness, including ethical standards and the limits of socially acceptable behaviour. Enthusiasm for political freedom and liberation from ideological dogmas has come up against an economic crisis, high unemployment and loss of social welfare. The essential moral ordeal for the population, and especially for older people, has been a deepening of social inequities, the loss of principles and standards, of cohesion and interrelations at the microsocial level, including within families, and changes in the customary system of values, and at the same time the impossibility of replacing them, rapidly and flexibly, with greater acceptance of the democratic principles of personal responsibility and individual decision-making.

Taking the Russian Federation as an example, it may be seen that these adverse trends are linked with each other or have developed roughly in parallel. The increase in alcohol abuse was accompanied by a peak in suicides, reaching a figure of 42 per 100 000 population in 1994. Despite a tendency towards social and economic stabilization, indicators of mental and general health in the countries of Eastern Europe have so far remained worse than they were in the 1970s and the 1980s, and also worse than current indicators in Western Europe and the USA (see Chapters 22 and 30).

The introduction of internationally recognized legislative standards into mental health service practice has undoubtedly been a positive development. Such standards ensure the protection of human rights during the delivery of mental health care and make it easier to organize new forms of care, especially in primary health care. There is also a move now to develop psychosocial methods of treating and rehabilitating people with mental disorders. An increasingly wide range of specialists in clinical psychology and social work, as well as former patients and carers, are now involved in providing care to people with mental disorders.

However there exist serious difficulties in the development of up-to-date psychiatric care. The first difficulty is connected with the rigid system of financing health care systems in general. It prevents the development of forms of care other than traditional hospitals and dispensaries. The budget of the national health care system has never exceeded 5 per cent of GDP and although a system of state medical insurance was introduced in 1993, it does not cover all medical services.

Psychiatric services have occupied an unusual position within the overall health care system developed over the last few decades. As a result, psychiatric care, along with medical care for patients with tuberculosis, contagious diseases and AIDS, are not included in the system of state medical insurance and are still only paid by a federal budget. At the same time, over the past few years the budgetary allocations given to psychiatric care services were about 4 per cent of the entire health care budget. Meanwhile expenditure on health care, including psychiatric care, was partly covered by local (regional, municipal) budgets.

To date the psychiatric care system in Russia has been based on local outpatient clinics, so-called psychiatric (psychoneurological) dispensaries and dispensary departments in psychiatric hospitals. Psychiatric dispensaries are complex institutions which include outpatient units, a day hospital, and remedial workshops. These dispensaries serve a given territory. This territory is divided into sections serving approximately 25 000 residents. A dispensary doctor offers outpatient therapeutic care, holds consultations, keeps in contact with psychiatric hospitals, and makes decisions regarding patients' hospitalization. In large dispensaries there are specialized units for geriatric psychiatry, epilepsy, sexology and psychotherapeutic units.

Along with psychiatric dispensaries and hospitals, there are so-called narcological dispensaries and hospitals (or, less often, narcological departments in psychiatric institutions) that provide care for alcoholics and drug addicts. Psychiatric (as well as narcological) hospitals have close connections with the dispensaries. When a patient is discharged from the hospital he or she receives a recommendation for an additional consultation with his or her doctor in the local dispensary or to continue the treatment as an outpatient in the local dispensary, in order to sustain continuity of psychiatric care.

Child and adolescent psychiatrists (child psychoneurologists) work under the same system of rendering psychiatric care which includes a network of institutions created for the needs of a given region. Each psychiatrist for children and adolescents administers psychiatric care over a catchment area of 15 000 children. As a rule, child psychoneurological units are situated not in the psychiatric dispensaries but in the local child primary care system.

As has been described above, during the 1970s and 1980s, the dispensary care system, which required the patient to be registered, was excessively inclusive and even covered those patients who did not need active or long-term care. As a result, it became possible to misuse psychiatry. In particular, the excessive expansion of criteria for legal involuntary examinations and hospitalization contributed to this misuse. Fear of social stigma caused by the previous registration system in psychiatric dispensaries led to a significant reduction in the number of patients who applied for care in the dispensary for the first time. Consequently, only 25–30 per cent of all mentally ill patients applied for psychiatric assistance in the dispensary. However, recently, the number of those patients asking for an initial psychiatric consultation has once again started to increase. At the same time, approximately 18–25 per cent of primary care patients need psychiatric consultations. The need has arisen to reform outpatient psychiatric care, including the development of various forms of care other than the dispensary.

Several important changes in the last decade may be noted, which mirror the direction and a sort of intrinsic regularity in the development of psychiatric care. First, a significant number of psychologists, psychotherapists, specialists in social work and social workers have been recruited into the staff of psychiatric institutions; this has created a basis for transition from a largely medical to a bio-psycho-social model of mental health care and a team approach to its provision.

The range of professionals providing mental health care has been significantly expanded (though still insufficiently) with a considerable number of psychologists and social workers (their numbers over the last five years have more than doubled). The ratio between doctors/psychiatrists and these professionals is now 4:1. There are two reasons for this lack of multidisciplinarity in health care provision. Firstly, low salaries, which make jobs unattractive, and secondly, a lack of leadership from the heads of the psychiatric institutions on the other hand. The number of doctors/psychotherapists has increased considerably. Unfortunately, the distribution of all these professionals between hospitals and out-of-hospital services still shows the dominance of inpatient care (Table 12.1).

Since 1990 there has been a reduction of 36 000 in the numbers of psychiatric beds in Russia, although bed numbers per population are still high. There has also been an apparent change in the incidence and prevalence of presentations for mental disorders. The number of people applying for psychiatric and psychological assistance gradually increased from 4.5 per cent of the population in 1995 to 5.2 per cent in 2004 (about 7.5 million from 143.1 million of the population). There are 958 109 people disabled due to mental disorders (on 1 January 2005).

Alcoholism is the dominating disorder among dependencies. The very high level of alcohol consumption in Russia (13–14 L per capita a year; Nemtsov, 2003) should be stressed. (This is an estimate of total alcohol consumption from sugar, including registered and non-registered sources, based on blood alcohol levels (Nemtsov, 2000). Some 75% of alcohol is consumed as vodka, and

**Table 12.1** *Resources available for the administration of psychiatric care in Russia*

|  | 1995 | 2004 |
| --- | --- | --- |
| Psychiatric dispensaries | 166 | 171 |
| Dispensary departments in hospitals | 125 | 110 |
| Narcological dispensaries (for alcoholics and drug addicts) | 220 | 208 |
| Dispensary units in general hospitals | 2 110 | 2 270 |
| Psychotherapeutic units in outpatient clinics | 1 090 | 1 170 |
| Psychiatric hospitals | 284 | 275 |
| Inpatient departments in psychiatric dispensaries | 103 | 111 |
| Total number of beds in hospitals | 183 100 | 163 179 |
| Psychiatric beds in somatic hospitals | 13 810 | 14 087 |
| The number of places in day hospitals | 13 260 | 15 495 |

there is controversy over methods of calculating consumption (Nemtsov, 2000).) The number of drug addicts reached 120 100 cases in 1995 and 230 000 in 2003. It is likely that if more diversified forms of mental health care were available the figures reported would be larger (Table 12.2).

Over the last few years, psychotherapeutic and consultative units have been created in general outpatient clinics in order to supplement dispensaries. The number of these units has tripled since 1987. More attention is now being paid to social issues and those of ecological psychiatry, and mental health problems associated with traumatic social events (forced emigration, unemployment, and others).

Recently, new forms of private outpatient psychiatric care, including special centres which provide medical, social and psychiatric assistance to victims of natural and technological (Chernobyl) disasters, war veterans (Afghanistan and Chechnya) and refugees and displaced peoples, have been created. These centres reflect the greater concern for social and psychological support of patients in the system of mental health care. As a result, the number of clinical psychologists and social workers in psychiatric institutions has increased. However, the shortage of such specialists in psychiatric clinics still exists. Currently (2004 figures) there are 16 378 psychiatrists and 2862 clinical psychologists and 509 specialists in social work (with higher education) and 1354 social workers in Russia (Table 12.3).

The reform of psychiatric care in hospitals has become an urgent priority. Excessive centralization is the main problem. Thirty-five per cent of hospitals have between 600 and 1000 beds. In 20 per cent of hospitals the number of beds exceeds 1000. In general hospitals, psychiatric units are almost non-existent. It should be noted that 90 per cent of the buildings in which psychiatric hospitals are located are in need of repair or reconstruction. It can be noted that the overall number of beds in psychiatric hospitals has gradually decreased: from 200 000 beds in 1990 to 163 179 beds by 1 January 2005.

One of psychiatry's most serious problems, the creation of a rehabilitation and social assistance system for patients, remains unsolved to this day. The number of socially maladapted mental patients, including the disabled, is increasing. Over the past few years, the total number of disabled has increased by 40 per cent. At the same time, only 4 per cent of them have been placed in jobs. Many of them have been in psychiatric institutions for a long time. Transitional forms of housing, such as 'half-way houses' and hostels for patients, exist only in some regions. Available nursing homes and protected jobs for the mentally ill do not meet the need. The number of disabled people who work in

**Table 12.2**   *Mental disorders in Russia (by the data of psychiatric and narcological dispensaries and psychotherapeutic units)*

|  | 1995 | 2004 |
|---|---|---|
| Number of people with mental disorders | 3 800 000 | 3 762 274 |
| Number of alcohol abusers | 4 350 000 | 3 771 100 |
| Number of drug addicts | 120 100 | 339 800 |

**Table 12.3**   *Specialists offering mental health care in Russia*

|  | 1997 | 2004 |
|---|---|---|
| Psychiatrists including | 15 860 | 16 378 |
| Psychotherapists | 1 715 | 3 510 |
| Child psychiatrists | 1 900 | 1 551 |
| Narcologists (physicians rendering care for alcoholics and drug addicts) | 4 470 | 4 820 |
| Clinical psychologists (in psychiatric and narcological institutions) | 1 380 | 2 862[a] |
| Specialists in social work (with higher education) | 50 | 509[a] |
| Social workers | 605 | 1 354[a] |

[a]This figure is increasing.

general society under special conditions and in remedial workshops has declined catastrophically.

The system of psychiatric care has shown contradictory tendencies in its development. On the one hand, taking into account the shortages in state budget allocations, psychiatric care on the basis of local psychiatric dispensaries that are open to the general public and connected to local psychiatric hospitals is expedient. On the other hand, psychiatric patients' stigma and societal prejudices against psychiatry and psychiatric institutions hinder the development of psychiatric dispensaries.

A certain number of psychiatric patients apply for care to private institutions which are not competent or are not ready to work with psychiatric patients. On the one hand, the decreasing number of beds in psychiatric hospitals reflects the process of decentralization of psychiatric care that is usual for developed countries. Thus, much more emphasis has been put on preventive measures and outpatient institutions. On the other hand, the number of vacancies in day hospitals located in dispensaries does not meet the needs of the population. As for psychiatric day departments in general hospitals, they are not yet developed. The need for clinical psychologists and social workers who would be able to take part in group psychotherapy for the mentally ill is becoming increasingly urgent. However, the number of such specialists is still insufficient and is growing very slowly. Disability among the mentally ill is growing due not only to the deterioration of their health condition, but also the increasing number of obstacles to be overcome for the social adaptation of the mentally ill. At the same time the number of sheltered working places for the mentally ill has significantly declined over the past few years.

In recent years in a number of regions the introduction of new developments in mental health care has led to changes in the very structure of the mental health service, with greater emphasis on the development of care in the community, involving a system of psychosocial rehabilitation, hostels and other types of protected housing, interaction with social services, assertive treatment departments (teams), and 'hospital at home', employment, psycho-education and psycho-social work with families (Gurovich, 2005). Non-governmental

organizations exist but are not yet sufficiently focused on mental health care, and require more capacity (contrast with the situation in Europe: Chapter 30).

## ETHNOCULTURAL APPROACHES IN MODERN RUSSIAN PSYCHIATRY

In Soviet Russia, ethnocultural investigations in psychology, sociology and psychiatry were almost totally absent because Soviet ideology denied any other important differences between persons other than ones of social class. It was only educational level that was allowed to be used for the explanation of some obvious differences, and the reason was that a high educational level of the population and obligatory secondary school education were considered state goals; ultimately these goals were reached for all, hence even differences in education were not explored.

At the end of the 1920s, practically all the population of Russia could read and write, and in the 1930s a similar goal was reached in all former republics of the Soviet Union. However, obvious differences in the parameters of mental health in different regions of the country (e.g. suicide rate, mental retardation and alcoholism) were interpreted as reflecting insufficient detection of cases or mental illness was recognized, but not considered in relation to ethnic or cultural risk factors and influences. The professional psychiatric community was aware of the fact that people living in Northern Caucasus were concealing serious mental disorders because in this region, and especially in rural areas, schizophrenia, epilepsy and mental retardation were considered a disgrace for the family or kin.

After the collapse of the Soviet Union in 1991 and the formation of new independent states, the importance of ethnocultural research became clear. However, ethnocultural psychiatry is still quite a new field and at the moment there are very few publications concerning regional differences in suicidal behaviour, alcohol abuse and behaviour disorders in Russia by ethnic or cultural groups (see Chapter 30 for discussion of how ethnicity is not a variable often used in European states, although it is commonly used in the UK and the USA; regional and country differences within the same racial group are more commonly investigated).

In the last 15 years, suicide rates in Russia have risen dramatically. Trends in Russia follow Lithuania in the suicide rate in the post-Soviet era. However, there are significant differences in the suicide rates in the country, varying from 3 per 100 000 population in Kabardin-Balkaria (Northern Caucasus) to 80 per 100 000 in some territories in the north of Russia (Komy Republic and Udmurtia, where the Finno-Ugric ethnic group dominates). Indications concerning the cultural acceptance of suicide as a way to resolve a domestic conflict in families belonging to Finno-Ugric peoples and other ethnic minorities need to be confirmed by further investigation based on strict methodology (Minevich, 1994; Minevich *et al.*, 1994; Dmitrieva and Polozhy, 2003; Kazharov, 2005; Nikolaev, 2005).

Another important factor that requires additional investigation is the combination of high rates of suicide and alcohol abuse, principally in northern regions of Russia, including those mentioned above (Nemtsov, 2003; Voitsekh, 2006).

The public health situation in Russia over the last two decades has been complicated by ethnic conflicts, military actions and terrorist acts. In turn, these have given rise to the problem of refugees, which is still causing internal migration, emigration and demographic imbalances. The crisis in transitional societies has revealed the vulnerability of people's mental health, as evidenced not only through changes in the incidence of the main mental disorders but also by the upward trend in alcohol and drug use, higher suicide rates and a fall in life expectancy, especially among men.

Recently, there have been a growing number of publications concerning the mental health of refugees and displaced persons who have had to move out of areas of military action in the Chechen Republic. The Chechens constitute a homogeneous ethnic group but their psychological health seems to reflect more their extreme and harsh living conditions rather than ethnocultural features (Akhmedova, 2002). Post-traumatic stress disorder can be detected better than other disorders such as depression and anxiety disorders. The findings of the above-mentioned investigations suggest a

kind of cultural taboo in this population against admitting and describing emotional disturbances. Similar psychological mechanisms have been reported among Afghan refugees (Soldatova, 2001). However, special methods used in the investigation of mental health of the population of the Chechen Republic exposed to a long-term emergency situation (Idrisov and Krasnov, 2005) suggest a variety of affective spectrum disorders, mainly of subsyndromal level. These disorders remain a problem though the number of patients with post-traumatic stress disorder has decreased over the last two years.

Our activities in the recognition and treatment of depression in primary health care (Krasnov, 1999b, 2000) have suggested that there were cultural limitations in the diagnostic instruments; such limitations become obvious in pilot studies. Diagnostic screening instruments borrowed from North American (Spitzer *et al.*, 1995) and West European (World Health Organization, 1996) sources seemed not to work well in Russia (see Chapter 4). In both the USA and Western Europe, the common instruments for diagnosing depression combine into one item such experiences and symptoms as 'losing interest in normal habits' and 'inability to experience pleasure'. While working with the clients of one local polyclinic, we also studied the interpretation of individual questions by patients and their verbalization of certain experiences, which could be associated with cultural characteristics of the Russian population. These characteristics include the following:

- insufficient 'sensitivity' to issues dealing with anhedonia, which could reflect low hedonistic motivation of their behaviour and relatively low position of hedonism as a life value in the population;
- increased (more than expected) sensitivity towards differences between 'losing the ability to experience pleasure' and 'losing interest'.

In the majority of Western questionnaires and commonly used diagnostic schedules these two phenomena are similar and presented as one question, while in our investigation the clients definitely separate them. Elderly people in particular hardly interpreted 'no enjoyment' as something outside of the normal human experience.

As a result, in the final screening form we separated these experiences in order to improve the sensitivity of the screening test. In the primary health care system, the proportion of clients with mild and moderate depression was close to the level established for the USA and Western Europe (Regier *et al.*, 1993; Ustun and Sartorius, 1995). For the city population this proportion was 6 per cent. These preliminary observations warrant further cultural investigations in Russia.

Cultural and transcultural psychiatry are in their infancy, but given the globalized future world, and greater levels of inter-country and intra-country migration, understanding the role of culture in the expression and management of mental distress is probably the most important knowledge and skills gap to be addressed. Furthermore, as our mental health services are developed, it is imperative to discern the effectiveness of new organizations of service or new interventions, taking account of the cultural context in Russia (see Chapter 9).

## REFERENCES

Akhmedova, Kh.B. 2003: Fanaticism and idea of revenge in persons with post-traumatic stress disorder (PTSD) (in Russian). *Social and Clinical Psychiatry* 13, 34–37.

Bekhterev, V.M. 1908: *Suggestion and its Role in Public Health* (in Russian). St Petersburg.

Dmitrieva, T.B. and Polozhy, B.S. 2003: *Ethnocultural Psychiatry* (in Russian). Moscow: Meditsina.

Gurovich, I.Y., Gusera, L.Y., Zaitser, D.A. and Prets, V.B. 1994: Psychiatric care in the Russian Federation. Current status and problems. *Journal of Russian and East European Psychiatry* 27, 19–36.

Gurovich, I.Y. 2005: Reform of psychiatric care system: organizational aspect (in Russian). *Social and Clinical Psychiatry* 15, 12–18.

Idrisov K.A. and Krasnov, V.N. 2005: Mental health in the Chechen population exposed to long-term emergency circumstances (in Russian). *Social and Clinical Psychiatry* 15, 5–11.

Kazharov, M.Kh. 2005: Sociocultural aspects of suicide in Kabardin-Balkaria (in Russian). *Social and Clinical Psychiatry* 15, 35–40.

Krasnov, V.N. 1999a: The provision of mental health care in Russian Federation – manage or perish? In Guimon, J. and Sartorius, N. (eds) *The Challenges of Managed Mental Health in Europe*. New York: Kluwer, 173–80.

Krasnov, V.N. 1999b: Recognition and treatment of depression in primary care settings. *Social and Clinical Psychiatry* 9, 5–8.

Krasnov, V.N. 2000: Depression as a general medical problem, *Common Health* 8, 19–23.

Krasnov, V.N. 2002: Ethical problems of contemporary Russian psychiatry (in Russian). *Independent Psychiatric Journal* 3, 12–17.

Krasnov, V.N. and Mosolov, S.N. 2002: Modern ethical and legislative problems of psychiatry (in Russian). In Pokrovsky, V. and Lopukhin, Y. (eds) *Biomedical Ethics*. Moscow: Meditsina, 146–53.

Minevich, V.B. 1994: Boloshin – endemic psychosis in buryat ethnos. *Ethnopsychiatry in Sybiria* (in Russian). Tomsk: Ulan-Ude, 164–70.

Minevich, V.B., Baranchik, G.M. and Rachmazova, L.D. 1994: Alcohol psychosis from point of view of the ethnonarcology. In *Ethnopsychiatry* (in Russian). Tomsk: Ulan-Ude, 171–79.

Nemtsov, A.V. 2000: Estimates of total alcohol consumption in Russia, 1980–1994. *Drug Alcohol Dependency* 58(1–2), 133–42.

Nemtsov, A.V. 2003: *Alcohol Loss of the Russian Regions* (in Russian). Moscow: Nalex.

Nikolaev, E.L. 2005: *Social and Cultural Determinants of Mental Health* (in Russian). Tcheboksary: Chuvash University Publishing.

Polubinskaya, S.V. 2000: Reform in psychiatry in post-Soviet countries. *Acta Psychiatrica Scandinavica* 399, S106–108.

Regier, D.A., Narrow, W.E., Rae, D.S., Manderscheid, R.W., Locke, B.Z. and Goodwin, F.K. 1993: The de facto US mental and addictive disorders service system. Epidemiologic catchment area prospective 1-year prevalence rates of disorders and services. *Archives of General Psychiatry* 50, 85–94.

Russian Society of Psychiatrists 1994: Code of professional ethics of psychiatrists (in Russian). *Social and Clinical Psychiatry* 4, 147–50.

Soldatova, G.U. 2001: *Psychology of Refugees and Displaced Persons* (in Russian). Moscow: Smysl.

Spitzer, R.L., Kroenke, K., Linzer, M., Hahn, S.R., Williams, J.B., deGruy, F.V., III, Brody, D. and Davies, M. 1995: Health-related quality of life in primary care patients with mental disorders. Results from the PRIME-MD 1000 Study. *Journal of the American Medical Association* 274, 1511–17.

Ustun, T.B. and Sartorius, N. 1995: *Mental Illness in General Health Care: An International Study*. Chichester: John Wiley & Sons.

Voitsekh V.F. 2006: Dynamics and structure of suicides in Russia. *Social and Clinical Psychiatry* 16, 22–27.

World Health Organization 1996: *Diagnostic and Management Guidelines for Mental Disorders in Primary Care*. Geneva: World Health Organization.

Yudin, T.I. 1951: *Sketches in the History of Fatherland's Psychiatry* (in Russian). Moscow: Medgiz.

# 13

# Culture and mental health in West Africa: Nigeria

Oyedeji Ayonrinde and Gbenga Okulate

## INTRODUCTION

West Africa consists of 15 independent and diverse countries: Benin, Burkina Faso, Cape Verde, Côte d'Ivoire, The Gambia, Ghana, Guinea, Guinea-Bissau, Liberia, Mali, Niger, Nigeria, Senegal, Sierra Leone and Togo. These countries occupy the westernmost region of Africa and comprise about one-fifth the continental land mass. Geographical diversity is marked; beyond the northern border is the Sahara desert, the southern border is made of tropical rainforest, the eastern border is mixed desert and savannah grasslands, and the western border is formed by the Atlantic Ocean. Apart from colonial and ethnic histories, geopolitical boundaries have significantly shaped West African cultures. There are notable similarities in diet, dress, music and spiritual beliefs across the region. Religion is influential in the northern and southern sectors of the region, with Islam predominating in the north and Christianity in the south.

Nigeria is the most populous country in West Africa and indeed the whole continent, with a population of approximately 130 million. This represents over half of the West African population, with the next most populous country being Ghana with a little more than 22 million. Situated at the western curvature of Africa, it is bordered by Benin to the west, Niger and Chad to the north and Cameroon to the east. South of Nigeria is the Atlantic Ocean. Although all Nigeria's neighbours are former French colonies (Francophone states) it shares ethnic and cultural similarities with them in many ways while sharing a British colonial identity with other (Anglophone) countries like Ghana.

Nigeria has a very diverse ethnic mix, with over 200 spoken and literate languages of which three (Yoruba, Hausa and Ibo) are spoken by about

60 per cent of the population. Interestingly some estimates suggest that originally there were 500 languages on record in Nigeria, of which many were only maintained by oral tradition and no written script. The rapid extinction, absorption or modification of some languages by larger or more predominant economic-political ethnic groups within the region is currently being observed (see Seibert, 2000 for a detailed appendix of Nigerian languages). The official language of government and educational instruction is English.

## HISTORY

The history of Nigeria and other West African countries is critical to understanding cultures, identities and challenges faced by this region. The history of Nigeria and other countries can be divided into the prehistoric period, the great empires, slavery and the colonial period and the post-colonial era.

In about 500 BC to AD 200, the Nok civilization thrived in central Nigeria. The profitable trans-Saharan trade routes were used for exports from West Africa, including gold, cotton cloth, metal ornaments and leather goods towards the north as far as the Mediterranean. These goods were exchanged for copper, horses, salt, textiles and, later ivory, slaves and kola nuts. Successful trade nurtured the growth of several kingdoms and by around 1000–1300 the Hausa states developed in north-western Nigeria. The Kanem-Bornu kingdom in north-east Nigeria introduced Islam to the region, while the Yoruba culture thrived around the Ife and Oyo empires.

In the fifteenth century, Portuguese sailors visited Nigeria and other sea ports, opening up sea routes and trade with the prosperous kingdom of Benin, which controlled the area between Lagos and the Niger Delta. Shortly afterwards the slave trade began and was accelerated by the demand for cheap labour in the Americas. In 1510 the Spanish crown legalized the slave trade and this was followed by similar English laws in 1562. Active slave trade led to a depletion of the region's economic prosperity and population. By the 1700s the British had begun to dominate the lucrative slave trade along the Nigerian and West African coast. Abolition of the slave trade was not achieved until 1808 when Britain discouraged other countries from trading in slaves with Nigerian kingdoms whilst establishing its colonial presence. In 1851 Britain seized Lagos to increase its influence and slowly expanded its control over the rest of the region.

British consolidation of West African territory began when Sierra Leone became an official British Protectorate in 1896; this was followed by The Gambia in 1889, Nigeria in 1901 and Ghana (formerly Gold Coast) in 1902. This later became known as British West Africa. In the colonial race for Africa, Portugal claimed Guinea-Bissau (formerly known as Portuguese Guinea), while Togoland (modern-day Togo) became a German colony in 1884. Modern-day Guinea, Senegal, Mali, Benin (formerly Dahomey), Burkina Faso (formerly Upper Volta), and Niger were consolidated into the federation of French West Africa.

Liberia managed to retain its independence despite extensive territorial losses. Liberia has a uniquely distinct history in West Africa dating back to 1821, when private societies in the United States began founding colonies for free black slaves. These 'Free Blacks' or freedmen were perceived as a burden on society as they attempted to achieve equality with the white population, or rebel, or even mix with whites, hence it was suggested that they would be better off in Africa. Returning Christian slaves were also felt to be able to spread Christianity in Africa, while opening trade routes with Africa (Kocher, 1984).

By 1914 Britain formed the colony of Nigeria, and then divided Nigeria into three regions based on the core tribal divisions by 1946. Western-style education, governance and economy were more widely established in the north than in the south, a factor that has had ramifications in Nigerian society from independence in 1960 until today. West African countries attained independence between 1957 (Ghana) and 1973 (Guinea-Bissau), led by French West Africa and followed by the remainder of the British colonies a decade later. This history has greatly defined and influenced the national identities, governance, religion and migration patterns of the region into the twenty-first century.

## DOMINANT LOCAL NATIVE CULTURAL GROUPS

Given the very large and diverse ethnic mix of Nigeria, it is neither possible nor practicable to discuss each group in detail in this text. However, a discussion of the three main groups in Nigeria (Yoruba, Ibo and Hausa) gives an insight into the cultural diversity of this West African subpopulation.

## The Yoruba

The Yoruba (pronounced 'yorooba') make up about 21 per cent of the population of Nigeria. They are the indigenous population inhabiting south-western Nigeria and parts of neighbouring Republic of Benin. Predominantly town dwellers, the traditional Yoruba practise small-scale, domestic agriculture. They are also traders and craftspeople. The Yoruba now chiefly live in the cities of Ibadan, Lagos, Abeokuta, Ife and Ondo, among others.

By the seventeenth century the Yoruba had established the kingdom of Oyo, between the then Dahomey (present-day Benin) and the river Niger. Oyo fragmented into smaller kingdoms during the first half of the nineteenth century and came under British rule at the end of the century. Inherent in Yoruba culture is the encouragement of artistic expression and academic achievement as the key to success. This is reinforced by sayings such as 'if you are studious and successful your shoes will resonate with authority, however, if lazy they will be silent or drag like shoddy footwear'.

### Language
The Yoruba language is spoken by around 22 million people, mainly in Nigeria and Benin, but also in Togo, the UK and the USA. Yoruba culture and language was further dispersed round the world during the West African slave trade. Yoruba slaves were sent to British, French, Spanish and Portuguese colonies, and in a number of these places Yoruba traditions still thrive. In Brazil, Cuba, Haiti and Trinidad, Yoruba religious rites, beliefs, music and myths are still evident in daily cultural practice. In Haiti the Yoruba were generally referred to as the Anagos. In this society, Yoruba religious rituals and beliefs still involve numerous deities of Yoruba origin. In Brazil, Yoruba religious practices are called Anago or Shango, while in Cuba they are referred to as Lucumi.

While Yoruba customs and rituals permeate parts of the Caribbean and South America, the language is not spoken in a recognizable form. A member of the Niger-Congo family of African languages, Yoruba has around 20 different dialects. It is a tonal language (unlike English which is a stress language), and the meaning of certain words is distinguished by the pitch alone. For example, changes in intonation with the word *ogun* have at least eight different meanings:

- *Ógùn* – medicine
- *Ogún* – twenty
- *Ògun* – war
- *Ògún* – god of iron/war
- *Ogun* – inheritance
- *Ògùn* – name of a river
- *Ōgun* – sweat
- *O gun* – the person was stabbed
- *Ogun* – it is long/s(he) is tall (Ayonrinde, 2003).

### Religious worship
Traditional Yoruba religious practice is animistic, with numerous gods and deities worshipped. These practices, while still present, are being rapidly eroded by Christian and Muslim faiths, particularly in urban areas. It is not uncommon to find Yoruba spiritual practices and beliefs amalgamated into contemporary society. Traditional Yoruba cosmology has striking similarities to that of Ancient Greece with a pantheon of deities known as *Orisha*.

Of the hundreds of recognized gods worshipped by the Yoruba, the most popular are Sango (god of thunder and lightning), Ifa (also known as Orunmila, god of divination), Eshu (the messenger and trickster god also referred to as the 'devi') and Ogun (god of iron and of war). In traditional Yoruba practice, when a child is born, a diviner, or *babalawo*, is consulted to determine which *orisha* the child should follow. This may also involve stressing specific totems and taboos the child must be aware of. These also bear some similarities to the Western concept of horoscopes. As adults, the

Yoruba often honour several of these deities depending on their circumstances. It is not uncommon among some Westernized Yoruba to reject these deities or even change family names, incorporating deities to reflect their current faiths.

### Significance of the 'head' in Yoruba culture

The head (*ori*) is both an important anatomical structure and psychic symbol in Yoruba culture. Shaving of the head is customary in a number of rituals as spirits are believed to enter and exit the body through the scalp. Furthermore, the customary belief is that every human being has been given a 'head', or destiny, prior to birth that can be foreseen and arbitrated by consultations with a diviner. It is also held that each person has the ability to engage the power of his or her 'inner or internalized head' (*ori inu*) in order to achieve optimum potential in life. Character and personality are believed to emanate from this inner head. It is therefore understandable that any insult to the head, whether physical, verbal or by supernatural force, is a cause of great concern.

### Folk diagnostic categories

Yoruba folk culture and traditional healers recognize a range of nosological categories and descriptions for difficulties with emotional distress and for neuropsychiatric disorders. Some of these are described below:

- *ode ori* – this is a disorder with the chief complaints being crawling sensations in the head and body, noises in the ears, palpitations and various other somatic complaints. Anxiety and depressive symptoms are prominent in this presentation.
- *were* – a mentally ill person (often used to refer to a psychotic illness). In contemporary use this description is pejorative and carries a lot of stigma.
- *were oja* (literally a mentally ill person found in the market) – suggests severity of the illness as the ill person is vagrant or begging for alms and food in the marketplace, stressing that the illness could no longer be discreetly contained in the home setting.

- *irewesi okan* (fatigue or 'tiredness of the heart') – often used to refer to a depressive illness and may include a range of fatigue syndromes.
- *warapa* – epilepsy (generalized tonic-clonic or grand mal type seizures).
- *didirin* – intellectually impaired.

As in many societies, abnormal or unfamiliar behaviours are associated with perplexity, anxiety, myth and occasionally stigma in West African society. There are also a wide range of aetiological models for these disorders as well as alternative therapeutic interventions. For instance, there are beliefs among some Yoruba that '*warapa*' can be caused by coming into direct physical contact with the agama lizard. There are also beliefs that the froth/foaming saliva following an epileptic fit can be infectious and cause others to convulse. These beliefs could be problematic during emergency situations following a convulsion as some people may be reluctant to assist. In some rural areas, cow's urine is offered as a treatment and prophylaxis for convulsions and in others the feet are placed on hot coals.

## The Ibo/Igbo

The Igbo (pronounced 'eebow') are the main ethnic group inhabiting the south-eastern region of Nigeria. They are one of the three largest ethnolinguistic groups in the country and play a prominent role in the economics and politics of Nigeria. Following independence in 1960, the attempted secession of the eastern region from the Federal Republic of Nigeria led to the Nigerian civil (Biafran) war of 1967–1970. Since the conflict, the Igbo are now a fully integrated and potent force in Nigerian society.

Igbo has around 18 million speakers and many dialects; that notwithstanding, Igbo speakers can usually adapt their speech to a more common form of the language (lingua franca) to communicate between groups. While the Igbo population is most dense in eastern Nigeria, many now live in other parts of Nigeria with an expanding diasporic population in Britain, North America, Japan and other African countries.

The Igbo have a long history of cultural achievement and are traditionally farmers, entrepreneurs and trades people. Resourceful engineering and industrial design is also a vocational interest. The Igbo have great pride in their business and commercial exploits and open expression of this achievement is encouraged.

## Religious worship

Historically, traditional Igbo religion includes a belief in an afterlife and reincarnation, sacrifice, spirits and ancestor worship. Elaborate community ceremonies are held to mark funerals and other rites of passage. The farming communities also hold annual rituals and sacrifices to promote good rains, crops and harvest, for example the 'yam festival'. Contemporary Igbo spiritual practice is mainly Christianity.

## Community structure

Igbo towns and villages were historically defined by family lineage, containing family living quarters, dance areas for public performances, marketplaces and shrines for local deities. By tradition, the Igbo lived in small village democracies with older men responsible for coordinating the affairs of the community, and decision making is by consensus, often after lengthy debates. These councils are headed by the *Ozo* title holders, the highest ranking being the *Ezeani*; a title reserved for honest, upright and prominent senior members of the community.

The geographically dispersed cities, towns and village settlements are united by the tradition of a single founding ancestor. These village groups are sometimes called 'clans'; for example, one clan includes members of the *Umueri* (descendants of *Eri*). Other communities are active through a network of oracles, for example, the *Arochukwu* (*Aro* a subgroup of the Igbo, *Chukwu* means 'God'). Where there is individual or communal conflict, attempts are initially made to settle these within the clan, however should this fail parties are brought to face the oracle for adjudication.

## Illness models/folk illness categories

In Igbo mythology the supreme god Chukwu created the world and a solar deity. Ala, sometimes referred to as Ani, the daughter or wife of Chukwu, is the earth goddess of fertility and death, divining over the beginning and end of life. The culture also believes in the role of retributive justice, where anyone guilty of an evil act faces the wrath of Amadioha (god of thunder and lightning). Some other deities include Ahia Njoku (god of yams), Agwu (god of medicine men) and Agwunsi (god of divination and healing).

Igbos believe that each person has their own personal god called Chi (like a guardian angel) who personifies the individual's fate and destiny including luck and misfortune. It is important the Chi is well catered for and deities may be called upon to support it.

Other supernatural forces, such as *mami wota* (mermaid) or *ogbanje* (ghost or reincarnated spirit children), may cause suffering and illness. There are beliefs that wellbeing is also associated with the extent of people's hidden and potentially destructive dealings with others through inflicting the 'evil eye', envy or jealousy, witchcraft (*ita amusu*) or sorcery (*nsi na aja*), curses (*ibu onu*) or invoking of supernatural wrath (*iku ofo na iju ogu*). Such malicious behaviour is believed to cause physical injury or insanity, as well as social misfortune like loss of property, income or employment. Slighted ancestors and evil spirits (*ajo mmuo*) are also thought to be capable of causing misfortune, illness and even death. To maintain homeostasis of the society and wellbeing, healers are often consulted (Iroegbu, 2005).

## Igbo traditional healers

While folk healing is accessible to all community members, the expert healers, called *dibia*, specialize in a variety of medical and psycho-social needs, providing healing skills and resources. The *dibia* is often an inherited role following a lengthy period of apprenticeship and then takes responsibility for prophylaxis, healing, neutralizing malevolent forces and rituals. Some examples of designated healer titles and specialist roles are as follows (Iroegbu, 2005):

- *Dibia afa, dibia ogba aja* – divination diagnosis
- *Dibia aja, or nchu aja, or anya odo* – priest, ritual expert
- *Dibia onye oha* – community matters, king making
- *Dibia mgborogwu* – root and herb expertise, herbalist

- *Dibia ara* – insanity (*ara* means 'insanity')
- *Dibia ogbaokpukpo* – bone-setting
- *Dibia ogbanje* – *ogbanje* healing, care for spirit children
- *Dibia amosu* – witchcraft healing
- *Dibia mmanwu* – masquerade guarding
- *Dibia amadioha* – rain and thunder matters
- *Dibia omumu* – fertility, healing and attending
- *Dibia owa ahu or okwochi* – surgical ailments
- *Dibia owu mmiri* – *mami wota* crisis.

## The Hausa

The Hausa (pronounced 'haoosa') are the main residents of northern Nigeria. While ethnically diverse in the region, they are culturally homogeneous, numbering about 10–15 million individuals.

### History

Originally a group living in feudal cities and states, the Hausa were conquered from the fourteenth century by a series of West African kingdoms including Mali, Songhai, Bornu and Fulani. In the early twentieth century, when the Hausa were in conflict with the Fulani, the British invaded northern Nigeria and the Hausa–Fulani ruling alliance, in northern Nigeria, was established. A large proportion of the Fulani have now become culturally and linguistically Hausa.

Although the earliest Hausa were animists, Islam is now the dominant religion among the majority of Hausa. Subsistence agriculture is the primary occupation of most, but other skills such as tanning, dyeing, weaving and metalworking are also highly developed. The Hausa have long been famous for trans-Saharan trade and pilgrimages. The travelling trading and wealthy merchants share the highest social positions with the politically powerful and the highly educated classes.

### Language

Hausa language has evolved over the centuries, absorbing from other languages; about a quarter derived from Arabic and the rest from Fulfulde and Kanuri languages. It has adapted well to the demands of contemporary cultural change and has become a common language for millions of non-Hausa West Africans in the northern areas of several countries.

Sizeable Hausa-speaking communities called *Sabo* exist in major West and North African cities (akin to Chinatowns in many parts of the world). Hausa names and titles are predominantly Arabic due to the historical influence of Islam, and indigenous or traditional Hausa names are uncommon.

### Family and social structures

Muslim Hausa social structure is a complex system of hierarchies, based on occupation, wealth, birth and 'patron–client' ties. Occupational specialties are ranked and tend to be hereditary; it is not uncommon for the first son to succeed his father in the same vocation. In many communities, wealth is often associated with prestige and power, and is beneficial in sociocultural interactions.

The traditional Hausa Muslim man may have up to four wives depending on his ability to support a larger family. Large family size in some communities, other than enhancing status, also provides additional farm hands, labour and keeps business in the family. Wives are ranked in seniority according to marriage order and are expected to show deference as part of their role.

Respect is fundamental to family relationships and discreet or secluded behaviour is encouraged amongst adult women. This varies in degree from the housebound women in 'purdah', the wearing of veils, to partial seclusion in the home or family compound. A few women in society exhibit no restrictions but this is frowned upon by traditionalists. Traditional gender-specific female roles include domestic and child care, craft specialties, and sometimes assisting in trade.

The city of Kano is the cultural and economic capital of northern Nigeria with a well-established Islamic culture including the promulgation of Islamic Sharia law. Sharia law, based on the tenets of Islam, defines all aspects of culture including diet, dress code, penalties, business and social hierarchies. Attempts to impose this on other groups have led to recurrent conflicts in the region.

## MIGRATION PATTERNS

As discussed in the sections above, West Africa has numerous homogeneous groups spread across geopolitical borders. Migration may present as intra-ethnic cross-border migration within groups divided by national boundaries, for example, migration between the Yoruba of Nigeria and Benin and the Hausa of northern Nigeria and Niger, has been going on for centuries.

Contemporary migration of displaced people within the same country may arise where there is movement to neighbouring regions as a result of communal conflicts. It is not uncommon for political, religious and ethnic misunderstandings, for example, between Muslim and Christian groups, or between security forces and militant groups, herdsmen and rural farming communities. This can culminate in the temporary or permanent displacement of inhabitants.

Immigration into Nigeria is mainly from the West African subregion. For example the flight of refugees from civil war zones led to the official migration of Liberians (about 7000), Sierra Leoneans (about 2000) and Chadians (over 3000) to Nigerian refugee camps (World Refugee Surveys, 2004/5). These figures are a very conservative estimate, as movement of groups is fluid and declaration of refugee status in a non-social welfare country has limited benefits.

Other established immigrant groups include employees of multinational petroleum, business and technology industries from Europe and North America, Asian employees of educational establishments, the well-established Lebanese community and, in recent years, a rapidly growing Chinese business sector.

Given Nigeria's relative regional wealth, there is also a steady stream of economic migrants from less affluent African states.

Conversely, emigration from Nigeria is predominantly to Europe and North America with a significant growth of diaspora populations (professional and unskilled) in these countries. Significantly less migration occurs between West Africa and the sub-Saharan continent and where this occurs it has mainly been to southern regions in the last decade. Migrations from West Africa to Europe are principally to former colonial 'master' nations based on imbibed identities and pre-existing cultural and linguistic awareness; for example Nigerian and Ghanaian migration to the UK, and migration from Benin or Côte D'Ivoire to France are common.

## EARLY PSYCHIATRIC SERVICES IN NIGERIA/MENTAL HEALTH CARE DELIVERY

Although the recognition and treatment of mental disorders predate written records, Western models of mental health care were not introduced until the early twentieth century. The first asylum was established in the south-eastern city of Calabar in 1904, followed in 1907 by the Yaba Asylum in Lagos, in the south-west. In 1954, the Aro Mental Hospital was established in Abeokuta by the British colonial government in response to the need for improved mental health care (Asuni, 1967). The hospital, later known as the Aro Neuropsychiatric Hospital, has played an important historic role in the development of psychiatry in Nigeria with a number community and World Health Organization initiatives.

## CURRENT PSYCHIATRIC PRACTICE/SERVICE DEVELOPMENT/HEALTH SERVICE CONSTRUCTION

The bulk of psychiatric service delivery in Nigeria is from the eight regional psychiatric hospitals and the departments of psychiatry in 12 medical schools. A number of general hospitals also provide psychiatric services of variable and often limited resource. Despite statutory facilities, mental health care remains inadequate nationally with the ratio of psychiatric beds being about 0.4 to 10 000 persons, while that for both psychologists and social workers is 0.02 to 100 000 persons (World Health Organization, 2001). The psychiatric medical workforce per head of the population numbers about 1 per million. Most orthodox psychiatric services are within urban centres in southern parts of the country with both a North–South and rural–urban skew in resource availability and accessibility. It is therefore understandable that this void is filled by a range of traditional, faith healing and complementary therapies in most communities. Traditional views of mental illness are often based on acceptable supernatural belief systems and indigenous illness models, so Western models of psychiatric care still struggle for acceptance in some sectors of society.

Psychiatric practice in Nigeria has been significantly influenced by the country's British colonial history. The majority of pioneering Nigerian psychiatrists trained in the UK in the 1960s. Since 1976, the National (Nigerian) and West African Postgraduate Colleges have been actively involved in training psychiatrists from Nigeria, Ghana, Liberia, Sierra Leone and Gambia.

## RESEARCH AND PRACTICE

Psychiatric research in Nigeria was initially spearheaded by the work of Aro Psychiatric Hospital (Aro village) in Abeokuta, which pioneered community epidemiologic studies among the Yoruba in collaboration with Cornell University, USA (Leighton et al., 1963). It is heartening that epidemiological research is laying a foundation for a range of interventions and service developments. Contemporary research is also evolving across the psychopharmacological, social science and neurobiological fields.

### Schizophrenia

Nigeria was one of the key centres for the landmark International Pilot Study of Schizophrenia (IPSS), the ten-country study of the incidence and manifestations of schizophrenia. Better prognosis was found in Nigeria and other developing countries than in others. In the past two decades, studies on brain neuroimaging, social outcomes, caregiver burden (Ohaeri, 2001) and cost of treatment (Suleiman et al., 1997) have explored the impact of this disorder. In Nigeria, there are no national social welfare and community rehabilitation programmes for the mentally ill, so families bear a major burden of care.

Disturbed behaviour has been identified as a greater determinant of severity of burden than psychiatric diagnosis itself (Ohaeri, 2001). There is increasing evidence of the acceptability of antipsychotic medication among people with schizophrenia; however, as identified in other regions of the world, symptom severity, side effects, lack of insight and being employed are a challenge to long-term care (Adewuya et al., 2006).

### Primary care

The majority of psychiatric presentations seen by clinicians in Nigeria are in primary care. A number of studies (Abiodun, 1993) have assessed psychological symptomatology and morbidity in both rural (21.3 per cent) and urban (27.8 per cent) primary care settings. These identified significant rates of disorders with unmet therapeutic need. Psychological symptoms that fall just below a diagnostic threshold were found to be associated with impaired functioning over 12 months (Gureje, 2002). A hidden area of morbidity such as the 7.4 per cent rate of geriatric depression in primary care was found to be significantly associated with low income and subjective poor health (Sokoya and Baiyewu, 2003). Programmes to improve the size and efficacy of the primary care workforce have met with mixed opinions and require a policy shift in training and resource initiatives (Omigbodun, 2001).

### Dementia

Collaborative research in dementia between researchers at the University of Ibadan and the Indiana University in the USA is yielding fascinating information. This longitudinal study has been going on for over a decade and among its major findings is the observation that both the prevalence and incidence of Alzheimer's disease are significantly less among the Yoruba in Nigeria than among African-Americans living in Indianapolis (Hendrie et al., 2001). Putative genetic and environmental factors that may underlie this difference, including the role of genetic polymorphisms for apolipoprotein E (apoE), are being explored.

## Substance misuse

Substance misuse research is a rapidly evolving field, reflecting changing patterns of drug use in Nigeria. The identification of user groups, their patterns of use, risk and harm minimization as well as the development of culturally acceptable treatment interventions are a current priority. Public interest in substance misuse was highlighted in the late 1980s with national concern about trafficking routes through West African countries. Invariably this introduced crack, cocaine and heroin to thriving urban areas with ensuing social problems including criminal behaviour.

A recent World Health Organization-sponsored evaluation of intravenous drug use in Lagos highlights the hitherto uncommon practice of intravenous drug use among cocaine and heroin users in cosmopolitan Lagos (Adelekan and Lawal, 2000). Non-sterile practice was not uncommon among the group as well as unprotected sexual activity with poor awareness of blood-borne viruses. These findings stress the need for major policy change from the current emphasis on supply control and demand reduction to harm reduction practices. Current research in this area also has far-reaching public health implications on the management of HIV transmission, health and criminal justice expenditures.

Health service research involving the evaluation of therapeutic interventions such as detoxification, group therapy sessions, occupational and vocational rehabilitation and relapse prevention initiatives are also in the process of dissemination.

## Eating disorders (anorexia nervosa and bulimia)

The prevailing cultural analysis of these disorders emphasizes a drive for thinness following a Western cultural ideal of feminine beauty. Conversely, in some parts of West Africa, a robust appearance is seen as 'evidence of good living' or affluence and slimness is viewed as unfortunate or a sign of poverty. In south-eastern Nigeria, prenuptial 'fattening houses' aim to encourage weight gain in the young bride preparing for marriage. It is understandable, therefore, that eating disorders are thought to be 'culture-bound' and that in the midst of hunger, bingeing followed by purging or induced vomiting would be unacceptable. In spite of these observations, a survey (Oyewumi and Kazarian, 1992) of female Nigerian youths in high school, college and university, revealed that 14.1 per cent of the female youths had eating disorders associated with anorexic behaviour and 20 per cent displayed bulimic behaviour and controlled their weight by vomiting, or using laxatives, diuretics and diet pills. Rapid transition in global youth culture with media images of slim models and the quest for foreign values may shift epidemiological trends within segments of the population over time.

## Perinatal mental health

The mental health of post-natal mothers has benefited from increasing interest in screening in some specialist centres where rates between 10.7 and 14.6 per cent have been found for post-natal depression. Given the high rates of traditional birth attendant use and the dearth of post-natal follow-up care, there is major scope for maternal and child health interventions to improve survival and quality of life (Fatoye and Fasubaa, 2002; Uwakwe and Okonkwe, 2003).

## FORENSIC MENTAL HEALTH

Forensic psychiatry has had a protracted incubation in Nigeria and other West African states. This has not been facilitated by equally protracted reviews of the colonial mental health legislation. Psychiatric morbidity surveys of a Nigerian prison population found a prevalence of schizophrenia in 2 per cent, major depression in 2 per cent and recurrent mild depression in 21 per cent, generalized anxiety disorder in 8 per cent and somatization disorder in 1 per cent of inmates. Six per cent had an antisocial personality disorder while another 1 per cent had a probable mild learning disability. Drug and alcohol misuse prior to detention included cannabis (11 per cent) and alcohol

(13 per cent). Significant psychiatric morbidity in the population emerged while in the prison setting (Agbahowe *et al.*, 1998). Other researchers (Mafullul *et al.*, 2001), exploring the prevalence of mental illness among convicted perpetrators of homicides, observed that 24 per cent had a psychotic disorder (mainly paranoid schizophrenia) and alcohol intoxication. However, psychiatric services were underutilized in legal processes. High rates (45 per cent) of substance use disorders preceded the homicides. Findings like these stress the need to improve mental health services in prisons as well as the need for legislative frameworks for the management of mentally disordered offenders.

## TRADITIONAL HEALERS

As the bulk (approximately 70 per cent) of mental health service provision is through non-orthodox means such as religious organizations and traditional healers, these services cannot be ignored. A number of researchers have assessed the role of traditional therapists in mental health interventions (Adelekan *et al.*, 2001). A common finding is that traditional healers recognize symptoms of severe mental illness, but they hold strong beliefs about supernatural causative factors. A study of Yoruba traditional healers with specific interest in mental disorders identified two main groups of mental disorders, namely *asinwin* (psychotic disorders) and *ode ori* (a less severe disorder with prominent somatic symptoms) (Makanjuola, 1987b). Further subcategorization of disorders was predominantly aetiological. These aetiological factors were considered to be the actions of enemies who often deployed supernatural forces; self-induced disorders (including cannabis misuse), *soponna* (smallpox) and 'hereditary' factors (Makanjuola, 1987a). Although beliefs regarding mode of hereditary transmission may seem at variance with those of modern medicine, it is not unusual for Yoruba families to investigate families of potential in-laws for mental disorders or disorderly character before approving marriage. Psychoeducation has been found to improve understanding of aetiology and reduce the use of

corporal punishments as intervention; for example, whipping and chaining. There remain numerous opportunities to work closely with healers who may be the first point of contact in some communities.

Therapeutic interventions employed by indigenous healers are predominantly paranormal and pharmacological; the use of structured psychological treatments being limited. Traditional medication can be further categorized into two groups, namely agents with active pharmacological influences and agents invested predominantly with paranormal expectations and influences. The healers' choice is often based on perceived causative factors as well as clinical presentation. Up to 163 plants have been referred to as being of benefit in the management of mental disorders. About a third of these plants and herbal prepar-ations are recognized by a quarter or more of healers. It is noteworthy that the bark of *Rauwolffia vomitoria* was universally prescribed by all healers (Makanjuola and Jaiyeola, 1987). The use of animal parts, sacrifices and other agents such as cowrie shells, feathers and beads plays an important role in these therapeutic processes.

Arguably, whilst therapeutic transactions are mainly directive in spartan settings, they involve a process of history taking, introspection by the healer and prescription of therapeutic options. The healer may take time to consult oracles directly through rituals or may invoke a trance state. The code of ethics also recognizes the importance of confidentiality in transactions. This may also ensure future patronage. Systems of fee collection are either in cash or in kind, such as farm produce or manual labour. It is a commonly held belief that failure to reward services is associated with a poor prognostic outcome unless fees are waived by the healer. Some of these therapeutic processes have a striking similarity to Western practice.

A health economics investigation compared orthodox and traditional mental health care per illness episode, taking account of duration of illness, duration of therapy, costs of consultation, medication, accommodation and feeding. Traditional mental health care was three times more expensive than orthodox mental health care (Makanjuola, 2003).

## SPIRITUAL AND FAITH ORGANIZATIONS

The role of faith and spiritual organizations in all tiers of mental health interventions cannot be underestimated in this religious society. With a rapidly expanding Pentecostal church influenced by African-American styles of worship and charismatic leadership, help-seeking behaviours and pathways to care frequently involve contact with a spiritual leader, pastor or representative of the church.

Interventions for emotional distress and mental health difficulties include advice on reading Bible passages when experiencing mild or common anxiety difficulties. More complex or enduring difficulties may be presented in front of a church congregation of several hundred people for spiritual cleansing or 'exorcism' of evil spirits. On occasion, this may involve the individual being encouraged to confess to past misgivings which may have 'brought on' the emotional problems, social adversity or mental illness with the support of the congregation in praying for forgiveness from God.

Healing processes in church settings may also involve 'the laying of hands', a process by which the spiritual healer and sometimes other church members place their hand on the person's head and pray for him or her. In some congregations this also involves 'speaking in tongues' (a spiritually filled trance-like state in which the individual speaks in what appears to be in an incoherent way to the unfamiliar). Following the healing process, the individual is informed they have been cured or healed. This can be exceptionally challenging in clinical situations should a patient be advised to stop using medication or advised that the problems experienced are spiritual in causation, so that pharmacological remedies are then seen to be unnecessary. In some extreme situations people are left feeling that orthodox medical interventions are associated with the 'devil' and are therefore declined.

In some situations 'holy water' is prescribed for consumption or sprinkling in conjunction with stipulated tasks or rituals. It is not unknown for psychotropic medication to be introduced into the holy water by dubious spiritual therapists. Group support and identification, testimonial confessions in a non-judgemental atmosphere, sleep deprivation in night vigils and use of ritualistic symbols are other well-recognized therapeutic processes in churches.

## PHARMACOTHERAPEUTICS

Like many countries in Africa there is restricted pharmaceutical industry support of mental health services such as funding of research and the subsidized cost of psychotropic medication (Lawal *et al.*, 2003). Ethically, even when used effectively in trials, lack of signifi-cant medication subsidies hinders the use beyond the clinical trial. This is all the more pertinent at a period of international concern about the dearth of drug trials across geographical, racial and ethnic groups. A common problem is the exorbitant cost of newer medications (atypical antipsychotics, non-tricyclic antidepressants and dementia therapies), thereby limiting access to wealthier patients (Amoo and Ogunlesi, 2005). National governments still have major roles in ensuring accessible, affordable and appropriate medication choices.

## PRIORITIES

### Legislation

No West African country has established mental health legislation. In Nigeria, the pre-independence legislation of the 1950s is still in place though rarely used. Concerted attempts have been made to push the revised draft legislation through legislative arms of the government over recent years. The main priority for Nigerian mental health service provision is the development of a contemporary mental health legislation. This is not an easily achieved task, and clinical practice has to comply, but also must have the capacity to comply (see Chapter 7 on mental health law, and Chapter 9 on mental health policy).

## Manpower – psychiatric workforce

Serious devaluation of national currencies have been partly responsible for poor remuneration of the clinical workforce, and the consequential emigration to other countries offering higher income and better quality of life. While a reversal of the trend is now emerging, emigration of trained professionals remains a daunting challenge; the establishment of the Postgraduate Medical Colleges in West African countries for the training of specialist doctors has minimized the unpalatable consequences of the 'brain drain'.

## Retention of specialist staff

A recurrent challenge faced by mental health services is the retention of experienced and highly specialized clinical staff (medical, nursing, psychology, occupational therapy and social work). The perennial 'brain drain' to Western countries of staff and depletion of clinical input through taking on senior management positions demonstrates the need for significant workforce growth.

## Training

Training in mental health care delivery at primary care level is an area of priority if the majority of citizens is to have access to care. Awareness of common mental disorders and emergency interventions, appropriate referrals and health promotion are greatly needed. Furthermore, collaboration with non-orthodox agencies such as spiritual healing homes and traditional healers taps into a vast and widely acceptable resource. Multidisciplinary training and supervision will encourage promotion of skill mix in areas of short supply.

## Funding

A universal challenge faced by West African countries is the national expenditure on health, of which HIV, malaria, maternal and child health trump mental health as areas of priority. The total expenditure on health as a percentage of the gross domestic product of West African countries ranges from 3.5 per cent (Sierra Leone) to 8.1 per cent (Gambia). Nigeria, on the other hand, spends 5 per cent of its GDP on health, of which only a small proportion is towards the provision of mental health care (compared with the health expenditures of the USA 15.2 per cent, the UK 8 per cent, India 4.8 per cent, China 5.6 per cent and Russia 5.6 per cent) (World Health Organization, 2006).

## Research

Expenditure in mental health research is quite small in relation to the burden of mental health problems, and the need for interventions and health services that are effective in this cultural context. Most research is undertaken with donor agencies. Even then, this is small compared with expenditure on malaria, HIV and other communicable diseases. Widespread poverty, resource limitations and rural–urban migration in the presence of tropical physical health disorders sets the stage for high rates of mental disorders. Improved training, African and international collaboration, funding and the enabling of opportunities should enhance research in this region (Ayonrinde *et al.*, 2004; Okulate *et al.*, 2004).

## CONCLUSIONS

In conclusion, this chapter has highlighted the wide cultural diversity of Nigerian and other West African societies. One cannot overemphasize the influence of historical experiences on the present sociocultural circumstances. The evolution and limitations of current orthodox and traditional clinical practice have been explored, including resource challenges, training and research.

## REFERENCES

Abiodun, O.A. 1993: A study of mental morbidity among primary care patients in Nigeria. *Comprehensive Psychiatry* 34, 10–13.

Adelekan, M.L., Lawal, R.A., Akinhanmi, A.O., Haruna, A.Y.A. *et al.* 2000: Injection drug use and associated health consequences in Lagos, Nigeria. *2000 Global Research Network Meeting on HIV Prevention in Drug Using Populations.* Baltimore, MD: National Institute on Drug Abuse, 27–41.

Adelekan, M.L., Makanjuola, A.B. and Ndom, R.J. 2001: Traditional mental health practitioners in Kwara State, Nigeria. *East African Medical Journal* 78, 190–96.

Adewuya, A.O., Ola, B.A., Mosaku, S.K., Fatoye, F.O. and Eegunranti, A.B. 2006: Attitude towards antipsychotics among out-patients with schizophrenia in Nigeria. *Acta Psychiatrica Scandinavica* 113, 207–11.

Agbahowe, S.A., Ohaeri, J.U., Ogunlesi, A.O. and Osahon, R. 1998: Prevalence of psychiatric morbidity among convicted inmates in a Nigerian prison community. *East African Medical Journal* 75, 19–26.

Amoo, G. and Ogunlesi, A.O. 2005: Financial cost of treating Nigerian in-patients with schizophrenia. *African Journal of Medicine and Medical Sciences* 34, 15–23.

Asuni, T. 1967: Aro Mental Hospital in perspective. *American Journal of Psychiatry* 124, 763–70.

Ayonrinde, O. 2003: Importance of cultural sensitivity in therapeutic transactions: considerations for healthcare providers. *Disease Management and Health Outcomes* 11(4), 233–48.

Ayonrinde, O., Gureje, O. and Lawal, R. 2004: Psychiatric research in Nigeria: bridging tradition and modernisation. *British Journal of Psychiatry* 184, 536–38.

Fatoye, F.O. and Fasubaa, O.B. 2002: Post-partum mental disorders: pattern and problems of management in Wesley Guild Hospital, Ilesa, Nigeria. *Journal of Obstetrics and Gynaecology* 22, 508–12.

Gureje, O. 2002: Psychological disorders and symptoms in primary care: association with disability and service use after 12 months. *Social Psychiatry and Psychiatric Epidemiology* 37, 220–24.

Hendrie, H.C., Ogunniyi, A., Hall, K.S., Baiyewu, O., Unverzagt, F.W., Gureje, O., Gao, S., Evans, RM., Ogunseyinde, A.O., Adeyinka, A.O., Musick, B. and Hui, S.L. 2001: Incidence of dementia and Alzheimer disease in 2 communities: Yoruba residing in Ibadan, Nigeria, and African Americans residing in Indianapolis, Indiana. *Journal of the American Medical Association* 285, 739–47.

Iroegbu, P. 2005: Healing insanity: skills and expert knowledge of Igbo healers. *Africa Development* XXX, 78–92.

Kocher, K.L. 1984: A duty to America and Africa: a history of the independent African colonization movement in Pennsylvania. *Pennsylvania History* 51, 118–53.

Lawal, R.A., Suleiman, G.T. and Onyenze, B. 2003: Risperidone in the treatment of schizophrenia. *Nigerian Medical Practitioner* 44, 11–18.

Leighton, A.H., Lambo, T.A., Hughes, C.C., Leighton, D.C., Murphy, J.M. and Maeklin, D.B. 1963: *Psychiatric Disorder Among the Yoruba – A Report from the Cornell-Aro Mental Health Research Project in the Western Region, Nigeria.* Ithaca, NY: Cornell University Press.

Mafullul, Y.M., Ogunlesi, O.A. and Sijuwola, O.A. 2001: Psychiatric aspects of criminal homicide in Nigeria. *East African Medical Journal* 78, 35–39.

Makanjuola, R.O. 1987a: Yoruba traditional healers in psychiatry I. Healers' concepts of the nature and aetiology of mental disorders. *African Journal of Medicine and Medical Science* 16, 53–59.

Makanjuola, R.O. 1987b: 'Ode Ori': a culture-bound disorder with prominent somatic features in Yoruba Nigerian patients. *Acta Psychiatrica Scandinavica* 75, 231–36.

Makanjuola, A.B. 2003: A cost comparison of traditional and orthodox mental health care. *Nigerian Postgraduate Medical Journal* 10, 157–61.

Makanjuola, R.O. and Jaiyeola, A.A. 1987: Yoruba traditional healers in psychiatry. II. Management of psychiatric disorders. *African Journal of Medicine and Medical Science* 16, 61–73.

Ohaeri, J.U. 2001: Caregiver burden and psychotic patients' perception of social support in a Nigerian setting. *Social Psychiatry and Psychiatric Epidemiology* 36, 86–93.

Okulate, G.T., Olayinka, M.O. and Jones, O.B. 2004: Somatic symptoms in depression: evaluation of their diagnostic weight in an African setting. *British Journal of Psychiatry* 184, 422–27.

Omigbodun, O.O. 2001: A cost-effective model for increasing access to mental health care at the primary care level in Nigeria. *Journal of Mental Health Policy and Economics* 4, 133–39.

Oyewumi, L.K. and Kazarian, S.S. 1992: Abnormal eating attitudes among a group of Nigerian youths: I Bulimic behaviour. *East African Medical Journal* 69, 663–66.

Seibert, U. 2000: *Nigerian Languages A-Z.* http://www.uiowa.edu/intlinet/unijos/nigonnet/nlp/list-abc.htm (accessed 31 July 2006).

Sokoya, O.O. and Baiyewu, O. 2003: Geriatric depression in Nigerian primary care attendees. *International Journal of Geriatric Psychiatry* 18, 506–10.

Suleiman, G.T., Ohaeri, J.U., Lawal, R.A., Haruna, A.Y. and Orija, O.B. 1997: Financial cost of treating out-patients with schizophrenia in Nigeria. *British Journal of Psychiatry* 171, 364–68.

Uwakwe, R. and Okonkwo, J.E. 2003: Affective (depressive) morbidity in puerperal Nigerian women: validation of the Edinburgh Postnatal Depression Scale. *Acta Psychiatrica Scandinavica* 107, 251–59.

World Health Organization 2001: *Atlas – Mental Health Resources in the World, Mental Health Determinants and Populations.* Department of Mental Health and Substance Dependence. Geneva: World Health Organization.

World Health Organization 2006: WHO Statistical Information System, 2006: http://www.who.int/health_financing (accessed October 2006).

World Refugee Surveys 2004/5: http://www.refugees.org/articles.aspx?id=1565&subm=19&ssm=29&area=Investigate (accessed 8 December 2006).

# 14

# North Africa: focus on psychiatry in Egypt

## Ahmed Okasha

## HISTORICAL BACKGROUND

Mental disorders have been recognized in Egypt for millennia; 5000 years ago they were considered to be physical ailments of the heart or uterus, as described in the Ebers and Kahun papyri (Okasha, 2001). These disorders carried no stigma, as there was no demarcation then between psyche and soma. In the fourteenth century – 600 years before similar institutions were founded in Europe – the first psychiatric unit was established, in Kalaoon Hospital in Cairo.

Egypt is central to the Arab world, which, despite its wealth and its natural and human resources, has fared poorly in many aspects of development. Important problems include illiteracy (especially among women), lack of job opportunities (especially for young people), and slow economic growth because of loss of traditional economies, low productivity, and lack of innovation and competitiveness. Military spending is triple that of other regions. Rapid expansion of Arab populations threatens progress, especially in countries with limited resources such as Egypt.

## PSYCHIATRIC EDUCATION IN EGYPT

Egypt has 17 medical schools; all of them have psychiatric departments, seven of which are departments of neuropsychiatry. They have offered a diploma of neuropsychiatry for more than 60 years, a master's degree in psychiatry for the past 25 years and a doctorate for the past 20 years. Students must complete a thesis and written, oral and clinical examinations.

## MENTAL HEALTH SERVICES

For its population of over 70 million inhabitants, Egypt has about 1000 psychiatrists (one psychiatrist for approximately 70 000 citizens), more than 1300 psychiatric nurses and about 200 clinical psychologists, with hundreds of general psychologists working in fields unrelated to mental health services. There are many social workers practising in all psychiatric facilities, but unfortunately they are general social workers with minimal graduate training in psychiatric social work. In 1960 there was an attempt to provide further training for psychiatric social workers at the Institute of Social Services in Cairo, but this lasted for only two years because of a shortage of applicants.

Egypt has about 9700 psychiatric beds, one bed for every 7000 citizens (15 beds per 100 000 population); this is less than 10 per cent of the total number of hospital beds (110 000). The two largest mental hospitals in Egypt were facing great difficulties regarding care, finances, treatment and rehabilitation while caring for 5000 patients. Three new hospitals, each providing 300 beds, have now been built on the premises of these two hospitals, with a view to providing sufficient mental health services of the highest quality (Okasha and Okasha, 2000).

The new policy of deinstitutionalization and the provision of community care may reduce the number of psychiatric inpatients, but will not solve the problem. Aftercare services in Egypt are still limited, owing to the poor understanding of most people of the need for follow-up care after initial improvement. Community care in the form of hostels, day centres, rehabilitation centres and health visitors is only available in major cities; otherwise it is provided by the family (Okasha and Karam, 1998).

## MENTAL HEALTH POLICY

The National Mental Health Programmes, running for the periods 1991 to 1996 and then 1997 to 2003, focused on the inclusion of mental health in primary health care, training family doctors to deal with the main bulk of mental disorders, and raising public awareness regarding recognition of mental disorders and encouraging appropriate referral routes. The future policy of psychiatric services in Egypt is to build medium-stay hospitals of 600 beds, which will serve three neighbouring governorates, and short-stay hospitals of 100 beds. The encouragement of intensive psychiatric outpatient treatment in all general hospitals is proposed.

Mental health legislation was introduced in Egypt in 1944, in advance of most other Arab and African countries. Most of the existing laws dealing with mental health are now old, having been written prior to the new concepts of community psychiatry and the integration of mental health into other health services (Okasha and Karam, 1998). An attempt to update them is now in progress.

## PROFILE OF PSYCHIATRIC DISORDERS IN EGYPT

### Hysteria (conversion or dissociative disorder)

Hysteria occupies a position at the top of the list of psychiatric diagnoses. There has been much controversy about its nosological status. In 1990, the first 1000 people presenting to the outpatient clinic of the Institute of Psychiatry of Ain Shams University in Cairo were screened to determine whether they fulfilled *Diagnostic and Statistical Manual of Mental Disorders* (DSM-III-R) criteria for either conversion or dissociation disorder (Okasha *et al.*, 1993a), replicating a study undertaken at an Egyptian university hospital 23 years earlier, where hysteria constituted 11.2 per cent of the sample (Okasha, 1967). The newer study aimed to test the relevance of the diagnosis of 'hysteria' (conversion and dissociative disorder). According to its results, many disorders that would formerly have been diagnosed as hysteria would now receive another diagnosis, mostly somatoform disorder. However, some disorders still require the diagnostic label of hysteria to reflect the symptoms and the underlying mechanisms (stress, primary gain, secondary gain, and motor or sensory symptoms that are culturally and symbolically specific for the stress). The prevalence of 5 per cent in that study is comparable with that of organic mental disorders (5.1 per cent), personality disorders (4.9 per cent) and anxiety disorders (7.9 per cent), indicating that hysteria cannot be ignored as a diagnostic category. Factors that might contribute to a real decline in the incidence of hysteria could be related to the industrialization of Egyptian society and its increasing complexity, for which the primitive mechanism of defence against frustration is no longer strong enough to ward off anxieties.

However, the decrease in the diagnosis of hysteria could also be attributed to the diagnostic system used. The International Classification of Diseases (ICD-10) and DSM-III-R, which do not favour the diagnosis of hysteria because of its dynamic character, contain a number of categories that would have been included under the previous diagnosis of hysteria. These categories include other somatoform disorders such as somatisation, psychogenic pain disorder, hypochondriasis, body dysmorphic disorder and undifferentiated somatoform disorder not otherwise specified.

## Anxiety disorders

Earlier studies of psychiatric morbidity among university students in Egypt showed that anxiety states were diagnosed in 36 per cent of the study sample (Okasha et al., 1977). In 1993 anxiety states represented about 22.6 per cent of diagnoses made in psychiatric outpatient clinics in a selective Egyptian sample (Okasha et al., 1993a). In 1981, the first study on sociodemographic aspects of anxiety disorders in Egypt was published; this applied the Arabic version of the Present State Examination in evaluating the profiles of clusters and symptoms of anxiety in a sample of 120 patients with anxiety (Okasha and Ashour, 1981). The findings revealed that the most common symptoms were worrying (82 per cent), irritability (73 per cent), free-floating anxiety (70 per cent), depressed mood (65 per cent), tiredness (64 per cent), restlessness (63 per cent), and anergia and retardation (61 per cent). Panic attacks were present in 30 per cent, situational anxiety in 35 per cent, specific phobias in 37 per cent and avoidance in 53 per cent of the sample. Male patients showed significantly more hypochondriasis and anxiety on meeting people than females. This can be explained by the fact that men in Egyptian culture tend to somatize their psychological symptoms, as the latter may lower their prestige and degrade their pride, because of the belief that 'real' men do not have psychological symptoms. In the same study, female patients showed significantly more increased free-floating anxiety, loss of weight and conversion symptoms.

## Obsessive–compulsive disorder

A study investigating the demographic profile and symptoms of Egyptian patients with obsessive–compulsive disorder found that more than two-thirds of the patients were males. The most commonly occurring obsessions were religious and contamination (60 per cent) and somatic obsessions (49 per cent), whereas the most commonly occurring compulsions were repeating rituals (68 per cent), cleaning and washing compulsions (63 per cent) and checking compulsions (58 per cent). A third of patients had a co-morbid depressive disorder. A comparison was drawn between the most prevalent symptoms in our sample and those of other studies performed in India, England and Jerusalem. Obsessions were found to be similar in content in Muslims and Jews, differing from those in Hindus and Christians, signifying the role of cultural and religious rituals in the presentation of obsessive–compulsive disorder. The obsessions of the patients from Egypt and Jerusalem were similar, dealing mainly with religious matters and matters related to cleanliness and dirt. Common themes between the Indian and British samples, on the other hand, were mostly related to orderliness and aggressive issues (Okasha et al., 1994).

## Depressive disorders

The prevalence rates of depression among selected samples from an urban and a rural population in Egypt were found to be 11.4 per cent and 19.7 per cent, respectively. Dysthymic disorder was the most common diagnostic category in the urban population (4.1 per cent), whereas adjustment disorder with depressed mood was more frequently encountered in the rural population (6.7 per cent). Major affective disorder according to DSM-III criteria was diagnosed in 1.9 per cent of the urban population compared with 3.3 per cent of the rural population; the total prevalence was 2.5 per cent (Okasha et al., 1988).

A cross-cultural comparison between Western and Egyptian patients with depressive illness reveals some differences. Depression among Egyptian patients is manifested mainly by agitation, somatic symptoms, hypochondriasis, physiological changes such as decreased libido, anorexia and insomnia, which is not characterized by early morning awakening. Egyptian patients mask their affect with multiple somatic symptoms, which occupy the foreground, and the affective component of their illness recedes to the background. This may be because of the greater social acceptance of physical complaints than of psychological complaints that are either not taken seriously or are believed to be cured by rest or extra praying. The increase in somatic symptoms can be explained by the seriousness with which people in a given culture view 'psychological stress' compared with physical illness. Non-Western cultures emphasize social integration rather than autonomy.

However, when affiliation is more important than achievement, how one appears to others is vital, and shame becomes more of a driving force than guilt. In the same way, physical illness and somatic manifestations of psychological distress are more acceptable and likely to evoke a caring response than vague complaints of psychological symptoms, which can be either disregarded or considered a stigma of being 'soft' – or, even worse, insane (Okasha et al., 1977; Gawad and Arafa, 1980).

Egyptians who are depressed either resort to their primary health care physician, who is likely to request unneeded and costly investigations, or ask traditional healers to alleviate their suffering. A considerable number do not ask for help at all, especially in rural populations, among which absenteeism from work or inability to face day-to-day affairs is largely tolerated by the community.

## Suicide and parasuicide

Feelings of hopelessness and the intention to kill oneself are not common among Muslims, for whom losing hope in anticipated relief by God and self-inflicted death are both blasphemous and punishable in the afterlife. However, the rates of suicide attempts (deliberate self-harm or parasuicide) that are intended to elicit care have no significant associations with religiousness among Arabs. Although the wish to die is not uncommon among people with depression in Arab cultures, it

usually remains at the level of wishing that God would terminate their life, and does not progress to the wish to kill themselves (Fakhr el Islam, 2000).

The crude rate of suicide attempts in Cairo was found to be 38.5 per 100 000. There was a high percentage in the age group 15–44 years, with no major difference between the genders. Single patients represented 53 per cent of the total, with the greatest risk being among students (40 per cent). Depressive illnesses, hysterical reactions and adjustment disorders (in that order of frequency) were the main causes of the attempt. Overdose by tablet ingestion was the most commonly used method (80 per cent). Official government reports are misleading and do not represent the true rate; assuming that one in ten suicide attempts ends with actual suicide, a crude estimate of suicide in Egypt would be about 3.5 per 100 000 (Okasha and Lotaief, 1979). A study in 1981–1982 showed that the majority of suicide attempters were young women living in large, overcrowded families. They showed a higher prevalence to be single, literate and unemployed than found in the corresponding age group in the general population. Drug overdose was the method most commonly used. The majority made their attempt at home when there was somebody nearby, and 31 per cent had made previous nonserious attempts. Dysthymic disorders and adjustment, affective and personality disorders were the most common diagnoses encountered (Okasha et al., 1986).

## Acute psychosis

The symptomatological and diagnostic differentiation and outcome of acute psychosis were studied in 50 Egyptian patients using the Schedule of Clinical Assessment of Acute Psychotic States (Wig and Parhee, 1984). The prevailing symptoms were delusions, worry, irritability, mood changes and disturbed behaviour. Almost two-thirds (64 per cent) of the patients were symptom-free when assessed one year later. The category of acute and transient polymorphic psychotic disorder with or without stress described in ICD-10 encompasses these clinical syndromes (Okasha et al., 1993a).

## Schizophrenia

In Egypt, schizophrenia is the most common chronic psychosis and accounts for the majority of inpatients in Egyptian mental hospitals. The nature of their delusions reflects the individual characteristics of the patients in relation to their identification and practice of Egyptian culture. What strikes one first and foremost in schizophrenia occurring among Egyptians from rural areas is the belief in the intervention of supernatural beings, occult forces or magic. Persecutory delusions with ideas of reference are the rule; religious, political, scientific and sexual delusions are frequent; financial, social, health-related, emotional and autistic delusions are less common, and delusions of grandeur are uncommon. Religious delusions are frequent, owing to the highly religious nature of Egyptian society. Political delusions are positively correlated with the level of political sanctions and pressure. Sexual delusions are more common in groups in whom sexual behaviour is severely suppressed, for example single and rural patients.

Our observations revealed that catatonic forms of the disorder are relatively common compared with other varieties, and more common than found in developed countries. The main symptoms are retardation, withdrawal, mutism and stupor, which may be interrupted by outbursts of excitement. Many patients present with an undifferentiated type of schizophrenia, exhibiting a wide variety of symptoms such as confused thinking and a turmoil of emotion manifested by perplexity, ideas of reference, fear, dream states and dissociative phenomena (Okasha *et al.*, 1993b).

## Child and adolescent psychiatry

Egyptian children under five years old (9.5 million) and those aged 5–16 years (14.5 million) constitute 14.8 per cent and 24.7 per cent of the total population, respectively (Ministry of Health, 1999). Thus, almost 40 per cent of the Egyptian population of 67 million are under 16 years old. The number of working children under 12 years of age is more than 1 million. Egyptian children constitute 7 per cent of the country's labour force (Central Agency for Public Mobilization and Statistics, 1992). The general public does not favour the inclusion of disorders of children and adolescents within the province of psychiatrists, although prevalence rates indicate that such disorders constitute a considerable percentage of the profile of psychiatric illness in Egypt.

### Emotional disorders

In the 1999 national survey of Egyptian children and adolescents ($n = 14271$, aged 10–18 years), 59 per cent of the sample reported experiencing feelings of fear or anxiety. Girls reported this more than boys, urban dwellers substantially more than rural dwellers (63.2 per cent versus 55.7 per cent), adolescents of higher socio-economic status more than those of middle to lower status, and working adolescents less than non-working ones. Fear was more reported by adolescents who were in school compared with those who were not (Ibrahim *et al.*, 1999). More than 35 per cent of high school students showed moderate anxiety on the Taylor Anxiety Scale and the majority of them had a history of exposure to chronic stress. The prevalence was higher among secondary school students (40.8 per cent) than among preparatory school students (32.8 per cent), showing significant correlation with older age, neurotic traits in childhood, larger family size, lower family income, a disturbed parental relationship and parental separation by divorce rather than death (Seif El Din, 2000). Psychiatric co-morbidity revealed a prevalence of 58.4 per cent, with neurotic stress-related disorders and somatoform disorders being the most common diagnoses (Okasha *et al.*, 1999a).

Anxiety disorders were diagnosed in 7.9 per cent and hyperkinetic disorder in 2.2 per cent of a sample of 8459 schoolchildren aged 6–12 years. Nocturnal enuresis was present in 1.9 per cent of children in Egyptian surveys. Bedwetting is tolerated in a child up to the age of 5–6 years; the age at which parents decide to do something about it is usually 7–10 years. The greatest prevalence of stammering was found in two age groups: 6–7 years and 11–12 years. At all ages stammering was more prevalent in males than in females, with a gender ratio of 3.2:1 (Okasha *et al.*, 1999b).

Another study revealed a 7.9 per cent prevalence rate of anxiety among Egyptian primary school children. Psychiatric co-morbidity was found in 89 per cent of the anxiety-positive sample, including mainly 'behavioural and emotional disorders with onset usually occurring in childhood' and 'neurotic, stress-related and somatoform disorders'. Forty per cent of children with anxiety disorders had a co-morbid depressive disorder (Okasha et al., 1999b).

In a governorate-wide study involving a representative sample of primary and preparatory schools in the city of Alexandria 10.3 per cent of pupils demonstrated depressive scores, which were highest among the oldest age group (20.3 per cent). Girls were highly represented among depression scores compared with boys. Lack of communication and presence of child–parent conflict ranked highest among predisposing factors (23.4 per cent), followed by parental conflicts (20.7 per cent) and scholastic problems (29.8 per cent). In 90.1 per cent of the depressed sample there were frequent complaints of physical symptoms for more than six months prior to the study (Abou Nazel, 1989). Adolescents who had a positive history of suicide attempts had significantly higher depression scores (93.7 per cent) (Abou Nazel et al., 1991). Egyptian children suffering from depressive episodes present to the clinic with other symptoms, such as nocturnal enuresis and headache. Ten per cent of them met conduct disorder criteria and 15 per cent had mixed anxiety and depressive disorder according to ICD-10 criteria (Seif El Din, 1990). Frequently they receive symptomatic treatment without identification of the underlying psychiatric disorder (Attia et al., 1991).

### Behavioural disorders

Behavioural problems in childhood are frequently interpreted as misbehaviour that can be managed by punishment or reward within the family. Within overcrowded schools, teachers are less likely to differentiate between children with a developmental disorder, adjustment disorder or mild learning diability. Behaviour disorders represented 5 per cent (in 1967) and 8.2 per cent (in 1990) of diagnoses in all children attending the outpatient psychiatric facilities of the Ain Shams University hospitals (Okasha et al., 1993a). The presenting symptoms were mainly hyperactivity, aggression, stealing and wandering. This problem was more common in patients from the cities; in Egyptian villages, conditions are conducive to the development of happy and socially secure children. Such children learn crafts and appropriate conduct smoothly from their everyday coexistence with parents and elders, and are gradually initiated into the fuller social responsibilities of the extended family community.

When villagers move to the cities, their work becomes mechanized, and mothers as well as fathers work away from home. They pass on to their children little knowledge and fewer skills which could earn them the children's respect. In such circumstances, it is difficult for parents to train their children in social responsibilities, so different from those with which the parents themselves grew up; hence, delinquency and behaviour disorders tend to develop out of lack of modelling and identity crises. Since compulsory schooling is more enforced in the cities, there is also a tendency to see more cases of educational problems there.

Temper tantrums are a common complaint in families with three-year-old children. Most of the time parents respond to a tantrum by giving their children what they want; this may aggravate this developmental problem, which constitutes 23 per cent of behavioural problems in preschool nurseries (Seif El Din et al., 1989).

Nocturnal enuresis, particularly secondary nocturnal enuresis, is the most common type of behaviour disorder presenting to urban primary health care facilities; it accounts for 63.9 per cent to 82.5 per cent of all behavioural disorders (Koura et al., 1993). Hyperactivity and attention-deficit symptoms are encountered significantly more often among children who are underachievers. Attention-deficit hyperactivity disorder is six times more common among boys than girls (Hassan, 1999). This disorder puts children under great pressure since they are usually treated as misbehaving both at home and at school, and most of them are exposed to corporal punishment (Youssef et al., 1998a,b). Violent behaviour was nearly 2.5 times more common among children and adolescents subjected to corporal punishment at school, and even higher among those who were subjected to this form of punishment by their caregivers. The condition is frequently associated with poor communication between adult carers and the child, leading to the use of verbal and physical punishment as a tool to control and shape the proper behaviour of the children (Youssef *et al.*, 1998b).

### Smoking and drug misuse

Smoking and drug misuse were found among 6 per cent of a large national sample. An additional 2 per cent of children reported having tried smoking only once. Boys report smoking at considerably higher incidence than girls (11.2 per cent versus 0.3 per cent) and more boys than girls have tried smoking once. Working boys smoke twice as much as non-working boys. Peer influence was reported by 41.1 per cent of the sample as the reason for starting smoking (Ibrahim *et al.*, 1999).

## Learning difficulties

The prevalence of scholastic under-achievement in a sample of pupils attending elementary schools was 42.8 per cent. Diagnoses made in this group included attention-deficit hyperactivity disorder, depression, anxiety, speech difficulties and elimination problems, none of which had been detected by their teachers. Underachievers also had significantly more physical disabilities leading to school backwardness, such as visual and hearing deficits (Hassan, 1999).

Parents are often over-demanding in relation to the academic achievement of their children, even in the earliest years, and this leads to an increase in the school drop-out rate. In an Egyptian national survey a quarter of boys aged 10–19 years and a third of girls are not at school, with the highest proportion coming from families of lower socio-economic status (Ibrahim *et al.*, 1999). The awareness of parents and school staff of children's needs at different phases of development is often inadequate. A child who is an under-achiever at school is usually labelled as 'mentally retarded' by the teachers and is referred to the student psychiatric clinic for psychological assessment. During the academic year 1998–1999 the number of children referred for this reason constituted 31.8 per cent of the total number of referred children; after complete assessment, the percentage of children with this diagnosis dropped to 18.9 per cent (Seif El Din, 2000).

Childhood disorders that have priority in Egyptian health planning are life-threatening conditions such as diarrhoea and acute respiratory infections. The country has few psychiatrists specializing in childhood problems. Figures from the Central Agency for Public Mobilization and Statistics indicate that mother and child care units are gradually being replaced by urban health centres, and the same is happening to the 305 school health units, which had incorporated 17 psychiatric units across the country. The problem is not only the lack of resources for providing mental health care facilities to children, but also the attitude of the community to child mental health problems. A small percentage of general psychiatrists have an interest in child psychiatry, but their knowledge and skill are based on expertise and education acquired abroad. Egyptian universities do not offer a degree in child psychiatry in spite of the magnitude and severity of mental health problems in childhood.

## Drug misuse

The 1980s witnessed a sharp rise in morbidity due to drug misuse. Since then, Egyptian community leaders at all levels have demonstrated intense concern over this problem. Estimates of the magnitude of substance addiction and the changing pattern of drug availability showed that the most commonly used drugs in the 1980s were cannabis, opium, solid and liquid hypnosedatives, heroin and finally cocaine, in descending order of frequency (Okasha, 1996a). Although epidemiological data on drug misuse in Egypt are scarce, health professionals report a multitude of reasons for such concern, including an increase in the rate of addicts seeking psychiatric treatment (Al Azayem and Ez Eldin, 1996), increases in drug-related health problems (mainly overdose toxicity; Salem, 1998) and an alarming drop in age at initiation of drug use, with a consequent rise in adolescent addicts (Amer *et al.*, 1986). The average amount of heroin seized annually is about 50 kg; this represents about 10 per cent of total consumption. Therefore, it is safe to assume that 500 kg are consumed annually. If we calculate that the average daily intake is 0.25–0.5 g per addict, we arrive at an estimate of about 7000–10 000 heroin users in Egypt (Okasha, 1996b).

During the 1990s synthetic psychoactive drug use increased exponentially to become the third most commonly available drug following cannabis and alcoholic beverages. Towards the second half of the 1990s cannabis became prevalent in the form of *bango*, which is prepared from leaves of *Cannabis sativa*. The plant is increasingly widely cultivated in Egypt, especially in the Sinai peninsula.

Epidemiological research and clinical studies of known addicts show that there are twice as many who use more than one drug compared with those who use one drug exclusively. Thus, experts estimate that drug seizures represent a fifth of the real drug use in society. Using this formula, one can safely estimate the rate of 'experimentation' with drugs to be about 10–12 per cent in the 15–25 age group; the rate for drug 'misuse' would be 2.5–3 per cent, whereas those identified as drug 'addicts' would constitute less than 1 per cent of the population (65 million in 1998). Such estimates are alarming, and are a warning to policy-makers and service providers.

The present scene in Egypt is characterized by an unprecedented shift towards 'demand reduction' at the primary prevention level, hand in hand with efforts to provide services at both secondary and tertiary health care levels. Supply control mechanisms are seriously implemented and enforced (Al Akabawi, 2001).

Soueif (1994) reports different reasons for the different user categories. For secondary school students the main reason for drug use was recreational, or entertainment on happy social occasions, and the substance mostly used was hashish. Sedatives and hypnotics were the next most frequently used substances; these substances were used in situations of physical exhaustion and fatigue, and to cope with psycho-social problems or difficult working conditions, as well as at times of studying and examinations.

Egyptian surveys have found a gradual increase in the consumption of alcohol, leading to the prediction that this will be the most common form of substance misuse in the coming years. It is interesting to note that despite the relative availability of alcohol in Egypt compared with the Gulf States, the incidence of alcohol misuse is much higher in the latter countries, where the sale of alcohol is strictly prohibited on religious grounds (Okasha, 1996b).

## Geriatric psychiatry

Health care systems in Egypt have largely ignored the needs of the elderly. There are only sporadic programmes of care for the elderly, mainly initiated by the community or within the private sector. Those above 65 years old represent 4.4 per cent of Egypt's population. The country has 34 old people's homes for over a million elderly people, and some homes have waiting lists of over 1000 persons (Abyad *et al.*, 2001).

An increasing number of elderly people live alone, or with elderly spouses and/or with only one or two other family members. The 'Care With Love' programme was established to create a sustainable, well-trained cadre of home health care providers in Egypt in order to staff units delivering such services. It was developed at the Centre for Geriatric Services in partnership with the Coptic Evangelical Organization for Social Services and As'salam Hospital in Cairo. The first training course was run in 1996, and about 500 trainees have joined the programme, taking various courses between 1996 and 2003. Ain Shams University in Cairo has started a series of courses on old age psychiatry; in addition, the Malta Institute on Ageing runs a course (in Egypt), and medical schools have started slowly to introduce lectures on ageing for undergraduates (Iskandar, 1999). Egyptian universities offer a master's degree and doctorates in geriatrics, focusing on psychogeriatrics, which is addressed as a multidisciplinary issue.

## THERAPIES

### Psychotherapy

Psychotherapy is an important element of psychiatric management in Egypt, with a strong religious (Muslim or Coptic) emphasis. The behaviour of individuals in Arab culture is determined more by group needs and thinking rather than by those of the individual, so that the source of control of behaviour is external rather than internal.

Sources of distress and suffering on the one hand, and happiness on the other, are related to personal failure or success to achieve the expectations of significant others or of society at large. The emphasis is on conformity rather than self-actualization. One of the objectives of psychotherapy with Arab patients is to improve adaptation by whatever means available and to focus the therapy on the manifest stress or disability. The strategy is to deal primarily with conscious problems, symptoms, thoughts, feelings and memories.

In contrast to Western cultures, Arab culture is based on shame rather than guilt, so that an important motivation in social interactions is to save face and avoid being shamed. Inner desires, wishes and conflicts that are socially unacceptable must be kept secret. Inner exploration may threaten the integrity of the psyche. At the same time, gaining insight and self-realization is socially isolating. Affects already consciously experienced by the patient should be expressed and dealt with. The therapeutic relationship should be maintained at a positive level of rapport, with deeper transference responses remaining unconscious and out of the patient's awareness. Negative transference is discussed early so that it can be dissipated as promptly as possible, allowing the patient to experience the therapist as accepting, permissive and comfortable with hostile feelings. If the patient's defences are useful and acceptable, they can be strengthened and acknowledged; if the defences are maladaptive, new ones are suggested. The therapist also tries to improve the patient's self-image by minimizing the discrepancy between the patient's expectations of himself or herself (derived from the expectations of significant others) and his or her ability to realize these expectations (El Leithy, 2000).

## Alternative therapies

In spite of rapid social change in Egypt, the majority of people – especially in rural areas – belong to an extended family hierarchy. It is considered shameful to care for an elderly person with dementia away from family surroundings. The parents of children with learning disabilities or hyperkinetic disorders accept primary responsibility for them, rather than having them looked after in an institution.

Traditional and religious healers play a major role in primary psychiatric care in Egypt. They deal with minor neurotic, psychosomatic and transitory psychotic states using religious and group psychotherapies, suggestion and devices such as amulets and incantations (Okasha, 1966). About 60 per cent of outpatients at the university clinic in Cairo serving a population of low socioeconomic status had consulted a traditional healer before coming to the psychiatrist (Okasha et al., 1968). In rural areas of Egypt, community care is implemented without the need for health care workers. Those living in the countryside have a special tolerance of people with mental disorders and an ability to assimilate them into their community. These people, and those with mild or moderate learning disabilities, are rehabilitated daily by cultivating and planting the countryside along with, and under the supervision of, family members.

The need to add mental health care to the traditional priorities for public health care services, bilharziasis (schistosomiasis), birth control, infectious diseases of children, smoking and illicit drug use, has been gradually attracting the attention of decision-makers. Programmes for community care in big cities have been introduced in the form of outpatient psychiatric clinics, hostels for the elderly, institutions for people with learning disabilities, centres for the treatment of drug misuse, and school and university mental health services.

The National Mental Health Programme for Egypt emphasizes the role of primary health care in looking after 80 per cent of psychiatric patients. Its focus is on decentralization of mental health care and community care in different governorates. Emphasis is on recruiting mental health teams, especially psychiatric nurses, psychiatric social workers, occupational therapists and clinical psychologists (Okasha, 1993).

## THE FUTURE

Egypt has made substantial progress since the 1950s in reducing infant and child mortality, improving life expectancy and increasing access to health care. Major problems, however, remain. Public health challenges include high rates of maternal mortality, malnutrition, wide disparities between rural and urban areas, emphasis on curative rather than preventive care, the relative weakness of public health institutions, the variable quality of health care, lack of capacity in policy-making, and unresponsive and inequitable health systems.

The Arab Human Development report (2002) links current development status with external and internal conditions. The main external factor is military spending as a direct impediment to development, channelling resources away from development priorities such as health (including mental health). Alternative strategies conducive to development would be greater spending on technological development, empowerment of vulnerable groups, such as women and children, and promotion of democracy and human rights. In view of the lack of human resources, mental health policies and legislation in the majority of the world's developing countries, such as Egypt, have developed in partnership with other community agencies agents such as non-governmental organizations and consumer groups. This process has to ensure relevance and improvements in standards of care for psychiatric patients.

## REFERENCES

Abou Nazel, M.W. 1989: Study of depression among preparatory school children. Doctoral degree thesis, University of Alexandria.

Abou Nazel, M., Fahmy, S., Younis, I., Seif El Din, A.G., Abdel Fatah, M., Mokhtar, S. and Ayoub, A.I. 1991: A study of depression among Alexandria preparatory school adolescents. *Journal of the Egyptian Public Health Association* 66, 6.

Abyad, A., Ashour, A.M. and Abou-Saleh, M.T. 2001: The scope of psychogeriatrics in the Arab world. In Okasha, A. and Maj, M. (eds) *Images in Psychiatry. An Arab Perspective.* Geneva: World Psychiatric Association, 175–88.

Al Akabawi, A. 2001: Drug abuse in the Arab world. A country profile of Egypt. In Okasha, A. and Maj, M. (eds) *Images in Psychiatry. An Arab Perspective.* Geneva: World Psychiatric Association, 143–50.

Al Azayem, A. and Ez Eldin, A.G. 1996: Changing pattern of substance abuse and its reflection on management programs. *Proceedings of First Egyptian International Conference on Addiction and Drug Abuse.* Cairo: Ministry of Health.

Amer, H., Saleh, H., Guirguis, W., Bassiouni, F. and Gueneldy, M. 1986: Use of Delphi technique in determining certain factors related to drug dependence among youth: part I. *Bulletin of the High Institute of Public Health* 16, 63–77.

Arab Human Development Report 2002: *Arab Human Development Report.* New York: United Nations Development Program, Regional Bureau for Arab States. 145–49.

Attia, M., Abou Nazel, M., Guirguis, W. and Seif El Din, A. 1991: Impact of a mental health program on the utilization of the psychiatric clinic in Sporting Students' Hospital. *Journal of the Egyptian Public Health Association* 66, 6.

Central Agency for Public Mobilization and Statistics 1992: *Annual Report.* Cairo: CAPMAS.

El Leithy, W. 2000: Arab psychotherapy. In Okasha, A. and Maj, M. (eds) *Images in Psychiatry. An Arab Perspective.* Geneva: World Psychiatric Association, 247–54.

Fakhr el Islam 2000: Social psychiatry and the impact of religion. In Okasha, A. and Maj, M. (eds) *Images in Psychiatry. An Arab Perspective.* Geneva: World Psychiatric Association, 21–36.

Gawad, M.S. and Arafa, M. 1980: Transcultural study of depressive symptomatology. *Egyptian Journal of Psychiatry* 3, 163–82.

Hassan, E. 1999: Epidemiological study of scholastic underachievement among primary school children in Alexandria: prevalence and causes. Thesis, Faculty of Nursing, University of Alexandria.

Ibrahim, B., Sallam, S., El Tawila, S., El Gibaly, O. and El Sahn, F. 1999: *Transitions to Adulthood. A National Survey of Egyptian Adolescents.* Cairo: Population Council.

Iskandar, M. 1999: Care With Love training programme for home health care providers. *Al-Raida* 16, 57–58.

Koura, M., Abdel Aal, N., Khairy, A. and Seif El Din, A. 1993: Study of the role of Alexandria Primary Health Care Program in the assessment of behaviour disorders of primary school children, part II: Appraisal of school mental health services provided by primary health care facilities. *Bulletin of the High Institute of Public Health* 23, 919–30.

Ministry of Health 1999: *Health Insurance of North West of Egypt. School Health Insurance Annual Statistics Report.* Alexandria: Ministry of Health.

Okasha, A. 1966: A cultural psychiatric study of El-Zar cult in UAR. *British Journal of Psychiatry* 112, 1217–21.

Okasha, A. 1967: Hysteria: its presentation and management in Egypt. *Ains Shams Medical Journal* 18, 13–20.

Okasha, A. 1993: Psychiatry in Egypt. *Psychiatric Bulletin* 17, 548–51.

Okasha, A. 1996a: Combat and management of drug abuse: means and challenges. An Egyptian perspective. In

*Proceedings of the First Egyptian International Conference on Addiction and Drug Abuse.* Cairo: Ministry of Health.

Okasha, A. 1996b: Substance use is a major public health hazard. In *Proceedings of the First Egyptian International Conference on Addiction and Drug Abuse.* Cairo: Ministry of Health.

Okasha, A. 2001: History of mental health in the Arab world. In Okasha, A. and Maj, M. (eds) *Images in Psychiatry: An Arab Perspective.* Geneva: World Psychiatric Association, 1–20.

Okasha, A. and Ashour, A. 1981: Psycho-demographic study of anxiety in Egypt: the PSE in its Arabic version. *British Journal of Psychiatry* 139, 70–73.

Okasha, A. and Karam, E. 1998: Mental health services and research in the Arab World. *Acta Psychiatrica Scandinavica* 98, 406–13.

Okasha, A. and Lotaief, F. 1979: Attempted suicide: an Egyptian investigation. *Acta Psychiatrica Scandinavica* 60, 69–75.

Okasha, A. and Okasha, T. 2000: Mental health in Cairo (Al-Qahira). *International Journal of Mental Health* 28, 62–68.

Okasha, A., Kamel, M. and Hassan, A.H. 1968: Preliminary psychiatric observations in Egypt. *British Journal of Psychiatry* 114, 949–55.

Okasha, A., Kamel, M., Sadek, A. and Lotaif, Z.B. 1977: Psychiatric morbidity among university students in Egypt. *British Journal of Psychiatry* 131, 149–54.

Okasha, A., Lotaief, F. and El Mahallawy, N. 1986: Descriptive study of attempted suicide in Cairo. *Egyptian Journal of Psychiatry* 9, 53–90.

Okasha, A., Khalil, A.H., El Fiky, M.R., Ghanem, M. and Hakeem, R.A. 1988: Prevalence of depressive disorders in a sample of rural and urban Egyptian communities. *Egyptian Journal of Psychiatry* 2, 167–81.

Okasha, A., Seif El Dawla, A. and Asaad, T. 1993a: Presentation of hysteria in a sample of Egyptian patients – an update. *Neurology, Psychiatry and Brain Research* 1, 155–59.

Okasha, A., Seif El Dawla, A., Khalil, A.H. and Saad, A. 1993b: Presentation of acute psychosis in an Egyptian sample: a transcultural comparison. *Comprehensive Psychiatry* 34, 4–9.

Okasha, A., Khalil, A.H., Seif El Dawla, A., Khalil, A.H. and Yehia, N. 1994: Phenomenology of obsessive–compulsive disorder: a transcultural study. *Comprehensive Psychiatry* 35, 191–97.

Okasha, A., Bishry, Z. and Ragheb, K. 1999a: Anxiety disorder in a sample of Egyptian adolescents: a psychodemographic study. *Current Psychiatry* 6, 342–54.

Okasha, A., Bishry, Z. and Seif El Dawla, A. 1999b: Anxiety symptoms in an Egyptian sample: children and adolescents. *Current Psychiatry* 6, 356–68.

Salem, S. 1998: *Annual Statistical Report.* Alexandria: Poison Center, Alexandria Main University Hospital.

Seif El Din, A. 1990: Evaluation of the training program for professionals working with school children in Alexandria. *Alexandria Journal of Pediatrics* 4, 61–68.

Seif El Din, A. 2000: Child psychiatry in the Arab world. In Okasha, A. and Maj, M. (eds) *Images in Psychiatry: An Arab Perspective.* Geneva: World Psychiatric Association, 151–66.

Seif El Din, A., Badawy, Y., Kader, E. and Kamel, M. 1989: Behavioural screening for pre-school children in Alexandria. *Bulletin of the High Institute of Public Health* 19, 363–77.

Soueif, M.I. 1994: *Extent and Patterns of Drug Use Among Students and Working Class Men in Egypt.* Cairo: National Centre for Social and Criminological Research.

Wig, N. and Parhee, R. 1984: Acute transient psychosis. A view from the developing countries. In Mezzich, J.E. and von Granach, M. (eds) *International Classification in Psychiatry.* Cambridge: Cambridge University Press, 1987, 115–21.

Youssef, R., Attia, M. and Kamel, M. 1998a: Children experiencing violence. I: Paternal use of corporal punishment. *Child Abuse and Neglect* 22, 959–73.

Youssef, R., Attia, M. and Kamel, M. 1998b: Children experiencing violence. II: Prevalence and determinants of corporal punishment in schools. *Child Abuse and Neglect* 22, 975–85.

# 15

# Culture and mental health services in the Horn of Africa: Ethiopia

## Daniel Fekadu

## INTRODUCTION

This chapter begins with a short account of the unique geography of Ethiopia and a history of the Ethiopian people with special reference to kinship, culture, social structure and immigration. The next two sections focus on mental disorders and the services available, both native and modern. The fourth section deals with systems issues such as policy, service development and research. Finally, I give some concluding thoughts. The major cultures and people are described in relative detail, as it is impossible to cover all ethnicities in the chapter. As there are also many languages in Ethiopia, the text refers to Amharic speakers throughout the chapter, unless it is stated otherwise.

## Geography

Ethiopia is located in what is commonly referred as the 'horn', in the north-eastern part of Africa. Its neighbours are Djibouti and Somalia to the east, the Sudan to the west, the Sudan and Kenya to the south, and Eritrea to the north.

The climate is mainly tropical, with long dry seasons from September to May, and a short wet season from June to August. The north is mainly a highland terrain. The south is mainly lowland with fertile green fields, the famous Rift Valley, and its lakes. There are islands in some of these lakes that are inhabited by isolated ethnic minority groups (Zewde, 1991, p. 1).

## The People

Ethiopia is an ancient and beautiful country with a rich history. It is best known for its prehistoric archaeological findings, such as *Dənk näsh* (*Australopithecus afarensis*, a.k.a. 'Lucy'), surviving as the only independent nation through the colonization era (except for five years of Italian occupation) and for its long-distance runners (Johanson and Taieb, 1976). Notable are the ancient civilizations of Meroe, Axum, Lalibela and Gondar. Both the ancient Christian and Muslim texts have records of its people and the rulers. In the Western media Ethiopia is notoriously portrayed in terms of harrowing images of its starving children and endless wars.

There are 70 languages and over 200 dialects (Zewde, 1991, p. 5). Almost all of these use the unique and ancient Geez script for writing. Neighbouring countries on the other hand use Arabic or Latin alphabets. Geez is now only used among the clergy of Orthodox Christians and its scholastic system. Each script represents a sound. It is a distant family to ancient South Yemen and Middle Eastern Semitic languages. Ethiopia, for example, is written as ኢትዮጵያ. Linguistically there are four parent languages that correspond to the natives and early migrants who inhabited the country, namely the Nilo-Saharan, Cushitic, Omotic, and Semitic groups. The main languages are Oromiffa, Amharic and Tigrigna. Official languages are Amharic and English; in addition some of the federal regions have started to use their preferred languages, and Latin alphabets for writing. People near the borders have more in common culturally than in the central highlands.

The population is estimated at 69.1 million, the second highest in sub-Saharan Africa. Children under 15 years old account for 44 per cent. It has one of the highest fertility rates at 5.9, and the life expectancy at birth is 54 (Ministry of Health, 2004).

The staple diet around the north and the centre is *ənjära*, soft and sour wrapping bread that is prepared from flour of the tiny indigenous grains of *teff* (*Eragrostis teff*). The equivalent in the south is *kocho* made from the roots of enset (*Enset ventricosum*), a false banana. People in the east use millet, maize, wheat or sorghum. Accompanying stews are cooked from different vegetables, cereals and meat (Zewde, 1991, p. 4). A local beer called *tälla*, mead (*täj*) and a distilled spirit called *aräki/katikala* are widely consumed. There are a number of beer, wine and spirit factories that have expanded recently.

## The state

Power transition was mainly through subterfuge and bloodshed among many dynasties and rulers. Ethiopia was ruled by different kings from the Axum dynasty in the first century to the Shoan dynasty in 1974. The State and the Church, or mosques, were closely linked through most of these kingdoms (Tamene, 1998). In 1974 the Derg, a group of armed forces, put an end to the Empire and put in place a Marxist–Leninist one-party rule.

The war with Eritrea intensified massively during the Derg regime. Thousands of people were killed, tortured and uprooted. The 'Red Terror' was a very long campaign against all forms of opposition. On a positive note the Derg put an end to the feudal system of land ownership, set up a literacy campaign and introduced basic units of administration called *käbäle*.

In 1991 a group of rebel fronts took over from the Derg. This government supports a multiparty democratic system and federalism based on ethnic groups, and has just won a third controversial term in office.

## Social structure

The end of the Empire signalled the end of the old dichotomous hierarchy of the mainly Amhara nobility or landlords versus peasantry, which was replaced by a land reform giving the rights to the poor peasants.

The main social structure at present is therefore between the urban and rural majority. Within the urban population this gap is expanding. The businesses in the towns and cities mainly thrive on trade, consumable-related activities and exports such as coffee, hides and skins.

In most Ethiopian cultures it is customary to show modesty and respect to others by exchanging greeting, shaking hands (two hands and bowing from the head, especially if older), standing up when adults arrive and saying 'näwor' whilst waiting until they have sat down or have given permission by saying 'bägzher' (by God, please be seated), avoiding eye gaze, not interrupting, addressing using titles such as *Ato/Woizero/Woizerit* (Mr/Mrs/Miss) or in the plural as *ərso* or *antu* (similar to the French *vous*) unless they are minors. Most Ethiopians use their first names and their father's (a paternal grandfather's first name may be added as necessary), so there is no surname or maiden name as such (Zewde, 1991, p. 235).

In spite of all the dynamic social changes in the last three decades, the following social and occupational groups still carry prestige to a varying extent: elders, parents, the clergy, professionals, officials, and the rich.

## Kinship

Ethiopians have a very close kinship system. They may address even distant relatives and close friends as their siblings or uncles, a metaphor indicating intimacy. The Oromo have a more elaborate and hierarchical democratic structure based on age groups, the *Gada* (Legesse, 1973, p. 8). Here everyone has a clear and defined role which is respected by the rest of the group, including women and children.

The typical Ethiopian family is extended and is a central unit of communal life. It is the duty of the young and the able-bodied to support the elderly. Children are mostly considered as a grace, a source of fortune and respect. Parents are often addressed through their eldest child, for example if the children are boys called Abebe, Miruts and a daughter called Derartu, in respective order, then the parents are known as 'father/mother of Abebe'.

In rural communities, children start helping their family early and get initiated into herding cattle and sheep, farming or domestic work often before 10 years of age (Central Statistical Authority, 2001). They marry young and claim their own piece of land, and then they all continue to live within huts built in close proximity to the parents. This means that a distinctive network of first-, second- and third-rank families, living closely is not uncommon. In urban areas life is often more competitive, materialistic and less cohesive; people tend to marry later and in some cases not at all (Kinfu, 2000).

Marriage and the number of spouses are influenced by religious and traditional factors. The Christians are monogamous, except in some parts of the Gurage (Shack, 1964). Polygamy is practised among the Muslims or some of the descendants of the indigenous inhabitants such as the Oromo and Gambella.

Neighbours, friends, acquaintances and colleagues have all-important, albeit equal roles as the extended family within the supportive network. They are part of the daily routine of life, and the immediate portal of call for good and bad times.

This is similar to the role played by social workers in developed Western countries.

## Migration

Over many years, there have been numerous conflicts internally and across borders, internal migration and intermarriage of its people. The most recognized and major recent event is the mass deportation following the Ethiopia–Eritrea border dispute (De Jong *et al.*, 2001). Similarly, it is not uncommon for people living in the border regions, who are probably more similar to those in neighbouring countries than people in the centre in many ways, to share the privileges of Ethiopian hospitality as 'migrants'.

There are a few hundred isolated Rastafarians from the Caribbean, mainly from Jamaica, who have been settled in Shashemene, a town 240 km south of the capital, since early 1940s, as part of Emperor Haile-Selassie's sign of gratitude for their support during the struggle against the Italian Occupation. Given the abundance of research among the African Caribbeans in the UK, it is surprising that there are no similar published studies describing the mental health of the first or second generation of this Caribbean origin group living in Ethiopia.

As a result of the various wars and persecutions, people have always moved about, either as groups, families or individuals. This has invariably affected all ethnic groups at one point or another. Others, such as the Gurage or Tigre, also immigrate for business. Importantly there were people from the respective ruling dynasties, mainly the Amhara soldier families, commonly known as the *näftäña*, who settled in other ethnic areas. The *näftäña* and their families were some of the major victims as a result of the ethnic clashes described above. Notable, but least publicized, recent interethnic carnages that resulted in mass immigration were those among peoples of the Arusi, Sidamo, Gambella and Borena regions of Ethiopia. There are very few published studies on the effects of immigration on Ethiopians' risk of mental illness, especially in relation to the most recent life events (Arieli *et al.*, 1996; Ponizovsky *et al.*, 1998; Fenta *et al.*, 2004; Halcon *et al.*, 2004).

## Culture

The indigenous inhabitants have their own religion and belief systems that have persisted in one way or another to the present day. This mainly includes animism and belief in the spirits. Most of the Tigrigna and Amharic speakers in the north are Christians, while most of the Oromiffa speakers are Muslims, but the natives also believe in Waaqa, also a monotheistic deity.

Whether it is due to its proximity to the Middle East, the positive attitudes of its rulers, the hospitality of its people, or a combination of all three, Judaism, Christianity and Islam found their way into Ethiopia earlier with relative ease and less conflict than that seen in other countries.

The various cultures of the people are therefore a colourful and harmonious blend of native values, traditions, and belief systems with those of the main Middle East religions. The spirits and the evil forces are widely accepted as causes and explanations for all sorts of misfortunes and ills, whether of the body or the soul. So it is legitimate among the Christians to simultaneously practise and believe in God, the *tabot* (replica of the Ark of the Covenant), circumcision, etc. It is acceptable to combine this with *adbar* (a protective spirit), exorcism, sorcery, auguries, *wuqabi* (a possession by spirits), witchcraft, and so on without a noticeable dissonance. Likewise, a Muslim could do the same by having a mixed belief in Allah and *shekoch* (the wise men). It is acceptable to acknowledge the central role of *khat* (leaves of a shrub plant with amphetamine-like effects)-chewing ceremonies for *dua* (intense prayer or intercession on behalf of someone) and of the beliefs stated above.

## MENTAL HEALTH CARE

This section will take a closer look on the impact of cultural factors on traditional practices and modern mental health services (Kortman, 1987; Alem, 2001).

## Traditional

The inextricable link between religion, culture and belief system that passes through oral or written traditions across generations have been welded to, among other things, the established practice of dealing with mental health problems. Therefore, most behavioural disturbances are considered as either arising from or somehow explained by the works of the supernatural (Hamer and Hamer, 1966; Giel et al., 1968; Uhlman and Minas, 1975; Kahana, 1985; Araya and Aboud, 1993, pp. 493–506; Alem et al., 1999). Although there is a significant overlap, these are classified as the works of numerous 'good', 'bad' and 'ugly' spirits for convenience in this chapter.

### The good spirits

In the first group of 'good spirits', problems attributed to God, Allah, the angels and saints or Waaqa (a traditional Oromo equivalent of God) are probably considered as deserved punishments. In some cases this could be atonement for the sins committed by previous generations extending to seventh-rank families. This is commonly known as *ərgəman* ('a curse'). This may either be considered as a cause of mental illness or in some cases is thought to explain why they have inherited certain conditions, such as *zar* or any heritable condition such as Down's syndrome or severe mental illness.

*Zar* has been described by many foreign writers as a 'culture-bound syndrome', and is classified as such in the *Diagnostic and Statistical Manual of Mental Disorders* (DSM-IV) (Kahana, 1985; Grisaru et al., 1997; Rahim, 2001). Although culturally tolerated and dealt with, *zar* is invariably a chronic state also seen in neighbouring countries extending to North Africa and the Middle East. The sufferer, commonly a female, presents with a typical episode manifested either with speaking in tongues or intense ritualistic dance and vocalization (*guria*), often in the company of an audience comprising family members, neighbours or a selected group of similarly affected people. Each episode lasts for minutes and at times hours. It then culminates when the possessed victim is exhausted and some of the demands of the possessing spirit to leave its victim ('the horse') are promised by a cajoling ritual from the audience. This is often a gift such as perfume, particular embroidered cloth or a slaughter of certain description of sheep or chicken. *Zar* results in enormous distress and dysfunction to the sufferers, and is more of a burden to the families than any of the non-psychotic disorders described in DSM-IV.

### The bad spirits

The commonest and widely dreaded 'bad spirit' is that perpetrated by other people, normally friends, and hence the saying *amläke käwädaj məqäña täbəkäñ* (My God protect me from my friends, for I know how to protect myself from known enemies). It is a basic common wisdom for the typical Ethiopian to be suspicious and exercise caution in his daily routines from any *yäsäw ayn* (a benign variant of evil eye) or *məkäña* (envy). Indeed, his Morning Prayer and mantra may include *amlake məkäña atasatäñ* (My God, don't deprive me of my envious neighbours, lest I would lose the motivation and aspiration to prosper). This is even worse if they fall out with their friend. If the person has not got the powers to cast spells on their enemies, they may not hesitate to consult the experts such as a *baləj* (a type of herbalist), *awaqi* (a wise man) or *tänquay* (wizard).

Also recognized and within the realms of the intrigues of the 'bad' or evil spirit are conditions that range from those carried out by ordinary individuals, such as the curses of the envious (*məkäña*) to *məch* (sudden exposure to sun), *yäsäw ayn*, *təla wägi*, *buda* (evil eye), and different descriptions of the Devil such as *mägaña*, *djinni*, *ganen* or *shäytan*. These are often related to an acute onset of loss of body function or mental disturbance. Hence *mägaña mätaw* (the Devil hit him) could be an alternative explanation for Bell's palsy or acute psychosis. Similarly, a fever blister or oral herpes could be a result of *mətch mätaw* (the sun hit him), exposure to midday sun after forgetting to wash the mouth after eating.

The most feared is probably *märz mablat or matätat* (poisoning through lacing someone's food or drink). This is thought to be fatal or result in loss of the faculties, such that the victim either gets bankrupt and wanders off in the streets, develops debilitating physical ailments, or an *absho*. The latter is described as a chronic state of mental poisoning complicated by alcohol idiosyncrasy. Therefore there will be a brief spell of relapse only when the subject imbibes some alcoholic drink. The commonest presentation of paranoid illness is poisoning of food, and often only a detailed history could uncover the delusional content. Perhaps the custom of initial tasting of food and drink by the host

is a reassurance to the guest that there is no malign intention, at least during the encounter. Other 'bad spirits' include *sänkala*, *dänkara*, *masakäl* and *mätät* (sorcery); *andärbi* and *asmat* (magic).

These various 'bad spirits' are believed to manifest in many ways. *Manzäfzäf* or *ləkəft* (convulsion), *manqätqät*, *yämitl bäshəta* (fits) could all mean seizure or pseudo-seizures (Tekle-Haimanot *et al.*, 1991). Alternatively, *gagərt* (stupor or mutism) could be a feature of depression, catatonia, aphonia, elective mutism, or even manic stupor. *əbdät* (madness) or *chärq mätal* (throwing off clothes) is a rather generic reference to all forms of agitation such as psychoses or mania, while *buda mäbälat* (to be devoured by the evil eyed, signifying the acute nature and severity of the spell from the ordinary evil eye or *yäsäw ayn*) might be a manifestation of a conversion disorder.

### The ugly spirits

In the third group is the widely held belief in superstition, common to many cultures including prophecy, omens and auguries (Pankhurst, 1990b, pp. 201–4). They are associated with rituals and are mainly a means of self-protection from illnesses and misfortunes. The omission of these rituals may be considered as an explanation of ill fate. They may also influence decisions and plans. In some cases of 'bad spirits' they could be deliberately placed as in *dänqara* or *mätät* to cast spells on others. The degree of conviction varies from individual to individual, but many people have one or more of their own. Consultations may be made from a wizard, or a fortune teller, for example, *Ayantu* among the Oromo. The annual traditional group rituals of sacrifices in *Adbar* (a protective spirit) held each May are still practised widely.

## Pathways to care

The typical response of families to an acute onset of behavioural disturbance is to call neighbours for opinion and assistance. If it is agreed to be *buda* (evil eye), they arrange for urgent exorcism aided by fumigation of *dign* (sulphur) or forcing the victim to sniff some other pungent substance. These coercive processes are so excruciating that it will not be more than a few minutes before the victim yields to the leading questions. Often an unfortunate neighbour may be named, with embarrassment, as the perpetrator of, for example, the evil eye. They would then be forced to acknowledge their act and spit on the victim, a sign of undoing the spell.

If it is considered as *Absho*, they would decide to let the victim get over the effects by gentle engagement over a few hours and give them space, and should that fail they would be subject to physical restraint. If there are convulsions or fits, someone will suggest lighting a match to let the victim smell the fumes or to sprinkle their face with *täbäl* (holy water). People may refrain from laying their hands on the victim until the crisis is completely over for fear of being possessed (Tekle-Haimanot *et al.*, 1991).

Some exaggerations of normal virtues such as being quiet and withdrawn are less likely to attract the family's attention. This may continue until the behaviour begins to have a significant effect on self-care and productivity or the family member starts to display severe behavioural disturbances.

All other forms of *əbdät*, characterized by psychomotor agitation such as being disruptive, destructive, assaulting, and abusive, singing incessantly, or being over-talkative, are often handled with physical restraint and isolation if engagement and reasoning with the person is unsatisfactory. Typically the patient's feet and arms are tied behind. The family would then try prayer or sprinkle them with holy water at home. If this fails he or she is usually taken to a priest or sheikh, for further prayer, and exorcism rituals, holy water or *dua* for a prescribed period, a minimum of a week or two. (Although not verified in Ethiopia, some holy water resorts are thought to have high salt contents including lithium; Moncrieff, 1997.) Similarly, all the types of case described above may find themselves at the healers if their conditions persist. It is only if these traditional healing methods fail that the family and the traditional healer may consider a visit to a modern health facility.

The rate at which this decision is made varies with the nature of the cases, the family's awareness, and the healer's attitude to modern health practices. By the time they reach modern health facilities they may have travelled for hours and sometimes days. They are often escorted by family, friends and colleagues. They are invariably dehydrated, and the site of rope ligature is often complicated with ulcers and infections.

Where the families were unable to restrain the victims, attend to them at the healers or bring them to modern mental health facilities, the victims may end as vagrants in nearby towns and cities; hence the saying '*əbd əna zənab kätäma yəwädal*' ('the mad and rain love the towns'). These vagrants live mainly by begging, stealing or feeding on leftovers and rubbish. Most learn to take substances such as *khat* or cigarettes, become settled, and achieve sustenance in urban areas, which further makes it unlikely for them to leave the towns, worsens their state of mind, or maintains their illness indefinitely (Alem and Shibre, 1997).

Although some recover spontaneously, others may find themselves in trouble with the law through their behaviour, such as severe self-neglect, wandering aimlessly and interfering with the traffic, violence to property and public. This is when the police may intervene and bring them to a modern mental facility. It is not also uncommon for some benevolent people to take the role of guardianship in getting them to a modern health facility. Some may perish from the poor living condition in towns as a result of starvation, car accidents or acquiring various forms of illnesses and infections.

Until about 50 years ago there was no Western model of psychiatry service in Ethiopia. However, detailed general records of the British diplomatic mission in 1841–1842 and the Russian Red Cross mission in 1896 included a range of diseases of the nervous system such as hysteria and mental derangement (Pankhurst, 1990a, pp. 197–8). This type of general medical service presumably continued until the establishment of Amanuel Hospital.

# MENTAL HEALTH SERVICES

## Amanuel Hospital

Amanuel is the only mental health hospital and one of the five specialist national hospitals in Addis Ababa. Apart from the grey literature, there is no published work on its establishment and early history. It is located in the western, deprived end of the city, where the inter-urban bus terminus, the noisy and dirty grain market with its large population of donkeys and the neighbouring Amanuel Church are all fascinating analogies of the chaos that is found in 'madness', as if to disguise, attract or at least be receptive to the experiences of the mentally ill.

During the Italian Occupation, the rulers segregated the natives to the western corner of Addis Ababa, and in 1938 opened the Hemanuel Ospedale per Indigeni de Tecla Haimanot (Emanuel Hospital for Natives of Tekle Haimanot) with four wards and 80–120 beds (Pankhurst, 1990a, p. 228). Towards the end of their rule, this served as an asylum, predominantly for the vagrant mentally ill, and this continued for many years with expansion of the wards. In 1947, when the Ministry of Health became independent, the budget and administrative staff were secured. In 1954 a British medical director, Dr Williams, was appointed to be the first psychiatrist and subsequently served at the hospital for five years (Fekadu *et al.*, 1999).

Dr Williams was later replaced consecutively by Dr Lee (South Korean) and then by Dr Pavicevic (Bulgarian). There was then a long period where a series of psychiatrists from Eastern Europe came in groups of 3–5 between the 1970s and late 1980s. Most did not know the local languages or culture, and routinely worked along with interpreters. Most patients were given a diagnosis of schizophrenia or manic depressive illness (Fekadu *et al.*, 2004). Almost everyone received a mixture of high-dose neuroleptics and unmodified bilateral electroconvulsive therapy (ECT). At times as many as 40 people received ECT daily so that the machine had to be dragged around the wards. It was left for the auxiliary and non-clinical staff to modify doses of medications and indeed administer ECT, shackle or handcuff people to bed railings or to put them inside metal-caged restraining beds.

In 1987, the Ethiopians Dr Mesfin Araya and Atalay Alem took over running the hospital consecutively. When they inherited this duty, the services were appalling and no doubt had inspired the plays *Amanuel därso mäls* (Return journey to Amanuel) and *Asra hulät əbdoch bäkätäma* (The 12 mad people in town). The 11 wards (three for women and eight for men) were so overcrowded that there were two patients per bed, and some had to sleep on the floor (Alem, 2004). Patients ate whilst sitting on the floor or in their beds. Most had their feet shackled and their hands cuffed. They spent the day idle. Most learnt to smoke cigarettes, and begged to supplement their habit. Some of the institutionalized patients sold cigarettes, leading many new patients to incur huge debts, paid for by their visitors.

It was not uncommon for some patients to improve whilst on a waiting list, but some were required to visit the hospital on a daily or twice daily basis to receive injections of neuroleptic and refills of oral medications. The hospital informally served as a sort of half-way hostel, like those now proposed in the developed world.

When Dr Menilik Desta took over in 1996, there had been many innovations in the administrative, clinical and academic aspects of the hospital, all run by indigenous staff. There were only 360 beds, and one patient per bed. The administrative staff had clearly defined roles. All clinical services were run by qualified personnel who received appropriate and close supervision. A matron and a nurse in charge ran the admission and allocation of outpatients to the clinics.

There was a well-stocked and efficient pharmacy run by a pharmacist and two technicians. An ECT suite with clear procedures, guidelines and a rota for each ward and psychiatrist was in place. Each ward had a designated psychiatrist, a resident psychiatrist, a psychiatric nurse, a nurse assistant and a psychologist. There was a library, a regular journal club run by the residents, a brief daily handover morning meeting of all doctors and a well-established psychiatry nursing school.

Apart from expanding the health manpower and consistency in the administration described above, the hospital has now been completely renovated at an estimated cost of £1 million. The barrack-like wards have been replaced with a concrete, single-storey complex building right in the middle of the premises, significantly reducing the risk of injuries to patients from absconding over the fence. The wards are still separated according to gender, but there is now a dining hall, modern facilities including offices and auditorium, library, internal telephone network and internet access. There is extensive space for various activities, sports, and occupational therapy. There is also a special addiction unit and a vibrant, generally academic atmosphere.

## Psychiatry units

These are clinics run by trained psychiatric nurses who often work in pairs. There are 43 active psychiatry units based in rural or regional hospitals throughout the country. By and large they work closely and smoothly with the other nurses and doctors however at times due to their perceived lower status they are subject to prejudice and contempt by the doctors. Overall they are successful in making mental health services accessible and are cost-effective alternatives. They have also reasonable retention rates due to the rigorous recruitment, job satisfaction and post training support systems (Alem, 2004).

## Training in mental health care

### Psychiatry nurse school

A World Health Organization workshop held in Nazareth in 1986 assessed the mental health service needs of Ethiopia. The recommendation was the setting up of a community psychiatry nurse school in Amanuel Hospital. The main objective was the decentralization of mental health services through the various hospitals and health centres in the country. Candidates were recruited from their local hospitals, and were experienced registered nurses. They were usually settled, mature and well versed in the local languages and culture. They received one year of intensive practice-based training at Amanuel Hospital on the assessment, recognition and psychopharmacotherapy of major psychiatric disorders. These are delivered through regular lectures, seminars, case discussion sessions and clinical placement. This is followed by one year of supervised internship in their respective units. They are capable of independent practice, including prescribing, and they can admit patients to their respective hospital. They follow up patients discharged from Amanuel Hospital, so reducing the burden and costs of travel for patients and their families. The psychiatry nurses all undergo

regular and periodic continuing medical education and get supervision twice a year. To date there are 107 active psychiatry nurses and Amanuel Hospital has greatly benefited from their excellent services.

### Postgraduate training in psychiatry

Postgraduate training in psychiatry has been through several major milestones (Giel, 1999). One of the pioneers was Professor Robert Giel, a Dutch social psychiatrist who came to Ethiopia in 1965 to set up a psychiatry unit, then Haile Selassie I University. The first Ethiopian psychiatrist, Dr Fikre Workeneh, joined him upon his return from his training in the USA in 1972. The Department of Psychiatry started in 1973. Dr Workeneh ran the outpatient clinic at St Paul's Hospital and taught in medical schools single handed, except for brief periods of assistance from overseas. He was joined 3 years later by Dr Abdulreshid Abdullahi who was first trained in Vienna, Austria and then in Scotland, UK. The Armed Forces also had a Yugoslavia-trained neuropsychiatrist exclusively to serve the Army and their families. Indigenous Ethiopian psychiatrists have trained in the UK, Austria, the Netherlands, Cuba, Germany, Bulgaria, Russia, Kenya, South Africa and the USA.

A postgraduate training programme was set up in 2003. This new beginning is the result of collaboration between the University of Toronto in Canada and three dedicated members from the Department of Psychiatry in Addis Ababa University. There are currently 23 residents. It is expected that seven will qualify for their finals in 2005/2006, joining the 11 overseas-trained psychiatrists. Upon graduation some will take on the duty of setting up psychiatry departments in the other three universities in Ethiopia. Another important milestone in this third phase is the foundation of an advocacy group, the Ethiopian Mental Health Society (EMHS) and the Ethiopian Psychiatrists Association (EPA). The latter currently has a growing membership of 14 psychiatrists in Ethiopia and abroad. It is an active member of the World Psychiatrists Association (WPA) and the Association of Allied African Psychiatrists and Associations (AAAPA).

## PSYCHIATRIC DISORDERS

### Common mental disorders

The prevalence of common mental disorders in Ethiopia is about 20 per cent (Alem, 2001). The commonest symptoms are mainly described as dysfunction of the body, such as *chənqəlaten/anaten yäqatelañal* (my head is burning), *anate lay wuha yəefässal* (cold water is flowing on my head), *majəraten yəchämädedäñal* (tightness behind my neck), *joroye wəstu yəchohal* or *yənkoshakoshal* (tinnitus), *tənfash eter eter yəläñal* (short of breath, cannot sigh enough), *ləbe əndä əsat yənädal* (my heart is burning like fire – pointing to the epigastrium), *säwnäten bämulu yəqorätatəmäñal* (generalized aches and pains), *yətäqätəqäñal* (tingling sensation), *yəwäräñal* (numbness), *däräten yəchämädədäñal* (tightness in the chest) or *əka yaräkubät yətäfañal* (forgetting where items were placed).

There are also common psychological symptoms of anxiety such as *ləbe* or *hode yəshäbäral* or *fərhat fərhat yəläñal* (I get frightened easily, I feel jumpy), *chənək chənək yəläñal* or *zəmbəye bäräba balräbaw əsägaləhu* (I feel easily worried and anxious), *mənəm salsära dəkəm yəläñal* (I get easily fatigued for no reason), *bäkälalu hod yəbsäñal* (I feel easily upset or tend to cry easily). Although there is no similar term for depression, the corresponding closer words are *dəbate* in Amharic or *tsəmona* in Tigrigna.

As can be seen from the above, Ethiopians have a range of diverse idioms to describe emotional distress. However they would not routinely seek help from modern health services for common mental disorders. Although they may recognize this as part of an imbalance of their soul, they are less likely to attribute the symptoms to psychiatric disorders. These subjective experiences are often not shared with others, probably to avoid the stigma of mental illness. Indeed some of the somatic features described above are seen in obviously reversible and prevalent differential diagnoses such as anaemia, peptic ulcer disease and pelvic inflammatory disease, and vitamin deficiencies.

There are a range of therapeutic options available in the management of common mental disorders such as anxiety and depression. This may involve consuming different herbs such as *tena adam* (*Ruta montana*), *tosəgn* (*Thymus schimperi* and *Thymus serrulatus*), garlic, or applying unrefined raw butter to the scalp for few days. Those affected may resort to visiting church regularly and praying outside the regular hours (routine church services and Mass are held daily at 6–8 am) or self-prescribing a course of holy water or *əmnet* (holy stone).

There is very limited experience of Western-style psychotherapies for common mental disorders. In addition to the treatment of reversible causes, the mainstay of treatment is pharmacological. The routine practice is to prescribe benzodiazepines or low doses of tricyclic antidepressants, sometimes with a small dose of benzodiazepine such as chlordiazepoxide. Some are known to respond to low doses of neuroleptics such as trifluperazine, or thiroridazine. Good listening, a firm professional approach and simple explanations of the symptoms is often sufficient.

### Psychoses

The prevalence of psychoses in Ethiopia is about 2 per cent (Alem, 2001). For instance, in Amanuel, there were 780 admissions in 2003, mainly for brief psychotic disorders, schizophrenia, major depression, bipolar affective disorder, and substance abuse disorder. Among the 63 147 outpatients seen, 30 per cent were due to psychoses (Amanuel Hospital, 2003).

Various studies show similarities in the incidence and prevalence of schizophrenia to those done elsewhere (Abdulahi *et al.*, 2000; Alem, 2001, 2004). The commonest presentation is mainly in the acute phase, with florid positive symptoms. Paranoid schizophrenia is the commonest, but hebephrenic and catatonic types are also seen. A wide range of passivity phenomena and perceptual disturbances such as hallucinations are also easily elicited. Isolated experiences of speaking in tongues (glossolalia) and apparition are normal and common experiences within certain sects of Christianity.

Most acute psychotic patients require admission for a few weeks to control the agitation and the abnormal experiences. Many respond well to surprisingly low doses of classic antipsychotics (chlorpromazine 100–500 mg per day or equivalent), and in the case of major depression to similar doses of tricyclic antidepressants (TCA) (75–100 mg per day of amitriptyline or equivalent). Although there is no local genetic or other similar explanatory research evidence, this could be due to a constitutional factor such as small body size and low fat reserves. In contrast, a study by Aklilu *et al.* (1996) showed that Ethiopians are ultra rapid metabolizers, implying that higher dose of the above medications may be needed (Aklilu *et al.*, 1996). This aspect of pharmacogenetics needs further study among Ethiopians.

Once calm, these patients are amenable to basic health education on relapse prevention and compliance. When they have reached this stage, families are capable of continuing home care. Psychiatry nurses in local units can refill medications and monitor the symptoms. There is no social security or benefit system, so the recovered patient is expected to resume his or her work as soon as possible. This limited sick role contributes to consolidating and the early establishment of remission. Family and friends are willing to step in for the care of the patient or their dependants.

## Folk illness

Etymologically, the Amharic word for disease, *bäshəta*, denotes a respiratory route to most illnesses. Mental illnesses are considered separately as *yäaəmro həmäm*. Causation and explanation of any misfortune, disease or illness, including mental illness, is either an omission of some of the rites or rituals, or a commission. There is a general sense of helplessness in this popular model. At best people will do everything possible to avoid transgressing the works of God, spirits, nature or people. Each Orthodox Christian family commonly has *yänäfs abat* (a confessor), who visits frequently and performs services, such as blessing the house and all its contents (Wondmagegnehu and Motoru, 1970, p. 104).

A common example of natural causes is *bərd* (cold draught, similar to the French *courant*). This is believed to affect mainly the lungs, but no organs are exempt, hence *yächənqəlat bərd* (a type of tension headache). It may loosely refer to some complex illnesses such as AIDS.

The influence of 'poisoning' is also well described above. A commonly used indigenous substance is *khat* (*Catha edulis*), an amphetamine-like green shrub, known to precipitate and perpetuate mental illness in vulnerable individuals (Kalix, 1996). It is widely grown and heavily consumed among the Gurage, Somali and Harari people, ethnic minorities known for their high use of mental health services. This presents a traditional aetiological model of drug-induced psychoses.

## HEALTH SERVICE CONSTRUCTION

Apart from sporadic contact with missionaries and travellers, Ethiopians entirely relied on traditional medicine until the reign of Menilik II (1889–1913). The first modern service was the Russian Red Cross Hospital in 1897. When the Empire was replaced by the Armed Forces in 1974, there were 82 hospitals.

Today the health services are organized in a four-tier system, starting from the health posts (1432), health stations (2396), health centres (451) and 119 hospitals (includes five central hospitals, of which Amanuel is one). The country's health budget in 2003 was under £100 million, which is just above 7 per cent of the total national budget (Ministry of Health, 2004).

In addition to psychiatry there are 11 postgraduate programmes. There are a host of other specialist nurse programmes too. There does not seem to be a clear liaison system of coordinating the various specialties for cross-referral and exchange of experiences.

There are three new hospitals, and five under construction. The opening of new universities and the need to expand psychiatry units in more hospitals and health centres is anticipated to absorb the indigenous specialist graduates, including psychiatrists.

## Mental health care delivery

This is primarily dealt with at Amanuel Hospital and the 43 psychiatric units. Last year 63 147 patients were seen at Amanuel, of whom 5617 (8.9 per cent) were new cases, and 749 (1.2 per cent) were inpatients. Given the size of the population and the general prevalence of psychiatric disorders, over 80 per cent of the cases must be receiving traditional help. At the current rate of postgraduate recruitment, unless clinical placements are spread across other hospitals and institutions, there could be a mismatch of demand and supply of services. This could manifest primarily through administrative problems of accommodating space, and abundant referrals and self-referrals to Amanuel Hospital. Second, it may create lack of clarity or over-rigidity about the roles of trainees and staff, which may impact on patient management, meeting the needs of trainees and job satisfaction of employees.

## Native traditional services and the interface

As described above, there is a lot to be said in favour of the partnership between statutory and traditional care services. There are many healers who are willing to acknowledge their limitations and refer severely disturbed, treatment-resistant psychotic patients to Amanuel (Bishaw, 1990). Equally the postgraduate training and services should put every effort into working closely with the healers. Some of the conditions might be best helped by the healers. They are respectful, understanding and charismatic figures; they provide an affordable and culturally acceptable group setting, similar to a therapeutic community (Workeneh and Giel, 1975; Kleinman and Sung, 1979).

## Policy

There is no mental health policy or mental health act to protect the rights of patients in Ethiopia. There is a nominal mental health desk within the Ministry of Health responsible for facilitating this. Although by law traditional healers should be registered, in practice this mainly focuses on herbalists and bonesetters. A good policy, especially in a developing country setting, should assess the needs of the community, accommodate the traditional less harmful practices, and provide a cost-effective, culturally acceptable and evidence-based

service with a reasonable expediency (Gureje and Alem, 2000).

## Priorities

Apart from consulting the community and the users, there should also be an assessment of the distribution of the scarce resources. Often planners in developing countries tend to neglect mental health, because more emphasis is given to curable and infectious causes that account for the top ten causes of mortality. Mental health affects a sizeable proportion of both fertile and dependent age groups at a ratio of 1:5. It contributes 12.45 per cent to the burden of disease, which is much higher than the World Bank global estimate of 8.1 per cent (World Bank, 1993; Abdulahi et al., 2000).

## Service development

The World Health Organization recently advised on regional mental health development (World Health Organization, 1999). According to an assessment of the needs of the predominantly rural populations, the services should be accessible and focus on both psychiatric and therapeutic approaches, whilst incorporating the existing community systems. Reason-able health and education services could be run using the existing systems of self-help social groups, such as ədər and mahbär (Pankhurst, 1990b, p. 190). With basic training and assistance, the community could integrate mental health care within their supportive network (Haile-Mariam, 2003).

Schools could also become the forum for a health education and stigma campaign. The numerous non-governmental organizations (NGOs) would welcome collaborative networks and support in delivering feasible mental health programmes. The media could also receive training to provide more responsible reporting and representation of mental health problems. A model that incorporates traditional thinking and folk therapeutic styles with modern services could accommodate most mental health problems, without the need to further stretch services that are mainly organized around treating mental illness.

## Research

One of the strengths of Ethiopia's mental health system is the prolific research activity that has taken place, especially in the last two decades (Fekadu *et al.*, 2000, 2004; De Jong *et al.*, 2001; Kebede *et al.*, 2003) Major collaborations are with Stanley Foundation Research Programs (USA), the University of Umeå (Sweden) and the Institute of Psychiatry (UK). Major research fields are the genetics and psychopharmacology of schizophrenia and bipolar disorders, epidemiology and correlates of substance abuse, schizophrenia, bipolar disorder, common mental disorders, and depression of post-natal onset, child labour and post-traumatic stress.

Of note is the Butajira cohort study that investigates the course and outcome of schizophrenia and major affective disorders in a large community sample. Butajira is better known as a DSS (demographic and surveillance system) site (Shamebo *et al.*, 1992; Byass *et al.*, 2002). It is a member of the INDEPTH consortium (International Network of Field Sites with Continuous Demographic Evaluation of Populations and their Health in Developing Countries). Future research should concentrate on international collaboration with prestigious institutions, especially among other African countries and similar population research centres of excellence. It should probably focus on the application of the epidemiology studies that have been undertaken already, and development of clinical trials, pharmacogenetic and neuroimaging studies that incorporate culturally acceptable therapeutic practices. Furthermore, studies should ensure the validity and adaptability of therapeutic techniques from overseas. There is also a need to improve the design of studies, assessment protocols and psychometric instruments; there is a need for appropriate services such as rehabilitation, alongside multi-agency and multidisciplinary skills improvement, and avenues of health care delivery that include health centre- and school-based primary mental health services. Given the stigma associated with mental illness, there is also a need for the appropriate use of the media, anti-stigma campaigns delivered in partnership with NGOs and agencies such as the Ethiopian Mental Health Society.

## FUTURE CHALLENGES

There have been significant socio-political changes in the last two decades that have affected the people, institutions and government of Ethiopia. The religious teachings and practices have had major reviews, highs and lows. The Ethiopian Orthodox Church, in using Amharic as a medium to access the laity, is determined to catch up with the rapid expansion of its rival evangelical churches. Most mosques have devoted tutors, sponsored missionaries from the Middle East, who provide a thorough textual basis to the traditional approach. There is an unprecedented Western cultural influence, especially from the USA. The diasporas and foreigners have easy to and fro access, thereby importing their new value standards and culture. The rapid expansion of information technology (IT) and Ethiopia's pioneering broadband internet networks have opened the door wide to the rest of the world.

The current government is also under pressure from the Western big powers, the International Monetary Fund (IMF) and the World Bank to comply with their conditions of aid and developmental programme packages. There are concerns that meeting these conditions might be at the expense of our heritage of traditional cultural values and the need for the establishment of centres of excellence.

Mental health in Ethiopia, therefore, may need to accommodate the pressure to conform to the rapid changes in Western psychiatry, while keeping an eye on the revival and intensification of religious experiences. There has also been a rise in the use of recreational and hard drugs. In the years to come the patterns of psychiatric disorders, detection rate, attitude and help-seeking behaviour may change dramatically.

Although the rate of innovation in psychiatry in Ethiopia in the last two decades is awesome, there remains a significant task to sustain quality and maintain the track record. The Ethiopian Psychiatric Association should therefore step up in its role. It should form tight networks and collaborate with neighbours, other Africans, and link with the rest of the world. It is time to establish a quality control mechanism such as a national mental health research council. There is also a paramount need to audit and appraise ethical standards and set benchmarks.

## CONCLUSION

This chapter has spanned the anthropological, cultural and social backgrounds of an ancient African nation and cradle of humanity. It has examined concepts of mental health and systems of care, taking account of local culture and challenges to social cohesion. Through recounting a number of remarkable milestones and gaps, the thoughts may encourage and raise the hopes of people in many developing countries. The chapter also aspired to provide a more balanced account than that usually given by most of the Western media and foreign visitors.

## REFERENCES

Abdulahi, H., Mariam, D.H. and Kebede, D. 2000: Burden of disease analysis in rural Ethiopia. *Ethiopian Medical Journal* 39, 271–81.

Aklilu, E., Persson, I., Bertilsson, L., Johanssen, I., Rodrigues, F. and Ingelman-Sundberg, M. 1996: Frequent distribution of ultrarapid metabolizers of debrisoquine in an Ethiopian population carrying duplicated and multiduplicated functional *CYP2D6* alleles. *Journal of Pharmacology and Experimental Therapeutics* 278, 441–46.

Alem, A. 2001: Mental health services and epidemiology of mental health problems in Ethiopia. *Ethiopian Medical Journal* 39, 153–65.

Alem, A. 2004: Psychiatry in Ethiopia. *International Psychiatry* 4, 8–10.

Alem, A., Jacobsson, L., Araya, M., Kebede, D. and Kullgren, G. 1999: How are mental disorders seen and where is help sought in a rural Ethiopian community? A key informant study in Butajira, Ethiopia. *Acta Psychiatrica Scandinavica Supplement* 397, 40–47.

Amanuel Hospital 2003: Amanuel Hospital Archives. Annual Statistics Report.

Arieli, A., Gilat, I. and Aycheh, S. 1996: Suicide among Ethiopian Jews: a survey conducted by means of a psychological autopsy. *Journal of Nervous and Mental Disorders* 184, 317–19.

Bishaw, M. 1990: Attitudes of modern and traditional medical practitioners toward cooperation. *Ethiopian Medical Journal* 28, 63–72.

Byass, P., Berhane, Y., Emmelin, A., Kebede, D., Andersson, T., Hogberg, U. and Wall, S. 2002: The role of demographic surveillance systems (DSS) in assessing the health of communities: an example from rural Ethiopia. *Public Health* 116, 145–50.

De Jong, J., Komproe, I.H., Van Ommeren, M., El Masri, M., Araya, M., Khaled, N., van De Put, W. and Somasundaram, D. 2001: Lifetime events and posttraumatic stress disorder in 4 post conflict settings. *Journal of the American Medical Association* 286, 555–62.

Fekadu, A., Kebede, D., Alem, A. and Shibre, T. 2000: Use of psychiatric rating instruments in Ethiopia. *Ethiopian Medical Journal* 38, 191–203.

Fekadu, A., Shibre, T., Alem, A., Kebede, D., Kebreab, S., Negash, A. and Owen, M.J. 2004: Bipolar disorder among an isolated island community in Ethiopia. *Journal of Affective Disorders* 80, 1–10.

Fenta, H., Hyman, I. and Noh, S. 2004: Determinants of depression among Ethiopian immigrants and refugees in Toronto. *Journal of Nervous and Mental Disease* 192, 363–72.

Giel, R. 1999: The prehistory of psychiatry in Ethiopia. *Acta Psychiatrica Scandinavica Supplement* 397, 5–10.

Grisaru, N., Budowski, D. and Witztum, E. 1997: Possession by the 'Zar' among Ethiopian immigrants to Israel: psychopathology or culture bound syndrome? *Psychopathology* 30, 223–33.

Gureje, O. and Alem, A. 2000: Mental health policy development in Africa. *Bulletin of the World Health Organization* 78, 475–82.

Haile-Mariam, D. 2003: Indigenous social insurance as an alternative financing mechanism for health care in Ethiopia (the case of elders). *Social Science and Medicine* 56, 1719–26.

Halcon, L.L., Robertson, C.L., Savik, K., Johnson, D.R., Spring, M.A., Butcher, J.N., Westermeyer, J.J. and Jaranson, J.M. 2004: Trauma and coping in Somali and Oromo refugee youth. *Journal of Adolescent Health* 35, 17–25.

Hamer, J. and Hamer, I. 1966: Spirit possession and its socio-psychological implications among the Sidamo of south-west Ethiopia. *Ethnology* 5(4), 392–408.

Kahana, Y. 1985: The zar spirits, a category of magic in the systems of mental health care in Ethiopia. *International Journal of Social Psychiatry* 31, 125–43.

Kalix, P. 1996: *Catha edulis* a plant that has amphetamine effects. *Pharmacy World and Science* 18, 69–73.

Kebede, D., Alem, A., Shibre, T., Negash, A., Fekadu, A., Fekadu, D., Deyassa, N., Jacobsson, L. and Kullgren, G. 2003: Onset and clinical course of schizophrenia in Butajira-Ethiopia: A community based study. *Social Psychiatry and Psychiatric Epidemiology* 38, 625–31.

Kleinman, A. and Sung, L.H. 1979: Why do indigenous practitioners successfully heal? *Social Science and Medicine* 13b(1), 7–26.

Kortman, F. 1987: Popular, traditional and professional mental health care in Ethiopia. *Transcultural Psychiatric Research Review* 24, 255–74.

Ministry of Health 2004: *Planning and Programming Department Health and Health Related Indicators.* Addis Ababa: Alpha Printers.

Moncrieff, J. 1997: Lithium revisited. *British Journal of Psychiatry* 171, 113–19.

Pankhurst, R. 1990a: *An Introduction to the Medical History of Ethiopia.* Lawrenceville, NJ: Red Sea Press.

Pankhurst, R. 1990b: *A Social History of Ethiopia.* Addis Ababa: Addis Ababa University Printing Press.

Ponizovsky, A., Ginath, Y., Durst, R., Wondimeneh, B., Safro, S., Minuchin-Itzigson, S. and Ritsner, M. 1998: Psychological distress among Ethiopian and Russian Jewish immigrants to Israel: a cross cultural study. *International Journal of Social Psychiatry* 44, 35–45.

Rahim, S.I.A. 2001: Zar and female psychopathology in Sudan. *Arab Journal of Psychiatry* 12, 20–32.

Shamebo, D., Sandstrom, A. and Wall, S. 1992: The Butajira rural health project in Ethiopia: epidemiological surveillance for research and intervention in primary health care. *Scandinavian Journal of Primary Health Care* 10, 198–205.

Tekle-Haimanot, R., Abebe, M., Forsgren, L., Gebre-Mariam, A., Heijbel, J., Holmgren, G. and Ekstedt, J. 1991: Attitudes of rural people in central Ethiopia towards epilepsy. *Social Science and Medicine* 32, 203–209.

Uhlman, G. and Minas, M. 1975: Perception of mental illness by rural high school students and parents. *Ethiopian Medical Journal* 13, 5–11.

Workeneh, F. and Giel, R. 1975: Medical dilemma: A survey of the healing practice of a Coptic priest and an Ethiopian Sheik. *Tropical and Geographical Medicine* 27, 431–39.

World Bank 1993: *World Development Report, Investing in Health.* New York: Oxford University Press.

World Health Organization 1999: *Regional Strategy for Mental Health 2000–2010.* Brazzaville: World Health Organization, Regional Office for Africa AFR/RC49/9.

Wondmagegnehu, A. and Motoru, J. 1970: *The Ethiopian Church.* Addis Ababa: Ethiopian Orthodox Mission.

Zewde, B. 1991: *A History of Modern Ethiopia, 1855–1974.* Addis Ababa: Addis Ababa University Press.

# 16

# Psychiatry in East Africa

## Frank G Njenga, Pius Kigamwa and Anna Nguithi

## HISTORICAL PERSPECTIVE

In writing about the history of medicine in Africa, it is always tempting to ignore the pre-colonial era for the superficial reason that there was no medicine in those days. It is now known, however, that an indigenous system of medicine existed in many African countries. Also it is common knowledge that in East Africa certain herbs were used in the treatment of insanity and epilepsy by traditional medicine-men and even a form of surgery known as *trepanation* (craniotomy) was performed by the Abagusii people in Kenya for centuries. There are also many traditional beliefs and customs with relevance to the mental health of the African. For example, according to the tribal legend of the Kikuyu people of Kenya, we are told that in the beginning of things, when humanity started to populate the earth, the man Gikuyu, the founder of the tribe, was called by the Mogai (the divider of the universe) and was given as his share of the land with ravines, the rivers, the forests, the game and all the gifts that the Lord of Nature bestowed on humanity (Kenyatta, 1995).

Gikuyu did as was commanded, and when he reached the spot, he found that the Mogai had provided him with a beautiful wife whom Gikuyu named Moombi (creator or moulder). Gikuyu and Moombi lived happily and had nine daughters and no sons. Gikuyu was very disturbed at not having a male heir, but in another 'miracle', nine young men just came to be. This story is the beginning of the gender 'wars' that exist within the tribe.

Many of the inequities between men and women in Africa have consequences for health and in particular mental health. Beyond the obvious high prevalence of depression (as in many parts of the world) and of conditions probably related to childbearing, African women suffer considerable stress relating to their gendered role and the expectations of husbands and in-laws, as well as children, economic adversity and discrimination.

Among the Gikuyu, a woman is referred to as *mundu wa nja* (a person from the outside of the clan) who by extension has no capacity to inherit. With increasing sophistication among young African women, issues of inheritance became matters of great contention.

In Tanzania (as in many other countries), mental illness has historically been considered an incurable curse. People feared and rejected the mentally ill and often resorted to witchcraft and traditional healers to remove the curses or supernatural forces behind the illness. With regard to services, the only mental hospital in Kenya for many years was Mathari Hospital, which has existed since 1910, operating under various names. Initially Mathari Hospital served the pressing needs of the colonial armed forces by admitting 'mad' soldiers during World Wars I and II.

Mental health services in East Africa have remained united in their apparent refusal to improve. A visit to the famous mental hospitals, Muhimbili (Tanzania), Butabika (Uganda) and Mathari (Kenya) in the late 1960s and early 1970s told the same story of neglected, dilapidated, overcrowded asylums located far from the centre of the city in areas not to be visited by those in any medical authority. Many of the patients spent years in these institutions, never visited by psychiatrists or relatives and often receiving chlorpromazine or barbiturates (when available) for sedation.

The first mental hospitals were set up under European rule, first the Germans in the late 1890s and then the British in 1935. In the 1960s and 1970s more regional psychiatric units were established around the country in an effort to take the services nearer to the people. It was also intended that each region would have a rehabilitation village and a few were built. However there was no systematic outline of the country's mental health policy.

More recently, some of the most remarkable changes in East Africa have taken place in Uganda recently, evidenced by the transformation of Butabika Hospital from the traditional, large neglected mental asylum of yesteryear, to a beautifully painted and manicured hospital serving the mental health needs of the local community as well as primary health care needs. This has been achieved by the creative use of available resources as well as dynamic, merit-based leadership. Makerere is showing definite signs of reclaiming her lost glory, with the re-establishment of a vibrant medical school, and a well-managed postgraduate training programme in psychiatry. Mental health is an integral part of primary health care policy in Uganda.

## EARLY LITERATURE

A notable early publication was the article 'Mental disorders in primary health care' (Harding *et al.*,

1980). This World Health Organization collaboration study was aimed at estimating the frequency of psychiatric disorders at primary health care level. It was also intended to assess the extent to which psychiatric morbidity is correctly identified by primary health workers. This multi-continental survey involving various cultures found that 15 per cent or more of primary health care attendees had a psychiatric disorder and that although they often presented themselves at the primary health care facility, in most instances they were not identified as 'psychiatric cases' by primary health care staff. It was also confirmed that many psychiatric disorders manifest themselves as somatic complaints and receive only symptomatic treatment.

Research on the relationship between culture and mental illness had become a topic of interest when Gordon (1936) expressed his views on this subject in a paper entitled: 'An inquiry into the correlation of civilisation and mental disorder in the Kenyan native'. The focus of enquiry had been the claim that 'primitive' societies are protected by traditional social and cultural values and that the incidence of mental illness would rise with progressive Westernization of the natives. Gordon feared that adolescent disorders would rise steeply in years to come and proved his point by demonstrating that the educated African was more susceptible to mental illness. There is some support for this fear. Depression seems more prevalent among the educated middle classes in East Africa (though no systematic studies have been done to establish this).

Although it is difficult to agree with some of the findings of Carothers (1951), the quality of his work for that time was remarkably high and worth noting. In support of his arguments he cited 33 examples of African behaviour based on his observations and stated that the 'African seldom uses his cortex'. Absence of depression was also attributed to this tendency, although it perhaps reflected a general attitude to the African by the colonial of the time. The debate raged on in scientific circles and, according to recently available evidence, was used by the colonial government to 'prove' that those Africans agitating for independence were psychopathic. This is an interesting instance of the abuse of psychiatry.

Smartt (1956) appears to have been one of the few earlier colonial psychiatrists who did not share the then prevailing general view that Africans generally showed some 'psychopathic' personality characteristics. Commenting on this controversial issue, Smartt (1956) stated, 'the personality traits in the African which appear psychopathic to the European may be due to the African simply lacking the physical means of monitoring behaviour'. He concludes his lengthy paper with a warning that 'there is no reason to suppose that the European does not appear equally psychopathic through the eyes of a rural African in the bush!'

## FACTORS INFLUENCING THE MENTAL HEALTH OF EAST AFRICANS

### Poverty

East Africans are some of the poorest people in the world. The World Bank ranks Kenya, Uganda and Tanzania among the poorest countries in the world. According to the World Health Report (World Health Organization, 2001)

*poverty and associated conditions of unemployment, low educational level, deprivation and homelessness are not only widespread in poor countries, but also affect a sizeable minority of rich countries. Data from cross-national surveys show that common mental disorders are about twice as frequent among the poor as among the rich. Depression is more common in the poor than in the rich.*

### Conflicts and disasters

East Africa is home to a large population of refugees (approximately 1.5 million; UN High Commissioner for Refugees, 2002) and survivors of myriad natural and man-made disasters. Somalia, Ethiopia, Sudan, Rwanda and Congo are the neighbours who are currently in armed conflict and provide the region with a large concentration of refugees and internally displaced persons. Conflicts

including wars and civil strife understandably result in an increase in mental problems. These situations place a heavy toll on the already overstretched health and social services of the region. According to the World Health Report 2001, between a third and a half of those affected suffer mental distress, including post-traumatic stress disorder (PTSD), depressive and anxiety disorders.

### AIDS

The human immunodeficiency virus (HIV) is spreading very rapidly in many parts of the world. In 16 countries of sub-Saharan Africa more than 10 per cent of the population of reproductive age are now infected with HIV (World Health Organization, 2001). The HIV/AIDS epidemic has slowed the pace of economic growth, with reduced life expectancy by up to 50 per cent. In many countries HIV/AIDS is now considered a threat to national security.

The mental health consequences of this epidemic are substantial. A proportion of individuals suffer psychological consequences (disorders as well as problems) as a result of their infection. The effects of intense stigma and discrimination against people with HIV/AIDS also play a major role in psychological stress. In addition, family members also suffer the consequences of stigma and, later, of the premature deaths of their infected family members. The psychological effects on members of broken families and on children orphaned by AIDS have not been studied in any detail, but are likely to be substantial. There is a need for further research in this area (World Health Organization, 2001).

## SPECIFIC SYNDROMES

### Schizophrenia

Schizophrenia is a chronic and severely disabling illness affecting the brain. It occurs worldwide and cross-culturally and does not discriminate by race or gender. Schizophrenia incapacitates a large number of people, and also negatively affects those living in close proximity to them: family and friends. In addition, it has a detrimental impact on the economy of every country and especially on health services.

Socio-economic factors appear to influence both the prevalence and the outcome of schizophrenia. A higher prevalence of schizophrenia has been found amongst lower socio-economic groups. There are several theories put forward to explain this phenomenon. The most widely accepted is the so-called 'social drift' or 'downward drift' hypothesis.

Schizophrenia is a chronic illness and, like any other chronic illness, its course will be affected by social factors. It is clear that psycho-social stressors have a detrimental effect on the course of the illness and can precipitate a relapse. Social phenomena such as industrialization and urbanization may give rise to an accumulation of stressors that can play a part in the timing of the onset and the severity of the illness. Organic factors, trauma and malnutrition all probably play a role in influencing the age of onset in East Africa.

The content of delusions can vary considerably according to the patient's educational and cultural background. The availability of television may give rise to an increase in delusions of reference concerning television programmes or broadcasters. Delusions with religious content are common in societies in which religion continues to play an important role. For example, patients from traditional South African backgrounds often have delusions concerning possession by spirits, bewitchment or special relationships with the ancestors. In some indigenous belief systems, psychotic symptoms may be interpreted as a calling to become a traditional healer and patients may undertake training as a result. It is extremely important that beliefs alone do not constitute the grounds on which a patient receives a diagnosis of any mental illness, unless the belief is patently bizarre and incongruent with any cultural context.

In parts of sub-Saharan Africa, several culturally defined afflictions may resemble psychotic disorders. The most likely to be confused with schizophrenia are *ukuthwasa*, a condition found amongst the Xhosa and some other Nguni peoples. A person who is called by the ancestors to become a traditional healer may present with hallucinations, agitated and disorganized behaviour, and *amafufunyana*, a condition occurring in the same groups, in which a person is possessed by a malign spirit which causes agitation, disordered behaviour and strange utterances or noises, often in an altered voice. Local variants of these as well as other conditions may be present in various regions of the continent.

Cultural factors may influence the presentation, the diagnostic assessment, the choice of treatment modality, the response to treatment, the course and the outcome of schizophrenia.

The choice of treatment modality (traditional versus Westernized) may be an issue, and sometimes a compromise will have to be reached whereby the patients may need to be temporarily released from hospital in order to attend prescribed rituals related to their illness. It should be borne in mind that Western medicine teaches clinicians to explain how an illness occurred, whereas in some cultures the more important question is why the illness occurred. Compliance, and consequently the course and prognosis of the illness, is greatly enhanced if the family is supportive of the chosen treatment.

## Mood disorders

Depression is a major cause of distress and disability, leading to impaired ability to work or to care for children, disruption to interpersonal relationships, alcohol abuse and slow recovery from physical illness. It affects around 8–12 per cent of people living in the community, around 20–25 per cent of people who attend primary care clinics and is commoner still amongst general hospital inpatients.

Malnutrition, vitamin deficiencies (such as B complex or folate), chronic infections and endocrine dysfunctions (such as hypothyroidism) may produce depression syndromes. In the African context, careful physical examination and medical history taking must be carried out to exclude them.

There is increasing evidence that many of the core symptoms of the depressive syndrome are common to human beings worldwide. However, the ways in which depressed people seek help and describe their unhappiness varies considerably depending on life experience, culture and education.

In East Africa, most depressed people do not seek help from modern health services but find solace within their family or from the church or visit traditional or religious healers. They may recognize their sadness as the result of a social, family or spiritual problem or as a result of thinking too much about such problems, and often do not consider it an issue with which a health clinic could help them.

Studies in western, eastern and southern Africa all indicate that between 10 and 15 per cent of patients who attend primary care clinics do so with a depressive illness associated with somatic symptoms.

This poses a considerable problem for health staff, who often fail to realize that such physical symptoms can be caused by a psychiatric condition. The physical symptoms are investigated unnecessarily and the patient is given analgesics or antacids which prove to be ineffective. This results in patients consulting other agencies in a further search for relief. They may be subjected to expensive and invasive procedures and have inappropriate surgery or long courses of medication. In the interest of the patients, and of effective running of health clinics, it is important that patients with depressive disorder are detected correctly. Training programmes on how to recognize mental illness in primary care are on-going in parts of East Africa including Kenya, Tanzania and Zanzibar.

## Neuropsychiatric syndromes

This section presents syndromes that are commonly seen in East Africa, but are less frequently seen in the West. Delirium is believed to be caused by pathophysiological changes in the brain secondary to systemic diseases or sometimes primary brain disease. The range of possible causes is extremely wide, but identifying the exact cause, if possible, is important in treating and reversing the harmful consequences of the condition.

The most common cause of delirium in sub-Saharan Africa is likely to be infectious. The next most common would be alcohol/drug intoxication and withdrawal states, followed by head trauma and complications of epilepsy. Cardiovascular diseases (including strokes and the various causes of hypoperfusion), respiratory diseases (causing cerebral hypoxaemia), hypoglycaemia, other endocrine disorders and electrolyte disturbances, focal cerebral cortical diseases such as neoplasms, and other systemic diseases are less common causes of delirium in East Africa.

It must always be remembered that pyrexia, by itself, can cause delirium. Septicaemia, as a complication of any bacterial infection, commonly causes delirium. Cerebral malaria is an important and treatable cause of delirium in East Africa, usually manifesting as pyrexia, severe headache, mental confusion, tonic-clonic fits, and frequently gross focal neurological signs. Cerebral malaria usually occurs a week or two after initial infection and these individuals have often just been treated for a bout of malaria and/or have travelled to an area in which malarial mosquitoes are endemic.

HIV infection, or full-blown AIDS, predisposes the individual to all of the above brain infections and to opportunistic infections of the brain, including cryptococcal meningitis and cerebral toxoplasmosis. HIV infection can also cause delirium from toxic-metabolic insults, neoplasms, or the direct infection of the brain with the virus.

Less common but important infectious causes of delirium include viral encephalitides, neurosyphilis and fungal and parasitic infections. Viral encephalitides often present in a non-specific fashion. Confusion, influenza-like symptoms and a low-grade pyrexia with focal neurological signs of cranial nerve palsies, fits or movement disorders should guide the physician to considering the possibility of a viral encephalitis.

Herpes simplex virus encephalitis is usually rapidly progressive. It presents with headache, stiff neck, behavioural disorders and focal signs such as hemiparesis, aphasia or focal seizures.

Neurosyphilis often presents in the form of a very chronic condition, general paresis, which appears decades after the primary acute infection with spirochaetes. Rarely, however, syphilis attacks the central nervous system to cause acute meningitis and occasionally, within 1–5 years of infection, syphilis causes meningovascular disease, both of which are important to consider in a differential diagnosis because they generally respond to aggressive treatment with parenteral penicillin.

The most important fungal infection to be aware of is cryptococcal meningitis, which occurs in immune-compromised individuals. Important parasitic infections include cerebral toxoplasmosis, which usually presents as a multifocal cerebral lesion in immunocompromised individuals, cysticercosis and amoebic meningoencephalitis. African trypanosomiasis (sleeping sickness) is another parasitic infection which can present with delirium.

Epilepsy, particularly postictal states, can present with delirium. Complex partial seizure phenomena cause confusional states that can appear to be very similar to delirium. Head injury should always be considered in a differential diagnosis of delirium, since road traffic accidents, violence and falls are serious causes of morbidity in sub-Saharan Africa.

Investigations to determine the aetiology of delirium must be guided by clinical clues based on the history and examination of the patient. Since the risk of death is substantial, these investigations must be performed expeditiously, preferably in a medical ward.

The majority of patients with dementia in Africa are never seen by medical services. Those who are seen are usually treated as outpatients unless behavioural problems or physical ill-health needs in-patient management. The management of dementia starts with a proper diagnosis to identify and then treat any reversible causes of dementia. For example, this management involves further investigations and treatment with thyroid hormone for cases of hypothyroidism, and appropriate nutritional supplements for dementia caused by nutritional deficiency. If chronic bilateral subdural haematomas, brain tumours or normal pressure hydrocephalus are identified, then neurosurgical consultation should be obtained. If neurosyphilis is identified, then a two-week course of parenteral penicillin should be given to the patient. Incidental physical disorders, however minor, should be actively treated.

Although it is necessary to exercise caution in elderly patients, they should not be denied medications, especially for the treatment of depressive disorders. Antidepressant medication should be started cautiously and increased gradually. Electroconvulsive therapy can be remarkably successful in treating serious depressive illness in the elderly, even in the presence of dementia. Because of poor sleep, elderly patients often need hypnotics at night. If a hypnotic is essential, the minimum effective dose should be used and the effects monitored carefully.

Education of the patient and relatives is essential to help them prepare for the course of the illness and to settle legal and financial matters if necessary. In some countries, self-help groups have been formed to provide support for family members. Support for the family is given in the form of discussion of problems and advice about care, as well as practical help.

The stigma of mental illness is compounded in East Africa because of a common cultural belief that epilepsy is derived from a sudden possession by a spirit or demon, which may take the form of avenging family spirits. Because of this belief in spiritual causation or witchcraft, many people with seizures consult a traditional healer before seeing a medical practitioner. Indeed, the majority of people suffering from epilepsy in Africa never consult a medical practitioner.

In addition to social stigma, people with epilepsy often suffer from associated psychological problems and significant medical morbidity, especially burns incurred from falling into cooking or warming fires. Recent studies suggest that the public and even people with epilepsy and their nearest relatives lack basic information about the condition. Research suggests that intensive education and providing a reliable service increase the rate of clinic attendance and medication compliance among people with epilepsy.

## Neurotic and related disorders

Whilst neuroses are the commonest psychiatric conditions in the community and in primary care populations, they form only a small proportion of patients seen in psychiatric clinics and are rarely admitted to psychiatric inpatient facilities. Thus, research in Africa has shown that up to a quarter of primary care clinic attendees suffer from emotional disorders, more than two-thirds of which are neurotic in nature, whereas the vast majority of patients in psychiatric clinics suffer from psychotic disorders. Furthermore, even if the primary cause is recognized, in many African cultures, these disorders are not considered to be psychiatric illnesses and are therefore not referred to such specialist services. Due to the heavy workload in many primary care settings, most patients with neurotic disorders tend to receive symptomatic or placebo treatments (such as vitamins and analgesics).

In these clinics, many complain of 'malaria' which in many parts of East Africa is a generic term for fever or generally feeling unwell. Because Africans do not expect European-trained doctors to understand the distress caused by, say, evil eyes, bewitchment or other African problems, the patient communicates in a language he or she expects the physician to understand.

A substantial proportion of these patients are also known to consult traditional medical practitioners, who are frequently ignored in studies of help-seeking and care provision although they cover the health needs of a substantial proportion of the African population.

Symptoms of neurotic disorder are often influenced by socio-cultural factors and some presenting complaints and idioms may also vary from region to region. However, many symptoms are found in different populations and may be considered as 'universal' symptoms of neuroses.

A diverse range of aetiological theories have been proposed to explain the cause of neurotic disorders. What is clear is that all neurotic disorders are multifactorial in origin and many factors play a role in each case. A significant proportion of patients with neurotic disorders believe that they have been victims of witchcraft. Conflicts, including wars and civil strife, result in an increase in mental health problems. These traumatic experiences conspire to give Africans some of the highest risk factors for mental disorder. They place a heavy toll on the already overstretched health and other social services of the region.

Other priorities include understanding the role of social factors in the causation of mental illness. In this regard one has to understand the context of the presentation, in particular as such factors may need to be addressed directly, for example, interpersonal issues within a marital situation potentially influenced by the specific expectations of spousal roles.

Phobias, though common in developed countries, were rarely diagnosed in Africa. In some settings, phobias are conceptualized not as illnesses but as social or spiritual problems and may therefore not be brought to health facilities for treatment.

Panic disorder runs a variable course, with many sufferers resolving spontaneously. An essential ingredient of treatment is to explain the cause of the symptoms to the patient since one of the key reasons why such severe anxiety is experienced is because patients misinterpret their bodily experiences as being abnormal and due to a more serious cause.

For most parts of Africa, drugs are the first and preferred mode of treatment. Although many other disorders, such as obsessive–compulsive disorder, somatoform disorders and their treatment will not differ much from the West, the health worker must give up the idea of achieving a 'cure' in the usual sense of relieving symptoms but should accept the symptoms as a manifestation of a chronic psychiatric disorder, which will hold multiple meanings in a culturally diverse context. Over time, one may attempt to gradually shift the focus of the patients' concerns from the body to the social or psychological factors that may underlie the disorder, and competing cultural explanations may hinder this process.

## An indigenous syndrome?

The 'brain-fag syndrome' was first described by African psychiatrists over 30 years ago. The main symptoms are unpleasant head symptoms such as pain or crawling sensations, visual problems such as dimness and tearing, cognitive impairments such as difficulty in concentration, the mind going blank and poor retention of information, and a variety of somatic symptoms such as abdominal and chest pains, palpitations, dizziness, fatigue and sleepiness. Occasionally, patients may exhibit a behavioural disturbance akin to a hysterical dissociative state characterized by sudden onset of disinhibited behaviour with vivid hallucinations. The term 'brain-fag' is derived from the fact that students often attribute their symptoms to overwork of the brain. Teachers, doctors, lawyers and other professionals often place undue pressure on their children and siblings to perform well in national examinations, leading to the disorder. It is commonest in the weeks and months leading to examinations.

## Personality disorders

The concept of personality disorders has been formulated most clearly in the West. An understanding of personality disorders is important for physicians because these individuals often become difficult patients: demanding, non-compliant, manipulative or dependent. Western-raised and Western-trained mental health clinicians who work in sub-Saharan Africa have noted that Western-defined personality disorders are much rarer in sub-Saharan Africa than they are in the West. In many psychiatric clinics in Africa, only a few cases that would be called borderline personality disorder in the West can be reliably diagnosed. The reasons for these differences remain unclear. Cultural norms and attitudes towards personality disorders that are found in developed and industrialized individualistic societies are less likely to be applied in socio-centric societies. In socio-centric and smaller societies there may be more tolerance of personality difficulties, and therefore less likelihood of labelling these as disease entities. In the circumstances no urgent need for the delivery of services is felt. After all, personality disorder services are only just developing with any sophistication in the developed world.

## Post-traumatic stress disorder

Terrorism is now a global concern. Every day there are headlines reporting terrorist activities in industrialized Western nations and elsewhere, including Africa. Despite the magnitude of this threat to worldwide mental health, there are few published studies that systematically determine the prevalence and risk factors for post-traumatic stress disorder (PTSD) following a terrorist attack.

Pfefferbaum et al. (2001) showed a close association between injury and post-traumatic stress in a directly exposed group of 21 individuals eight months after the US embassy bombing in Dar es Salaam, Tanzania, in which 11 people were killed and 80 wounded. Njenga et al. (2004a) undertook a similar study following the bombings in Nairobi in Kenya. They found that the following factors were associated with post-traumatic stress: a) pre-incident demographic factors: female gender, unmarried status and less previous education; b) incident-related factors: being outside during the blast, seeing the blast, injury, not fully recovering from injury, feeling afraid, helpless, or threatened at the time of the blast; c) post-incident factors: not talking with a friend or workmate about the blast, bereavement, experiencing or anticipating financial difficulty after the blast, inability to work because of injury, and receiving material or financial assistance. There was no significant association with PTSD symptomatology for age, number of children, religion, assessment of hospital care or immediate medical response, receiving counselling or the relationship of the person mourned.

The 35 per cent prevalence of significant PTSD symptomatology in this highly exposed sample a few months after the Nairobi US embassy bombing is comparable to the prevalence found in studies of Western populations affected by terrorism. Likewise, frequently reported predictors of PTSD, for example female gender, injury, peri-traumatic response, financial sequelae were confirmed in this large non-Western sample. These findings provide fertile grounds for collaborative research as the fact of terrorism continues to impact mental health service delivery.

## Depression and cardiovascular disease

Dramatic changes in the overall health needs of the world's populations are occurring. It has been generally assumed that in the developing regions, where four-fifths of the world's people live, the leading causes of disease burden are communicable diseases. In fact, non-communicable diseases such as depression and heart disease are replacing the traditional enemies such as infectious diseases and malnutrition as the leading causes of disability and premature death. Diabetes, obesity and hypertension are all risk factors for coronary artery disease, and are all on the increase, as is the incidence of coronary heart disease in East Africa (Schneider and Bezabih, 2001; Jablonski-Cohen *et al.*, 2003; Njenga *et al.*, 2004b). Similar trends have been reported from Japan and Australia. Their results suggest that depressive symptoms are an important factor in the health care of patients with coronary disease; although it is still hypothesized without firm conclusions that depression is an antecedent of coronary heart disease, it is much clearer that the treatment of depressive symptoms among those with cardiac disorders improves the quality of life and adherence to a healthier lifestyle and prescribed treatments. For example, depressed post-infarction patients are more often re-admitted for cardiac reasons and their work resumption is delayed. African scientists must not be caught unawares by this emerging epidemic.

## Anorexia nervosa

Anorexia nervosa is probably a very rare condition in Africa (Njenga and Kangethe, 2004). The first case in a black child was described nearly 300 years after Morton's first case report. A MEDLINE search (for anorexia nervosa, Africa) carried out by the authors in 2001 revealed four possible cases (Nwaefuna, 1981; Buchan and Gregory, 1984, Famuyiwa, 1988; Binitie *et al.*, 2000). Nwaefuma's case is described in a letter to the editor that does not give sufficient detail to enable *Diagnostic and Statistical Manual of Mental Disorders* (DSM-IV) diagnosis but nonetheless emphasizes the rarity of the condition. Buchan and Gregory (1984) reported one case in a black Zimbabwean woman that satisfied Feighner's diagnostic criteria but which showed unusual features in the clinical symptoms, including the role of a traditional healer in her recovery.

In 1988, Famuyiwa reported two cases of anorexia nervosa in two Nigerian girls. He states:

*the relatively low prevalence of the disorder that has been observed might be due to the protective influence of the Nigerian extended kinship system, the customary passion for plumpness as an attribute of physical attractiveness, carbohydrate-diet and the non-inclusion of cases in hospital records because of consultation with unorthodox healers.*

The usual explanation for anorexia is that it is an abnormal response to immense social pressures exerted by peers and the media to be slim. However, if this were the case, one would expect rates in Africa to be rising rapidly with increasing globalization. Twenty-first-century African girls in urban settings share magazines, television, universities and future with their sisters in the West. There is no longer room for the mistaken perception that Africans still hold that fat women are more desirable. The twenty-first-century African is health conscious, goes to the gym, exercises and carefully watches his or her diet. The pressure on the girl to be slim is now evident, but no corresponding increase in cases of anorexia nervosa has yet been seen. There is still no reliable explanation for these observations, and this may reflect a need for research at the interface of social and genetic paradigms.

## PRIMARY CARE

The development of health care guidelines for primary health care workers remains a priority since 20–30 per cent of those attending primary health facilities suffer primarily from psychiatric disorder (Ndetei and Muhangi, 1979). Training in the treatment of mental disorders is a priority as Kenyan doctors have indicated their own need for further training in psychiatry (Othieno *et al.*, 2001).

## MENTAL HEALTH LEGISLATION

In 1933, the British Government applied the Indian Mental Health Act in Kenya. In 1949, the colonial parliament enacted a law, the Mental Treatment Act, based on a prototype borrowed from Britain (see Chapter 7). This Act determined patients' care until 1959 when the Mental Treatment Act was replaced with a more humane Mental Health Act. This placed emphasis on community mental health services. The current Mental Health Act came into operation in 1989 and for the first time provides for the voluntary treatment of people with mental illness. It also creates a regulatory board to oversee the implementation of the Act.

Kenya is one of the earliest countries in Africa to implement a mental health act. Whereas the former legislation covered only the handling of patients with mental illness (their hospitalization, discharge, repatriation and the management of their property), the new legislation is also concerned with efforts to decriminalize, demystify and destigmatize mental illness. It is concerned with making mental health care more 'communal' and less centralized, simplifying admissions and integrating mental health services within the national framework.

As a result of the 1989 Mental Health Act, over half of all state-owned general hospitals began to accept psychiatric patients. This led to the deployment of psychiatric nurses to general hospitals around the country; general medical officers became involved in mental health care; outpatient mental health clinics were set up in general hospitals; and some outreach services were established. In addition, the Kenya Board of Mental Health has begun to regulate the administration of the Act. The application of mental health legislation in rural and traditional practice settings is uncertain.

## TRADITIONAL HEALERS IN MENTAL HEALTH CARE

Formally trained doctors have finally begun to consider traditional healers as potential allies in the battle to prevent the spread of HIV/AIDS by recognizing that the longstanding trust and credibility of these healers in the communities can facilitate change in sexual behaviour.

Traditional healers have a potential role as change agents in AIDS prevention and mental health promotion, given their authority to urge senior members of kin groups to relax their objections to condoms. They can also play a role as change agents in the programme against the stigma of mental illness.

Some Tanzanian biomedical practitioners tend to view this communication as a one-way street, aiming only to train poorly educated traditional healers and recruit their support in the pursuit of public health goals. True collaboration will occur when each is ready and willing to learn from the best of the others' practices.

A law to regulate traditional healers in South Africa has been passed by Parliament to acclaim from the predominantly black parliamentarians, who believe that a widely practised form of health care in the country will be officially recognized (see Chapter 13d).

The law seeks to regulate the practice and practitioners in much the same way as doctors and other health practitioners are now. Other countries in the region are watching with keen interest to see how the system works.

In Africa, traditional healers are generally more accessible than biomedical practitioners; in rural Tanzania the ratio of doctors to population is 1:20 000 whereas that of traditional healers is 1:350 (Tanzania Development Gateway). Another report suggests one doctor to 33 000 people and one traditional healer to 156 people (Integrated Regional Information Networks, 2006).

Doctors must accept, respect and collaborate with traditional healers, who have much to teach and can be employed in prevention and health promotion programmes, as for example in HIV programmes.

## REFERENCES

Binitie, A., Osaghae and Akenzua, O.A. 2000: A case report of anorexia nervosa. *African Journal of Medicine and Medical Sciences* 29, 175–77.

Buchan, T. and Gregory, L.D. 1984: Anorexia in a black Zimbabwean. *British Journal of Psychiatry* 145, 326–30.

Carothers, J.C. 1951: Frontal lobe function and the African. *Journal of Mental Science* 97, 12–48.

Famuyiwa, O.O. 1988: Anorexia nervosa in two Nigerians. *Acta Psychiatrica Scandinavica* 78, 550–54.

Gordon, H.L. 1936: An enquiry into the correlation of civilization and mental disorders in the Kenyan native. *East African Medical Journal* 12, 327–35.

Harding, T.W., de Arango, M.V., Baltazur, J., Climent, C.E., Ibrahim, H.H., Ladrido-Ignacio, L., Murthy, R.S. and Wig, N.N. 1980: Mental disorders in primary health care: a study of their frequency and diagnosis in four developing countries. *Psychological Medicine* 10(2), 231–41.

Integrated Regional Information Networks 2006: Tanzania: Focus on drawing on traditional remedies to fight HIV/AIDS. *PlusNews*. http://www.plusnews.org/AIDSreport.asp?ReportID= 2715& SelectRegion= Great_Lakes (accessed 8 January 2007).

Jablonski-Cohen, M.S., Kosgei, R.J., Rerimoi, A.J. and Mamlin, J.J. 2003: The emerging problem of coronary heart disease in Kenya. *East African Medical Journal* 80, 293–97.

Kenyatta, J. 1995: *Facing Mount Kenya. The Traditional Life of the Gikuyu.* Nairobi: East African Educational Publishers.

Ndetei, D.M. and Muhangi, J. 1979: The prevalence and clinical presentation of psychiatric illness in a rural setting in Kenya. *British Journal of Psychiatry* 135, 269–72.

Njenga, F.G. and Kangethe, R.K. 2004: Anorexia nervosa in Kenya. *East African Medical Journal* 81, 188.

Njenga, F.G., Nicholls, P.J., Nyamai, C., Kigamwa, P. and Davidson, J.R. 2004a: Post-traumatic stress after terrorist attack: psychological reactions following the US embassy bombing in Nairobi: Naturalistic study. *British Journal of Psychiatry* 185, 328–33.

Njenga, F.G., Kamotho, C.G., Joshi, M.D., Gikonyo, D.K. and Wanyoike, M. 2004b: Coronary artery disease and depression: the silent African epidemics. *East African Medical Journal* 81, 611–15.

Nwaefuna, A. 1981: Anorexia nervosa in a developing country. *British Journal of Psychiatry* 138, 270–71.

Othieno, C.J., Okech, V.C., Omondi, J.A. and Makanyengo, M.A. 2001: How Kenyan physicians treat psychiatric disorders. *East African Medical Journal* 78, 204–71.

Pfefferbaum, B., North, C.S., Flynn, B.W., Ursano, R.J., McCoy, G., DeMartino, R., Julian, W.E., Dumont, C.E., Holloway, H.C. and Norwood, A.E. 2001: The emotional impact of injury following an international terrorist incident. *Public Health Reviews* 29, 271–80.

Schneider, J. and Bezabih, K. 2001: Causes of sudden death in Addis Ababa, Ethiopia. *Ethiopian Medical Journal* 39, 323–40.

Smartt, C.G.F. 1956: Mental adjustment in the East African. *Journal of Mental Science* 102, 441–66.

Tanzania Development Gateway http://www.tanzaniagateway.org (accessed 11 December 2006).

World Health Organization 2001: The World Health Report: *Mental Health: New Understanding, New Hope.* Geneva: World Health Organization.

UN High Commissioner for Refugees (UNHCR) 2002: www.unhcr.org (accessed October 2006).

# 17

# Culture and the mental health of African refugees: Somali help-seeking and healing

Nasir Warfa

## INTRODUCTION

Somalia is situated on the north-east coast of the Horn of Africa. It has borders with Djibouti, Ethiopia and Kenya. The population was estimated to be between 7 and 9 million in 1997, with an annual growth rate of 3 per cent (United Nations Development Programme, 2001). The people are divided into three main types: nomadic or semi-nomadic, agricultural and urban. In 1979, the nomadic group represented 70 per cent of the whole population (Warsame, 1979). The country has been without an effective government since the start of the civil war in 1990. Many factors were blamed for the collapse of Somalia as a modern state. Social and political analysts agree among themselves that these factors overlap but that the collapse was largely due to the legacy of colonialism, human rights abuses and the impact of a war with Ethiopia in 1977 (Amnesty International, 1997). The failure to shape cohesive and independent economic policies, overcentralized and unsustainable

government structures, clanism, nepotism and corruption on a wide scale were all mentioned as key factors contributing to the destruction of the Somali state in 1991 (Issa-Salwe, 1996; Mubarak, 1996). The civil war has also led Somalia's mass population movements (both internal and international displacement). Nearly a million and half Somalis have fled their country to neighbouring states such as Kenya, Ethiopia and Djibouti and as many as 50 000 Somalis have gone to North America and Western Europe.

An increasing body of literature has examined and explored the mental health consequences of pre-migration traumatic events and post-migration life stressors among African refugee populations. These studies found that refugee populations have a wide range of social problems, and have higher levels of unmet need and severe levels of mental health problems, including depression, panic attacks, social phobia, general anxiety, suicidal ideation and post-traumatic stress disorder (PTSD) (Warfa and Bhui, 2003; McCrone et al., 2005; Bhui et al., 2003,

2006). For example, McCrone *et al.* (2005) found significant common mental health problems and low levels of mental health service uptake among Somali refugees living in London. Yet it is not clear what other strategies Somalis use to cope with these mental health problems. This chapter explores the findings of focus group discussions exploring Somali concepts and narratives of psychological problems and coping strategies, including spiritual services and traditional ritual ceremonies.

## FOCUS GROUPS

A total of 59 male and female professional and lay Somalis from varied socio-economic backgrounds were invited to participate in eight focus groups in London (UK) and Minneapolis (USA). Participants were recruited from local Somali professional networks, and lay Somalis from places such as cafes, community centres and call centres. In London, the discussion group meetings of the Somali professionals were held at the Institute of Community Health Sciences and the British Refugee Council. The lay focus group discussions were held at Somali Community Centres, except one lay session where the discussion took place, at the request of the lay male group, in a lay participant's residential setting. In Minneapolis, the lay and professional focus group discussions were held at Akmal Educational Centre, which is located within a popular Somali shopping centre. The focus group participants explored Somali perceptions and meanings of health and illness and risks to health. A topic guide framed the domains of interest but participants were allowed to discuss the specific areas of interest in their own terms.

## MENTAL DISORDERS

The professional participants from both cities discussed a wide range of common mental health problems including depression, PTSD, anxiety and suicide in considerable detail and thought these were critical issues that warrant the immediate attention of health care providers:

> *Madness is now widespread in the Community. Though the* waali *(madness) they are talking about is 'buufis' as they call it. We did not have depression back home! We did not know this name and you couldn't find it in the person because they were not crazy.*
> **Professional, male, Minneapolis**

> *I deal with mental health issues of Somalis as part of my work every day. I have also been trained on how to detect when abnormality appears. There are over 30 Somalis who are not normal, women and men.*
> **Professional, female, Minneapolis**

> *How many times I have seen people who have recently arrived from Kenya, they looked healthy, their skin was shining and they looked good. They stay here for six months and the same people have changed completely. All of a sudden, they look gloomy and are depressed.*
> **Professional, female, Minneapolis**

The above professional participants regarded these core themes of *buufis* (depression), PTSD and *waali* (madness) as the most profound health problems among Somalis in London and Minneapolis. The London professional participants were more worried about these problems than the Minneapolis focus groups. The observation that the Somali refugees in Minneapolis looked healthy and had shiny skin when they first arrived in the USA but looked gloomy and depressed six months later, suggests an adverse interaction between social stressors and mental health. Nevertheless, it does not state what factors or social problems are interacting with the lives of the newcomers to make their mental health poor.

Lay participants also discussed mental health problems but used less clinical descriptions than the professional groups:

> *I see a lot of people who talk to themselves.*
> **Lay, female, London**

*When someone has* buufis, *things are not working out for him.*

**Lay, male, London**

*It is another form of mini madness.*

**Lay, male, Minneapolis**

*I think* buufis *is frustration because the person may be unemployed or he may be suspicious. If someone is arrested, he usually has* buufis. *If somebody has no job, he gets* buufis. *You think this* buufis *is everywhere.*

**Lay, male, Minneapolis**

It is not apparent from these lay views whether they regarded 'talking to yourself', worries, stress, anxiety and *buufis* as mental disorders or if they see them as the early symptoms of a mental breakdown. Patterns of behaviour such as not talking with people, not making sense when talking or hanging around places alone with no apparent reason were regarded as strange behaviour which suggests the presence of some form of mental illness, whereas the statement 'it is another form of mini madness' appears to be referring to the severity of *buufis*. To some extent these lay participants were in agreement with the professional views about increasing mental health problems among the Somali refugees. The main difference between the professional and the lay participants was the language they used to describe these problems, with the professional participants using more clinical terms. For instance, the professional participants used depression to describe *buufis* whereas the lay participants were not quite sure how to define *buufis*, even in Somali terms.

Some of the lay participants equated *buufis* with frustration or with life failures. In contrast to the professional participants, the lay groups were divided over these issues. Some lay Somalis proposed that the discourse on mental health issues was not a top priority for them. Paradoxically, it was for this reason that some of the professional participants were more concerned about mental health issues than the lay Somalis. They felt people with mental health problems were not seeking treatment early enough or that they neglected their

health care needs, leading to the development of more serious mental disorders:

*We as a community have mentally ill people who have never been diagnosed because they have other priorities and responsibilities they need to take care of.*

**Professional, female, Minneapolis**

*This guy had an argument with another Somali when he dialled 911 and said to the police 'Bin Laden is here', the police asked him, 'Bin Laden was there?', and the guy said, 'Yes, right here'. The police came to see him very quickly and said where is Bin Laden and the guy said, 'Here he is!'. The police said, 'This is not Bin Laden. OK what kind of medication are you on?' The guy said, 'I am not taking anything'. Then they arrested him and realized he was mentally ill so they called me and said to me 'There is a mentally ill guy who needs help' and then I went to see him. People don't know about their illness or if they do they are ignoring their medical needs until it is too late to do anything about it.*

**Professional, female, Minneapolis**

Moreover, there was some reluctance among the lay groups to identify common mental health problems as serious health conditions worth seeking medical treatments. This may be because of the distinct cultural ways in which Somalis measure the severity of an illness. For instance, the lay views described earlier also acknowledged *waali* (madness) to be a serious mental illness and *buufis* (depression) and *isla hadlid* (talking to oneself) as the early symptoms of madness or 'mini madness'. The general perception among the lay groups was that *buufis* and 'talking to yourself' are mild conditions but that they could eventually progress into madness:

*There are many Somalis who had* buufis *who eventually became mad. There was this guy who had* buufis *and one day he left his home and didn't come back. His body was found in the lakeside.*

**Lay, male, Minneapolis**

*I have seen about ten people who gone mad, four men and six women and some of the men were in and out of hospital. These were people who have been in Minneapolis for sometime and they were doing fine. They started talking to themselves before they were taken to the hospital for mental people.*

**Lay, female, Minneapolis**

For these lay views, 'madness' is a severe mental health problem and it is only when the person becomes 'mad' that they are regarded as someone with a severe mental disorder. As described in the previous paragraphs, this is amongst the most common Somali traditional method of both perceiving and constructing folk illnesses and psychiatric symptoms.

## COPING STRATEGIES AND TREATMENT METHODS

Professional and lay focus groups cited a number of strategies for coping with ill-health, including traditional healing practices, spiritual services and the use of modern medical services. They often commented on the use of spiritual services for the treatment of mental illnesses:

*If your relatives think that there is something wrong about you, they would look after you and would ask a Mullah to read Quran on you, it really works.*

**Lay, male, Minneapolis**

*When it comes to* buufis (waali), *we have our own culture and religion to deal with it. Religion is the best medicine for* buufis.

**Lay, female, Minneapolis**

*Quran is the most important treatment.*

**Lay, male, Minneapolis**

*I know the Sheikhs have been very busy, much busier than they were in Somalia. A friend of mine is a Sheikh and he is visiting a family for whatever reasons on every Friday. Believe me or not, every weekend he is either*

*doing 'Meher' or reading Quran on someone who lost it. They never had it so good but no one at least complains about them.*

**Professional, male, Minneapolis**

These lay and professional views demonstrate that religious acts are frequently accessed for the treatment of health problems, specifically for mental health problems. 'Something is wrong about you' and 'lost it' have dormant meanings, possibly referring to psychiatric symptoms and/or mental disorders. *Meher* is a Somali word for 'engagement', as in when a man and a woman agree to marry. Spiritual leaders often must perform *meher* on behalf of the man and woman who are about to marry in order to validate their marriage according to Sharia law (Islamic law). In this context, *meher* is used to highlight the different religious activities the Sheikhs (Mullahs) offer to the Somali community. The statements 'Sheikhs . . . were busier than they were in Somalia' and 'they never had it so good' partly elaborate the popularity of the spiritual services used by some Somalis for social and medical reasons. This also indicates (unlike other Somali professional participants, like the doctors who viewed their skills and talents as wasted) the ability of spiritual leaders to utilize these religious services in the host nation, withstanding social pressures emerging from life in a new environment.

Professional participants acknowledged and agreed with the lay views on the positive way in which religion is used to counteract mental health problems. Nevertheless, they were worried that some people with severe mental health problems were heavily relying on religious treatments to the point where they were not seeking treatment with modern medical professionals for mental disorders:

*There is this woman if you do not read the Quran on her once in every month, there will be a fight in her house. If you say to her 'I would take you to the doctors', it would not work. So, there are still people who believe that Quran alone will treat them 100 per cent.*

**Professional, male, Minneapolis**

*Exactly. That is why people are not going to see their family doctors when they are depressed.*

**Professional, female, Minneapolis**

*We need to let them know the results of the kind of fatalistic attitudes they have or whatever you call it. If they are not feeling well and you tell them to see a doctor, they say things like, 'Oh we know the best' or 'God knows the best'. They say, 'I will die when my time is up', 'I will be safe, remain sound and healthy until then'. So it's that fatalism attitude which needs dispelling. They have to seek out what they need to improve their health.*

**Professional, female, London**

These last quotes offer some explanation for the adverse effects of using religious remedies to the exclusion of health services. These professional participants were concerned that people with mental health problems were not seeking treatment for their health problems partly because Somalis prefer the use of spiritual services to modern medicine. Fatalistic attitudes and beliefs about the existence of life in which God predetermines all future life events were among other reasons stated for the lack of service uptake by Somalis with mental health problems. Here, the professional participants were not dismissive of the role of religion and spirituality in the treatment of health problems but merely emphasizing how people with health problems could benefit both from traditional treatments and modern medical services:

*If the person has an illness, he would be taken to a famous healer who would listen to his problems and then cure him. The healer would release bloated air (naqaska kaa sii daaya) from him that was definitely a good therapy. I know most people got help in this way in Somalia. 60 per cent of people in America are depressed but they are on Prozac and there is no one who is mad, of course, they are chemically imbalanced. But in our community, if people go to hospital and they start taking medication for depression, you*

*would be counted like the crazy people in Malikooniya. Next thing, you hear people saying, 'Oh he is gone mad'.*

**Professional, female, Minneapolis**

Again, this professional view highlighted the way in which traditional healers diagnosed and treated psychological problems in Somalia. The traditional healer would listen to the ill person and by doing so the healer was understood as easing accumulated pressures (*naqas*) from the patient. The statement: 'I know most people got help in this way in Somalia' suggests traditional healers were popular and therefore were used to treating mental illnesses. However, it is not apparent if the healers were popular because they were seen as traditional healers who knew how to diagnose and treat medical problems or because there was no alternative way of seeking treatment for mental illnesses in Somalia. Although this professional view seems to be suggesting that the traditional healers in Somalia were more effective in treating psychological problems, it offers a compromise in which the traditional and modern medical practices both play a crucial role in the treatment of psychological problems.

Another view presented by the participants is that some Somalis have folk illnesses that only health care professionals familiar with the Somali culture can manage:

*People with these illnesses are usually fine. Mentally, they are stable so you can't say they are suffering from schizophrenia. So there are folk illnesses like that people just believe in them, which you can't label them. Boorane and* saar *are related to spiritual beliefs. People believe that there are things in their body that are acting against their will. If you tell these things to a medical doctor, the best thing he will say is that you have a psychological problem. But the person may be healthy and may be working but from time to time they experience these problems.*

**Professional, female, Minneapolis**

*It is often women who say that I have* boorane, wadaado *or* mingis. *Now, can they tell that to their doctors? No chance, they just buy nice perfumes and cosmetics like* hine and catar *from Somali malls. If you see women buying these things from the shops they must be in for a great occasion. You also want to be at the house of the woman who would be treated for* mingis. *Who knows, she may feel better afterwards, whatever, it is great fun.*

**Professional, female, Minneapolis**

However, male professionals thought that innocent women were being manipulated into paying money to unscrupulous middle-aged women:

*I assume the victim pays for these expensive cosmetics.*

**Professional, male, Minneapolis**

This suggests that the professional participants were not convinced by Somali women's luxury use of super perfumes and cosmetics and the money spent on the treatment of *boorane* and *mingis*. Alternatively, this may indicate that Somali men may not necessarily have the same beliefs as women when it comes to some folk illnesses like *boorane* and *mingis*.

## THE ROLE OF THE FAMILY IN THE TREATMENT OF MENTAL DISTRESS

The pivotal role of the family in the mentally ill individual was also explored. Family members were seen as the main carers for people with mental illnesses. They carry out what they see as the right course of action to help the ill person feel better even if that means sending him or her back to Somalia for folk treatments, if all others fail (i.e. spiritual treatments):

*Yes, a lot of them are now sick in the head and they are all going back to Somalia.*

**Lay, female, London**

*They took them back to Somalia to get proper treatment and to get married and when they returned to Minneapolis, they are very healthy.*

**Professional, male, Minneapolis**

*When someone is ill, he goes back home and comes back with a wife, you have to think of what made the difference.*

**Professional, male, Minneapolis**

These professional quotes described some of the reasons why Somalis with mental health problems are sent back home by their family members. A common agreement was that it is easier for the family of an individual with mental illnesses to arrange marriage for him or her in Somalia than abroad. Here, an 'arranged marriage' is discussed in a context that is different from when a family arranges a marriage for a healthy young couple. The professional participants are not merely describing the cultural way in which lay Somalis understand and deal with psychiatric disorders but they, too, like lay Somalis, hinted that arranged marriage was a successful treatment for mental illness.

Individuals with mental health difficulties are sent back to Somalia to get married so they can get back to 'normal'. The professional participants, however, hardly discussed the mechanism through which 'marriage' cures mental illness. The statement 'you have to think of what made the difference' can be interpreted in different ways: that sexual frustration was the main cause for poor mental health among this group and therefore marriage acts as a sex therapy, or that the arranged marriage not only supports the sick person but also rehabilitates him or her back into the community. Thus, marriage may be seen to build up self-esteem, minimize social isolation and reduce stigma and stereotyping.

## DISCUSSION

There was some evidence that some Somalis use spiritual healers and traditional ceremonies to cope with psychological problems, including culture-specific illnesses such as *jin*, *boorane* and *saar*. This may explain the low-level service update often reported among Somali refugees with both mild and severe mental health problems. *Boorane* and *saar* were thought to be unique to Somali women. It was also evident in the focus group discussions that some Somalis do not distinguish various types of mental disorders, for example, depression, dysthymia, general anxiety, stress, distress, mood swings and psychotic disorders. For most Somalis, the demarcation line between sanity and insanity was clear: one would either be labelled 'mad' or 'not mad'. Nevertheless, 'madness' is considered to be a serious mental disorder worthy of seeking modern medical treatments, in addition to spiritual services. The symptoms of 'madness', from a Somali perspective, include being out of control and being a nuisance to other people constantly, as well as being violent.

As in many other cultures, Somalis construct and conceptualize mental illnesses through cultural symptoms and culturally perceived deviant behaviours. Somalis recognize when an individual deviates from his or her known behaviour. These deviant behaviours are then observed, conceptualized and described using culturally coded phrases (Table 17.1).

It is important to note that many of these culturally coded symptoms of mental illness are not perceived as serious conditions that require medical attention. It is only when the person goes beyond the threshold of insanity that spiritual and medical interventions are sought.

In the focus group discussions, the lay participants were more likely to talk about these culturally specific psychological problems such as *buufis*, *roohaan*, *mingis* and *jini*. The professional participants were more likely to discuss depression, PTSD, suicide and anxiety. Some of the lay focus group participants also stated that Somalis were using heavily religious and traditional services that were available to them, while some of the professional participants thought that these traditional methods of treatments were not as effective as modern medicine. The different emphasis on the descriptions and use of spiritual and cultural services between the lay and professional groups could be a reflection of their different models of illness, with the Somali lay models of mental illness more typically expressed in terms of bodily complaints than emotional or mental distress (Warfa *et al.*, 2006).

**Table 17.1**  *Culturally coded phrases used to describe deviant behaviours*

| | |
|---|---|
| Aad buu u walwelaa | He worries excessively |
| Way rafaadsan tahay | She is suffering/rough |
| Aad buu u fakaraa | He thinks too much |
| Sidii hore ma aha | He is not like he used to be before |
| Wuu wareeray | He became confused |
| Neerfoos ayuu noqday | He became nervous |
| Wey isla hadashaa | She talks to herself |
| Ma dhana | He is incomplete |
| Wuu murugoday | He became sad |
| Wuu niyad jabsan yahay | He is dejected |
| Qulub baa haya | He is depressed |
| Wuu waalan rabaa | He is going mad |
| Wuu dhar dhigtay | He is gone naked (mad) |
| Wuu waashay | He became mad |
| Gini baa waalay | Geni made him mad |

To this end, language, conceptual and cultural differences complicate Western psychological interventions for refugee populations. The poor emphasis on descriptions of depression and PTSD by the Somali lay groups, compared with the professional participants, supports the thesis that mental health problems are not perceived to be important among refugee populations (Warfa *et al.*, 2006). Therefore, recommending pharmacological treatments to a Somali patient presenting with psychosomatic symptoms and social problems, including loneliness, immigration, housing and legal issues is not always straightforward. It was clear that not many lay Somalis were familiar with Western methods of psychological treatments. This demands a holistic approach to the problem. More than this, if public services give less attention to the complex health and social care needs of refugees, they may hinder the engagement of vulnerable patients in a system that provides adequate care, particularly since these vulnerable refugees with mental health problems may have already experienced numerous system failures (Warfa and Bhui, 2003). Social and health care providers should work together more closely and in partnership with community groups and refugee groups.

Crucial to a holistic approach is education, health promotion and support to negotiate multiple barriers that many of us might have taken for granted. Health professionals treating Somali refugees with poor mental status need to be sensitive to Somali ways of expressing illness and distress (Warfa *et al.*, 2006) and to be aware that Somalis with severe mental disorders may require more than the standard Western psychiatric interventions, including psycho-social and health promotional work using practical solutions and local ethnographic knowledge.

## REFERENCES

Amnesty International 1997: *Country Report on Somalia. 1997.* London: Amnesty International.

Bhui, K., Mohamud, S., Warfa, N., Craig, T. and Stansfeld, S. 2003: Cultural adaptation of mental health measures: improving the quality of clinical practice and research. Editorial. *British Journal of Psychiatry* 183, 184–86.

Bhui, K., Craig, T., Mohamud, S., Warfa, N., Stansfeld, S.A., Thornicroft, G., Curtis, S. and McCrone, P. 2006: Mental disorders among Somali refugees: Developing culturally appropriate measures and assessing socio-cultural risk factors. *Social Psychiatry and Psychiatric Epidemiology* 41, 4008.

Issa-Salwe, A.M. 1996: *The Collapse of the Somali State.* London: Haan Publishing.

McCrone, P., Bhui, K., Craig, T., Mohamud. S., Warfa, N., Stansfeld, S., Thornicroft, G. and Curtis, S. 2005: Mental health needs, service use and costs among Somali refugees in the UK. *Acta Psychiatrica Scandinavica* 111, 351–57.

Mubarak, J.B. 1996: *From Bad Policy to Chaos in Somalia: How an Economy Fell Apart.* London: Praeger Publications.

United Nations Development Programme (UNDP) 2001: National Human Development Report on Somalia: http://www.so.undp.org/hdr.htm (accessed October 2006).

Warfa, N. and Bhui, K. 2003: Refugees and mental healthcare. *Psychiatry*, Special Topics, Vol. 2.6. London: The Medicine Publishing Company, 26.

Warfa, N., Bhui, K., Craig, T., Curtis, S., Mohamud, S., Stansfeld, S., McCrone, P. and Thornicroft, T. 2006: Post-migration geographical mobility, mental health and health service utilisation among Somali refugees in the UK: a qualitative study. *Health and Place* 12, 503–15.

Warsame M. 1979: Early marriage and teen age deliveries in Somalia. Background papers to the WHO Khartoum Seminar, Sudan.

# 18

# Culture and mental health in South Africa and neighbouring countries

## Leslie Swartz

## INTRODUCTION

Southern Africa as a region is diverse, generally very poor, and still strongly affected by the aftermath of colonialism. Since the fifteenth century when Portuguese sailors rounded the Cape of Good Hope at the foot of Africa, there has been a long and complex history of conquest, domination, resistance and political realignment. A mere few decades ago white minorities controlled political and economic life in all southern African countries; since the 1960s decolonization has occurred, culminating in the demise of apartheid and the inception of democracy in South Africa in 1994. In the post-colonial period, there have been three central challenges which have an important impact on mental health.

First, the question of economic development and redistribution of wealth and resources remains a challenge. Southern African countries in general are poor and very unequal, and attempts to enforce redistribution have had complex results, including the disastrous land reform programme which continues to rack Zimbabwe. A second and related issue is that of governance in the region – there have

been wars both for independence (as in Zimbabwe) and as part of civil conflict (as in Angola and Mozambique), concern about safety and security more generally, and large numbers of internal displacements and refugees as a result of political and economic problems and violence. The third major issue, and one which dominates health concerns in the region, is the rapid and devastating spread of the HIV/AIDS epidemic. Sub-Saharan African currently bears the brunt of the epidemic world-wide, with some estimates suggesting that Botswana has the highest estimated HIV prevalence, and that South Africa has the highest absolute number of HIV-positive people of any country worldwide (UNAIDS, 2005a,b).

South Africa is the economic powerhouse in the region, and has moved from being the pariah it was during the apartheid era, to its current role as dominant regional power since 1994. A recent report for the Global Forum for Health Research, of which the author of the present chapter was principal investigator, shows how this dominance is reflected in literature on mental health – by far the most research into mental health issues of all kinds has been conducted in South Africa (Child,

Youth and Family Development, Human Sciences Research Council, 2005). For this reason, the emphasis in the current chapter will be on research conducted in South Africa, with some references to work from other countries.

Like other countries in the region, South Africa has historically been dominated by a white minority group who were originally settlers. Over 80 per cent of the population is of indigenous African origin. There are also smaller groups of mixed and Asian origin, some of whom can trace their history back to slavery or indentured labour; for example, some of the population of Indian origin in the KwaZulu-Natal province are descendants of people who were brought across from India by white farmers to work on sugar plantations. South Africa is culturally and linguistically diverse; there are 11 official languages in the country. By far the dominant religion is Christianity, but there are also adherents of other religions, including Islam and Hinduism. There are indigenous systems of animistic religion, and spiritual healing takes place in the context of many religious groups, including the context of the syncretic African indigenous churches. These churches combine aspects of Christianity and indigenous religion.

In indigenous religions, there are healers of various kinds, including *amagqirha* or *izangoma* (indigenous healers or diviners, who engage in spiritual healing and are commonly concerned with social ecology, and relationships amongst living people and between the living and their ancestors who have gone before them) and *amaxwhele* (herbalists, sometimes styled as indigenous pharmacists). Within the syncretic religions, healing functions are often taken on by *amaprofita*, or prophets, who use the relationships between people and the Holy Spirit as a key explanatory device for misfortune and a key tool in healing (Swartz, 1998).

Though South Africa is far better supplied with formal health and mental health services than neighbouring countries (Child, Youth and Family Development, 2005), the country is still grossly underserved in terms of mental health services when compared with wealthier countries (Foster *et al.*, 1997; Freeman, 2000).

Although the picture is changing to some degree, by far the majority of professionals in the upper echelons of mental health care (psychiatrists and psychologists in particular) are white and do not speak an indigenous language apart from Afrikaans. This language is related to Dutch, and Afrikaans was extensively promoted by the apartheid regime, as white Afrikaners were dominant in the party of apartheid.

In addition, about 60 per cent of expenditure on health is in the private sector, which is accessed by less than 20 per cent of the population, there are enormous differences in access to care between urban centres, where access can be excellent, and rural areas, where access is commonly very poor. South Africa, like many of her neighbours, also faces a huge exodus of skilled health workers to wealthier countries (Health Systems Trust, 2005). Given South Africa's diversity, and the maldistribution and inaccessibility of resources, it is hardly surprising that many, if not most, South Africans access a range of health resources in a range of healing systems, and in spite of policies designed to bring mental health services into primary and community care, it remains true that state mental health services tend to be accessed primarily by people with serious mental disorder (Swartz and MacGregor, 2002; K and Duncan, 2006).

## THE EXPRESSION AND EXPERIENCE OF DISORDER

### Depression and anxiety

As in many other parts of the world, Western psychiatrists have historically expended considerable energy in southern Africa in attempting to determine whether depression exists and how it is expressed in indigenous African people. As McCulloch puts it:

*During the 1960s there was a flood of publications on depressive illness in Africa, and Western-trained psychiatrists who for two generations had been unable to find any evidence of depression now found it in abundance. . . . The symptoms presented by patients had not changed, nor had the nosology; what had changed was the capacity of clinicians to recognize them.*

McCulloch (1995, p. 113)

The racist view that depression does not occur in African populations because African people lack the insight and sophistication to experience such distress has been replaced with a more sober view, supported by evidence, that anxiety disorders are at least as common in the region as elsewhere, and that there may even be very high rates of depression and anxiety in certain populations, because of social conditions. For example, Cooper *et al.* (1999) found a rate of depression in the puerperium of almost 35 per cent amongst women living in severe poverty in an informal settlement close to Cape Town, roughly three times the rate that would be expected from studies in wealthier countries.

Part of the reason for the underdiagnosis of depression and anxiety in Africa relates to difficulties in finding appropriate assessment methods. Challenges may arise from all or any of the following:

- language and translation difficulties,
- a tendency to express distress in somatic rather than psychological terms (fuelled, possibly, partly by inaccessibility of mental health services),
- the use of spiritual idioms of distress, and
- a possible acceptance of unpleasant but non-disruptive mood states as 'part of life' on the part of oppressed and marginalized people with little access to help (Swartz, 1998).

It is increasingly accepted that when symptoms of anxiety and depression are carefully probed by clinicians, and not assumed to be absent, it may be fairly easy to elicit these symptoms. Two-stage studies of rates of disorder in communities have shown that through some modifications it is possible to use standard international assessment tools to assess common mental disorders (Rumble *et al.*, 1996; Bhagwanjee *et al.*, 1998). The internal consistency of instruments to assess prevalence estimates using certain standard assessment tools can be good when used in southern African contexts (De Bruin *et al.*, 2004).

There is also some interest in ways in which indigenous idioms of distress can be usefully applied by mental health professionals in their work in the field of common mental disorders. For example, Patel *et al.* (1995a,b) describe the use of the term *kufungisisa* (thinking too much) as an idiom for distress associated with common mental disorder amongst Shona-speaking people in Zimbabwe. They suggest that use of this term may assist both in the diagnosis of depression and anxiety and in designing appropriate treatments.

## Psychoses

A central concern about the assessment of psychoses in southern Africa links very closely to issues discussed about depression and anxiety. Whereas depression in particular was at one time erroneously thought to be rare in southern Africa, it appears that psychosis was at one time excessively diagnosed in this context. Belief in the spirit world and the world of the ancestors has historically been seen as a symptom of psychosis – a delusion – instead of a widely held cultural belief. There is now a large literature alerting clinicians to the importance of taking culture into account when making a diagnosis (Swartz, 1998). An additional feature of presentation of mental disorder in the region seems to be a tendency to ascribe misfortune to interpersonal difficulties, including a belief about being bewitched by others. The view that personal distress, illness and symptoms may be caused by malevolent deeds of others is reported to be widely held and not an indication of illness at all. In the study by Rumble *et al.* (1996) mentioned above, the authors had to reanalyse data which had been collected through use of the Present State Examination (PSE) because respondents' reports that they were experiencing emotional distress as a result of harm wished to them by others were incorrectly recorded as psychiatric symptoms, and led to computer-generated tentative diagnoses of psychoses when in fact depression and anxiety were more likely to be correct diagnoses.

In similar vein, there has been extensive concern in southern Africa with patterns of psychosis which appear to be florid but which show atypical features and which may remit quickly. Apart from the question of misdiagnosis of psychosis, there has also been discussion of the question to which social conditions may predispose people to a psychotic presentation (similar to non-affective remitting psychosis in Asia and elsewhere in Africa – see, for example, Collins *et al.*, 1996). There are high rates of substance abuse (including alcohol abuse) in the region (Parry *et al.*, 2004, 2005) and in fact an early contribution to the literature on the possibility of a circumscribed cannabis psychosis comes from a South African team (Rottanburg *et al.*, 1982). There are also, of course, major challenges in the region in terms of nutrition, physical health and parasites, all of which may be implicated in the presentation of serious mental disorder (Petersen *et al.*, 2004; Richter and Norris, 2004). As with common mental disorders, though, there is evidence that when other factors are excluded, the presentation and factor structure of psychosis may appear rather similar to other places in the world (Emsley *et al.*, 2001).

## Folk categories

In many parts of the region, the process of being 'called' to be an indigenous healer is associated with a period of emotional turmoil very similar to that reported in processes of initiation into shamanic roles and states in many other countries. This process, known as *ukuthwasa* in Xhosa and Zulu, has in the past mistakenly been viewed as a form of psychopathology. *Ukuthwasa* may be experienced as very unpleasant, and may be resisted, but is a valued state which can lead to an esteemed role as an indigenous healer. This state is to be differentiated from *amafufunyane*, a form of negative spirit possession which is not wished for and not socially sanctioned and is thought to have a poor outcome. *Phambana*, by contrast, is a term used for mental disorder which is thought to 'just happen' and not to have any spiritual basis.

A huge range of symptoms have been described for *ukuthwasa*, *amafufunyane* and *phambana*, and there are a host of other terms used for folk categories for mental disorders. The key issue to understand, though, is that terms such as these are used to describe the presumed aetiology of disorder and distress rather than a specific set of symptoms. Positive and negative spirit possession have been viewed as responsible for a wide range of physical and mental symptoms and disorders, and the indigenous categories are essentially models of explanation, rather than taxonomies in the sense that categories in Western diagnostic systems are empirical codifications of patterns of behaviour (Swartz, 1998).

## MENTAL HEALTH SERVICES AND OTHER SYSTEMS OF HEALING

It is commonly the case that the idea of the 'cultural' in mental health and disorder is often associated with beliefs that we may have about primordial, unchanging cultures and links to a pre-colonial past. The fact is that culture is a dynamic concept which has very important contemporary political overtones. South Africa in particular has long been a case study in showing how the idea of culture can be manipulated for political ends (as was seen in the apartheid era). In the post-colonial context, the question of what, if any, the relationships between different systems of healing should be, including Western and indigenous healing systems, is only partly a question of what is good for patients. It is also a question of the way in which independent African states wish to present themselves and their relationships with real or imagined indigenous traditions. In both Zimbabwe and South Africa, there has been increasing official recognition of indigenous healing as part of a complex set of interacting health systems; it is even possible in South Africa for some medical insurance systems to be billed for consultations with indigenous healing. There are numerous reports of cross-referral across different healing systems in the region, but the question of how best to use all that different systems have to offer is commonly obscured by the reality that formal health services are difficult to access. People then do not have a choice between different services, but are often forced to use whatever services they can access (Health Systems Trust, 2005).

## FURTHER CHALLENGES

Both the volatile political landscape and the HIV/AIDS epidemic hold challenges for mental health in southern Africa (Kaminer *et al.*, 2001; Smit *et al.*, 2005). It is simply impossible to separate issues of culture and mental health in the region from the broader health context and questions of human rights, governance, violence, and displacement of large numbers of people (Gibson *et al.*, 2001). Though it is certainly the case that mental health issues are intertwined with all other quality-of-life issues throughout the world, this is especially clear in a region of the world which is beset by many difficulties and in the grip of a devastating pandemic.

This leads to a key dilemma for those serious about mental health issues in the region. People concerned with culture and mental health issues can argue their case from a uniquely mental health platform, from a broader public health platform, or even more broadly from the position that health and mental health issues are embedded in national political questions and questions of the kinds of lives that many poor people live. All these positions are useful, and all require attention, but in a situation where there are many claims on national coffers and on the energies of professionals it is by no means clear whether there is any one correct strategy to follow (Freeman, 2000). On the one hand, for mental health workers to focus narrowly on disorders is to ignore much of the evidence relating the aetiology and course of these disorders to contextual factors. On the other hand, to focus on the big picture may lead to abandonment of the particular contribution that mental health can make to the wellbeing of individuals, communities and nations. Case studies quoted by the Child, Youth and Family Development team of the Human Sciences Research Council (2005) indicate that successful mental health practitioners and researchers in these countries are required to play multiple, demanding roles. It is not unheard of, for example, for a single person to be delivering services, making national policy, participating in university administration, and contributing substantially to the research output of a discipline in a country.

As far as research is concerned, the same challenges facing provision of mental health service personnel apply to the development and sustainability of research careers in the region. There is no question that good-quality mental health research can and does emerge from the region, but global initiatives such as that currently under way under the auspices of the Global Forum for Health Research in collaboration with partners such as the World Health Organization are urgently needed. Good researchers, if they are to build long-term careers in the region, need considerable support and access to international networks. The attractions and comforts of the international research environment are considerable, and need to be considered as realities in the planning of research careers. Similarly, though international researchers' interests in the region are admirable and can lead to useful research outputs, multinational research teams need to think carefully about the international dynamics and politics of research (Tomlinson and Swartz, in press). Increasingly, there are models about how to work together across divides in ways which are mutually beneficial and not exploitative.

There is enormous vitality in the culture and mental health field in southern Africa. The challenges are enormous but there are opportunities to make differences to people's lives and to how we understand mental health and disorder. Nowhere in the world is it more clear how interlocked mental health issues are with politics and culture on the one hand and with physical health on the other. This makes the region a very exciting place to work and to develop ideas.

## REFERENCES

Bhagwanjee, A., Parekh, A., Paruk, Z., Petersen, I. and Subedar, H. 1998: Prevalence of minor psychiatric disorders in an adult African rural community in South Africa. *Psychological Medicine* 28, 1137–47.

Child, Youth and Family Development, Human Sciences Research Council 2005: Mental health: Mapping of research capacity in low- and middle-income countries. Final report by the Cape Town team for the Global Forum for Health Research. Cape Town: Human Sciences Research Council.

Collins, P.Y., Wig, N.N., Day, R., Varma, V.K., Malhotra, S., Misra, A.K., Schanzer, B. and Susser, E. 1996: Psychosocial and biological aspects of acute brief psychoses in three developing country sites. *Psychiatric Quarterly* 67, 177–93.

Cooper, P.J., Tomlinson, M., Swartz, L., Woolgar, M., Murray, L. and Molteno, C. 1999: Post-partum depression and the mother-infant relationship in a South African peri-urban settlement. *British Journal of Psychiatry* 175, 554–58.

De Bruin, G., Swartz, L., Tomlinson, M., Cooper, P. and Molteno, C. 2004: The factor structure of the Edinburgh Postnatal Depression Scale in a South African peri-urban settlement. *South African Journal of Psychology* 34, 113–21.

Emsley, R.A., Niehaus, D.J., Mbanga, N.I., Oosthuizen, P.P., Stein, D.J., Maritz, J.S., Pimstone, S.N., Hayden, M.R., Laurent, C., Deleuze, J.F. and Mallet, J. 2001: The factor structure for positive and negative symptoms in South African Xhosa patients with schizophrenia. *Schizophrenia Research* 47, 149–57.

Foster, D., Freeman, M. and Pillay, Y (eds) 1997: *Mental Health Policy Issues for South Africa*. Cape Town: MASA Multimedia.

Freeman, M. 2000: Using all opportunities for improving mental health – examples from South Africa. *Bulletin of the World Health Organization* 78, 508–10.

Gibson, K., Swartz, L. and Sandenbergh, R. 2001: *Counselling and Coping*. Cape Town: Oxford University Press.

Health Systems Trust. 2005: *The South African Equity Gauge*. http://www.hst.org.za/generic/28 (accessed 27 May 2006).

K, S. (pseudonym) and Duncan, M. 2006: Psychiatric disability and social change: an insider perspective. In Watermeyer, B., Swartz, L., Lorenzo, T., Schneider, M. and Priestley, M. (eds) *Disability and Social Change: A South African Agenda*. Cape Town: HSRC Press, 290–310.

Kaminer, D., Stein, D.J., Mbanga, I. and Zungu-Dirwayi, N. 2001: The Truth and Reconciliation Commission in South Africa: relation to psychiatric status and forgiveness among survivors of human rights abuses. *British Journal of Psychiatry* 178, 373–77.

McCulloch, J. 1995: *Colonial Psychiatry and the African Mind*. Cambridge: Cambridge University Press.

Parry, C.D., Myers, B., Morojele, N.K., Flisher, A.J., Bhana, A., Donson, H. and Plüddemann, A. 2004: Trends in adolescent alcohol and other drug use: findings from three sentinel sites in South Africa (1997–2001). *Journal of Adolescence* 27, 429–40.

Parry, C.D., Plüddemann, A., Donson, H., Sukhai, A., Marais, S. and Lombard, C. 2005: Cannabis and other drug use among trauma patients in three South African cities, 1999–2001. *South African Medical Journal* 95, 429–32.

Patel., V., Gwanzura, F., Simunyu., E., Lloyd, K. and Mann, A. 1995a: The phenomenology and explanatory models of common mental disorder: a study in primary care in Harare, Zimbabwe. *Psychological Medicine* 25, 1191–99.

Patel, V., Simunyu, E. and Gwanzura, F. 1995b: Kufungisisa (thinking too much): a Shona idiom for non-psychotic mental illness. *Central African Medical Journal* 41, 209–15.

Petersen, I., Bhana, A., Kvalsvig, J., Allen, S. and Swartz, L. 2004: HIV/AIDS, tuberculosis and parasites. In Swartz, L., de la Rey, C. and Duncan, N. (eds) *Psychology: An Introduction*. Cape Town: Oxford University Press, 449–63.

Richter, L. and Norris, S. 2004: Nutrition. In Swartz, L., de la Rey, C. and Duncan, N. (eds) *Psychology: An Introduction*. Cape Town: Oxford University Press, 437–48.

Rottanburg, D., Robins, A.H., Ben-Arie, O., Teggin, A. and Elk, R. 1982: Cannabis-associated psychosis with hypomanic features. *Lancet* 18, 1364–66.

Rumble, S., Swartz, L., Parry, C. and Zwarenstein, M. 1996: Prevalence of psychiatric morbidity in the adult population of a rural South African village. *Psychological Medicine* 26, 997–1007.

Smit, J., Middelkoop, K., Myer, L., Lindegger, G., Swartz, L., Seedat, S., Tucker, T., Wood, R., Bekker, L. and Stein, D.J. 2005: Socio-behavioural challenges to phase III HIV vaccine trials in sub-Saharan Africa. *African Health Sciences Journal* 5(3), 198–206.

Swartz, L. (1998). *Culture and Mental Health: A Southern African View*. Cape Town: Oxford University Press.

Swartz, L. and MacGregor, H. 2002: Integrating services, marginalising patients: psychiatric patients and primary health care in South Africa. *Transcultural Psychiatry* 39, 155–72.

Tomlinson, M. and Swartz, L. in press: Insiders and outsiders: levels of collaboration in research partnerships across resource divides. *Infant Mental Health Journal*.

UNAIDS 2005a: *Botswana*. http://www.unaids.org/en/Regions_Countries/Countries/botswana.asp (accessed 27 May 2006).

UNAIDS 2005b: *South Africa*. http://www.unaids.org/en/Regions_Countries/Countries/south_africa.asp (accessed 27 May 2006).

# 19

# Indigenous peoples of South America – inequalities in mental health care

## Mario Incayawar

## INTRODUCTION

The scarcity of information and psychiatric research for the South American region is alarming (Seale *et al.*, 2002). Although there are pioneering studies of psychiatric disorders using conventional instruments (see Chapter 20), these do not always ensure validity across cultures; for example, there is very little information on indigenous illness categories or indigenous healing practices. According to reports from the 1970s and 1980s, comprehensive mental health services are lacking in Latin America and often have the lowest priority both politically and socially (Argandoña and Kiev, 1972; Alarcon, 1986). A transition now under way in these countries involves a move away from the use of large urban psychiatric hospitals towards establishing psychiatric beds in general hospitals, and ultimately towards the integration of mental health care with primary health care (Murthy, 1998; Larrobla and Botega, 2001; Saldivia *et al.*, 2004). The process of restructuring psychiatric care in South America began in the 1980s and escalated during the 1990s. Although these structural developments in mental health care are laudable, they neglect the mental health care needs of the indigenous peoples of South America. In the context of limited resources,

resource-starved mental health services, and social indifference to the mentally ill, it is ironic to attempt to describe South American mental health services for the indigenous peoples.

The fact is that 30 million indigenous people in South America, forming up to 10 per cent of the general population, live in outrageous conditions of human misery and neglect. Conventional Western-type mental health care for them is just non-existent. This chapter adopts a specific way of documenting the mental health status of indigenous peoples by reviewing some of the socio-economic and health indicators of this forgotten and voiceless people.

## POVERTY AND SOCIAL EXCLUSION

Poverty and social exclusion plague the indigenous peoples of the Americas. Many international organizations, including the Pan American Health Organization (PAHO), the United Nations (UN), the World Bank, and the Inter-American Development Bank, among others, have produced numerous technical reports revealing their misery. What is striking is the consistently higher poverty rates (defined as living on US$2 per day or less) found among the indigenous population. In some South American countries, the poverty rates are three to four times the national average. There is a clear-cut geographical distribution of misery in South America. The highest rates of poverty and extreme poverty are found precisely in regions with the highest indexes of indigenous population (Psacharopoulos and Patrinos, 1994). A strong poverty–ethnicity correlation exists in rural and urban areas among different countries of the region. The World Bank's 1995 poverty assessment for Ecuador, for instance, found that households in which an indigenous language is spoken are more likely to be poor than are Spanish-speaking house-holds, and strongly indigenous populated regions are worse off with respect to social and service vari-ables, such as education, nutrition, housing, water and sewerage. In areas with an indigenous popula-tion majority, the poverty rate (including those highly vulnerable to poverty) is approximately 85 per cent (Van Nieuwkoop and Uquillas, 2000). Latin America in general and South America in particular demonstrates the greatest disparities in income as well as other socio-economic determin-ants of health in the world (Pan American Health Organization, 1999). Brazil has the highest income disparity in the world, and in some countries, the richest 10 per cent of the population receive 84 times the income received by the poorest (Duncan *et al.*, 1995). Table 19.1 shows some details of the estimated indigenous population in several countries of South America.

The United Nations, in its World Population Prospects for 1998, noted the dramatic nature of the socio-economic conditions of South America's indigenous peoples. Recently, the United Nations Economic Commission for Latin America and the Caribbean confirmed their deplorable status of being the poorest among the poor. Fortunately, in the last couple of years, the word is spreading pub-licly. Nils Kastberg, UNICEF's Regional Director for Latin America and the Caribbean, said at the Foro Iberoamericano sobre la Niñez, held in Madrid in 2005: 'in Latin America, discrimination is a structural problem, between 88% to 95% of the Indigenous Peoples continue to live in exclusion'.

In this continental context of extreme socio-economic inequality, we can expect dramatic health

**Table 19.1** *Estimated indigenous population in South America countries and selected territories (by millions of inhabitants)*

| Country | National population | Indigenous population | Per cent |
|---|---|---|---|
| Bolivia | 6.9 | 4.9 | 71 |
| Peru | 20.0 | 9.3 | 47 |
| Ecuador | 9.5 | 4.1 | 43 |
| French Guiana | 0.1 | 0.004 | 4 |
| Paraguay | 3.5 | 0.10 | 3 |
| Colombia | 30.0 | 0.60 | 2 |
| Venezuela | 18.0 | 0.40 | 2 |
| Argentina | 31.9 | 0.35 | 1 |
| Brazil | 140.0 | 0.3 | 0.20 |

Adapted to show data for South America.
Source: Pan American Health Organization (1993).

and mental health service disparities. Moreover, often the indigenous peoples in South America are treated as outsiders and as inferiors (Cohen, 1999) and consequently they are literally excluded from the conventional Western mental health services.

## INDIGENOUS PEOPLES' POOR HEALTH

The poor health status of the indigenous peoples of South America is believed to result from social exclusion, alienation of health and mental health services, genetic vulnerabilities and colonial oppres-sion (Duran and Duran, 1995; Durie, 2003). The Pan American Health Organization Report on Health Disparities in Latin America and the Caribbean concludes that there are direct ties between the indigenous people, extreme poverty and disproportionately high mortality/morbidity rates (Pan American Health Organization, 1999).

Indigenous peoples generally have high mortal-ity rates, lower life expectancy, malnutrition and higher incidence of most diseases than non-indigenous populations. The infant mortality among the Quichuas of northern Ecuador was 211 per 1000 in 1986, while the national average was 38. The infant mortality in the region is 2–3.5 times higher for the indigenous children. In Honduras, life expectancy was 29 years lower for men and 27 years lower for women than the national average. A 1993/94 survey in Colombia found a life expectancy of 57.8 for women and 55.4 for men while the national average for the country was 67–65 years (Pan American Health Organization, 1999, p. 10). According to a 2004 Mission Report for the World Food Program in Guatemala, malnutrition affects 69.5 per cent of the indigenous population compared with 35.7 per cent in non-indigenous populations; in some areas this figure increases to 88 per cent (World Food Program, 2004). It is estimated that 95 per cent of indigenous people aged 14 years or less are malnourished.

We are going to close this section of health indicators by mentioning the consistent lack of basic public services such as water, sanitation, housing, electricity, etc. available for the indigenous communities (Van Nieuwkoop and Uquillas, 2000).

There is a scarcity of research on mental health among the indigenous peoples of South America. There is a very limited knowledge about the prevalence, incidence, risk factors and protective factors for mental disorders among this population (Seale *et al.*, 2002). We do not have mental health services data related to gender, the elderly, children, adolescents, migrants, displaced communities and other vulnerable groups.

## THE SOUTH AMERICAN COUNTRIES' RESPONSE

Following 180 years of independent life as nation-states, the countries of South America have done little or nothing for the wellbeing of the indigenous peoples. Only in 1978, the World Health Organization conference in Alma Ata, URSS proposed the implementation of primary care as a priority in which the indigenous medicine was mentioned for the first time 'with the support of formal health systems, the agents of Traditional Medicine can become important allies in organizing efforts to improve community health'. This proposal was welcomed with great enthusiasm by the Asian and African countries, but not by those in South America (Pan American Health

Organization, 1996). The official sources in most of the countries of the region have little or no information on the health status and living conditions of their indigenous peoples. Then, in 1995 the United Nations launched the International Decade of the World's Indigenous People (1995–2004), aimed at increasing international cooperation to tackle their human rights, environmental, educational and health problems (United Nations, 1994).

Other regional and continental meetings followed, such as the First Continental Meeting, Five Hundred Years of Indigenous Resistance, held in Quito, Ecuador in 1990; the Continental Campaign, 500 Years of Indigenous, Black, and Popular Resistance, held in Esteli, Nicaragua in 1992; and finally, the First Hemispheric Working Meeting on the Health of the Indigenous People, held in Winnipeg, Canada in 1993. Those efforts culminated with the approval of Resolution V at the XXXVII Meeting of the Directing Council of the PAHO, on 28 September 1993. Resolution V reflects the higher ranking political will of the member governments of the PAHO in promoting the Initiative on the Health of Indigenous Peoples of the Americas (Pan American Health Organization, 1993).

Despite the goodwill and high-profile signing of the PAHO Initiative by the member states, the follow-up of the programme is poor, and its impact on the health status and wellbeing of the members of the indigenous nations of South America has been hardly noticeable. PAHO has even created the Health of the Indigenous Peoples Unit. Several countries have created specific units that are meant to deal with indigenous peoples' health in general, with no mention of mental health.

One last, yet interesting workshop called 'Programas y Servicios de Salud Mental en Communidades Indígenas' (Mental Health Programmes and Services for the Indigenous Communities) was held on 16–18 July 1998 in Santa Cruz city in Bolivia (Pan American Health Organization, 1998). The goal of this meeting, sponsored by PAHO and the Government of Bolivia, was to outline the basis for the implementation of mental health programmes and services for the indigenous peoples of the region. Many countries participated in this unique and small workshop, including: Bolivia, Brazil, Chile, Ecuador, the USA, Guatemala, Mexico, Nicaragua, Peru and nine PAHO officials. Seven years later, however, no particular programmes of mental health designed for indigenous peoples exist in South America.

As recently stated by Health Unlimited (a British non-governmental organization) and the London School of Hygiene and Tropical Medicine, indigenous peoples are unable to access routine health care and are dying prematurely, despite efforts by the United Nations and PAHO, and their member states (Tayal, 2003). Although the above-mentioned initiatives are commendable, legitimate and full participation of indigenous peoples in controlling their own future remains contentious. Organizations such as PAHO, and regionally the ministries of health and mental health care services, remain hermetic and distant to the indigenous people. For example, the author himself was repeatedly unsuccessful in even getting an appointment to meet the Ecuador Representative of PAHO when attempting to invite PAHO to participate in the World Psychiatric Association's Transcultural Psychiatry Section Symposium entitled 'Psychiatrists and Healers: Unwitting Partners – A Challenge for Transcultural Psychiatry in Times of Globalization', held in Quito, Ecuador, in May 2005. The Runajambi – Institute for the Study of Quichua Culture and Health hosted this meeting.

To further put local human faces to this situation, in 1986, we were the first two Quichua physicians in Ecuador to graduate from the medical school in Quito. Today, almost 20 years later, there are five Quichua physicians for an estimated population of 5 million indigenous people in Ecuador. With this pace of change, the existing staff, the available psychiatric services, and the mental health of our communities will not improve in the foreseeable future.

## TRADITIONAL MENTAL HEALTH RESOURCES – THE FUTURE

The indigenous peoples view themselves as invisible, voiceless, dispossessed nations subdued by the nation-states of South America. The global neglect and exploitation is viewed as the perpetuation of centuries-long colonial oppression. The lack of mental health services and the outrageous health disparities are interpreted as the consequence of their status of subjugated nations. Furthermore, it is striking to see how much conventional health care systems and professionals end up overlooking the extensive indigenous systems of health care that carry the trust of indigenous peoples.

Fortunately, a widespread traditional health and mental health care network exists within the indigenous peoples communities, composed of traditional healers, bonesetters, midwives, the community, families and elderly women. Traditional healers, of which there are tens of thousands, still enjoy high prestige in their communities, and they are often considered by indigenous patients to be their trusted doctors (Incayawar, 1995). According to the World Health Organization's World Mental Health Surveys, 75–85 per cent of the world population relies on local healers when in need of medical care (Demyttenaere et al., 2004). At the same time, only a fraction of the world population has access to Western psychological and psychiatric services. In Ecuador, we have only one Quichua psychiatrist for 5 million indigenous people. If mainstream conventional services neglect the needs of these peoples, and there are insufficient numbers of Quichua psychiatrists, then the problems of indigenous peoples are clearly likely to be neglected for generations to come.

Indigenous peoples-led health institutions are proposing some alternative approaches. Although the majority of them are located in the USA and Canada (Aboriginal Healing Foundation, 2004; Royal Commission on Aboriginal Peoples, Canada, 1993; Walters et al., 2002), there are at least two formal projects in South America that deserve attention. One is the Jambihuasi project in Otavalo, Ecuador, which was founded in 1984, with the support of Quichua professionals, Quichua healers, community leaders and a provincial political organization. Jambihuasi offers an integrated Western and Quichua medical service, and referral to medical specialists. The patients are free to choose the provider, either a traditional healer, a biomedically trained physician, or both. The levels of acceptance and satisfaction of this integrated service by the Quichua patients and families is very good. Another project is Runajambi – Institute for the Study of Quichua Culture and Health, created in 1990, which was the first Quichua institution created in Ecuador. It is devoted to the betterment, through research, of the health of the indigenous peoples of the Andes. Runajambi promotes the collaboration of healers and doctors as the key element for achieving a good health for the Quichuas.

Traditional healers are helping to reduce the disparities in life expectancy and health among indigenous peoples of South America. As stated in the *World Health Report 2001 – Mental Health: New Understanding, New Hope* (World Health Organization, 2001), traditional healers could help in the global efforts to improve health through the following activities: (a) as active case finders; (b) facilitators of referrals; (c) providing counselling; monitoring and in the follow-up of cases. Their role is viewed as essential for increasing access, identification of psychiatric cases in the community (Incayawar, 2001) and successful treatment of psychiatric patients.

In closing, we can conclude that mental health care for indigenous peoples remains a low priority for health and social care agencies and local governments. From the indigenous perspective, global exclusion is a direct result of a policy of internal colonialism that has continued for centuries (see Chapters 2 and 5). The indigenous nations and their members are treated as second-class or vanquished individuals. In this context of consistent neglect throughout South America, the indigenous peoples remain encouraged by the active role of traditional medicine in the provision of health services but not by the plans and reports of the South American states and governments. Culturally insensitive mental health services, programmes designed without the participation of Amerindian people and experts, services that emphasize greater influence of Western-trained mental health professionals and expensive Western health service infrastructures, can only perpetuate the misery and suffering of the indigenous people. Our communities and organizations are proposing to take control of our own destiny, promoting self-determination, having our own voice, taking a legitimate place within the Western-dominated institutions, requesting a fair

sharing of allocation of funds, heightening the capacities of traditional health systems, overall, becoming less invisible and voiceless. This kind of socio-political transformation is important in helping to improve the health and mental health of the indigenous people of South America.

## REFERENCES

Aboriginal Healing Foundation 2004: *Historic Trauma and Aboriginal Healing*. Ottawa, Canada: Aboriginal Healing Foundation.

Alarcon, R.D. 1986: Mental health in Latin America, 1970–1985. *Bulletin of the Pan-American Sanitary Office* 101, 567–92.

Argandoña, M. and Kiev, A. 1972: *Mental Health in the Developing World. A Case Study in Latin America*. New York: Free Press.

Cohen, A. 1999: *The Mental Health of Indigenous Peoples: An International Overview*. Geneva: Nations for Mental Health, Department of Mental Health, World Health Organization.

Demyttenaere, K., Bruffaerts, R., Posada-Villa, J., Gasquet, I., Kovess, V., Lepine, J.P., Angermeyer, M.C., Bernert, S., de Girolamo, G., Morosini, P., Polidori, G., Kikkawa, T., Kawakami, N., Ono, Y., Takeshima, T., Uda, H., Karam, E.G., Fayyad, J.A., Karam, A.N., Mneimneh, Z.N., Medina-Mora, M.E., Borges, G., Lara, C., de Graaf, R., Ormel, J., Gureje, O., Shen, Y., Huang, Y., Zhang, M., Alonso, J., Haro, J.M., Vilagut, G., Bromet, E.J., Gluzman, S., Webb, C., Kessler, R.C., Merikangas, K.R., Anthony, J.C., Von Korff, M.R., Wang, P.S., Brugha, T.S., Aguilar-Gaxiola, S., Lee, S., Heeringa, S., Pennell, B.E., Zaslavsky, A.M., Ustun, T.B. and Chatterji, S. 2004: Prevalence, severity, and unmet need for treatment of mental disorders in the World Health Organization World Mental Health Surveys. *Journal of the American Medical Association* 291, 2581–90.

Duncan, B.B., Rumel, D., Zelmanowicz, A., Mengue, S.S., dos Santos S. and Dalmaz, A. 1995: Social inequality in mortality in Sao Paulo State, Brazil. *International Journal of Epidemiology* 24, 359–65.

Duran, E. and Duran, B. 1995: *Native American Postcolonial Psychology*. Albany: State University of New York Press.

Durie, M.H. 2003: The health of indigenous peoples. *British Medical Journal* 326, 510–11.

Incayawar, M. 1995: *Llaqui* and depression: exploration of a Quichua (Ecuador) folk illness cluster. Presented at the 148th Meeting of the American Psychiatric Association, Symposium on Culture Bound Syndromes, Miami, Florida, 20–25 May.

Incayawar, M. 2001: Psychiatric case identification skills of *yachactaita* (Quichua healers). Presented at the Symposium

Andorra 2001, Transcultural Psychiatry Section, World Psychiatric Association, Principality of Andorra, 23–26 May.

Larrobla, C. and Botega, N.J. 2001: Restructuring mental health: a South American survey. *Social Psychiatry and Psychiatric Epidemiology* 36, 256–59.

Murthy, R.S. 1998: Rural psychiatry in developing countries. *Psychiatric Services* 49, 967–69.

Pan American Health Organization 1993: *Resolution V – Health of the Indigenous People*. Washington DC: PAHO.

Pan American Health Organization 1996: *Initiative on the Health of Indigenous Peoples Toward a Comprehensive Approach to Health*. Washington DC: PAHO and World Health Organization, 1.

Pan American Health Organization 1998: *10. Programas y Servicios de Salud Mental en Comunidades Indigenas, Grupo de Trabajo*. Washington DC: PAHO, 10.

Pan American Health Organization 1999: *Health disparities in Latin America and the Caribbean: the role of social and economic determinants*. Washington, DC: Division of Health and Human Development, PAHO/WHO.

Psacharopoulos, G. and Patrinos, H. 1994: *Indigenous People and Poverty in Latin America: An Empirical Analysis*. Washington, DC: World Bank.

Royal Commission on Aboriginal Peoples, Canada 1993: *The Path to Healing Report of the National Round Table on Aboriginal Health and Social Issues*. Ottawa: Royal Commission on Aboriginal Peoples.

Saldivia, S., Vicente, B., Kohn, R., Rioseco, P. and Torres, S. 2004: Use of mental health services in Chile. *Psychiatric Services* 55, 71–76.

Seale, J.P., Seale, J.D., Alvarado, M., Vogel, R.L. and Terry, N.E. 2002: Prevalence of problem drinking in a Venezuelan Native American population. *Alcohol and Alcoholism* 37, 198–204.

Tayal, U. 2003: UN policy fails to tackle health needs of indigenous people. *British Medical Journal* 327, 413.

United Nations 1994: Statement by the President of the General Assembly at the Commencement of the International Decade of the World's Indigenous People. UN Information Co-ordinator GA/8842, 9 December 1994, New York.

Van Nieuwkoop, M. and Uquillas, J.E. 2000: *Defining Ethnodevelopment in Operational Terms: Lessons from the Ecuador Indigenous and Afro-Ecuadoran Peoples Development Project*. Washington, DC: World Bank, 6.

Walters, K.L., Simoni, J.M. and Evans-Campbell, T. 2002: Substance use among American Indians and Alaska natives: incorporating culture in an 'indigenist' stress-coping paradigm. *Public Health Reports* 117, S104–S117.

World Food Program 2004: Mission Report – Guatemala, 10–17 February.

World Health Organization 2001: *The World Health Report 2001. Mental Health: New Understanding, New Hope*. Geneva: World Health Organization.

# 20

# Mental health and cultural psychiatry in Latin America

## Robert Kohn

## INTRODUCTION

The Latin American region consists of 18 countries that are divided into five subregions: Andean Area, Brazil, Central America, Mexico and Southern Cone. The Andean Area is made up of Bolivia, Colombia, Ecuador, Peru and Venezuela. The Central American countries include Belize, Costa Rica, El Salvador, Guatemala, Honduras, Nicaragua and Panama. The Southern Cone constitutes Argentina, Chile, Paraguay and Uruguay. These countries are quite varied in regards to their demographics, health and economies. Although all have Spanish as one of their official languages with the exception of Brazil (Portuguese) and Belize (English), large segments of the population only speak their indigenous language.

In many Latin American countries a high proportion of the population are under 15 years of age, in particular in Central America. In Guatemala 42.3 per cent of the population are under age 15 (see Table 20.1). One in five households in Latin America are headed by women, many of whom have children under the age of 18 (Economic Commission for Latin America and the Caribbean, 1997). In 1998, in Costa Rica, 21 per cent of households were headed by women, and 44 per cent of births were registered as 'father unknown' (Núñez et al., 2000); in El Salvador, 35 per cent of households were headed by women.

Nearly all countries in the region have a negative migratory balance with the exception of Argentina and Costa Rica, with Mexico having the largest population migrating to the USA. In 2002, 300 000 people left Mexico. Segments of the region continue to have high rates of illiteracy, such as in Nicaragua where 42 per cent of the population cannot read or write. More than half of the nations in Latin America have greater than 10 per cent of their population below the international poverty line. In addition, large economic disparities exist in many of the countries between the wealthy and the poor. None of the countries has an income distribution ratio of less than 10 per cent, and Brazil has the largest disparity, 32.2 per cent. Fourteen of the countries still have life expectancies from birth less than 75 years.

**Table 20.1**   *Demographic data on Latin American countries*

| Country | Population (thousands) | Urban population (%) | Age <15 (%) | Age >60 (%) | Population below the international poverty line[a] (%) | Income ratio[b] | Literacy rate (%) | Life expectancy at birth (years) |
|---|---|---|---|---|---|---|---|---|
| Argentina | 38 871 | 90.3 | 26.9 | 13.7 | 3.3 | 18.2 | 97.2 | 74.6 |
| Belize | 261 | 48.5 | 37.0 | 5.9 | – | – | 94.4 | 71.3 |
| Bolivia | 8 973 | 63.9 | 38.2 | 6.7 | 14.4 | 12.3 | 87.7 | 64.6 |
| Brazil | 180 654 | 83.6 | 27.5 | 8.4 | 8.2 | 32.2 | 88.5 | 68.7 |
| Chile | 15 996 | 87.3 | 27.0 | 11.1 | 2.0 | 18.8 | 96.3 | 76.3 |
| Colombia | 44 914 | 76.9 | 31.4 | 7.4 | 14.4 | 22.9 | 92.7 | 72.7 |
| Costa Rica | 4 250 | 61.2 | 29.0 | 8.1 | 2.0 | 12.3 | 96.1 | 78.4 |
| Ecuador | 13 192 | 62.3 | 32.2 | 7.6 | 17.7 | 17.6 | 92.7 | 71.2 |
| El Salvador | 6 614 | 59.8 | 34.5 | 7.7 | 31.1 | 19.7 | 80.6 | 71.2 |
| Guatemala | 12 661 | 46.8 | 42.3 | 5.3 | 16.0 | 24.7 | 71.2 | 66.5 |
| Honduras | 7 099 | 46.0 | 39.7 | 5.5 | 23.8 | 21.8 | 77.4 | 68.8 |
| Mexico | 104 931 | 75.8 | 31.8 | 7.6 | 9.9 | 19.1 | 92.3 | 73.8 |
| Nicaragua | 5 597 | 57.7 | 41.2 | 4.7 | 45.1 | 16.6 | 67.8 | 70.1 |
| Panama | 3 177 | 57.5 | 30.6 | 8.6 | 7.2 | 25.1 | 92.8 | 75.0 |
| Paraguay | 6 018 | 57.9 | 38.0 | 5.6 | 14.9 | 27.4 | 94.2 | 71.3 |
| Peru | 27 567 | 74.2 | 32.7 | 7.6 | 18.1 | 18.3 | 91.2 | 70.4 |
| Uruguay | 3 439 | 92.7 | 24.4 | 17.4 | 2.0 | 10.4 | 97.9 | 75.7 |
| Venezuela | 26 170 | 87.9 | 32.0 | 7.2 | 15.0 | 17.8 | 93.7 | 74.1 |

[a]Defined as less than $1.08 a day at 1993 international prices.
[b]Highest 20 per cent minus lowest 20 per cent income ratio.
Source: Pan American Health Organization website based on most recent data available as of 2004.

The indigenous population of Latin America is estimated to be between 45 and 50 million, of whom 90 per cent are concentrated in Central America and the Andean subregion. The countries with the highest indigenous population, at 40–70 per cent, are Bolivia, Ecuador, Guatemala and Peru. In Belize, Chile, El Salvador, Honduras, Mexico, Nicaragua and Panama indigenous people account for 5–20 per cent of the total population (Pan American Health Organization, 2002) (Table 20.2). The countries with the largest proportion of people of African descent are Brazil (45 per cent), Colombia and Venezuela. The indigenous populations and those of African descent in the region are disproportionately poor and illiterate in comparison with the rest of the population. For example, in Brazil the lowest income quartile are found among Mulattos (29.5 per cent), indigenous people (27.9 per cent), blacks (23 per cent), and only 13.4 per cent of the

whites and 8.1 per cent of the Asians are to be found in the lowest income quartile (Torres, 1996). In Bolivia, Brazil, Guatemala and Peru those individuals who are indigenous or of African descent have wages that are less than half of the rest of the population and will receive from 3 to 4 years less schooling (Zoninsein, 2002). These populations also have higher infant mortality rates, higher maternal mortality rates, higher mortality from external causes and poorer health outcomes.

## DISABILITY ADJUSTED LIFE YEARS (DALYS) AND YEARS LIVED WITH DISABILITY (YLDS)

Neuropsychiatric conditions in 1990 were estimated to account for 8.8 per cent of disability

**Table 20.2**   *Estimated indigenous, Mestizo, and black populations in Latin America (ranked by per cent indigenous) and percentage of indigenous population living in poverty compared with the general population*

| Indigenous ranking | Country | Indigenous population in thousands | Percentage of total population | | | Percentage living in poverty | |
|---|---|---|---|---|---|---|---|
| | | | Indigenous | Mestizo | African origin | General | Indigenous |
| Group 1 Over 40% | Bolivia | 5 662 | 71 | | | 52.5 | 64.3 |
| | Guatemala | 7 129 | 66 | | | 65.6 | 86.6 |
| | Peru | 11 655 | 47 | 37 | 3 | 53.0 | 79.0 |
| | Ecuador | 5 235 | 43 | 65 | 3 | | |
| Group 2 5–20% | Belize | 44 | 19 | 44 | 7 | | |
| | Honduras | 922 | 15 | 90 | | | |
| | Mexico | 13 416 | 14 | 60 | | 22.6 | 80.6 |
| | Chile | 1 186 | 8 | | | | |
| | El Salvador | 422 | 7 | 90 | | | |
| | Panama | 132 | 6 | 70 | | | |
| | Nicaragua | 240 | 5 | 69 | 9 | | |
| Group 3 1–4% | Paraguay | 157 | 3 | 95 | | 20.5 | 36.8 |
| | Colombia | 816 | 2 | 71 | 5 | | |
| | Venezuela | 465 | 2 | 65 | 10 | | |
| | Costa Rica | 38 | 1 | | 3 | | |
| | Argentina | 361 | 1 | 3 | | | |
| Group 4 Less than 1% | Brazil | 332 | 0.2 | 40 | 5 | | |
| | Uruguay | 1 | 0.016 | 8 | 4 | | |

Source: Pan American Health Organization (2002) for indigenous population; People Please Almanac for missing data on the Mestizo (white–indigenous mix) and African origin population. Note, as data came from a variety of sources some population figures are more than 100 per cent. The percentage living in poverty from Bolivia is based on urban populations only and for Paraguay only the non-bilingual Guarani-speaking population.

adjusted life years (DALYs) (Murray and Lopez, 1996). In the year 2002, the contribution of neuropsychiatric conditions to overall disability rose to 22.2 per cent (World Health Organization, 2002). In part, the excess disability due to mental disorders is a result of their early age of onset compared with other chronic conditions (WHO ICPE, 2000). In 2002 for those between the ages of 15 and 59, 29.3 per cent of the DALYs were accounted for by neuropsychiatric conditions. This increasing burden in Latin America and the Caribbean may be a result of the epidemiological transition from infectious diseases to chronic illness, an increased focus on emergent disorders, such as violence and AIDS, as well as the changing population structure leading to a relative older population at increased risk for mental disorders (Pan American Health Organization, 2002; see Chapters 31 and 32). Unipolar depressive

disorder alone accounts for 6.9 per cent of all DALYs for the region across all age groups, and 10.3 per cent among the 15–59 age group. Table 20.3 lists the 20 most significant causes of DALYs in the region.

Neuropsychiatric disorders account for 40.4 per cent of all years lived with disability (YLDs) irrespective of age, and 47.1 per cent for those 15–59 years of age. Unipolar depressive disorder accounts for 13.2 per cent of all YLDs, and 17.3 per cent among those aged 15–59. Unipolar depressive disorder, schizophrenia and alcohol use disorders are the three top causes of YLD in women aged 15–59. For men aged 15–59 it is alcohol use disorders, unipolar depressive disorders and violence. The number of years lost (in thousands) from depression-related death and disability in Latin America and the Caribbean (2000) was estimated at 1815 in men and

**Table 20.3**   *Year 2002 disability adjusted life years (DALYs) for Latin America and Caribbean by top 20 causes*

| | All ages | | | Ages 15–59 | | |
|---|---|---|---|---|---|---|
| | T | M | F | T | M | F |
| Unipolar depressive disorders | 1 | 4 | 1 | 1 | 3 | 1 |
| Violence | 2 | 1 | | 2 | 1 | 13 |
| Birth asphyxia and birth trauma | 3 | 6 | 2 | | | |
| Alcohol use disorders | 4 | 2 | | 3 | 2 | 7 |
| Other unintentional injuries | 5 | 3 | 10 | 5 | 5 | 14 |
| Ischaemic heart disease | 6 | 7 | 7 | 9 | 7 | 12 |
| Road traffic accidents | 7 | 5 | 20 | 4 | 4 | 11 |
| Cerebrovascular disease | 8 | 10 | 3 | 8 | 10 | 6 |
| HIV/AIDS | 9 | 8 | 9 | 6 | 6 | 2 |
| Lower respiratory infection | 10 | 9 | 4 | | | |
| Other digestive diseases | 11 | 11 | 5 | 7 | 11 | 4 |
| Diarrhoeal diseases | 12 | 12 | 8 | | | |
| Diabetes mellitus | 13 | 17 | 6 | 12 | 14 | 8 |
| Asthma | 14 | 16 | 11 | 17 | 15 | |
| Other perinatal conditions | 15 | 14 | 15 | | | |
| Other infectious diseases | 16 | 13 | 19 | | 18 | |
| Mental retardation, lead-caused | 17 | 18 | 12 | | | |
| Chronic obstructive pulmonary disease | 18 | 19 | 13 | 15 | 19 | 10 |
| Schizophrenia | 19 | | 17 | 10 | 12 | 5 |
| Cataracts | 20 | | 14 | 16 | | 16 |
| Cirrhosis of the liver | | 15 | | 14 | 8 | |
| Drug use disorders | | 20 | | 13 | 9 | |
| Other maternal conditions | | | | 19 | | 3 |
| Endocrine disorders | | | 16 | | | 19 |
| Bipolar disorder | | | 18 | 11 | 13 | 9 |
| Hearing loss, adult onset | | | | 18 | 17 | |
| Vision disorders, age-related | | | | 20 | | |
| Self-inflicted injuries | | | | | 16 | |
| Tuberculosis | | | | | 20 | |
| Maternal sepsis | | | | | | 15 |
| Rheumatoid arthritis | | | | | | 17 |
| Panic disorder | | | | | | 18 |
| Breast cancer | | | | | | 20 |

3423 in women. Men, on the other hand, exhibited a higher incidence of dependency on substances such as alcohol and drugs. The figure for years lost due to alcohol consumption was 11 times higher for men than for women (4321 compared with 389); males' loss of years due to drug consumption was nearly double that of females (881 compared with 472) (World Bank, 2001). Table 20.4 has a summary of the rankings for YLDs.

## SUICIDE, HOMICIDE AND VIOLENCE

Suicide is the only external cause of death for which men did not always rank higher than women in Latin America. In the past completed suicide tended to be higher in males, in contrast with suicide attempts, which were more prevalent in females. Recent data, however, indicate that the suicide rates among female adolescents have surpassed those for

**Table 20.4** *Year 2002 years lived with disability (YLDs) for Latin America and Caribbean by top 20 causes*

| | All ages | | | Ages 15–59 | | |
|---|---|---|---|---|---|---|
| | T | M | F | T | M | F |
| Unipolar depressive disorders | 1 | 2 | 1 | 1 | 2 | 1 |
| Alcohol use disorders | 2 | 1 | 8 | 2 | 1 | 3 |
| Violence | 3 | 3 | | 3 | 3 | |
| Other unintentional injuries | 4 | 4 | 17 | 5 | 4 | 17 |
| Asthma | 5 | 5 | 4 | 12 | 8 | 18 |
| Mental retardation, lead-caused | 6 | 6 | 2 | | | |
| Schizophrenia | 7 | 9 | 6 | 4 | 6 | 2 |
| Cataracts | 8 | 10 | 3 | 9 | 11 | 8 |
| Other digestive diseases | 9 | 12 | 5 | 8 | 13 | 6 |
| Hearing loss, adult onset | 10 | 8 | 12 | 10 | 9 | 12 |
| Vision disorders, age-related | 11 | 13 | 7 | 13 | 12 | 14 |
| Bipolar disorder | 12 | 11 | 11 | 6 | 7 | 5 |
| Birth asphyxia and birth trauma | 13 | 14 | 14 | | | |
| Drug use disorders | 14 | 7 | | 7 | 5 | |
| Chronic obstructive pulmonary disease | 15 | 16 | 15 | 11 | 14 | 7 |
| Osteoarthritis | 16 | 19 | 13 | 17 | 17 | 16 |
| Endocrine disorders | 17 | 17 | 16 | | | 20 |
| Migraine | 18 | | 9 | 20 | | 15 |
| Other neuropsychiatric disorders | 19 | | 19 | | | |
| Dental caries | 20 | 18 | | | | |
| Road traffic accidents | | 15 | | 16 | 10 | |
| Cerebrovascular disease | | 20 | | | | |
| Other maternal conditions | | | 10 | 14 | | 4 |
| Rheumatoid arthritis | | | 18 | 19 | | 10 |
| Maternal sepsis | | | 20 | | | 9 |
| Obsessive–compulsive disorder | | | | 15 | 15 | 13 |
| Panic disorder | | | | 18 | | 11 |
| HIV/AIDS | | | | 16 | | |
| Chagas disease | | | | 18 | | |
| Falls | | | | 19 | | |
| Epilepsy | | | | 20 | | |
| Diabetes mellitus | | | | | | 19 |

male adolescents in Ecuador (1996), El Salvador (1996) and Nicaragua (1996). Suicide is among the top three causes of death among the youth (Espejo and Sandoval, 2001). The rates of suicide and homicide for each of the countries are presented in Table 20.5.

The leading causes of death among adolescents aged 10–19 years are external, and include violence and homicide (Pan American Health Organization, 2002). Violence in adolescence is not limited to physical trauma, but also includes sexual aggression, emotional and verbal abuse, threats, and other types of psychological abuse. Youths in this age group represent 29 per cent of all homicides in Latin America. Colombia and El Salvador are two of the countries hardest hit by violence. In Colombia, an important contributing factor to this epidemic is drug trafficking. In countries such as El Salvador and Brazil, the emergence and growth of youth gangs is a key factor. Youth gang violence has contributed to the rise in homicides, particularly in El Salvador, which has one of the

**Table 20.5**   *Mortality from suicide and homicide per 100 000 population*

| Country | Suicide | | | Homicide | | |
|---|---|---|---|---|---|---|
| | T | M | F | T | M | F |
| Argentina | 8.2 | 13.0 | 3.5 | 7.0 | 12.0 | 1.9 |
| Belize | 4.7 | 9.0 | 0.4 | 10.3 | 17.6 | 2.7 |
| Bolivia | – | – | – | – | – | – |
| Brazil | 4.9 | 7.9 | 2.0 | 29.3 | 54.0 | 5.1 |
| Chile | 10.9 | 18.3 | 3.2 | 5.7 | 10.0 | 1.3 |
| Colombia | 5.2 | 7.8 | 2.5 | 80.4 | 143.5 | 12.7 |
| Costa Rica | 6.7 | 11.3 | 1.9 | 6.7 | 11.2 | 1.9 |
| Ecuador | 5.9 | 7.9 | 3.8 | 21.2 | 37.6 | 3.9 |
| El Salvador | 11.5 | 14.7 | 8.2 | 50.5 | 87.6 | 9.1 |
| Guatemala | 1.9 | 2.9 | 0.8 | 22.8 | 41.6 | 3.7 |
| Honduras | – | – | – | – | – | – |
| Mexico | 4.1 | 7.0 | 1.3 | 11.3 | 20.5 | 2.7 |
| Nicaragua | 13.2 | 17.8 | 8.5 | 12.8 | 22.3 | 2.9 |
| Panama | 6.3 | 10.3 | 2.0 | 13.5 | 23.7 | 2.7 |
| Paraguay | 3.7 | 4.8 | 2.5 | 15.8 | 26.8 | 3.6 |
| Peru | 2.3 | 2.8 | 1.7 | 4.4 | 7.8 | 1.2 |
| Uruguay | 13.9 | 22.8 | 5.6 | 5.0 | 8.3 | 2.0 |
| Venezuela | 4.8 | 8.0 | 1.7 | 14.7 | 27.1 | 2.2 |

Source: Pan American Health Organization website based on most recent data available as of 2004.

highest homicide rates. Young poor urban males are the most affected group.

Intimate partner violence against women is highly prevalent in many Latin American countries. A series of studies were carried out examining serious assaults by partners against women aged 15–29 in Colombia (1995), Nicaragua (1998), Santiago, Chile (1997), and Metropolitan Lima, Peru in middle and low income areas (1997). These studies found 20 per cent, 21 per cent, 23 per cent and 31 per cent of the women were assaulted by their partners respectively in the past 12 months (Heise *et al.*, 1999). In a study of ten countries in Latin America most of the women who suffered sexual violence considered forced sex to be part of their domestic obligation (Pan American Health Organization, 2003). This same study found that intimate partners also subject the women frequently to economic violence by limiting, withholding or withdrawing financial support from them and their children, by threatening or actually throwing them out of the house, or controlling any income the women brought into the home, as well as breaking objects of value to the family.

In indigenous communities the most significant cause of domestic violence is gender inequality (Hughes, 2004). Indigenous men often claim that they are entitled to use sexual, physical and/or psychological violence to control their partners' behaviour if they suspect them of having an affair (Center of Studies and Information of the Multiethnic Woman, 2002). In Nicaragua, 32 per cent of rural women believe it is acceptable for a husband to beat his wife if he even suspects that she has been cheating on him. Three-quarters of married Nicaraguan women have been beaten, coerced into sex or abused in some way (Correia and Pena, 2002). Violence may be one avenue that indigenous men use to reaffirm their masculinity as they find fulfilling their role as a financial provider more difficult with growing unemployment in their communities and higher fertility rates (Hughes, 2004).

Hughes describes how changing values among the indigenous populations may influence domestic violence:

*In Paraguay, indigenous women argue that domestic violence in their communities has resulted from them adopting the chauvinist manners of the Paraguayan man. In the old times, among the Nivaklé, women were the owners of all sexual initiative in their relationships. Invested with a certain aggressiveness for love, she could choose the man she preferred. Nowadays, the kinds of romantic relationships among white people have influenced the relationships among the indigenous people. It is no longer the woman who takes the initiative in sexual relations; it is the man. Imitating the white patron, now he dares to compel women for love.*

## ADULT PSYCHIATRIC DISORDERS

Numerous community-based epidemiological studies examining the rates of specific mental disorders in adults have been conducted in Latin America. The first, in 1979, was conducted in a series of stratified districts in the region of Buenos Aires, Argentina (Di Marco, 1982; Larraya *et al.*, 1982; Aszkenazi and Casullo, 1984) using the Present State Examination (PSE) (Wing *et al.*, 1977). This study found an exceptionally high prevalence rate for schizophrenia of 3.0 per cent. Other than schizophrenia, the rates in this study cannot be compared with those in other countries as it used *International Classification of Diseases, version 9* (ICD-9) diagnoses: affective psychosis 4.0 per cent; paranoia 0.2 per cent; neurotic depression 3.5 per cent; and neurotic disorders 14.5 per cent.

In Brazil three studies have been conducted. One in Bambui, a town in the state of Minas Gerias, using the Composite International Diagnostic Interview (CIDI) (Robins *et al.*, 1988) limited to only the diagnosis of depression (Vorcaro *et al.*, 2001). Another CIDI study was conducted in São Paulo in a middle and upper socio-economic class catchment area (Andrade *et al.*, 1999, 2002; WHO International Consortium, 2000). The third study consisted of surveys of three major urban areas: Brasilia, São Paulo and Porto Alegre; they used a two-stage cross-sectional design. The first stage was a screening interview using the Questionnaire for Psychiatric Morbidity in Adults (QMPA) (Santana,

1982). Each family member above the age of 14 completed the screening interview. The second stage consisted of a structured diagnostic interview developed by the Brazilian team based on *Diagnostic and Statistical Manual of Mental Disorders III* (DSM-III) conducted on 30 per cent of the screened positives and 10 per cent of the screened negatives (Almeida-Filho *et al.*, 1992, 1997).

Two surveys have been completed in Chile. One used the Clinical Interview Schedule (CIS-R) (Lewis and Pelosi, 1990) and the other the CIDI. The former was limited to the metropolitan area of Santiago (Araya *et al.*, 2001). The latter was a multistage sample from four catchment areas in Chile, representing each of the major geographic regions of the country (Rioseco *et al.*, 1994; Vicente *et al.*, 2002, 2004, 2006; Bjil *et al.*, 2003; Saldivia *et al.*, 2004). In Colombia two nationally representative studies have been conducted using the CIDI to investigate the prevalence of mental disorders (Torres de Galvis and Montoya, 1997; Demyttenaere *et al.*, 2004; Posada-Villa *et al.*, 2004). A third national study using the CIDI was limited to affective disorders (Gómez-Restrepo *et al.*, 2004).

Mexico has produced four surveys. Two studies were based on nationally representative samples: one was limited to urban areas of the country (Caraveo-Anduaga *et al.*, 1996) using the PSE supplemented by the Diagnostic Interview Schedule (DIS) (Robins *et al.*, 1981) and the other used the CIDI in a representative national sample (Medina-Mora *et al.*, 2003; Demyttenaere *et al.*, 2004; Borges *et al.*, 2006). Another CIDI study conducted in Mexico was limited to Mexico City (Caraveo-Anduaga, 1995; Caraveo-Anduaga *et al.*, 1997, 1999; Merikangas *et al.*, 1998; Andrade *et al.*, 2003, Caraveo-Anduaga and Bermúndez, 2004), and the fourth study was one of rural regions in two Mexican states also using the CIDI (Salgado de Snyder and Diaz-Pérez, 1999).

In Peru a study using the DIS was conducted in Independencia, a poor northern district of Lima (Hayashi *et al.*, 1985; Minobe *et al.*, 1990; Yamamoto *et al.*, 1993; Perales and Sogi, 1995).

Table 20.6 provides a summary of the methods used in these studies, and in Tables 20.7–20.9 the prevalence rates by disorder across studies are provided. The rates across countries cannot be

**Table 20.6** *Psychiatric epidemiologic prevalence studies conducted in Latin America and the Caribbean*

| Study | Field dates | Sample size | Age | Instrument | Diagnosis |
|---|---|---|---|---|---|
| AR1: Argentina | 1979 | 3 410 | 17+ | PSE | CATEGO/ICD-9 |
| BR1: Brazil, Bambuí | 1996–1997 | 1 041 | 18+ | CIDI | DSM-III-R |
| Multicenter, Brazil (BR2: Brasilia; BR3: Porto Alegre; BR4: São Paulo) | 1991 | 6 476 | 15+ | QMPA/DSM | DSM-III |
| BR5: Brazil, São Paulo | 1994–1996 | 1 464 | 18+ | CIDI 1.1 | DSM-III-R |
| CH1: Chile, Santiago | 1996–1998 | 3 870 | 16–64 | CIS-R | ICD-10 |
| CH2: Chile, National | 1992–1999 | 2 978 | 15+ | CIDI 1.1 | DSM-III-R |
| CO1: Colombia | 1997 | 15 048 | 12+ | CIDI 2.0 | DSM-IV |
| CO2: Colombia WMH | 2003 | 4 544 | 18–65 | CIDI-CAPI 15 | DSM-IV |
| CO3: Colombia depression | 2000–2001 | 6 610 | 18+ | CIDI 2.1 | ICD-10 |
| ME1: Mexico ENEP | 2001–2002 | 5 826 | 18–65 | CIDI-CAPI 15 | DSM-IV |
| ME2: Mexico PSE | 1988 | 1 984 | 18–64 | PSE | ICD-9 |
| ME3: Mexico City | 1995 | 1 937 | 18–64 | CIDI 1.1 | DSM-III-R |
| ME4: Rural, Mexico | 1996–1997 | 945 | 15–89 | CIDI 1.1 | ICD-10 |
| PE1: Peru, Lima | 1983 | 815 | 18+ | DIS | DSM-III |

PSE, Present State Examination; CIDI, Composite International Diagnostic Interview; QMPA,Questionnaire for Psychiatric Morbidity in Adults; DSM, *Diagnostic and Statistical Manual*; CIS-R, Clinical Interview Schedule; ICD, *International Classification of Diseases*.

contrasted due to the widely differing methodologies used, such as diagnostic criteria, diagnostic instruments and sampling frame.

However, as a composite these studies do provide insight into the overall rate of mental disorders in the region. Using the median rate across studies, non-affective psychosis was found in approximately 1.7 per cent of the population across their lifetime and in 0.7 per cent currently. As for the affective disorders, major depression had a lifetime prevalence of 9.5 per cent and a current prevalence of 3.7 per cent; dysthymia had a lifetime prevalence of 3.4 per cent and a current prevalence of 0.2 per cent; and bipolar disorder had a lifetime prevalence of 1.5 per cent and a current prevalence of 0.5 per cent. The lifetime prevalence rates of the anxiety disorders were generalized anxiety disorder 2.6 per cent, panic disorder 1.6 per cent, and obsessive compulsive disorder 1.4 per cent. The anxiety disorders had a current prevalence of generalized anxiety disorder 0.7 per cent, panic disorder 0.5 per cent, and obsessive compulsive disorder 1.3 per cent. Alcohol and drug use disorders were highly prevalent: 9.2 per cent had a lifetime history of alcohol abuse and dependence while 1.5 per cent had history of drug abuse and dependence. The one-year

prevalence of alcohol abuse and dependence was 5.2 per cent and for drug abuse and dependence.0.5 per cent. These studies for the most part did not explore rates across ethnic groups.

*Nervios* is a syndrome that has been described among Mexicans, El Salvadorians, Costa Ricans, Ecuadorians and Guatemalans (see Chapters 2 and 11). This is considered to be a generalized condition of distress that is expressed with both somatic and psychological symptoms. Only one study based in rural Mexico has specifically looked at the prevalence of *nervios* in the community and found it to be present in 15.5 per cent of the population. The disorder is twice as frequent in women than men (Salgado de Snyder *et al.*, 2000).

## STUDIES OF CHILD PSYCHIATRIC DISORDERS

Studies specifically examining child mental health are few in Latin America. All of the available studies used screening scales to determine which children were potential cases or not, often with a second stage confirmatory assessment. These studies rarely

**Table 20.7**  *Lifetime prevalence rates (per cent) in community-based Latin American surveys*

| | | BR1 | BR2 | BR3 | BR4 | BR5 | CH2 | CO1 | CO2 | ME1 | ME3 | ME4 | PE1 | Mean | Median |
|---|---|---|---|---|---|---|---|---|---|---|---|---|---|---|---|
| NAP | T | | 0.3 | 2.4 | 0.9 | 1.9 | 1.8 | 1.4 | | | | | 0.6 | 1.3 | 1.4 |
| | M | | 0.0 | 2.4 | 0.0 | 1.7 | 1.6 | 1.3 | | | | | 0.3 | 1.0 | 1.3 |
| | F | | 0.5 | 2.5 | 1.2 | 2.0 | 1.8 | 1.4 | | | | | 1.0 | 1.5 | 1.4 |
| MDD | T | 12.8 | 2.8 | 10.2 | 1.9 | 12.6 | 9.2 | 19.6 | 12.1 | 3.3 | 8.1 | 6.2 | 9.7 | 9.0 | 9.5 |
| | M | 7.3 | 1.9 | 5.9 | 0.0 | 8.8 | 6.8 | 18.3 | 8.6 | 2.0 | 5.5 | 2.9 | 6.1 | 6.2 | 6.0 |
| | F | 17.0 | 3.8 | 14.5 | 3.8 | 15.3 | 11.5 | 20.7 | 14.9 | 4.5 | 10.1 | 9.1 | 13.5 | 11.6 | 12.5 |
| DYS | T | | | | | 4.9 | 8.0 | | 0.7 | 0.9 | 1.4 | 3.4 | 3.6 | 3.3 | 3.4 |
| | M | | | | | 4.2 | 3.5 | | 0.6 | 0.5 | 0.9 | 1.4 | 1.0 | 1.7 | 1.0 |
| | F | | | | | 5.5 | 12.1 | | 0.7 | 1.1 | 1.8 | 5.2 | 5.9 | 4.6 | 5.2 |
| BIP | T | | 0.4 | 1.1 | 0.3 | 1.3 | 1.9 | 1.7 | 2.0 | 3.3 | 1.4 | 2.1 | 0.5 | 1.5 | 1.4 |
| | M | | 0.9 | 0.5 | 0.0 | 1.1 | 1.5 | 1.9 | 2.3 | 4.0 | 2.1 | 1.6 | 0.7 | 1.5 | 1.5 |
| | F | | 0.0 | 1.7 | 0.6 | 1.4 | 2.2 | 1.6 | 1.7 | 0.7 | 0.9 | 2.5 | 1.0 | 1.3 | 1.4 |
| GAD | T | | 17.6 | 9.6 | 10.6 | 2.5 | 2.6 | 3.1 | 1.3 | 1.2 | 0.9 | | | 5.5 | 2.6 |
| | M | | 13.6 | 5.2 | 7.3 | 1.8 | 0.9 | 2.6 | 1.5 | 0.7 | 0.8 | | | 3.8 | 1.8 |
| | F | | 21.6 | 14.0 | 13.9 | 3.0 | 4.1 | 3.5 | 1.2 | 1.6 | 1.0 | | | 7.1 | 3.5 |
| PAN | T | | | | | 1.3 | 1.6 | 0.3 | 1.2 | 2.1 | 2.9 | | 1.6 | 1.6 | 1.6 |
| | M | | | | | 0.2 | 0.7 | 0.3 | 0.6 | 1.3 | 2.1 | | 1.2 | 0.9 | 0.7 |
| | F | | | | | 2.2 | 2.5 | 0.2 | 1.7 | 2.9 | 3.8 | | 2.9 | 2.3 | 2.5 |
| OCD | T | | 0.9 | 2.1 | | 0.6 | 1.2 | 3.6 | | | 1.4 | | 2.2 | 1.7 | 1.4 |
| | M | | 0.7 | 1.7 | | 0.4 | 0.7 | 3.3 | | | 0.8 | | 2.0 | 1.4 | 0.8 |
| | F | | 0.5 | 2.5 | | 0.8 | 1.6 | 3.9 | | | 1.7 | | 2.9 | 2.0 | 1.7 |
| ALC | T | | 8.0 | 9.2 | 7.6 | 14.9 | 10.0 | 16.6 | 9.0 | 8.3 | 9.1 | | 18.7 | 11.1 | 9.2 |
| | M | | 15.0 | 16.0 | 15.2 | 24.4 | 17.3 | 25.8 | 17.9 | 16.4 | 19.4 | | 34.8 | 20.2 | 17.6 |
| | F | | 1.1 | 2.5 | 0.0 | 7.9 | 3.3 | 7.8 | 1.9 | 1.3 | 1.3 | | 2.5 | 3.0 | 2.2 |
| DRG | T | | | | | 1.0 | 3.5 | | 1.6 | 1.5 | 0.7 | | 1.5 | 1.6 | 1.5 |
| | M | | | | | 1.9 | 3.4 | | 2.3 | 3.1 | | | 2.2 | 2.6 | 2.3 |
| | F | | | | | 0.6 | 3.5 | | 0.3 | 0.2 | | | 0.7 | 1.1 | 0.6 |

T, Total; M, Male; F, Female; NAP, non-affective psychosis; MDD, major depressive disorder; DYS, dysthymia; BIP, bipolar disorder; GAD, generalized anxiety disorder; PAN, panic disorder; OCD, obsessive–compulsive disorder; ALC, alcohol abuse and dependence; DRG, drug abuse and dependence. For an explanation of the study codes see Table 20.6.

**Table 20.8** *One-year prevalence rates (per cent) in community-based Latin American surveys*

| | | BR1 | BR2 | BR3 | BR4 | BR5 | CH2 | CO1 | CO2 | CO3 | ME1 | ME3 | PE1[a] | Mean | Median |
|---|---|---|---|---|---|---|---|---|---|---|---|---|---|---|---|
| NAP | T | | 0.2 | 2.0 | 0.6 | 0.8 | 1.1 | 0.6 | | | | | 0.6 | 0.8 | 0.6 |
| | M | | 0.0 | 2.4 | 0.0 | 0.8 | 0.8 | 0.5 | | | | | 0.2 | 0.7 | 0.5 |
| | F | | 0.4 | 2.0 | 1.2 | 0.9 | 1.3 | 0.6 | | | | | 1.0 | 1.1 | 1.0 |
| MDD | T | 9.1 | 1.5 | 1.3 | 6.7 | 5.8 | 5.7 | 1.9 | 5.6 | 10.0 | 1.4 | 4.4 | 5.2 | 4.9 | 5.4 |
| | M | 5.1 | 1.1 | 0.0 | 5.9 | 3.6 | 3.7 | 0.7 | 3.5 | 6.2 | 0.9 | 3.1 | 3.4 | 3.1 | 3.5 |
| | F | 12.2 | 2.9 | 3.6 | 7.6 | 7.5 | 7.5 | 3.0 | 7.3 | 12.0 | 2.1 | 5.6 | 6.9 | 6.5 | 7.1 |
| DYS | T | | | | | 1.9 | 3.9 | | 0.5 | | 0.4 | 0.3 | 3.3 | 1.7 | 1.2 |
| | M | | | | | 1.8 | 1.6 | | 0.5 | | 0.4 | 0.3 | 1.0 | 0.9 | 0.8 |
| | F | | | | | 2.1 | 5.9 | | 0.5 | | 0.5 | 0.4 | 5.9 | 2.6 | 1.3 |
| BIP | T | | 0.3 | 0.2 | 1.0 | 0.6 | 1.4 | | 0.9 | | 2.0 | 0.7 | 0.1 | 0.8 | 0.7 |
| | M | | 0.5 | 0.0 | 1.7 | 0.3 | 0.7 | | 0.8 | | 1.8 | 1.3 | 0.0 | 0.8 | 0.7 |
| | F | | 0.0 | 0.4 | 0.3 | 0.8 | 2.1 | | 1.0 | | 2.0 | 0.3 | 0.2 | 0.8 | 0.4 |
| GAD | T | | 12.1 | 5.4 | 6.9 | 1.0 | 1.6 | 1.3 | 0.7 | | 0.7 | 0.6 | | 3.4 | 1.3 |
| | M | | 7.8 | 5.2 | 4.3 | 0.7 | 0.7 | 1.7 | 0.9 | | 0.6 | 0.7 | | 2.5 | 0.9 |
| | F | | 16.4 | 5.6 | 9.6 | 1.3 | 2.4 | 0.9 | 0.5 | | 0.8 | 0.4 | | 4.2 | 1.3 |
| PAN | T | | | | | 1.0 | 0.9 | 0.1 | 0.6 | | 1.1 | 1.6 | 1.6 | 1.0 | 1.0 |
| | M | | | | | 0.2 | 0.5 | 0.2 | 0.3 | | 0.4 | 0.8 | 1.0 | 0.5 | 0.4 |
| | F | | | | | 1.6 | 1.2 | 0.1 | 0.9 | | 1.7 | 1.9 | 2.2 | 1.4 | 1.6 |
| OCD | T | | 0.5 | 1.2 | | 0.6 | 1.2 | 3.1 | | | | 1.0 | 1.5 | 1.3 | 1.2 |
| | M | | 0.5 | 1.7 | | 0.4 | 0.7 | 2.4 | | | | 0.7 | 1.5 | 1.1 | 0.7 |
| | F | | 0.4 | 0.7 | | 0.7 | 1.6 | 3.8 | | | | 1.2 | 1.5 | 1.4 | 1.2 |
| ALC | T | | 4.7 | 8.7 | 4.3 | 9.9 | 6.9 | 4.7 | 2.2 | | 2.3 | 5.6 | 6.9 | 5.6 | 5.2 |
| | M | | 8.6 | 15.9 | 8.6 | 15.9 | 12.1 | 4.3 | 4.6 | | 4.7 | 10.9 | 12.5 | 9.8 | 9.8 |
| | F | | 0.8 | 1.6 | 0.0 | 5.4 | 2.2 | 5.1 | 0.4 | | 0.2 | 2.2 | 1.2 | 1.9 | 1.4 |
| DRG | T | | | | | 0.6 | 1.8 | | 0.5 | | 0.5 | | 0.2 | 0.7 | 0.5 |
| | M | | | | | 1.1 | 1.7 | | 0.9 | | 1.0 | | 0.2 | 1.0 | 1.0 |
| | F | | | | | 0.2 | 2.1 | | 0.2 | | 0.0 | | 0.2 | 0.5 | 0.2 |

T, Total; M, Male; F, Female; NAP, non-affective psychosis; MDD, major depressive disorder; DYS, dysthymia; BIP, bipolar disorder; GAD, generalized anxiety disorder; PAN, panic disorder; OCD, obsessive–compulsive disorder; ALC, alcohol abuse and dependence; DRG, drug abuse and dependence. For an explanation of the study codes see Table 20.6.
[a]PE1 – six-month prevalence.

**Table 20.9**  *Current prevalence rates (per cent) in community-based Latin American surveys*

| | | AR1 | BR1 | BR5 | CH1 | CH2 | CO2 | CO3 | ME1 | ME2 | ME3 | Mean | Median |
|---|---|---|---|---|---|---|---|---|---|---|---|---|---|
| NAP | T | 4.0 | | 0.7 | | 0.6 | | | | 0.7 | | 1.5 | 0.7 |
| | M | 3.0 | | 0.5 | | 0.4 | | | | 0.7 | | 1.2 | 0.6 |
| | F | 4.3 | | 0.8 | | 0.8 | | | | 0.7 | | 1.7 | 0.8 |
| MDD | T | 6.0 | 7.5 | 3.9 | 5.5 | 3.4 | 1.9 | 8.5 | 0.6 | 3.2 | 2.2 | 4.3 | 3.7 |
| | M | 6.0 | 5.1 | 2.7 | 2.7 | 2.3 | 0.7 | 5.3 | 0.3 | 2.2 | 1.4 | 2.9 | 2.5 |
| | F | 6.0 | 10.2 | 4.8 | 8.0 | 4.5 | 2.8 | 10.2 | 0.8 | 3.9 | 2.8 | 5.4 | 4.7 |
| DYS | T | | | 1.6 | | 2.9 | 0.1 | | 0.2 | | 0.2 | 1.0 | 0.2 |
| | M | | | 1.6 | | 1.5 | 0.1 | | 0.2 | | 0.0 | 0.7 | 0.2 |
| | F | | | 1.5 | | 4.2 | 0.2 | | 0.2 | | 0.3 | 1.3 | 0.3 |
| BIP | T | | | 0.4 | | 1.0 | 0.1 | | 0.8 | 0.5 | 0.3 | 0.5 | 0.5 |
| | M | | | 0.3 | | 0.5 | 0.1 | | 0.8 | 0.4 | 0.5 | 0.4 | 0.5 |
| | F | | | 0.4 | | 1.3 | 0.1 | | 0.8 | 0.6 | 0.1 | 0.6 | 0.5 |
| GAD | T | | | 0.9 | 5.1 | 0.9 | 0.3 | | 0.4 | | 0.2 | 1.3 | 0.7 |
| | M | | | 0.7 | 3.2 | 0.3 | 0.5 | | 0.6 | | 0.0 | 0.9 | 0.6 |
| | F | | | 1.1 | 6.9 | 1.5 | 0.2 | | 0.3 | | 0.3 | 1.7 | 0.7 |
| PAN | T | | | 0.5 | 1.3 | 0.6 | 0.3 | | 0.4 | | 0.4 | 0.6 | 0.5 |
| | M | | | 0.0 | 1.1 | 0.3 | 0.1 | | 0.2 | | 0.1 | 0.3 | 0.2 |
| | F | | | 0.9 | 1.5 | 0.8 | 0.5 | | 0.5 | | 0.7 | 0.8 | 0.8 |
| OCD | T | | | 0.5 | 1.3 | 1.2 | | | | 3.0 | | 1.5 | 1.3 |
| | M | | | 0.4 | 1.4 | 0.7 | | | | 1.3 | | 1.0 | 1.0 |
| | F | | | 0.5 | 1.1 | 1.6 | | | | 4.3 | | 1.9 | 1.4 |
| ALC | T | | | 7.5 | | 5.4 | 0.7 | | 0.6 | | 2.6 | 3.4 | 2.6 |
| | M | | | 12.0 | | 9.1 | 1.6 | | 1.3 | | 5.7 | 5.9 | 5.7 |
| | F | | | 4.1 | | 2.0 | 0.1 | | 0.1 | | 0.3 | 1.3 | 0.3 |

T, Total; M, Male; F, Female; NAP, non-affective psychosis; MDD, major depressive disorder; DYS, dysthymia; BIP, bipolar disorder; GAD, generalized anxiety disorder; PAN, panic disorder; OCD, obsessive–compulsive disorder; ALC, alcohol abuse and dependence. For an explanation of the study codes see Table 20.6.

utilized diagnostic instruments to evaluate specific disorders.

In Brazil Almeida-Filho *et al.* (1985) conducted studies among middle-class sections of Salvador, Bahia, using a household probability sample of 829 children between the ages of 5 and 14. The evaluation of psychopathology was done using a two-stage screen. The first stage consisted of the Questionário de Morbidade Psiquiátrica Infantil (QMPI) (Almeida-Filho, 1981). All the screen positives and a subsample of the screen negatives underwent a second-phase diagnostic interview. Some type of psychopathology was noted in 23.2 per cent of the children; however, moderate behavioural problems were noted in 6.9 per cent of cases and serious problems in 3.1 per cent.

Another study conducted in Brazil attempted to evaluate the relationship between social problem and mental health in children (Fleitlich and Goodman, 2001) aged 7 to 14 using lists from compulsory school enrolment. They evaluated children in three different communities: an urban slum ($N = 488$), a rural community ($N = 64$) and a stable urban community ($N = 346$). Psychopathology was assessed by interviewing teachers and parents using the Strength and Difficulties Questionnaire (SDQ) (Goodman *et al.*, 1998; Fleitlich *et al.*, 2000). The rate of psychopathology was highest in the children from the slums (22 per cent) compared with the stable urban community (12 per cent) or the rural community (13 per cent). However, in a regression analysis the type of community was no longer significant, but rather low socio-economic class, psychiatric problems in the parent, and corporal or very strict disciplining of the child. Another study conducted in Brazil found that 12.7 per cent of children age 7–14 had a DSM-IV disorder (Fleitlich-Bilyk and Goodman, 2004). This was a study of 1251 children using the Development and Well-Being Assessment.

A small sample study of 89 children aged 4–17 was evaluated in a low-income neighbourhood in São Paulo, Brazil (Bordin *et al.*, 2002) using the Child Behavioral Checklist and the Self-Report Questionnaire (20-item version) (SRQ-20) on the children and mother, respectively. The rate of child behavioural problems found in interviews of the child and mother was 22.4 per cent. A strong relationship was noted between pathology in the mothers and children.

Several reports have been published on child and maternal mental health from Embu in Brazil. One study noted that infant malnutrition was linked to maternal mental health (Miranda *et al.*, 1996). Bordin *et al.* (1995) studied 83 primary school age children, 6–9 years old, and found that 16.9 per cent of the children had externalizing behavioural problems. Other studies from this catchment area have found that being born to a mother without a husband, loss of contact with the father, and family conflict increased risk of developmental delays in three-year-old children (Paula *et al.*, 2002). There is a very high rate of domestic violence in the Embu community, with 74.2 per cent of the children having been abused physically (Bordin *et al.*, 2002).

More recently Anselmi *et al.* (2004) examined 634 four-year-old children from a birth cohort of 5304 in Brazil administering the Child Behavior Checklist (CBCL) and the SRQ in the mothers. They found that 24 per cent of the children had behavioural problems. Predictive factors for behavioural problems included maternal psychiatric disorder, education and age, number of younger siblings and quality of the home environment. When the Beck Depression Inventory was administered to a sample of 1555 Brazilian children aged 13–17, using a cut-off of 20, 7.6 per cent of the sample was felt to have clinically significant depression.

In Bucaramanga, Colombia 239 schoolchildren aged 8–11 were administered the Child Depression Inventory (CDI) (Mantilla Mendoza *et al.*, 2004). This study found that 9.2 per cent of the children had clinically significant depressive symptoms, being greater in older children, girls, and those in lower grades. The investigators found no association with social class. In Latin America, 13.8 million people suffer from mental retardation (Pan American Health Organization, 2002).

## STUDIES OF SUBSTANCE ABUSE

A number of studies on tobacco, drug and alcohol use have been carried out across Latin America. An urban study in Bolivia with 3003 subjects provided data on individuals aged 12–50 (Alcaraz del Castillo *et al.*, 1993). In Mexico, a national survey (Secretaria de Salud, 1993) on substance use of 2005 people aged 12–65 was utilized for the projections for that country. A community study of 6085 individuals aged 10 and older in Ecuador provided data on alcohol, tobacco and illicit drug consumption (Aguilar, 1992). For Colombia, information was obtained from the National Household Survey on Drug Abuse (Ospina *et al.*, 1993), a study of 8975 people aged 12–60. The Panamanian study (Jutkowitz and Day, 1992) was a household survey of 911 respondents limited to the population ages 12–45 in three regions: Panama City, San Miguelito and Colón. A study of three cities in Guatemala (Guatemala City, Quezaltenango and Escuintala) limited to individuals 12–45 years of age with a sample of 1807 was conducted in 1990 (Development Associates, 1990). This same group also conducted a nationwide survey of substance use in Peru on 7425 individuals aged 12–45 (Jutkowitz *et al.*, 1989). Another community study limited to individuals aged 12–45 was also conducted using 2484 respondents in Paraguay (Ministerio de Salud Publica y Bienestar Social, 1991); however, data only by gender distribution and not by age distribution were available. A report from Venezuela gave results from a study of individuals aged 12 and older on their tobacco use (Domador, 1991). A household study of 512 persons limited to teenagers and young adults aged 14–30 in Belize City was the source of data in Belize (Pride Belize, 1993).

The community epidemiologic prevalence studies focusing on substance abuse and dependence do not fully capture the extent of the problem, especially among the teenage population. Tables 20.10 and 20.11 highlight the results of these studies standardized to the 1990 estimated population of each of the countries surveyed. Most striking is the high rates of tobacco usage, alcohol use and use of inhalants in the teenage population. Marijuana use is highly prevalent across many segments of the population, and cocaine and cocaine paste (*basuca*) are commonly used among adults in a number of countries. Brazil was not included in the tables, as data were not available in the format provided as in the other reports; however, a recent study conducted in Brazil found that 19.4 per cent

of the population between 12 and 64 had a lifetime use of illicit substances and 4.6 per cent in the past year. In Brazil 68.7 per cent had a lifetime use of alcohol and 41.1 per cent tobacco; the corresponding past year rates were 50.5 per cent and 19.5 per cent respectively (Galduróz *et al.*, 2005).

## MENTAL HEALTH OF INDIGENOUS POPULATIONS

Few data exist on the mental health of the indigenous population in Latin America (see Chapters 2 and 19). A recent study using the CIDI in a household survey of 75 Mapuche and non-Mapuche in Chile found few significant differences between the two groups; however, generalized anxiety disorder, simple phobia and drug dependence were less prevalent among the Mapuche (Vicente *et al.*, 2005). Earlier reports have suggested an increased risk for psychosis among the Mapuche (Muñoz *et al.*, 1966; Biedermann *et al.*, 1983). A study of another indigenous group in Chile, Pehuenches, using screening among 57 individuals found a suspected ICD-10 prevalence rate of 40.4 per cent (Vicente *et al.*, 1992).

## REFUGEES

Little is known about refugee populations despite the fact that sizeable populations have been displaced during war and internal political conflicts over the past several decades. According to the United Nations High Commission for Refugees (2005) in 2004 there were over 36 000 refugees in Latin America with approximately 2 million internally displaced people. Currently Colombia accounts for nearly all the internal displaced population of Latin America. Of the populations of concern to the UN over 2500 reside in camps primarily in Mexico, 58 per cent.

A few studies have been conducted on the mental health of the Mayan refugees who fled to Mexico during the 36-year Guatemalan civil war that ended

**Table 20.10** Lifetime drug use rates in selected Latin American countries by age

| | | Marijuana | Cocaine | Basuca | Hallucinogen | Inhalants | Stimulants | Tobacco | Alcohol |
|---|---|---|---|---|---|---|---|---|---|
| Belize | 14–19 | 0.0 | 1.0 | | | | | 17.1 | 47.7 |
| | 20–30 | 15.2 | 2.7 | | | | | 27.4 | 68.0 |
| | Male | 16.1 | 2.5 | | | | | 12.0 | 70.5 |
| | Female | 1.8 | 1.5 | | | | | 34.4 | 48.7 |
| Bolivia | 12–17 | 0.5 | 0.4 | 0.3 | 0.3 | 9.1 | 0.8 | 20.0 | 34.5 |
| | 18–50 | 3.2 | 1.6 | 1.7 | 0.4 | 4.5 | 2.4 | 55.6 | 80.4 |
| | Male | 4.7 | 2.2 | 2.4 | 0.6 | 5.9 | 2.2 | 64.5 | 76.4 |
| | Female | 0.7 | 0.4 | 0.3 | 0.2 | 5.7 | 1.8 | 32.7 | 62.7 |
| Colombia | 12–17 | 0.9 | 0.1 | 0.2 | | 6.6 | 0.4 | 15.1 | 81.2 |
| | 18–60 | 6.7 | 1.9 | 2.0 | | 3.0 | 0.7 | 53.9 | 93.1 |
| | Male | 10.4 | 2.9 | 3.0 | | 3.8 | 0.5 | 58.1 | 94.6 |
| | Female | 1.7 | 0.4 | 0.5 | | 3.8 | 0.7 | 36.4 | 87.7 |
| Ecuador | 10–19 | 0.4 | | | | | 10.9 | 4.1 | 7.6 |
| | 20–70 | 29.5 | | | | | 26.9 | 26.7 | 25.9 |
| | Male | 7.8 | 1.7 | 2.1 | | 2.0 | 0.8 | 69.5 | 79.8 |
| | Female | 0.6 | 0.3 | 0.1 | | 1.4 | 1.3 | 39.3 | 69.8 |
| Guatemala | 12–19 | 3.8 | 1.0 | | 1.4 | 5.3 | 8.7 | 15.3 | 34.6 |
| | 20–45 | 8.9 | 1.4 | | 1.9 | 2.5 | 12.4 | 41.6 | 65.8 |
| | Male | 13.3 | 2.2 | | 3.2 | 6.1 | 14.6 | 50.1 | 65.9 |
| | Female | 1.8 | 0.6 | | 0.5 | 1.0 | 8.1 | 19.0 | 48.3 |
| Mexico | 12–18 | 1.8 | 0.3 | | 0.1 | 0.3 | | 25.9 | |
| | 19–65 | 3.8 | 0.6 | | 0.2 | 0.5 | | 51.4 | |
| | Male | 6.6 | 1.1 | | 0.4 | 1.0 | | 63.0 | 82.2 |
| | Female | 0.6 | 0.1 | | 0.1 | 0.1 | | 30.8 | 61.6 |
| Panama | 12–19 | 1.8 | 0.3 | 0.0 | | 3.8 | 1.7 | 12.7 | 69.4 |
| | 20–45 | 8.1 | 6.3 | 2.5 | | 3.0 | 3.3 | 47.7 | 82.5 |
| | Male | 8.9 | 5.4 | 1.9 | | 4.5 | 3.1 | 45.8 | 85.8 |
| | Female | 2.4 | 1.6 | 1.2 | | 2.1 | 2.2 | 23.2 | 69.0 |
| Paraguay | 12–45 | 1.4 | 0.3 | | 0.1 | 1.9 | 4.6 | 32.4 | 79.5 |
| | Male | 2.6 | 0.4 | | 0.2 | 2.5 | 2.1 | 48.9 | 88.3 |
| | Female | 0.3 | 0.1 | | 0.0 | 1.7 | 6.3 | 22.7 | 75.7 |
| Peru | 12–18 | 2.4 | 0.6 | 0.0 | 0.6 | | 1.1 | 39.6 | 67.3 |
| | 19–45 | 10.4 | 3.3 | 5.6 | 3.7 | | 4.1 | 78.2 | 95.0 |
| | Male | 14.1 | 4.2 | 7.3 | 3.6 | 3.7 | 3.2 | 79.9 | 90.3 |
| | Female | 1.8 | 0.8 | 0.4 | 1.8 | 3.0 | 3.2 | 54.7 | 84.0 |
| Venezuela | 12–15 | | | | | | | 20.0 | |
| | 16–74 | | | | | | | 57.7 | |

**Table 20.11**  Current drug use rates in selected Latin American countries by age

| | | Marijuana | Cocaine | Basuca | Hallucinogen | Inhalants | Stimulants | Tobacco | Alcohol |
|---|---|---|---|---|---|---|---|---|---|
| Belize | 14–19 | 6.6 | 1.3 | | | | | 17.1 | 33.3 |
| | 20–30 | 8.1 | 0.7 | | | | | 27.4 | 49.8 |
| | Male | 14.2 | 1.9 | | | | | 34.3 | 57.4 |
| | Female | 0.8 | 0.0 | | | | | 12.0 | 28.4 |
| Bolivia | 12–17 | 0.1 | 0.1 | 0.1 | 0.1 | 2.0 | 0.1 | 8.6 | 16.7 |
| | 18–50 | 0.3 | 0.1 | 0.2 | 0.0 | 1.1 | 0.1 | 30.6 | 51.3 |
| | Male | 0.3 | 0.1 | 0.3 | 0.0 | 1.3 | 0.0 | 38.2 | 52.9 |
| | Female | 0.1 | 0.0 | 0.1 | 0.0 | 1.4 | 0.2 | 14.3 | 33.6 |
| Colombia | 12–17 | | | | | | | 3.7 | 26.9 |
| | 18–60 | | | | | | | 26.1 | 44.1 |
| | Male | | | | | | | 29.2 | 55.1 |
| | Female | | | | | | | 15.5 | 29.6 |
| Guatemala | 12–19 | 1.6 | 0.4 | | 0.4 | 1.9 | 2.9 | | 14.9 |
| | 20–45 | 3.5 | 0.3 | | 0.4 | 0.9 | 4.1 | | 32.2 |
| | Male | 5.4 | 0.4 | | 0.9 | 1.9 | 4.8 | | 34.9 |
| | Female | 0.5 | 0.3 | | 0.0 | 0.6 | 2.7 | | 19.7 |
| Mexico | 12–18 | 0.2 | 0.0 | | 0.0 | 0.1 | | 10.0 | 46.9 |
| | 19–65 | 0.3 | 0.1 | | 0.0 | 0.1 | | 29.9 | 67.2 |
| | Male | 0.7 | 0.2 | | 0.5 | 0.2 | | 38.3 | 75.0 |
| | Female | 0.0 | 0.0 | | 0.0 | 0.0 | | 14.2 | 52.7 |
| Panama | 12–19 | 1.0 | 0.3 | 0.0 | | 0.5 | 0.0 | 3.0 | 18.6 |
| | 20–45 | 1.6 | 2.3 | 1.2 | | 0.8 | 0.5 | 18.8 | 46.0 |
| | Male | 1.8 | 2.3 | 0.7 | | 0.8 | 0.6 | 19.3 | 49.7 |
| | Female | 0.9 | 0.8 | 0.8 | | 0.7 | 0.1 | 6.2 | 21.4 |
| Paraguay | 12–45 | 0.1 | 0.0 | | 0.0 | | 1.9 | | |
| | Male | 0.2 | 0.0 | | 0.0 | | 0.8 | | |
| | Female | 0.0 | 0.0 | | 0.0 | | 2.6 | | |

**Table 20.12**   *Selected results from countries that provided data for the WHO Project Atlas 2005*

| Country | Mental health care budget (% of total health care budget) | Psychiatric beds/10 000 | Psychiatrists/ 100 000 | Psychologists/ 100 000 | Social workers/ 100 000 | Psychiatric nurses/100 000 |
|---|---|---|---|---|---|---|
| Argentina | 2.0 | 6.0 | 13.3 | 106.0 | 11.0 | |
| Belize | 1.0 | 2.3 | 1.3 | 0.0 | 4.3 | 0.5 |
| Bolivia | 0.2 | 0.8 | 0.9 | 5.0 | | |
| Brazil | 2.5 | 2.6 | 4.8 | 31.8 | | |
| Chile | 2.3 | 1.3 | 4.0 | 15.7 | 1.5 | 1.1 |
| Colombia | 0.1 | 1.3[a] | 2.0 | | | 0.1[a] |
| Costa Rica | 8.0 | 2.6 | 2.0 | 2.0 | 0.5 | 2.0 |
| Cuba | 5.0 | 7.4 | 10.0 | 9.0 | 12.0 | 2.7 |
| Ecuador | | 1.7 | 2.1 | 29.1 | 0.1 | 0.5 |
| El Salvador | | 0.7 | 0.5 | 31.2 | | 0.0 |
| Guatemala | 0.9 | 0.4 | 0.5 | 0.7 | 0.1 | 0.1 |
| Guyana | | 3.0 | 0.2 | 0.0 | 0.4 | 0.6 |
| Honduras | 2.3 | 0.6 | 0.8 | 0.5 | 0.3 | 0.0 |
| Mexico | 1.0 | 0.7 | 2.7 | | 0.2 | 0.1 |
| Nicaragua | 1.0 | 0.3 | 0.6 | 1.5 | 0.7 | 0.1 |
| Panama | | 2.6 | 3.7 | 2.6 | 0.1 | 5.0 |
| Paraguay | 0.1 | 0.7 | 1.8 | | | 0.1 |
| Peru | 2.0 | 0.5 | 2.1 | 4.0 | 1.0 | 6.0 |
| Suriname | 4.2 | 5.2 | 1.3 | 0.2 | 0.6 | 15.0 |
| Uruguay | 8.0 | 5.4 | 22.9 | 15.1 | 62.0 | 0.9 |
| Venezuela | | 2.5 | 24.0 | | | |

[a] Data not available in Mental Health Atlas 2005; data taken from World Health Organization (WHO, 2005).

in 1996 and resulted in over 200 000 displaced persons. A study of 170 adults over the age of 16 showed that 20 years later 11.8 per cent had symptoms consistent with a diagnosis of post-traumatic stress disorder. Anxiety and depressive symptoms were also highly prevalent (Sabin *et al.*, 2003). However, a study of 58 children in two refugee camps in Chiapas found minimal evidence of psychological trauma, but did find a relationship between the child's mental health and the physical and mental health of their mothers (Miller, 1996).

Political repression also has been present in a number of Latin American countries. A study of Honduran children who experienced disappearance and assassination of their parents showed that psychological effects remained present for many years, with symptoms of traumatic stress, depression, anxiety and aggression (Munczek and Tuber, 1998).

## SERVICE UTILIZATION

In Guatemala, only 30 per cent of indigenous peoples are estimated to be employed and to have access to health services, compared with 60 per cent of the general population (Pan American Health Organization, 2001). In Ecuador, nearly 90 per cent of indigenous peoples lack sufficient social coverage needed to access basic services (Encalada *et al.*, 1999). Table 20.12 lists the current resources available for mental health care in each of the Latin American countries.

Five studies examining mental health service utilization among those with psychiatric problems have been conducted in Latin America (see Table 20.13). The treatment gap for mental health service utilization ranged from 44 per cent for non-affective psychosis to 80 per cent for alcohol abuse

**Table 20.13**  *Service gap in Latin America*

|  | BR5 | CH2 | ME1 | ME3 | ME4 | Mean | Median |
|---|---|---|---|---|---|---|---|
| Non-affective psychosis | 58.0 | 44.4 |  |  |  | 46.1 | 44.4 |
| Major depression | 49.4 | 46.2 | 78.2 | 43.4 | 66.3 | 55.2 | 52.3 |
| Dysthymia | 43.8 | 32.4 | 81.5 | 78.5 | 58.0 | 57.8 | 56.9 |
| Bipolar disorder | 46.0 | 50.2 | 85.7 | 74.1 |  | 61.7 | 57.0 |
| Generalized anxiety | 41.1 | 44.2 | 94.7 | 72.2 |  | 59.8 | 53.3 |
| Panic disorder | 47.8 | 22.7 | 71.2 | 70.0 |  | 51.8 | 49.5 |
| Obsessive–compulsive |  | 27.6 |  | 92.1 |  | 59.9 | 59.9 |
| Alcohol abuse/dependence | 53.3 | 84.8 | 80.2 |  |  | 72.8 | 80.2 |

For an explanation of the study codes see Table 20.6.
Note: Colombia WMH has published data only on any affective disorders 82.4 per cent; any anxiety disorder 95.4 per cent; any substance use disorder 92.5 per cent.

or dependence. This may be an underestimation of the treatment gap in Latin America. In Belize about 63 per cent of individuals with schizophrenia were untreated; 89 per cent with affective disorders; and 99 per cent of those with anxiety disorders (Bonander *et al.*, 2000). In the study conducted in Mexico (Borges *et al.*, 2006) only 57 per cent of those who were receiving treatment, whether from a mental health professional or not, received treatment deemed minimally adequate; and using more stringent criteria for adequacy of treatment this fell to 19.2 per cent.

The use of *espiritista* for mental health treatment was not as common a modality in Mexico or Chile as the use of the established health care system. In Mexico 1.7 per cent of those with an ICD-10 diagnosis went to an *espiritista* compared with 11.7 per cent for the established medical system (Medina-Mora *et al.*, 2003). In a study in Chile where respondents were asked what type of treatment they would seek if they required mental health care only 1.2 per cent endorsed a *curandero* (Saldivia *et al.*, 2004). In a meta-analysis conducted of studies examining community perceptions regarding mental health in Latin America there was little evidence to support the use of traditional medicine or religion over the established medical model (de Toledo Piza Peluso and Blay, 2004; see Chapter 19 for a different view, and Chapters 2, 18 and 21 for examples of indigenous practitioners in other countries).

## REFERENCES

Aguilar Zambrano E. 1992: *La Farmacodependencia en el Ecuador, 1992*. Ministerio de Salud Publica Division Nacional Salud Mental Programma Alcoholismo Y Farmacodependencia: Ecuador.

Alcaraz del Castillo, F., Salinas, N.F., Villarroel, E.F. and Jutkowitz, J.M. 1993: *La Prevalencia del Uso Indebido de Drogas en Bolivia*. Bolivia: Ministerio de Prevision Social y Salud Publica.

Almeida-Filho, N. 1981: Development and assessment of the QMPI: a Brazilian children's behaviour questionnaire for completion by parents. *Social Psychiatry* 16, 205–11.

Almeida-Filho, N., Souza-Santana, V., Souza, A.L. and Jacobina, R.R. 1985: Relações entre a saúde mental dos pais e a saúde mental das crianças em uma população urbana de Salvador-Bahia. *Acta Psiquiatrica y Psicologica de America Latina* 31, 211–21.

Almeida-Filho, N., Mari, J.J., Coutinho, E., França, J.F., Fernandes, J.G., Andreoli, S.B. and Busnello, E.D.A. 1992: Estudo mulicêntrico de morbidade psiquiátrica em áreas urbanas brasileiros (Brasília, São Paulo, Porto Alegre). *Revista da Associação Brasileira de Psiquiatria – Asociacion Psiquiatrica de la America Latina (ABP-APAL)* 14, 93–104.

Almeida-Filho, N., Mari J.J., Coutinho, E., França, J.F., Fernandes, J., Andreoli, S.B. and Busnello, E.D. 1997: Brazilian multicentric study of psychiatric morbidity. *British Journal of Psychiatry* 171, 524–29.

Andrade, L.H., Lolio, C.A., Gentil, V. and Laurenti, R. 1999: Epidemiologia dos trastornos mentais em uma area definida de captação da cidade de São Paulo, Brasil. *Revista de Psiquiatra Clínica* 26, 257–62.

Andrade, L., Walters, E.E., Gentil, V. and Laurenti, R. 2002: Prevalence of ICD-10 mental disorders in a catchment area in the city of São Paulo, Brazil. *Social Psychiatry and Psychiatric Epidemiology* 37, 316–25.

Andrade, L., Caraveo-Anduaga, J.J., Berglund, P., Bijl, R.V., De Graaf, R., Vollebergh, W., Dragomirecka, E., Kohn, R., Keller, M., Kessler, R.C., Kawakami, N., Kilic, C., Offord, D., Ustun, T.B., Vicente, B. and Wittchen, H.U. 2003: The epidemiology of major depressive episodes: results from the International Consortium of Psychiatric Epidemiology (ICPE) Surveys. *International Journal of Methods in Psychiatric Research* 12, 3–21.

Anselmi, L., Picinini, C., Barros, F.C. and Lopes, R.S. 2004: Psychosocial determinants of behaviour problems in Brazilian preschool children. *Journal of Child Psychology and Psychiatry* 45, 779–88.

Araya, R., Rojas, G., Fritsch, R., Acuña, J. and Lewis, G. 2001: Common mental disorders in Santiago, Chile: prevalence and socio-demographic correlates. *British Journal of Psychiatry* 178, 228–33.

Aszkenazi, M. and Casullo, M.M. 1984: Factores socioculturales y presencia de psicopatologías en poblaciones de distintas localidades argentinas. *Acta Psiquiatrica y Psicologica de America Latina (Buenos Aires)* 30, 11–20.

Biedermann, N., Barria, C., Maass, J. and Steil, W. 1983: Estudio de diez casos de psicosis en mapuches. *Acta Psiquiatrica y Psicologica America Latina* 29, 294–300.

Bjil, R.V., de Graff, R., Hiripi, E., Kessler, R.C., Kohn, R., Offord, D.R., Ustun, T.B., Vicente, B., Vollebergh, W.A.M., Walters, E.E. and Wittchen, H.U. 2003: The prevalence of treated and untreated mental disorders in five countries. *Health Affairs (Millwood, VA)* 22, 122–33.

Bonander, J., Kohn, R., Arana, B. and Levav, I. 2000: An anthropological and epidemiological overview of mental health in Belize. *Transcultural Psychiatry* 37, 57–72.

Bordin, I.A.S., Mari, J.J. and Caeiro, M.F. 1995: Validação da Versão Brasileira do Child Behavior Checklist (CBCL) (Inventário de Comportamentos da Infância e Adolescência): Dados Preliminares. *Revista da Associação Brasileira de Psiquiatria – Asociacion Psiquiatrica de la America Latina (ABP-APAL)* 17, 55–66.

Bordin, I.A.S., Paula, C.S. and Duarte, C.S. 2002: Domestic violence against children in a Brazilian urban poor community: Brazil SAFE Pilot Findings. Program and Abstracts: Eighteenth Global Meeting of the International Clinical Epidemiology Network (INCLEN XVIII), Sharm El-Sheikh, Egypt, 78.

Borges, G., Medina-Mora, M.E., Wang, P.S., Lara, C., Berglund, P. and Walters, E. 2006: Treatment and adequacy of treatment of mental disorders among respondents to the Mexico National Comorbidity Survey. *American Journal of Psychiatry* 163, 1371–78.

Caraveo-Anduaga, J.J. 1995: *Epidemiologia de la Morbilidad Psiquiátrica en la Ciudad de México*. Mexico City: Instituto Mexicano de Psiquiatria.

Caraveo-Anduaga, J.J. and Bermúndez, E.C. 2004: The epidemiology of obsessive-compulsive disorder in México City. *Salud Mental* 27, 1–6.

Caraveo-Anduaga, J., Medina-Mora, M.E., Rascón, M.L., Villatoro, J., Martinez-Vélez, A. and Gómez, M. 1996: La prevalencia de los trastornos psiquiátricos en la población urbana adulta en México. *Salud Mental* 19, 14–21.

Caraveo-Anduaga, J.J., Martinez Vélez, N.A., Rivera Guevara, B.E. and Dayan, A.P. 1997: Prevalencia en la vida de episodios depresivos y utilización de servicios especializados. *Salud Mental* 20, s15–23.

Caraveo-Anduaga. J.J., Colmenares, E. and Saldivar, G.J. 1999: Morbilidad psiquiátrica en la ciudad de México: prevalencia y comorbilidad a lo largo de la vida. *Salud Mental* 22, 62–67.

Center of Studies and Information of the Multiethnic Woman (CEIMM) of the University of the Autonomous Regions of the Caribbean Nicaraguan Coast, Uraccan 2002: Background paper on gender from the indigenous women's perspective. Presented at First Indigenous Women's Summit of the Americas, Oaxaca, Mexico 30 November–4 December 2002, 22.

Correia, M. and Pena, V. 2002: *Panorama de Género en América Central Washington, D.C.: Región de América Latina y el Caribe.* Washington, DC: World Bank.

Demyttenaere, K., Bruffaerts, R., Posada-Villa, J., Gasquet, I., Kovess, V., Lepine, J.P., Angermeyer, M.C., Bernert, S., de Girolamo, G., Morosini, P., Polidori, G., Kikkawa, T., Kawakami, N., Ono, Y., Takeshima, T., Uda, H., Karam, E.G., Fayyad, J.A., Karam, A.N., Mneimneh, Z.N., Medina-Mora, M.E., Borges, G., Lara, C., de Graaf. R., Ormel, J., Gureje, O., Shen, Y., Huang, Y., Zhang, M., Alonso, J., Haro, J.M., Vilagut, G., Bromet, E.J., Gluzman, S., Webb, C., Kessler, R.C., Merikangas, K.R., Anthony, J.C., Von Korff, M.R., Wang, P.S., Brugha, T.S., Aguilar-Gaxiola, S., Lee, S., Heeringa, S., Pennell, B.E., Zaslavsky, A.M., Ustun, T.B., Chatterji, S. and the WHO World Mental Health Survey Consortium 2004: Prevalence, severity, and unmet need for treatment of mental disorders in the World Health Organization World Mental Health Surveys. *Journal of the American Medical Association* 291, 2581–90.

de Toledo Piza Peluso, E. and Blay, S.L. 2004: Community perception of mental disorders – a systematic review of Latin American and Caribbean studies. *Social Psychiatry and Psychiatric Epidemiology* 39, 955–61.

Development Associates 1990: *Drug Awareness Needs Assessment for Guatemala.* Alexandria, Virginia: Development Associates for US Agency for International Development – Bureau for Research and Development – Narcotics Awareness and Education Project.

Di Marco, G. 1982: Prevalencia de desórdenes mentales en el área metropolitana de la República Argentina. *ACTA Psiquiatrica y Psicologica de America Latina (Buenos Aires)* 28, 93–102.

Domador, M.P. 1991. *Trafico y Consumo de Substancias Psioactivas en Venezuela*. Caracas: Ministerio de Sanidad y Asistencia Social Division de Salud Mental Organizacion Panamericana de Salud.

Economic Commission for Latin America and the Caribbean 1997: *Social Panorama of Latin America*. Santiago: ECLAC.

Encalada, E., García, F. and Ivarsdotter, K. 1999: La participación de los pueblos indígenas y negros en el desarrollo de Ecuador. Washington, DC: Banco Interamericano de Desarrollo. www.iadb.org/sds/ind/publication/publication_133_2171_e.htm (accessed 23 July 2005).

Espejo, F. and Sandoval, G. 2001: *Salud mental del adolescente en Latinoamérica y el Caribe*. Washington, DC: Pan American Health Organization.

Fleitlich, B. and Goodman, R. 2001: Social factors associated with child mental health problems in Brazil: cross sectional survey. *British Medical Journal* 323, 599–600.

Fleitlich, B.W., Cortazar, P.G. and Goodman, R. 2000: Questionário de Capacidades e Dificuldades (SDQ). *Infanto* 8, 44–50.

Fleitlich-Bilyk, B. and Goodman, R. 2004: Prevalence of child and adolescent psychiatric disorders in southeast Brazil. *Journal of the American Academy of Child and Adolescent Psychiatry* 43, 727–34.

Galduróz, J.C., Noto, A.R., Nappo, S.A. and Carlini, E.A. 2005: Household survey on drug abuse in Brazil: study involving the 107 major cities of the country – 2001. *Addictive Behaviors* 30, 545–56.

Gómez-Restrepo, C., Bohóquez, A., Pinto Masis, D., Gil Laverde, J.F.A., Rondón Sepúlveda, M. and Díaz-Granados, N. 2004: Prevalencia de depresión y factores asociados con ella en la población colombiana. *Revista Panamericana de Salud Pública/Pan American Journal of Public Health* 16, 378–386.

Goodman, R., Meltzer, H. and Bailey, V. 1998: The Strengths and Difficulties Questionnaire: a pilot study on the validity of the self-report version. *European Child and Adolescent Psychiatry* 7, 125–30.

Gorenstein, C., Andrade, L., Zanolo, E. and Artes, R. 2005: Expression of depressive symptoms in a nonclinical Brazilian adolescent sample. *Canadian Journal of Psychiatry* 50, 129–37.

Hayashi, S., Perales, A., Sogi, C., Warthon, D., Llanos, R. and Novara, J. 1985: Prevalencia de vida de trastornos mentales en Independencia (Lima, Peru). *Anales de Salud Mental* 1, 206–22.

Heise, L., Ellsberg, M. and Gottemoeller, M. 1999: *Ending Violence against Women* (Population Reports, Series L, Number 11). Baltimore: Johns Hopkins University, School of Public Health.

Hughes, J. 2004: *Gender, Equity, and Indigenous Women's Health in the Americas*. Washington, DC: Pan American Health Organization.

Jutkowitz, J.M, and Day, H.R. 1992: *Survey on Drug Prevalence and Attitudes in Urban Panama*. Arlington, VA: Development Associates for US Agency for International Development – Bureau for Research and Development – Narcotics Awareness and Education Project.

Jutkowitz, J.M., Arellano, R., Castro de la Mata, R., Davis, P.B., Elinson, J., Jeri, F. R., Shaycoft, M. and Timana, J. 1989: *Monografia de Investigacion-Uso y Abuso de Drogas en el Peru*. Lima: Centro de Informacion y Educacion para la Prevencion del Abuso de Drogas.

Kohn, R., Levav, I., Alterwain, P., Ruocco, G., Contrera, M. and Della Grotta, S. 2001: Factores de riesgo de trastornos conductauales y emocionales en la niñez: estudio communitario en el Uruguay. *Revista Panamericana de Salud Pública/Pan American Journal of Public Health* 9, 211–18.

Kohn, R., Alterwain, P., Levav, I., Ruocco, G., Murillo. N., Contrera, M., Carzoli, L., Della Grotta, S. and Kim, S. 2001: Trastornos mentales y uso indebido de alcohol en dos comunidades del Uruguay. *Acta Psiquiátrica y Psicológica de América Latina* 47, 221–28.

Larraya, F.P., Casullo, M.M. and Viola, F.P. 1982: *Prevalencia de la Patologia Mental en la Megalopolis de Buenos Aires*. Buenos Aires: Consejo Nacional de Investigaciones Cientificas y Técnicas.

Lewis, G. and Pelosi, A.J. 1990: *Manual of the Revised Clinical Interview Schedule (CIS-R)*. London: MRC Institute of Psychiatry.

Mantilla Mendoza, L.F., Sabalza Peinado, L.P., Diaz Martinez, L.A. and Camp-Arias, A. 2004: Prevalencia de sintomatología depresiva en niños y niñas escolares de Bucaramanga, Colombia. *Revista Colombiana de Psiquiatría* 33, 163–71.

Medina-Mora, M.E., Borges, G., Muñoz, C.L., Benjet, C., Jaimes, J.B., Bautista, C.F., Velázquez, J.V., Guiot, E.R., Ruíz, J.Z., Rodas, L.C. and Aguilar-Gaxiola, S. 2003: Prevalencia de trastornos mentales y uso de servicios: resultados de la encuesta nacional de epidemiología psiquiátrica en México. *Salud Mental* 26, 1–16.

Merikangas, K.R., Mehta, R.L., Mohar, B.E., Walters, E.E., Swendsen, J.D., Aguilar-Gaxiola, S., Bijil, R., Borges, G., Caraveo-Anduaga, J.J., DeWit, D.J., Kolody, B., Vega W.A., Wittchen, H.U. and Kessler, R.C. 1998: Comorbidity of substance use disorders with mood and anxiety disorders: results of the International Consortium in Psychiatric Epidemiology. *Addictive Behaviors* 23, 893–907.

Miller, K.E. 1996: The effect of state terrorism and exile on indigenous Guatemalan refugee children: a mental health assessment and analysis of children's narratives. *Child Development* 67, 89–106.

Ministerio de Salud Publica y Bienestar Social 1991: *Estudio Sobre Salud Mental y Habitos Toxicos en el Paraguay*. Asuncion, Paraguay: Comite Paraguay-Kansas.

Minobe, K., Perales, A., Sogi, C., Warthon, D., Llanos, R. and Sato, T. 1990: Prevalencia de vida de trastornos mentales en Independencia (Lima, Peru). *Anales de Salud Mental* 6, 9–20.

Miranda, C.T., Turecki, G., Mari, J.J., Andreoli, S.B., Marcolim, M.A., Goihman, S., Puccini, R., Strom, B.L. and Berlin, J.A. 1996: Mental health of the mothers of malnourished children. *International Journal of Epidemiology* 25, 128–33.

Miranda, M.P., Bordin, I.A.S. and Miranda, C.T. 1999: Psychosocial stress and child mental health problems at elementary school entrance in a Brazilian urban poor community. Scientific Abstracts and CEU Executive Summaries: Sixteenth Annual Meeting of the International Clinical Epidemiology Network (INCLEN XVI), Bangkok, Thailand.

Munczek, D.S. and Tuber, S. 1998: Political repression and its psychological effects on Honduran children. *Social Science and Medicine* 47, 1699–713.

Muñoz, L., Marconi, J., Horwitz, J. and Naveillan, P. 1996: Crosscultural definitions applied to the study of functional psychoses in Chilean Mapuches. *British Journal of Psychiatry* 112, 1205–15.

Murray, C.J.L. and Lopez, A.D. (eds) 1996: *The Global Burden of Disease: A Comprehensive Assessment of Mortality and Disability from Diseases, Injuries, and Risk Factors in 1990 and Projected to 2020*. Cambridge, MA: Harvard School of Public Health (published on behalf of the World Health Organization and the World Bank, distributed by Harvard University Press).

Núñez, J.G., Martínez, M.A., Maynard-Tucker, G. and Murray, N. 2000: *Proyecto Servicios Integrales para Adolescentes en Condiciones de Pobreza*. Informe final. San José: Banco Interamericano de Desarrollo, Pan American Health Organization, Paniamor.

Ospina, E.R., Ramirez, L.F.D. and Garcia, J.R. 1993: *National Household Survey on Drug Abuse – Colombia – Highlights 1992*. Santafé de Bogotá: Direccion Nacional de Estupefacientes.

Pan American Health Organization 2001: *Equity in Health from an Ethnic Perspective*. Washington, DC: PAHO. www.paho.org/English/HDP/HDD/etnia.pdf (accessed 23 July 2005).

Pan American Health Organization 2002: *Health in the Americas 2002*. Washington, DC: PAHO.

Pan American Health Organization 2003: Violence Against Women: The Health Sector Responds. Washington, DC: PAHO.

Paula, C.S., Bordin, I.A.S., Santos, L.C. and Miranda, C.T. 2002: Mental and motor delays in daycare children from an urban poor community. Program and Abstracts: Eighteenth Global Meeting of the International Clinical Epidemiology Network (INCLEN XVIII), Sharm El-Sheikh, Egypt, 109.

Perales, A. and Sogi, C. 1995: Epidemiologia psiquiatrica en el Peru. *Anales de Salud Mental* 11, 9–29.

Posada-Villa, J.A., Aguilar-Gaxiola, S.A., Magaña, C.G. and Gómez, L.C. 2004: Prevalencia de trastornos mentales y uso de servicios: resultados preliminaries del estudio nacional de salud mental. Colombia 2003. *Revista Colombiana de Psiquiatría* 33, 241–62.

Pride Belize 1993: *Survey of Drug Prevalence and Attitudes in Belize City*. Belize City: United States Agency for International Development.

Rioseco, P., Escobar, B., Vicente, B., Vielma, M., Saldivia, S., Cruzat, M., Medina, E., Cordero, M.L. and Vicente, M. 1994: Prevalencia de vida de algunos trastornos psiquiátricos en la provincia de Santiago. *Revista de Psiquiatria* 11, 186–93.

Robins, L.N., Helzer, J.E., Croughan, J. and Ratcliff, K.S. 1981: National Institute of Mental Health Diagnostic Interview Schedule: its history, characteristics, and validity. *Archives of General Psychiatry* 38, 381–89.

Robins, L.N., Wing, J., Wittchen, H.U., Helzer, J.E., Babor, T.F., Burke, J., Farmer, A., Jablenski, A., Pickens, R., Regier, D.A., Sartorius, N. and Towle, L.H. 1988: The Composite International Diagnostic Interview: an epidemiologic instrument suitable for use in conjunction with different diagnostic systems and in different cultures. *Archives of General Psychiatry* 45, 1069–77.

Sabin, M., Lopes Cardozo, B., Nackerud, L., Kaiser, R. and Varese, L. 2003: Factors associated with poor mental health among Guatemalan refugees living in Mexico 20 years after civil conflict. *Journal of the American Medical Association* 290, 635–42.

Saldivia, S., Vicente, B., Kohn, R., Rioseco, P. and Torres, S. 2004: Use of mental health services in Chile. *Psychiatric Services* 55, 7–6.

Salgado de Snyder, V.N. and Diaz-Pérez, M. 1999: Los trastornos afectivos en la población rural. *Salud Mental* 22, 68–74.

Salgado de Snyder, V.N., Diaz-Pérez, M. and Ojeda, V.D. 2000: The prevalence of nervios and associated symptomatology among inhabitants of Mexican rural communities. *Culture, Medicine and Psychiatry* 24, 453–70.

Santana, V. 1982: Estudo epidemiológica das doencas mentais em um bairro de Salvador. *Série de Estudos em Saúde (Secretaria de Saúde da Bahia)* 2, 122.

Secretaria de Salud 1993: *Encuesta Nacional de Adicciones. Tome I – Alcohol. Tome II – Tabaco. Tome IV – Drogas Illegales*. Mexico City: Secretaria de Salud.

Torres, C. 1996: *Una mirada desde la perspectiva de la etnicidad*. Washington, DC: Pan American Health Organization; 2001. Based on data from the National Household Sample Survey (Pesquisa Nacional por Amostra de Domicilios – PNAD).

Torres de Galvis, Y. and Montoya, I.D. 1997: *Segundo Estudo Nacional de Salud Mental y Consumo de Sustancias Psicoactivas*. Colombia: Ministerio de Salud.

United Nations High Commission for Refugees 2005: *2004 Global Refugee Trends*. Geneva: UNHCR.

Vicente, B., Rioseco, P., Medina, E., River, B., Velma, M. and Saldivia, S. 1988: Estudio exporatorio de la salud mental de los pehuenches de alto bío-bío. *Acta Psiquiatrica y Psicologica America Latina* 44, 169–76.

Vicente, B., Rioseco, P., Vielma, M., Uribe, M., Boggiano, G. and Torres, S. 1992: Prevalencia de vida de algunos trastornos psiquiátricos en la provincia de Concepción. *Revista de Psiquiatria* 9, 1050–60.

Vicente, B., Rioseco, P., Saldivia, S., Kohn, R. and Torres, S. 2002: Estudio chileno de prevalencia de patología psiquiátrica (DSM-III-R/CIDI) (ECPP). *Revista Médica de Chile* 130, 527–36.

Vicente, B., Kohn, R., Rioseco, P., Saldivia, S., Baker, C. and Torres, S. 2004: Population prevalence of psychiatric disorders in Chile: 6-month and 1-month rates. *British Journal of Psychiatry* 184, 299–305.

Vicente, B., Kohn, R., Rioseco, P., Saldivia, S. and Torres, S. 2005: Psychiatric disorders among the Mapuche in Chile. *International Journal of Social Psychiatry* 51, 119–27.

Vicente, B., Kohn, R., Rioseco, P., Saldivia, S., Levav, I. and Torres, S. 2006. Lifetime and 12-month prevalence in the Chile Psychiatric Prevalence Study. *American Journal of Psychiatry* 163, 1362–70.

Vorcaro, C.M., Lima-Costa, M.F., Barreto, S.M. and Uchoa, E. 2001: Unexpected high prevalence of 1-month depression in a small Brazilian community: the Bambuí Study. *Acta Psychiatrica Scandinavica* 104, 257–63.

Wing, J.H., Nixon, J., Mann, S.A. and Leff, J.P. 1977: Reliability of the PSE (ninth edition) used in a population survey. *Psychological Medicine* 7, 505–16.

World Bank 2001: *World Development Indicators 2001.* Washington, DC: World Bank.

World Health Organization International Consortium in Psychiatric Epidemiology 2000: Cross-national comparisons of the prevalences and correlates of mental disorders. *Bulletin of the World Health Organization* 78, 413–25.

World Health Organization 2002: *Global Burden of Disease Project.* http://www.who.int/healthinfo/bodabout/en/index.html (accessed 23 July 2005).

World Health Organization 2005: *Mental Health Atlas.* Geneva: WHO. www.who.intglobalatlas/DataQuery/default.asp

Yamamoto, J., Silva, J.A., Sasao, T., Wang, C. and Nguyen, L. 1993: Alcoholism in Peru. *American Journal of Psychiatry* 150, 1059–62.

Zoninsein, J. 2002: *El caso económico para combatir la exclusión racial y étnica en América Latina y el Caribe.* Washington, DC: Banco Interamericano de Desarrollo.

# 21

# South Asian region

Vikram Patel, Athula Sumathipala, Murad M Khan, Suraj B Thapa and
Omar Rahman

## INTRODUCTION

The South Asian region is one of the most populous and at the same time one of the poorest regions in the world. The region faces enormous social, economic and health challenges, including pervasive poverty, inequality, violence, political instability and a high burden of communicable diseases. There is evidence of a demographic and epidemiological transition in most parts of the region; thus, populations are gradually ageing, and non-communicable diseases contribute to a growing share of the burden of disease. There is also considerable evidence of the high burden of mental disorders. Thus in the South Asian region, 11 per cent of disability adjusted life years (DALYs) and 27 per cent of years lived with disability (YLDs) are attributed to neuropsychiatric disease. Furthermore, rates of disorders such as depression and anxiety reported from the region are amongst the highest in the world.

This chapter will mainly focus on mental health in India, Nepal, Bangladesh, Pakistan and Sri Lanka. Within the scope of this chapter on mental health in South Asia the important limitation of averages must be recognized at the outset. For example, India, the largest and most populous country in the region, is characterized by huge diversity within and between its over 30 states and union territories.

Thus, the variation in infant mortality rates in India ranges from a low of 16.3 in Kerala to a high of 86.7 in Uttar Pradesh, a fivefold difference (International Institute for Population Sciences, 2001). Nepal, on the other hand, has a population of more than 25 million with a growth rate of 2.3 per cent and an infant mortality rate of 71 per 1000 live births. Its per capita income is among the lowest in the world. The literacy rates for men and women are 63 per cent and 28 per cent, respectively. Almost 90 per cent of the total population live in rural areas of Nepal. The average life expectancy is 60 years (World Health Organization, 2003; Care Nepal, 2005). The country has been badly affected by an armed conflict between Maoist insurgents and state forces for the last ten years (Informal Service Centre, 2005). The latest political developments have pushed an already unstable nation into further crisis.

Seventy per cent of Pakistan's population of 140 million live in the rural areas where access to health facilities is abysmally low. Pakistan's overall literacy rate is around 35 per cent, but there is a great variation between urban (up to 70 per cent) and rural (8 per cent for women) areas. As elsewhere in the region, men's literacy rates are much higher than women's literacy rates.

Bangladesh has undergone some dramatic sociodemographic improvements (Demographic and

Health Surveys, Macro International Inc. 2004) over the last two decades. Total fertility rates have declined from a high of 7 in 1970–1975 to a low of 3 births per woman in 2004 – similar to current levels in India; infant mortality rates are now 66/1000; maternal mortality rates have declined from around 6/1000 in 1970–1975 to about 3.2/1000 in 2004, lower than in Pakistan or India. Primary school enrolments now exceed 95 per cent and gender parity has been reached in both primary and secondary school enrolments, a better performance than either Pakistan or India. Despite these laudable achievements, morbidity and mortality remain high: life expectancy at birth is around 62 for both men and women, with wide disparities in access between urban (now 20 per cent of the population) and rural areas.

Although Sri Lanka is a developing country its social indicators, particularly on health and education, are much more advanced than those of its South Asian neighbours. Thus, the literacy rate is 92.5 per cent for men and 87.9 per cent for women, life expectancy is about 74 years, and infant mortality rate is 15.4 per 1000 live births (Ministry of Health, Sri Lanka 2000). Whereas a substantial proportion of health care in the region is delivered in the private sector – some estimates put this at above 75 per cent of all health consultations in India and Bangladesh – in Sri Lanka the majority of heath care is provided in the public sector.

In all South Asian countries, biomedical systems coexist with strong indigenous medical systems, such as Ayurveda, Tibetan and Unani, as well as traditional, religious healing systems, particularly in rural areas.

## THE STATE OF MENTAL HEALTH CARE

There are an estimated 4000 psychiatrists in India, which represents a ratio of approximately 1 psychiatrist for 250 000 people (World Health Organization, 2005). In Bangladesh there are approximately 140 'psychiatrists' for 140 million people. This is perhaps a generous estimate as this represents the membership of the Bangladesh Association of Psychiatrists, which focuses on professionals' interests rather than specific credentials to cover the span

of health care needs (personal communication from the Bangladesh Association of Psychiatrists, March 2005). If one were to use the criteria of international level professional psychiatric training in an organized residency programme to gauge the number of trained psychiatrists, there would be between 30 and 50 trained psychiatrists. In Nepal, there are only five psychiatric beds allocated per million people in Nepal and less than 25 psychiatrists. About 3 per cent of total GDP is spent on health and 1 per cent of that goes to mental health. There is no mental health act and the National Mental Health Policy formulated in 1997 is not yet fully operational (Regmi et al., 2002). The ongoing civil war has made a large proportion of the population flee their homes due to the fear of persecution, torture and threats from both the state and rebels, which may worsen the mental wellbeing of the displaced and general population as well. In Pakistan, there are only 150–200 qualified psychiatrists, while Sri Lanka has about 28 psychiatrists, an alarming ratio of one psychiatrist to about a million people.

The number of trained psychologists, social workers and psychiatric nurses is even lower. Throughout the region, the vast majority of mental health specialists are located in cities. Thus the ratio of numbers of providers to the population is even greater in rural areas. Consequently, large numbers of people with mental health problems remain either without care or seek treatment from alternative health systems.

Formal psychological services are non-existent in the public sector. About 80 per cent of these beds are situated in mental hospitals where the quality of care has been found to be characterized by violation of even basic human rights (National Human Rights Commission, 1999). Recent newspaper reports have highlighted the very poor conditions (Ali and Saha, 2004; Plamandon, 2004) under which patients are treated in the major psychiatric hospital in Bangladesh. Links between the psychiatric services and general hospital services are very limited except in some university teaching units and larger provincial hospitals. However, over the last two years, in Sri Lanka, 36 medical officers were appointed to general hospitals under the designation of Medical Officer (Mental Health) with some limited supervision by the psychiatrists.

If one considers that the estimated number of people with schizophrenia alone is in excess of 10 million, it is obvious that the vast majority of people with mental disorders will not have access to a mental health professional in South Asia (Begum, 2003; Plamandon, 2004). The numbers of professionals in specialized areas of psychiatry such as child, substance abuse or elderly mental health cannot even be estimated because, barring a few academic centres, these specialties do not exist as distinct from general services. Thus, it may be fair to say that the primary provider of mental health care in South Asia is the general or primary health sector, with its wide (though uneven) network of primary health centres and general hospitals, both in the private and public sectors. The traditional and complementary medical sector is also a vibrant player in mental health care. For instance, it was found that about 7 per cent of male and 1 per cent of female refugees were working as traditional healers among Bhutanese refugees living in Nepal (van Ommeren *et al.*, 2002). This sector includes an array of religious, spiritual and alternative healing systems such as Ayurvedic, faith-healing and Unani medicine. Recently, there has been a renaissance of traditional systems of health promotion such as yoga.

The non-governmental organization sector also plays a key role in mental health care, in particular by filling in niche areas of need such as addictions, child mental health care, and by developing innovative community-based models of care (Patel and Thara, 2003). A large, mostly indigenous pharmaceutical industry ensures that most psychotropic drugs are available in India and Bangladesh, often at a fraction of the costs found in high income countries; however, this low cost does not translate into consistent availability at government-run primary and general health care settings (Patel and Andrade, 2003). In spite of prolonged ethnic conflict and war in recent decades, and one of the highest suicide rates in the world in Sri Lanka, mental health was not treated as a priority until recently. Only 1 per cent of the health budget is allocated to mental health.

However, across South Asia, mental health has been receiving increasing attention in national health policy and programming, best illustrated by a specific mention of mental health as a priority area for the new National Health Plan in India, drafted for the coming decade. The National Mental Health Program was formulated in 1982 with the objective of ensuring availability and accessibility of basic mental health care, particularly to the most vulnerable and underprivileged sections of the population. The programme, though visionary in its conceptualization, had slow progress due mainly to lack of dedicated finances. It is implemented at present in 22 districts (out of 593) and will be extended to over 100 districts in the next few years. The key approaches used are the training of primary health care personnel, the provision of neuropsychiatric drugs in peripheral institutions, establishing psychiatric units at the district level with streamlined referrals, and encouraging community participation. However, it is worth noting that, despite this programme, less than 1 per cent of the total health budget is devoted to mental health.

The Mental Health Act of 1987 replaced the Indian Lunacy Act of 1912. The Act has provided new definitions, simplified admission and discharge procedures, introduced licensing of psychiatric hospitals, set up central and state mental health authorities and promoted human rights for the mentally ill. However, the implementation of this law is very uneven across the states. Another key legislation has been the Persons with Disabilities Act which includes mental disabilities and provides access to social welfare and employment schemes. The Narcotic Drugs and Psychotropic Substances Act (amended in 2001) deals with the prevention, treatment and rehabilitation of drug-dependent people. In Sri Lanka, the Mental Diseases Ordinance, enacted in 1873, uses the vague term 'persons of unsound mind' to define mental illness. Despite some amendments in 1956 these ancient laws are clearly in need of a major revision. New draft laws to replace the existing regulations have been doing the rounds since 1973 but have not succeeded because of the lack of agreement among psychiatrists.

## SPECIFIC DISORDERS

Psychiatric disorders are profoundly influenced by regional factors such as cultural beliefs and socio-economic factors, and data from Western studies may not be entirely applicable to the South Asian context. This section summarizes the research and clinical evidence from South Asia on major categories of mental disorders.

## Severe mental disorders

While some work has been done on schizophrenia (for example in epidemiology and outcome) and dementia (diagnosis and prevalence), there is little information on bipolar disorders from South Asia. The World Health Organization's Global Burden of Disease 2000 reports a prevalence of 0.4–1 per cent for schizophrenia (World Health Organization, 2000), which leads to an estimate of about 6–12 million people with schizophrenia in South Asia. In contrast to the findings regarding the earlier age of onset in men, age at onset of the first psychotic symptom did not differ between the sexes, regardless of whether schizophrenia was diagnosed by the *Diagnostic and Statistical Manual of Mental Disorders* (DSM-IV) or by one of various alternative systems (Murthy *et al.*, 1998).

It has been repeatedly demonstrated that the course followed by schizophrenia in developing countries is less severe than that in developed countries (Thara and Eaton, 1996). For example, in the World Health Organization multisite international studies (which included centres in South Asia), the proportion of patients showing full remission at two years was 63 per cent in developing countries compared with 37 per cent in developed countries (Jablensky *et al.*, 1992). Although attempts have been made to explain this better outcome on the basis of stronger family support and fewer demands on patients, the exact reasons are not clear. There are also new concerns regarding the validity of the longitudinal studies, showing superior outcome in developing countries, given the fact that a substantial proportion of the cohort of subjects in these countries were lost to follow-up.

Dementia is a rapidly growing problem in all parts of the developing world, including South Asia (Prince, 1997). The prevalence rate of dementia among those aged 65 years old or more in urban India was 2.44 per cent (Vas *et al.*, 2001), while that for rural India was 3.24 per cent (Chandra *et al.*, 2001). Prevalence rates in a semi-urban area in Sri Lanka have been found to be 3.98 per cent (de Silva *et al.*, 2003). There is low awareness about dementia as a medical diagnosis; most persons with the condition are not considered to be ill, and consequently care is rarely sought or provided (Patel and Prince, 2001). There is heavy reliance on families as the cornerstone of support and care. Recent research from the region has demonstrated the validity of a one-step diagnostic interview for dementia in community studies, the high degree of sensitivity with which community health workers can identify community cases based on a simple training protocol, and the enormous burden on carers in terms of mental health and health care costs for caring for dementia (Shaji *et al.*, 2002; Prince *et al.*, 2003; Dias *et al.*, 2004).

Most formal care for severe mental disorders is focused on institutions; non-governmental organizations are at the forefront of developing community care and rehabilitation. One such programme evaluated a community-based rehabilitation intervention in a rural region of India and demonstrated the superiority of such care, compared with routine outpatient care, on clinical and disability outcomes (Chatterjee *et al.*, 2003).

## Common mental disorders

The typical presenting complaints of common mental disorders (CMDs) are somatic, in particular tiredness and weakness, multiple aches and pains, dizziness, palpitations and sleep disturbances (Chaturvedi, 1993). However, psychological symptoms are often elicited on inquiry (Patel *et al.*, 1998a). Diagnostic labels such as 'depression' and 'phobias' have no conceptually equivalent term in many South Asian languages, and may be used less precisely by lay people who are familiar with them. Thus, generic terms which perhaps most closely approximate the concept of 'nerves' or neuroses are in colloquial use. 'Depression' in medicine is seen as being closely linked to mood changes. Using such labels in South Asian cultures often leads to the mistaken belief that sadness is an essential presenting feature of the disorder.

Patients with emotional symptoms of depression have higher levels of perceived stigma than those with physical symptoms (Raguram *et al.*, 1996); as a result, many patients may prefer to use somatic idioms. Alternatively, this preference may be inevitable if there are cultural sanctions that are implicit in illness behaviours in this region, to give greater significance to physical complaints than emotional or psychological ones.

There have been a number of studies of the prevalence in community and primary or general health care settings in South Asia (for a full review, see Patel, 1999; Mirza and Jenkins, 2004). The rates range considerable from 5 per cent to over 50 per cent. As might be expected, rates of CMD are higher in primary care settings. A review of eight epidemiological studies of CMD in South Asia (Patel, 1999) found that the prevalence in primary care was 26.3 per cent (95 per cent confidence interval 25.3–27.4 per cent). Furthermore, the prevalence of depression and anxiety among displaced persons in Nepal due to the armed conflict was found to be as high as 80 per cent (Thapa and Hauff, 2005). A number of studies have examined the associations and risk factors for CMD. Three major themes emerge from these studies. First, the relationship between female gender and CMD has been shown in both primary care and community settings. Second, there is a relationship between economic impoverishment and CMD. For example, a primary care study reported a strong association between indicators of poverty such as being in debt and being unable to buy food with CMD (Patel et al., 1998b). The third association is that between low education and high risk for CMD. Thus, women, the poor and the less educated, already the most vulnerable sections of South Asian society, are at greatest risk of CMD. CMDs are strongly associated with disability. Thus, primary care attenders with a CMD spent twice the number of days in the previous month being unable to work as usual due to their illness and twice the number of days bedridden as a result of their illness compared with those without CMD (Patel et al., 1998b). A recent study in primary care in South Asia estimated the cost of an episode of CMD to be equivalent to three weeks' wages for agricultural workers (Chisholm et al., 2000).

A World Health Organization multinational study described the clinical practice of the primary care doctors and found that most common mental disorders were not recognized (World Health Organization, 1995). Nearly 10 per cent of primary care attenders in the Indian centre were prescribed psychotropic drugs. However, the majority of prescriptions were for tranquillizers rather than antidepressant drugs; for example, while 50 per cent of patients with anxiety disorders received tranquillizers, none received antidepressants. A similar, if less marked, imbalance was also recorded for patients with depressive syndromes. Psycho-social and psychotherapeutic interventions were rarely used. A recent study from Bangladesh in the outpatient department of a district hospital (Hamid et al., 2003) found that 1.53 per cent of all outpatients had primarily psychiatric problems, with 54.6 per cent of these patients being female. As per DSM-IV criteria, mood and anxiety disorders accounted for over 80 per cent of cases.

There is a small body of evidence relating to treatments. A review of research on the use of yoga for neurotic disorders suggests that some yoga-based exercises such as breathing exercises may be valuable in the management of CMD (Grover et al., 1996). A recent randomized controlled trial of cognitive behaviour therapy for medically unexplained symptoms in patients attending general medical clinics in Sri Lanka reported significant improvements in psychiatric morbidity and a number of medical consultations (Sumathipala et al., 2000). A trial from Goa (India), demonstrated the efficacy and cost-effectiveness of antidepressants (fluoxetine) in a general health care setting (Patel et al., 2003a). A trial in Karachi, Pakistan has shown that counselling provided by minimally trained counsellors to women of their own community resulted in a significant reduction in the levels of anxiety and/or depression (Ali et al., 2003).

## Substance abuse disorders

This section will focus on alcohol use disorders, which are the commonest of the substance abuse disorders in the region. However, we acknowledge that drug abuse is an important cause of morbidity and mortality, in particular, in the light of the risk for HIV/AIDS amongst injecting drug users in specific areas of the region. For example, in predominantly Muslim countries (Bangladesh and Pakistan), alcohol consumption is uncommon and the major focus of substance abuse is opiates.

The production of alcohol occurs in many settings, across the organized (commercial) and the unorganized (non-commercial) sector. A third category is that of illicit or illegal alcohol. In some countries or states, the production and sale of all types of alcohol are illegal, whereas in others only alcohol which is produced outside the official alcohol revenue system is illegal. Traditional alcohols are those which have been brewed using local produce such as rice, wheat, potatoes, sap from different types of palms and locally available fruit. These alcohols may be either fermented or distilled. Another, frequently used variety of beverage is illicit alcohol, a term usually used to describe alcoholic beverages which evade quality and tax controls. As a result, the alcohol content varies and can be as high as 60 per cent. The common characteristic of these alcoholic beverages is their low cost, which makes them attractive for use by poorer people. The lack of regulations makes these beverages hazardous to health, as evidenced by the regular occurrences of methanol poisoning leading to mortality, blindness and other morbidity. Distilled spirits are also freely available in many parts of the region.

Data on treatment-seeking populations suggest a remarkable rise in consultation for alcohol-related problems from almost all parts of the region. Thus, the number of people seeking help for alcohol use problems has been reported to be on the rise since the early 1980s and more so in the 1990s, in psychiatric hospitals as well as psychiatric services of general hospitals in the public and the private sector. There are few population-based studies of alcohol abuse in the region (for a more detailed review on studies from India, refer to Saxena, 1999). Most community-based studies have examined the prevalence of drinking alcohol as an event, rather than alcohol abuse or alcohol-related health or social problems. These surveys have revealed highly variable patterns of use. The one consistent finding in general population surveys has been the very low rates for alcohol use in females. Alcohol use in men (in the past year) varies from 20 per cent to 75 per cent. A few surveys have examined the prevalence of alcohol dependence; as might be expected, the rates are low, ranging from 0.5–3.4 per cent of the population.

Hazardous drinking is defined as a level of alcohol consumption that could prove harmful in the future. A study of male industrial workers in Goa reported a prevalence of 21 per cent (Silva *et al.*, 2003). A subsequent study on the impact and patterns of drinking reported that hazardous drinkers had significantly poorer physical and mental health and showed trends for adverse social outcomes such as violence. Casual drinkers, on the other hand, were no different from abstinent subjects on any of the key outcomes. As compared to casual drinkers, hazardous drinkers tended to drink alone, in bars, and preferred non-commercial alcoholic beverages which are cheaper and have high alcohol concentrations (Gaunekar *et al.*, 2005). Apart from male gender, other risk factors reported for substance use disorders are unemployment, less education and low socio-economic status.

The role of gender factors as a determinant of the male excess of drinking problems has been pointed out in many cultures and is likely to be a key reason for this excess in this region (Pyne *et al.*, 2002). To the best of our knowledge, there are no clinical trials of the treatment of drinking problems in non-psychiatric settings from the region.

## Suicide

Suicide is one of the hidden tragedies in South Asia. It is estimated that approximately 10 per cent of the estimated one million annual global suicides take place in South Asia. Negative attitudes towards mental illness, lack of recognition and of timely intervention of mental disorders, the relatively easy availability of lethal methods of suicide (particularly pesticides), punitive laws and religious and socio-cultural condemnation of suicidal behaviour has led to suicide remaining outside the public health agenda in South Asia. In terms of actual numbers, India, with more than 100 000 suicides annually, is second only to China (Girdhar *et al.*, 2003). In a verbal autopsy study in Vellore, South India, Aaron *et al.* (2004) showed that suicides accounted for about a quarter of all deaths in young men and for between 50 per cent and 75 per cent of all deaths in young women. The average suicide rate for young women was 148 per 100 000, which is one of the highest in the world. Sri Lanka's rate of more than 40/100 000 remains one of the highest national rates in the world (Ratnayeke, 1996). Pakistan, a Muslim country with traditionally low rates of suicide, has in recent years seen an alarming increase in suicides from a few hundred to more than 3000 at present (Khan and Prince, 2003). Data from other countries in the region are scarce but data from a rural subdistrict in Bangladesh, from 1980 to 1996, showed rates of 7.0/100 000 for men and 8.6/100 000 for women, while those for 15- to 24-year-old men and women for the same period were 9.3/100 000 and 19.5/100 000 respectively (Fauveau et al., 1988). A study of suicides in a district of Nepal showed annual rates of 3.7/100 000, with a mean age of 33.9 years (Thapa, 2000).

Several points need to be kept in mind in the context of suicides in South Asia.

- The choice of methods in suicides: organophosphate insecticides and pesticides are the most common methods employed. They are easily available and accessible in both rural and urban areas and their high lethality make them particularly dangerous as a method in attempts at suicide. Public awareness programmes and proper storage are important preventive steps (Eddleston et al., 1998).
- The role of mental illness as a risk factor for suicides in Asian countries: one of the common perceptions has been that in South Asian suicides, interpersonal relationship problems and financial problems are more important as risk factors than mental illness. This was no doubt given credence by earlier reports, based on retrospective reviews of police or forensic medicine data, neither of which studied the psychological factors in suicides in depth (Patel and Gaw, 1996). A recent psychological autopsy study from India, however, found mental illness to be present in 88 per cent of the victims (Vijayakumar and Rajkumar, 1999). Another recently completed psychological autopsy study of risk factors for suicides in Karachi, Pakistan, found psychiatric disorders in more than 90 per cent of the victims (Khan, personal communication). The relative lack of psychological sophistication among families

and investigating agencies, the stigma attached to mental illness, and limited psychological treatment resources may lead to underestimation of psychiatric illnesses that predispose to suicide.

- The issue of marital status and suicide: most studies show a higher proportion of married as compared with single women among suicides in South Asia. Similarly prevalence studies on psychological morbidity also show a higher proportion of married compared with single women (Mumford et al., 1997). Some of the associated factors are early marriage and motherhood, infertility or absence of male offspring, lack of autonomy in choosing marital partner and economic dependence on husband (Khan and Reza, 1998). Studies from the region have also highlighted the problem of domestic violence towards women, an important risk factor for mental illness and suicide (Fikree and Bhatti, 1999). It is important to note that in the largely patriarchal societies of South Asia there is some concern about potential misclassification of homicide of married women (usually by husbands and the husbands' family members) as suicide, especially with regard to conflicts about dowry.

There is little documented work on the prevention of suicide in South Asia. In India, Nepal and Sri Lanka a handful of suicide prevention centres, mainly in the non-governmental organization sector, are operating with encouraging results. Sumithrayo Befrienders in Sri Lanka, Sathi and Center for Victims of Torture in Nepal, and Sneha in Chennai in India are examples of such centres. However, much work needs to be done in the area of suicide prevention, particularly at the level of national health policy and programmes. While governments and policy-makers need to establish social policies which are equitable and just, which will improve the socio-economic situation of the countries of the region, health professionals in South Asia need to be proactive in early detection and appropriate management of mental disorders.

## FUTURE STRATEGIES

Given the enormous burden of mental disorders, the increased risk for vulnerable groups in the population (such as women and the poor) and the relative paucity of mental health services in the region, the most important policy implication of the evidence is to emphasize the importance of prevention. Given the enormous unmet need for care for people with mental disorders, it is arguable that secondary and tertiary prevention strategies must be the immediate priority of the mental health policy.

## Secondary and tertiary prevention

The key to secondary and tertiary prevention is to strengthen the availability of appropriate treatment and rehabilitation strategies for mental disorders in the community and primary health care. The sheer numbers of people with severe mental disorders implies that existing specialist mental health services will be unable to deal with them for the foreseeable future. Thus, there is a need to develop alternative ways of tackling mental disorders using, as far as possible, existing human resources or relying on new human resources which are cost-effective.

### Integration of mental health in primary health care

The integration of mental health into primary health care has been the mantra of the World Health Organization for over a decade. There needs to be greater emphasis on training general health workers to recognize and effectively treat CMD and alcohol abuse. Several manuals have been developed with recommendations on the management of CMD using a combination of psycho-educational and pharmacological interventions (Patel, 2003). An Indian Council of Medical Research (ICMR) multi-centre study reported the efficacy of a training package consisting of a manual and about 20 hours of face-to-face sessions in raising knowledge in general practitioners about mental disorders; however, the gain was not uniform either for diagnostic skills or interventions (Shamasundar et al., 1989). Significantly, the maximum gain was for depression, which was partly accounted for by the fact

that the GPs had low pretraining knowledge. A similar exercise for multipurpose health workers showed a significant increase in skills and knowledge after a one-week training programme.

Training is not a sufficient intervention to improve primary mental health care. Additional human resources are needed in primary care, and services must be linked with mental health professionals, where feasible, to ensure support, supervision and referral networks. Apart from the public primary care system, there is an important role to be played by the private sector, traditional and religious healers, non-governmental and voluntary organizations and families.

### Integration of mental health into other health and social programmes

There are several examples of existing public health priorities in which mental disorders are of great relevance, such as maternal and child health (see Box 21.1), reproductive and sexual health, adolescent health and violence prevention. Such programmes provide an ideal opportunity to 'piggyback' mental health interventions. Similarly, school health programmes are being implemented in many areas: mental health issues such as learning disabilities can be integrated in these programmes. Programmes aimed at helping people who have suffered disasters or societal violence, not infrequent in the region, should include a mental health component; such initiatives have been described following recent disasters such as the earthquake and the communal riots in Gujarat (Sekar et al., 2002). 'Piggybacking' mental health interventions would imply using existing resources and staff and providing more comprehensive care. Such integration can thus be implemented with minimal additional cost and would have the advantage of greater access to patients as a result of the lower level of stigma than would be attached to seeking help from mental health services.

### Community-based rehabilitation models for severe mental disorders

A recent study in a rural region of India has provided preliminary evidence that community-based rehabilitation, which has been widely implemented in the region for the management of physical disabilities, is a feasible model of rehabilitation for people with

Several recent studies from South Asia have documented significant rates of post-natal depression (Patel *et al.,* 2004). Depressed mothers had significantly higher levels of disability, and more than half remained ill for at least six months. Consistent risk factors for post-natal depression were antenatal psychiatric morbidity, economic deprivation, low education and marital disharmony. Education, support from extended family members and employment were protective factors. While most of these risk factors have also been demonstrated in developed countries, the studies have shown the importance of the gender of the newborn infant as a determinant of post-natal depression. The preference for male children is deeply rooted in South Asia. Women are often blamed for the birth of girls, especially in situations where the woman already has a girl child. Such bias and the limited ability of women to control their reproductive health can make pregnancy and the birth of a daughter a very stressful event contributing to the risk for depression. The continuous care and attention of children is a demanding task, and poor mental health in mothers might be expected to have adverse consequences on their children's health and development. In low-income countries, maternal competence in child care is likely to play a greater role in the child's physical wellbeing and survival, especially in the first year of life, as the environment is frequently more hostile than in the wealthy countries. Recent studies from South Asia have provided new evidence to demonstrate that this is the case. For example, in a cohort study of babies born in a district general hospital in Goa, India, babies who were under the fifth centile for weight at six months were 2.3 times more likely to have a mother with post-natal depression at six weeks ($P$ 0.01; Patel *et al.,* 2003b). In a community cohort study from Pakistan, it was reported that antenatal depression was associated with low birth weight, and poorer infant growth in the first year; post-natal depression independently increased the risk for poor infant growth and childhood physical health problems (Rahman *et al.,* 2004).

schizophrenia, even in deprived economic settings, and that outcomes are best for those who are treatment compliant (Chatterjee *et al.,* 2003). Since the lack of professional resources is the reality in rural settings, the community-based rehabilitation method offers a model which involves active local community participation and low levels of technical expertise to deliver services. Mental health professionals can contribute to capacity building of non-governmental organizations that have an existing grassroots foundation to initiate services that draw upon the resources of the community.

### Improvement in quality of care for the mentally ill

There is urgent need to improve the quality of care for the mentally ill at all levels of care. The National Human Rights Commission report on the quality of care in mental hospitals paints a sorry picture of neglect and human rights abuse in many hospitals (National Human Rights Commission, 1999). The major role of these hospitals is custodial rather than therapeutic. Since many of the hospitals were functioning with closed wards without any psycho-social intervention, the report concluded that the three basic rights for personal liberty, right to appropriate treatment and rehabilitation and the right to community and family life were being violated. The World Health Report has strongly advocated the need to replace mental hospitals with community care and general hospital psychiatric units, as well as to strengthen the community network of general physicians skilled in mental health care (World Health Organization, 2001). It is also important to regulate the practice of private psychiatric nursing homes and traditional or religious carers. The tragedy in Tamil Nadu, south India, in 2001 where more than 20 patients with mental illness were burned to death because they were chained to their beds at the time a fire swept through their traditional healing centre, is a reminder that the human rights of the mentally ill may be violated in traditional medical care settings as well.

### Primary prevention

The evidence to support the efficacy of primary prevention interventions is weak, mainly because few if any interventions have been tried and/or evaluated in terms of their impact on mental disorders. However, based on the evidence of risk factors, it is likely that programmes aiming to reduce poverty, enhance educational achievement, combat gender-related discrimination, reduce the impact of natural disasters and build social cohesion to eliminate the risk of conflict would all have an impact in reducing the population burden of mental disorders. A key strategy towards implementation of primary prevention programmes is the recognition that mental health outcomes are integral to many development initiatives. Thus, intersectoral collaborations should begin by representation of mental health perspectives in forums for development planning, and representation of development planners in developing mental health policies. Three examples of primary preventive and promotive strategies are considered below:

- Being in debt is a major cause of stress, particularly to the poorest and the illiterate who do not have access to bank credit. This is perhaps most vividly illustrated by the suicides of farmers in central regions of India as a result of recurrent failure of crops because of monsoons (Sundar, 1999). Radical community banks and loan facilities which are providing microcredit, such as those run by SEWA in Gujarat could be involved in setting up such loan facilities in areas where they do not exist. In Bangladesh, the experience of the Grameen Bank, an international pioneer in microcredit schemes for rural women is well recognized. Microcredit schemes are now increasingly available all over Bangladesh, administered both by non-governmental organizations and government financial institutions. Thus, microcredit may be a primary preventive strategy for common mental disorders and suicide.
- Public health campaigns such as the World Health Organization's Stop Exclusion: Dare to Care campaign have generally aimed to increase awareness of mental illness, and increase knowledge about the effectiveness of interventions available in health services. Health promotion and education is the key to

reducing the population burden of substance abuse disorders. Health promotion through schoolchildren has been shown to be an effective way or raising awareness regarding mental illness (Rahman et al., 1998). Mental health promotion in schools must be integrated into general school health programmes and should include greater awareness about mental health problems amongst teachers and parents.
- Despite a long history of prohibition, alcohol abuse does occur across the region and rates in men are high. Thus, alcohol is available even when prohibition is in place; instead of reducing the burden of alcohol use disorders, prohibition pushes the alcohol supply into the illegal sector, fuelling a criminal network of people engaged in bootlegging and smuggling. The human toll of these criminal activities is evident from the cases of illicit alcohol poisoning. Prohibition, as a legislative policy to reduce the burden of alcohol-related problems, should be replaced by enforcement of controlled distribution and sale of alcohol and provision of education about the dangers of drinking.

## Research strategies

A recent review of the contribution of non-Western countries to the international psychiatric literature found that 14 per cent of the papers published over a three-year period in six high-impact journals were from India, a figure second only to Japan (Patel and Sumathipala, 2001). There are more than a dozen journals in psychiatry and allied specialties in the region. However, despite a continuous publication record of several decades, journals such as the *Indian Journal of Psychiatry* are still not indexed on major international citation databases, limiting its impact on world psychiatry. Not surprisingly, some of the best scientific studies from the region still go to international journals. The region is the home of some leading universities and academic institutions and an array of non-governmental organizations which are pioneering service and research innovations in mental health. There is a thriving private medical sector, a strong pharmaceutical industry, and a limited number of funding agencies that are supporting research. Thus, there is a considerable potential, in terms of human resources, institutions and sources of funding, to implement a regional programme of research in mental and neurological disorders. Given the wide range of health systems in the region, from urban metropolises to remote rural regions, it is likely that data generated from the region may be beneficial to a number of other developing countries. It is worth noting, however, that despite this potential, mental health research is very much in its infancy in South Asia. On the whole there are relatively few mental health researchers, and very little funding for mental health.

Despite the evidence of an association between mental disorders and socio-economic problems, it is important to recognize that the majority of people living even in squalid poverty or having faced terrible traumas, remain well, cope with the daily grind of existence and do not succumb to the stressors they face in their lives. Research is required to investigate the factors that promote mental health and prevent mental disorders in people who face socio-economic or other adversities. There is little evidence available on the effectiveness of various models of interventions for mental disorders. Health services research and randomized controlled trials which evaluate the delivery, outcome and quality of various models of mental health care, including traditional health care, are required. The interface between mental health and other public health priorities, in particular reproductive and child health, is an important way of generating evidence that will facilitate the integration of mental health into existing public health programmes.

# REFERENCES

Aaron, R., Joseph, A., Abraham, S., Muliyil, J., George, K., Prasad, J., Minz, S., Abraham, V.J. and Bose, A. 2004: Suicides in young people in rural southern India. *Lancet* 363, 1117–18.

Ali, A. and Saha, B. 2004: Pabna Mental Hospital reels under drug crisis. *The Daily Star* 8 January, 11, 12.

Ali, B.S., Rahbar, M.H., Naeem, S., Gul, A., Mubeen, S. and Iqbal, A. 2003: The effectiveness of counseling on anxiety and depression by minimally trained counselors. *American Journal of Psychotherapy* 57, 324–36.

Begum, Roquia 2003: Mental hospital. In *Banglapedia*. Bangladesh: Asiatic Society of Bangladesh, Vol. 6.

Care Nepal 2005: Country background. Available at: http://www.careusa.org/vft/nepal/country_background.asp/ (accessed 3 November 2006).

Chandra, V., Pandav, R., Dodge, H.H., Johnston, J.M., Belle, S.H., DeKosky, S.T. and Ganguli, M. 2001: Incidence of Alzheimer's disease in a rural community in India: the Indo-US study. *Neurology* 25, 985–89.

Chatterjee, S., Patel, V., Chatterjee, A. and Weiss, H. 2003: Evaluation of a community based rehabilitation model for chronic schizophrenia in a rural region of India. *British Journal of Psychiatry* 182, 57–62.

Chaturvedi, S. 1993: Neurosis across cultures. *International Review of Psychiatry* 5, 179–91.

Chisholm, D., Sekar, K., Kumar, K., Saeed, S., James, S., Mubbashar, M. and Murthy, R.S. 2000: Integration of mental health care into primary care. Demonstration cost-outcome study in India and Pakistan. *British Journal of Psychiatry* 176, 581–88.

de Silva, H.A., Gunatilake, S.B. and Smith, A.D. 2003: Prevalence of dementia in a semi-urban population in Sri Lanka: report from a regional survey. *International Journal of Geriatric Psychiatry* 18, 711–15.

Demographic and Health Surveys, Macro International Inc., 2004: *Bangladesh Demographic and Health Survey, 2001–2004 (Preliminary Report).* National Institute of Population Research and Training, Bangladesh, Ministry of Health and Family Welfare; Mitra and Associates; Demographic and Health Surveys, Macro International Inc.

Dias, A., Samuel, R., Patel, V., Prince, M., Parameshwaran, R. and Krishnamoorthy, E.S. 2004: The impact associated with caring for a person with dementia. *International Journal of Geriatric Psychiatry* 19, 182–84.

Eddleston, M., Rezvi Sheriff, M.H. and Hawton, K. 1998: Deliberate self-harm in Sri Lanka: an overlooked tradgedy in the developing world. *British Medical Journal* 317, 133–35.

Fauveau, V., Koenig, M.A., Chakraborti, J. and Choudhury, A.I. 1988: Causes of maternal mortality in rural Bangladesh. *Bulletin of the World Health Organization* 66, 643–51.

Fikree, F.F. and Bhatti, L.I. 1999: Domestic violence and health of Pakistani women. *International Journal of Gynecology and Obstetrics* 65, 195–201.

Gaunekar, G., Patel, V. and Rane, A. 2005: The impact and patterns of hazardous drinking amongst male industrial workers in Goa, India. *Social Psychiatry and Psychiatric Epidemiology* 40, 267–75.

Girdhar, S., Dogra, A.T. and Leenaars, A. 2003: Suicide in India, 1995–1999. *Archives of Suicide Research* 7, 398–93.

Grover, P., Varma, V., Pershad, D. and Verma, S. 1996: Role of yoga in the treatment of neurotic disorders: current status and future directions. *Indian Journal of Psychiatry*, 36, 153–62.

Hamid, M.A., Choudhury, S., Nizamuddin, M. and Mohit, M.A. 2003: Comparative study of patients in different outpatient departments (OPDS) and pattern of psychiatric disorders in a district hospital. *Bangladesh Journal of Psychiatry* 17, 5–13.

Informal Service Centre 2005: *Nepal, Human Rights Year Book 2005*. Kathmnadu: INSEC, Nepal.

International Institute for Population Sciences 2001: *National Family Health Survey-2, 1998–99: India*. Mumbai: IIPS.

Jablensky, A., Sartorius, N., Emberg, N., Anker, M., Korten, A., Cooper, J.E., Day, R. and Bertelsen, A. 1992: Schizophrenia: manifestations, incidence and course in different cultures: a WHO 10 country study. *Psychological Medicine* Suppl 20.

Khan, M.M. and Prince, M. 2003: Beyond rates: the tragedy of suicide in Pakistan. *Tropical Doctor* 33, 67–69.

Khan, M.M. and Reza, H. 1998: Gender differences in nonfatal suicidal behaviour in Pakistan: significance of sociocultural factors. *Suicide and Life-Threatening Behaviour* 28, 62–68.

Ministry of Health, Sri Lanka 2000: *Annual Health Bulletin*. Colombo.

Mirza, I. and Jenkins, R. 2004: Risk factors, prevalence, and treatment of anxiety and depressive disorders in Pakistan: systematic review. *British Medical Journal* 328, 794–90.

Mumford, D.B., Saeed, K., Ahmad, I., Latif, S. and Mubbashar, M. 1997: Stress and psychiatric disorder in rural Punjab. A community survey. *British Journal of Psychiatry* 170, 473–78.

Murthy, G.V., Janakiramaiah, N., Gangadhar, B.N. and Subbakrishna, D.K. 1998: Sex difference in age at onset of schizophrenia: discrepant findings from India. *Acta Psychiatrica Scandinavica* 97, 321–25.

National Human Rights Commission 1999: *Quality Assurance in Mental Health*. New Delhi: NHRC.

Patel, V. 1999: The epidemiology of Common Mental Disorders in South Asia. *NIMHANS Journal* 17, 307–27.

Patel, V. 2003: *Where There is No Psychiatrist*. London: Gaskell.

Patel, V. and Andrade, C. 2003: Pharmacological treatment of severe psychiatric disorders in the developing world: lessons from India. *CNS Drugs* 17, 1071–80.

Patel, S.P. and Gaw, A.C. 1996: Suicide among immigrants from the Indian sub-continent: a review. *Psychiatric Services* 47, 517–21.

Patel, V. and Prince, M. 2001: Ageing and mental health in developing countries: Who cares? Qualitative studies from Goa, India. *Psychological Medicine* 31, 29–38.

Patel, V. and Sumathipala, A. 2001: International representation in psychiatric journals: a survey of 6 leading journals. *British Journal of Psychiatry* 178, 406–409.

Patel, V. and Thara, R. 2003: *Meeting Mental Health Needs in Developing Countries: NGO Innovations in India*. New Delhi: Sage (India).

Patel, V., Pereira, J. and Mann, A. 1998a: Somatic and psychological models of common mental disorders in India. *Psychological Medicine* 28, 135–43.

Patel, V., Pereira, J., Coutinho, L., Fernandes, R., Fernandes, J. and Mann, A. 1998b: Poverty, psychological disorder and disability in primary care attenders in Goa, India. *British Journal of Psychiatry* 171, 533–36.

Patel, V., Chisholm, D., Rabe-Hesketh, S., Dias-Saxena, F., Andrew, G. and Mann, A. 2003a: The efficacy and cost-effectiveness of a drug and psychological treatment for common mental disorders in general health care in Goa, India: a randomised controlled trial. *Lancet* 361, 33–39.

Patel, V., De Souza, N. and Rodrigues, M. 2003b: Postnatal depression and infant growth & development in low-income countries: a cohort study from Goa, India. *Archives of Disease in Childhood* 88, 34–37.

Patel, V., Rahman, A., Jacob, K.S. and Hughes, M. 2004: Effect of maternal mental health on infant growth in low income countries: new evidence from South Asia. *British Medical Journal* 328, 820–23.

Plamandon, L. 2004: The importance of education in improving mental health in Bangladesh. http://www.aishaka.net/School_Library/Senior per cent20Projects/04_Plamondon_mentalhealth.pdf (accessed 5 November 2006).

Prince, M. 1997: The need for research on dementia in developing countries. *Tropical Medicine and International Health* 2, 993–1000.

Prince, M., Acosta, D., Chiu, H., Scazufca, M. and Varghese, M. 2003: Dementia diagnosis in developing countries: a cross-cultural validation study. *Lancet* 361, 909–17.

Pyne, H.H., Claeson, M. and Correia, M. 2002: *Gender Dimensions of Alcohol Consumption and Alcohol-related Problems in Latin America and the Caribbean*. Washington, DC: The World Bank.

Raguram, R., Weiss, M.G., Channabasavanna, S.M. and Devins, G.M. 1996: Stigma, depression, and somatization in South India. *American Journal of Psychiatry* 153, 1043–49.

Rahman, A., Mubbashar, M., Gater, R. and Goldberg, D. 1998: Randomised Trial Impact of School Mental-Health Programme in Rural Rawalpindi, Pakistan. *Lancet*, 352, 1022–26.

Rahman, A., Lovel, H., Bunn, J., Lovel, H. and Harrington, R. 2004: Impact of material depression on infant nutritional status and illness: a cohort study. *Archives of General Psychiatry* 61(9), 946–52.

Ratnayeke, L. 1996: Suicide and crisis intervention in rural communities in Sri Lanka. *Crisis* 17, 149–51.

Regmi, S., Sligl, W., Carter, D., Grut, W. and Sear, M. 2002: A controlled study of postpartum depression among Nepalese women: a validation of the Edinburgh Postpartum Depression Scale in Kathmandu. *Tropical Medicine & International Health* 7(4), 378–82.

Saxena, S. 1999: Country profile on alcohol in India. In Riley, L. and Marshall, M. (eds) *Alcohol and Public Health in Developing Countries*. Geneva: World Health Organization, 37–60.

Sekar, K., Dave, A.S., Bhadra, S., Rajashekar, G.P., Kumar, K. and Murthy, R.S. 2002: *Riots: Psychosocial Care by Community Level Helpers for Survivors*. Bangalore: Books for Change.

Shaji, K.S., Arun Kishore, N.R. and Prince, M. 2002: Revealing a hidden problem. An evaluation of a community dementia case-finding program from the Indian 10/66 dementia research network. *International Journal of Geriatric Psychiatry* 17, 222–25.

Shamasundar, C., John, J., Reddy, P.R., Verghese, A., Chandramauli, M., Isaac, M.K. and Kaliaperumal, V. 1989: Training general practitioners in psychiatry – An ICMR multi-centre study. *Indian Journal of Psychiatry* 31, 271–79.

Silva, M.C., Gaunekar, G., Patel, V., Kukalekar, D. and Fernandes, J. 2003: The prevalence and correlates of hazardous drinking in industrial workers: a study from Goa, India. *Alcohol and Alcoholism* 38, 79–83.

Sumathipala, A., Hewege, S., Hanwella, R. and Mann, H. 2000: Randomized controlled trial of cognitive behaviour therapy for repeated consultations for medically unexplained complaints: a feasibility study in Sri Lanka. *Psychological Medicine* 30, 747–57.

Sumathipala, A., Siribaddana, S.H. and Bhugra, D. 2004: Culture-bound syndromes: the story of dhat syndrome. *British Journal of Psychiatry* 184, 200–209.

Sundar, M. 1999: Suicide in farmers in India (letter). *British Journal of Psychiatry* 175, 585–86.

Thapa, B.C.M. 2000: Suicide incidence in the Lalitpur district of Cental Nepal. *Tropical Doctor* 30, 200–203.

Thapa, S.B. and Hauff, E. 2005: Psychological distress among displaced persons during an armed conflict in Nepal. *Social Psychiatry and Psychiatric Epidemiology* 40, 672–79.

Thara R. and Eaton, W.W. 1996: Outcome of schizophrenia: the Madras longitudinal study. *Australia and New Zealand Journal of Psychiatry* 30, 516–22.

Van Ommeren, M., Sharma, B. and Sharma, G.K. 2002: The relationship between somatic and PTSD symptoms among Bhutanese refugee torture survivors: examination of comorbidity with anxiety and depression. *Journal of Traumatic Stress* 15, 415–21.

Vas, C.J., Pinto, C., Panikker, D., Noronha, S., Deshpande, N., Kulkarni, L. and Sachdeva, S. 2001: Prevalence of dementia in an urban Indian population. *International Psychogeriatrics* 13, 439–50.

Vijayakumar, L. and Rajkumar, S. 1999: Are risk factors for suicide universal? A case-control study from India. *Acta Psychiatrica Scandinavica* 99, 407–11.

World Health Organization 1995: *Mental Illness in General Health Care: an International Study*. Chichester: John Wiley & Sons.

World Health Organization 2000: *Burden of Disease 2000*. www.who.int/healthinfo/bodproject/en/index.html (accessed October 2006).

World Health Organization 2001: *The World Health Report 2001: Mental Health: New Understanding, New Hope*. Geneva: World Health Organization.

World Health Organization 2003: Nepal, selected indicators. pp. http://www.who.int/countries/npl/en/ (accessed 17 August 2005).

World Health Organization 2005: *Mental Health Atlas*. Geneva: World Health Organization.

# 22

# Mental health and cultural psychiatry in the United States and Canada

Robert Kohn

## INTRODUCTION

The USA is a country with a population of approximately 294 million. Immigrants account for 11.1 per cent of the US population, of which 42.4 per cent entered the country after 1990. Mexico accounts for the largest number of immigrants known as Hispanic migrants. A sizeable proportion of the population, 17.5 per cent, speaks a language other than English at home. The US is an ethnically heterogeneous nation with a population consisting of African Americans (12.3 per cent), American Indian or Alaska native persons (0.9 per cent), Native Hawaiian and other Pacific Islanders (0.1 per cent), Asian (3.6 per cent) and Hispanic or Latino origin (12.5 per cent). About 12.7 per cent of the population lives in poverty (data for 2004); however, one-quarter of African Americans live in poverty and over one-fifth of Hispanics. African Americans are disproportionately represented among the homeless population, with some estimating as much as 44 per cent of the homeless are African Americans (Jencks, 1994).

Canada has a population of over 30 million. English and French are the two principal languages; 59.3 per cent of people consider English and 22.7 per cent consider French to be their mother tongue. Immigrants make up 18.4 per cent of the Canadian population. One-third of the immigrant population of the country arrived after 1991. Ethnic minorities constitute 13.4 per cent of the Canadian population. The largest groups are of Chinese origin (3.5 per cent), South-East Asian (3.1 per cent), Black (2.2 per cent) and Filipino (1 per cent). The indigenous population of Canada makes up 3.3 per cent of the population; nearly two-thirds are North American Indians, 30 per cent are Métis and less than 5 per cent are Inuits.

## DISABILITY ADJUSTED LIFE YEARS AND YEARS LIVED WITH DISABILITY

In Canada and the USA neuropsychiatric conditions account for much of the overall burden of

**Table 22.1**   *Year 2002 disability adjusted life years (DALYs) for Canada and the United States by top 20 causes*

| | All ages | | | Ages 15–59 | | |
| --- | --- | --- | --- | --- | --- | --- |
| | Total | Male | Female | Total | Male | Female |
| Unipolar depressive disorders | 1 | 3 | 1 | 1 | 2 | 1 |
| Ischaemic heart disease | 2 | 1 | 2 | 3 | 3 | 7 |
| Alcohol use disorders | 3 | 2 | 12 | 2 | 1 | 2 |
| Chronic obstructive pulmonary disease | 4 | 5 | 5 | 5 | 7 | 4 |
| Cerebrovascular disease | 5 | 7 | 3 | 10 | 12 | 8 |
| Diabetes mellitus | 6 | 9 | 6 | 6 | 8 | 5 |
| Trachea, bronchus, lung cancers | 7 | 6 | 9 | 16 | 14 | 17 |
| Hearing loss, adult onset | 8 | 8 | 8 | 7 | 10 | 9 |
| Road traffic accidents | 9 | 4 | 16 | 4 | 4 | 6 |
| Alzheimer's and other dementias | 10 | 16 | 4 | | | |
| Other cardiovascular diseases | 11 | 11 | 11 | 18 | 15 | 18 |
| Other digestive diseases | 12 | 15 | 10 | 11 | 16 | 11 |
| Other neuropsychiatric disorders | 13 | 18 | 15 | 15 | 17 | 12 |
| Osteoarthritis | 14 | | 13 | | | 16 |
| Endocrine disorders | 15 | | 14 | 12 | 20 | 10 |
| Other unintentional injuries | 16 | 13 | | 14 | 11 | |
| Asthma | 17 | 19 | 17 | | | |
| Drug use disorders | 18 | 12 | | 8 | 5 | 20 |
| Self-inflicted injuries | 19 | 10 | | 9 | 6 | |
| Other malignant neoplasms | 20 | 17 | 20 | | | |
| Other respiratory diseases | | 20 | 19 | | | |
| Breast cancer | | | 7 | 20 | | 3 |
| Violence | | 14 | | 13 | 9 | |
| Schizophrenia | | | | 19 | | 15 |
| Bipolar disorder | | | | 17 | 19 | 14 |
| Migraine | | | 18 | | | 13 |
| Cirrhosis of the liver | | | | | 18 | |
| HIV/AIDS | | | | | 13 | |
| Iron-deficiency anaemia | | | | | | 19 |

Note: The estimates include Cuba.

disease or disability adjusted life years (DALYs) (29.6 per cent), with unipolar depression alone accounting for 11.2 per cent of the overall burden and alcohol-related disorders for 5.4 per cent. Among all diseases, unipolar depression is the number one cause of disability and alcoholism is number three. Among those aged 15–59 years of age 38.2 per cent of all DALYs are due to neuropsychiatric conditions, 16.2 per cent are a result of unipolar depression and 8.5 per cent result from alcoholism. Table 22.1 lists the 20 most significant causes of DALYs in the region (World Health Organization, 2002).

Neuropsychiatric disorders account for nearly half (48.1 per cent) of all years lived with disability (YLDs) across all age groups. Unipolar depression was the number one cause of YLDs across all diseases, accounting for 19.4 per cent of YLDs; alcoholism was the number two cause of disability and accounted for 8.8 per cent of YLDs. Among those at the age of greatest risk for developing psychiatric disorders (15–59 years old), neuropsychiatric disorders accounted for 55.4 per cent of the YLDs. The percentages for unipolar depression and alcohol-related disorders were 24.6 per cent and 12.3 per

**Table 22.2**   *Year 2002 years lived with disability (YLDs) for Canada and the United States by top 20 causes*

| | All ages | | | Ages 15–59 | | |
|---|---|---|---|---|---|---|
| | Total | Male | Female | Total | Male | Female |
| Unipolar depressive disorders | 1 | 1 | 1 | 1 | 2 | 1 |
| Alcohol use disorders | 2 | 2 | 4 | 2 | 1 | 2 |
| Hearing loss, adult onset | 3 | 3 | 3 | 4 | 5 | 4 |
| Chronic obstructive pulmonary disease | 4 | 4 | 6 | 3 | 4 | 3 |
| Alzheimer's and other dementias | 5 | 9 | 2 | | | |
| Diabetes mellitus | 6 | 6 | 7 | 6 | 6 | 5 |
| Osteoarthritis | 7 | 10 | 5 | 9 | 9 | 10 |
| Cerebrovascular disease | 8 | 8 | 8 | 11 | 11 | 14 |
| Asthma | 9 | 7 | 12 | 15 | 10 | |
| Drug use disorders | 10 | 5 | | 5 | 3 | 16 |
| Other digestive diseases | 11 | 15 | 10 | 13 | 15 | 11 |
| Other neuropsychiatric disorders | 12 | 13 | 11 | 12 | 13 | 12 |
| Endocrine disorders | 13 | 17 | 13 | 10 | 14 | 9 |
| Schizophrenia | 14 | 11 | 16 | 8 | 8 | 8 |
| Bipolar disorder | 15 | 14 | 14 | 7 | 7 | 7 |
| Migraine | 16 | | 9 | 16 | | 6 |
| Other unintentional injuries | 17 | 12 | 19 | 17 | 11 | |
| Iron-deficiency anaemia | 18 | 18 | 17 | 14 | 12 | 13 |
| Other respiratory diseases | 19 | 16 | | 19 | 18 | |
| Vision disorders, age-related | 20 | | 15 | | | |
| Ischaemic heart disease | | 19 | | | | |
| Rheumatoid arthritis | | | 18 | | | 17 |
| Panic disorder | | | | 18 | | 15 |
| Insomnia (primary) | | | | 20 | | |
| Falls | | 20 | | | | |
| Road traffic accidents | | | | | 20 | |
| Obsessive–compulsive disorder | | | | | | 20 |
| Breast cancer | | | 20 | | | 18 |
| Violence | | | | | 16 | |
| HIV/AIDS | | | | | 17 | |
| Gout | | | | | 19 | |
| Other maternal conditions | | | | | | 19 |

Note: The estimates include Cuba.

cent, respectively. Table 22.2 lists the 20 most significant causes of YLDs for Canada and the USA.

## RACISM AND MENTAL HEALTH

Racism and racial inequality has been linked to poorer mental health both in the USA and Canada. For example, perceived discrimination in African Americans was shown to be associated with increased psychological distress, lower wellbeing, poor self-reported health, and increased number of days confined to bed (Williams *et al.*, 1997; Kessler *et al.*, 1999; Ren *et al.*, 1999). Perceived discrimination has also been shown to increase depressive symptoms among children of Asian, Latin American and Caribbean immigrant (Rumbaut, 1994), as well as adults of Mexican (Finch *et al.*, 2000) and Asian origin (Noh *et al.*, 1999).

## INDIGENOUS PEOPLES IN CANADA AND THE USA

The indigenous population of Canada is relatively young, due in part to their higher birth rate; over half are under the age of 24. Their life expectancy is lower than the general population of the country by 6.9 and 4.8 years for females and males, respectively (Pan American Health Organization, 2002). The leading cause of death among the population is injuries and poisoning. Infant mortality is three times higher than in the national population. Indigenous children are at higher risk for disability, have more unintentional injuries, and are more likely to die from drowning. In addition, the children of indigenous people begin to smoke, drink alcohol and take drugs at an earlier age; their smoking prevalence is two to three times greater than in the non-indigenous population. The suicide rate among the indigenous population of Canada is two to seven times greater than in the general population, in particular among men in the Inuit communities. Unemployment in the indigenous population is high; estimates for 1996 suggest unemployment rates of 26–29 per cent.

The indigenous population in the USA consists of 561 recognized tribes with over 200 spoken languages. The words 'depressed' and 'anxious' are absent in some of these languages (Manson et al., 1985). Indigenous peoples in the USA have early mortality, and as a result a younger population. American Indians and Alaskan natives are five times more likely to die of alcoholism from liver disease, and twice as likely to have diabetes mellitus compared with whites. The indigenous population of the USA is also more likely to experience accidents, violence, suicide and homicide. One-third of this population does not receive regular health care (Brown et al., 2000). The Indian Health service only provides care to about 20 per cent of the target population.

## ADULT PSYCHIATRIC DISORDERS

A number of studies of adult psychiatric disorders have been conducted in the USA and Canada (see Table 22.3). In Canada there have been four studies. The earliest Canadian study was called the Stirling County Survey; this had three waves of representative cross-sectional surveys beginning in 1952, 1970 and 1992 (Murphy et al., 2000). In the last wave depression was evaluated using the Diagnostic Interview Schedule (DIS; Robins et al., 1981). The psychiatric epidemiological study of the province of Edmonton based on the DIS was the first study to try to provide Canada with estimates for a broad range of psychiatric disorders (Bland et al., 1988a,b). Subsequently, rates for the province of Ontario (Offord et al., 1996) were estimated using the Composite International Diagnostic Interview (CIDI) (Robins et al., 1988). Regional studies also have been conducted in Calgary (Patten, 2000), Montreal (Fournier et al., 1997) and Toronto (De Marco, 2000).

The first nationally representative sample was limited to examining the rates of major depression and alcohol use disorders across Canada in the National Population Health Survey (NPHS) (Patten and Charney, 1998). Only recently, a second national study examined the rates of different psychiatric disorders in a Canadian national sample, the Statistics Canada Canadian Community Health Survey: Mental Health and Well-Being (CCHS 1.2) (Patten et al., 2006). The prevalence rates for specific psychiatric disorders in Canada are presented in Table 22.4.

There have been a number of community-based psychiatric epidemiological studies including large representative samples in the USA. The Epidemiological Catchment Area Study (ECA) used the DIS as a diagnostic measure; this was the first and largest study to examine a broad spectrum of psychiatric disorders in five sites in the USA (Robins and Regier, 1991). The National Comorbidity Study used the CIDI as a diagnostic measure; this study examined disorders in a representative sample from 48 states in the USA (Kessler et al., 1994). The participants in this study were re-interviewed ten years later with the sample augmented to also represent the elderly population of the USA in the National Comorbidity Study Replication (NCS-R) (Kessler et al., 2005). Two other national surveys were conducted primarily to examine the rate of substance abuse, the National Longitudinal

**Table 22.3** *Psychiatric epidemiologic prevalence studies conducted in Canada and the USA*

| Study | Field dates | Sample size | Age | Instrument | Diagnosis |
|---|---|---|---|---|---|
| *Canadian studies* | | | | | |
| Edmonton | 1983–1986 | 3 258 | 18+ | DIS | DSM-III |
| Calgary | 1998–1999 | 2 542 | 18+ | CIDI-SF | DSM-III-R |
| CCHS 1.2 | 2002 | 36 984 | 15+ | CIDI-SF | DSM-IV |
| Montreal | 1992–1993 | 893 | 18+ | CIDIS | DSM-III-R |
| NPHS | 1994 | 17 626 | 12+ | CIDI-SF | DSM-III-R |
| Ontario | 1990–1991 | 6 261 | 15–64 | UM-CIDI | DSM-III-R |
| Stirling County | 1992 | 1 396 | 18+ | DIS | DSM-III |
| Toronto | 1991 | 1 393 | 18–55 | CIDI | DSM-III-R |
| *USA studies* | | | | | |
| AHDSOO | 1999 | 6 133 | 70+ | CIDI-SF | DSM-III-R |
| African Americans | 1993 | 865 | 20+ | DIS | DSM-III |
| AI-SUPERPFP, Northern Plains Indians | 1997–2000 | 1 638 | 15–54 | UM-CIDI | DSM-IV |
| AI-SUPERPFP, Southwest Indians | 1997–2000 | 1 446 | 15–54 | UM-CIDI | DSM-IV |
| Cache County Utah | 1995–1996 | 4 559 | 65+ | DIS | DSM-IV |
| California SADS | | | 20+ | SADS-L | RDC |
| Chinese Americans | 1993–1994 | 1 747 | 18–65 | UM-CIDI | DSM-III-R |
| ECA | 1980–1984 | 17 803 | 18+ | DIS | DSM-III |
| Florida | 1998–2000 | 1 803 | 19–20 | CIDI | DSM-IV |
| MAPSS | 1996 | 3 012 | 18–59 | CIDI 1.1 | DSM-III-R |
| NCS | 1990–1992 | 8 098 | 15–54 | UM-CIDI | DSM-III-R |
| NCS-R | 2001–2003 | 9 282 | 18+ | WHO-CIDI | DSM-IV |
| NESARC | 2001–2002 | 43 093 | 18+ | AUDASIS-IV | DSM-IV |
| New Haven | 1975–1976 | 511 | 26+ | SADS | RDC |
| NHANES III | 1988–1994 | 7 968 | 17–39 | DIS | DSM-III-R |
| NLAES | 1991–1992 | 42 862 | 18+ | AUDADIS-IV | DSM-IV |
| North East | 1990 | 386 | 18 | DIS | DSM-III-R |
| Pacific Northwest Indians | 1988 | 131 | 20+ | SADS-L | DSM-III-R |
| Southwest California Indians | 2003 | 483 | 18–70 | SSAGA | DSM-III-R |

CCHS, Canadian Community Health Survey; NPHS, National Population Health Survey; AHDSOO, Asset and Health Dynamics Study of the Oldest Old; AI-SUPERPFP, American Indian Service Utilization, Psychiatric Epidemiology, Risk and Protective Factors Project; SADS, Schedule for Affective Disorders and Schizophrenia; ECA, Epidemiological Catchment Area Study; MAPSS, Mexican American Prevalence and Services Survey; NCS, National Comordity Study; NCS-R, National Comorbidity Study Replication; NESARC, National Epidemiologic Survey on Alcohol and Related Conditions; NHANES, National Health and Nutrition Examination Survey; NLAES, National Longitudinal Alcohol Epidemiologic Survey; DIS, Diagnostic Interview Schedule; CIDI-SF, Composite International Diagnostic Interview – short form; CIDIS,Composite International Diagnostic Interview Simplified; UM-CIDI, University of Michigan Composite International Diagnostic Interview; SSAGA, Semi-Structured Assessment for the Genetics of Alcoholism.

Alcohol Epidemiologic Survey (NLAES) (Grant, 1995) and the National Epidemiologic Survey on Alcohol and Related Conditions (NESARC) (Grant *et al.*, 2004). The Third National Health and Nutrition Examination Survey (NHANES-III) included national estimates of affective disorders (Jonas *et al.*, 2003). Table 22.5 provides a summary of the rates from these studies.

A number of regional studies have also been conducted in the USA (Table 22.6). Weissman and

colleagues (1978) conducted one of the earliest community-based epidemiological studies in the USA using specific diagnostic criteria. Only two studies were limited to young adults. One study was a small study of 18 year olds conducted in northeastern USA (Reinherz *et al.*, 1993); the other was a study of 19–20 years olds in Florida (Turner and Gil, 2002). Two other studies were limited to the elderly population and both only examined affective disorders, the Asset and Health Dynamics Study of

**Table 22.4** Prevalence rates (per cent) in community-based Canadian surveys

| | | Edmonton | | Ontario | | Sterling | | NPHS | Calgary | Montreal | | Toronto | | CCHS | |
|---|---|---|---|---|---|---|---|---|---|---|---|---|---|---|---|
| | | L | Y | L | Y | L | C | Y | Y | L | S | L | Y | L | Y |
| NAP | T | 0.6 | 0.4 | | | | | | | | | | | | |
| | M | 0.5 | | | | | | | | | | | | | |
| | F | 0.7 | | | | | | | | | | | | | |
| MDD | T | 8.6 | 4.6 | 8.3 | 4.1 | 7.9 | 5.7 | 5.6 | 11.0 | 29.6 | 7.7 | 24.4 | 10.4 | 10.8 | 4.0 |
| | M | 5.9 | 3.4 | | 2.8 | 4.4 | 4.2 | 3.7 | | | 7.7 | | 7.4 | | 2.9 |
| | F | 11.4 | 5.9 | | 5.4 | 11.5 | 7.1 | 7.4 | | | 7.7 | | 13.2 | | 5.0 |
| DYS | T | 3.7 | 3.7 | | 0.8 | | | | | 14.0 | 5.2 | | | | |
| | M | 2.2 | 2.2 | | 0.0 | | | | | | 5.3 | | | | |
| | F | 5.2 | 5.2 | | 0.8 | | | | | | 5.0 | | | | |
| BIP | T | 0.6 | 0.1 | | 0.6 | | | | | | | | | 2.2 | |
| | M | 0.7 | 0.2 | | 0.0 | | | | | | | | | 2.2 | |
| | F | 0.4 | 0.1 | | 0.6 | | | | | | | | | 2.1 | |
| GAD | T | | | | 1.1 | | | | | | | | | | |
| | M | | | | 0.9 | | | | | | | | | | |
| | F | | | | 1.2 | | | | | | | | | | |
| PAN | T | 1.2 | 0.7s | | 1.1 | | | | | 3.3 | 1.4 | | | 2.1 | 1.5 |
| | M | 0.8 | 0.4s | | 0.0 | | | | | | 0.2 | | | | |
| | F | 1.7 | 1.0s | | 1.5 | | | | | | 2.5 | | | | |
| OCD | T | 3.0 | 1.6s | | | | | | | | | | | | |
| | M | 2.8 | 1.6s | | | | | | | | | | | | |
| | F | 3.1 | 1.6s | | | | | | | | | | | | |
| ALC | T | 18.0 | 7.9 | 12.0 | 4.4 | | | | | 11.5 | 3.1 | | | | 2.6* |
| | M | 29.3 | 13.5 | 19.2 | 7.1 | | | | | | 4.5 | | | | |
| | F | 6.7 | 2.4 | 4.8 | 1.8 | | | | | | 1.8 | | | | |
| DRG | T | 6.9 | 2.6 | | 1.1 | | | | | 5.4 | 0.8 | | | | 0.8* |
| | M | 10.6 | 4.3 | | 1.7 | | | | | | 1.1 | | | | |
| | F | 3.2 | 0.9 | | 0.4 | | | | | | 0.5 | | | | |

NAP, non-affective psychosis; MDD, major depressive disorder; DYS, dysthymia; BIP, bipolar disorder; GAD, generalized anxiety disorder; PAN, panic disorder; OCD, obsessive–compulsive disorder; ALC, alcohol abuse/dependence; DRG, drug abuse/dependence; L, lifetime prevalence; Y, one-year prevalence; S and s, six-month prevalence; C, current prevalence; * dependence only.

Table 22.5  Prevalence rates (per cent) in nationally based USA surveys

| | | ECA | | NCS | | NCS-R | | NLAES | | NESARC | NHANES-III |
|---|---|---|---|---|---|---|---|---|---|---|---|
| | | L | Y | L | Y | L | Y | L | Y | Y | L |
| NAP | T | 1.5 | 1.0 | 0.7 | 0.5 | | | | | | |
| | M | 1.2 | 0.9 | 0.6 | 0.5 | | | | | | |
| | F | 1.7 | 1.1 | 0.8 | 0.6 | | | | | | |
| MDD | T | 4.9 | 2.7 | 17.9 | 10.3 | 16.6 | 6.7 | 9.9 | 3.3 | | 8.6 |
| | M | 2.6 | 1.4 | 12.7 | 7.7 | | | 8.6 | 2.7 | | 6.0 |
| | F | 7.0 | 4.0 | 21.3 | 12.9 | | | 11.0 | 3.9 | | 11.2 |
| DYS | T | 3.2 | | 6.4 | 2.5 | 2.5 | 1.5 | | | | 6.2 |
| | M | 2.2 | | 4.8 | 2.1 | | | | | | 4.7 |
| | F | 4.1 | | 8.0 | 3.0 | 3.9 | | | | | 7.7 |
| BIP | T | 1.3 | 1.0 | 1.6 | 1.3 | | 2.6 | | | | 1.6 |
| | M | 1.1 | 0.9 | 1.6 | 1.4 | | | | | | 1.5 |
| | F | 1.4 | 1.1 | 1.7 | 1.3 | | | | | | 1.7 |
| GAD | T | | 3.8 | 5.1 | 3.1 | 5.7 | 3.1 | | | | |
| | M | | 2.4 | 3.6 | 2 | | | | | | |
| | F | | 5.0 | 6.6 | 4.3 | | | | | | |
| PAN | T | 1.6 | 0.9 | 3.5 | 2.3 | 4.7 | 2.7 | | | | |
| | M | 1.0 | 0.6 | 2.0 | 1.3 | | | | | | |
| | F | 2.1 | 1.2 | 5.0 | 3.2 | | | | | | |
| OCD | T | 2.6 | 1.7 | | | 1.6 | 1.0 | | | | |
| | M | 2.0 | 1.4 | | | | | | | | |
| | F | 3.0 | 1.9 | | | | | | | | |
| ALC | T | 13.8 | 6.8 | 23.5 | 9.7 | 18.6 | 4.4 | 18.2 | 7.4 | 8.5 | |
| | M | 23.8 | 11.9 | 32.6 | 14.1 | | | 25.5 | 11.0 | 12.4 | |
| | F | 4.6 | 2.2 | 14.6 | 5.3 | | | 11.4 | 4.1 | 4.9 | |
| DRG | T | 6.2 | 2.7 | 11.9 | 3.6 | 10.9 | 1.8 | 6.1 | 1.5 | | |
| | M | 7.7 | 4.1 | 14.6 | 5.1 | | | 8.1 | 1.8 | | |
| | F | 4.8 | 1.4 | 8.4 | 2.2 | | | 4.2 | 0.5 | | |

NAP, non-affective psychosis; MDD, major depressive disorder; DYS, dysthymia; BIP, bipolar disorder; GAD, generalized anxiety disorder; PAN, panic disorder; OCD, obsessive–compulsive disorder; ALC, alcohol abuse/dependence; DRG, drug abuse/dependence; ECA, Epidemiological Catchment Area Study; NCS, National Comorbidity Study; NCS-R, National Comorbidity Study Replication; NLAES, National Longitudinal Alcohol Epidemiologic Survey; NESARC, National Epidemiologic Survey on Alcohol and Related Conditions; NHANES-III, Third National Health and Nutrition Examination Survey; L, lifetime prevalence; Y, one-year prevalence.

the Oldest Old (AHDSOO) (Turvey et al., 1999) and the Cache County study (Steffens et al., 2000).

A number of community-based epidemiological studies in the USA have focused on the rates of disorders in specific ethnic groups (Table 22.7). Affective disorders have been examined among African Americans (Brown et al., 1995) and Chinese Americans (Takeuchi et al., 1998). An early study of Cuban Americans used the DIS and found relatively low rates of major depression of around 3.2 per cent for a lifetime prevalence estimate (Narrow et al., 1990). A more recent study has focused on

the mental health of Mexican Americans and was conducted in California: The Mexican American Prevalence and Services Survey (MAPSS) (Vega et al., 1998). Several studies have focused on the rates of disorders among American Indian populations, the Pacific Norwest Indians (Kinzie et al., 1992), the Southwest California Indians (Gilder et al., 2004), the Southwest Indians (Beals et al., 2005a), and the Northern Plains Indians (Beals et al., 2005a). Studies of specific ethnic groups are difficult to interpret and compare with other ethnic groups or other studies with the same ethnic

**Table 22.6**   *Prevalence rates (per cent) in regionally based USA surveys*

| | | Florida | | Northeast | | New Haven | | Cache | | AAHSOO |
|---|---|---|---|---|---|---|---|---|---|---|
| | | L | Y | L | S | L | C | L | C | L |
| MDD | T | 17.4 | 11.6 | 9.4 | 6.0 | 20.0 | 4.3 | 15.8 | 4.1 | 3.6 |
| | M | 12.4 | 7.2 | 5.1 | | 12.3 | 3.2 | 9.6 | 3.0 | 2.5 |
| | F | 23.1 | 15.8 | 13.7 | | 25.8 | 5.2 | 20.4 | 4.9 | 4.2 |
| DYS | T | 0.5 | 0.1 | | | | | | 0.2 | |
| | M | 0.6 | 0.1 | | | | | | 0.2 | |
| | F | 0.5 | 0.0 | | | | | | 0.2 | |
| BIP | T | | | | | 1.2 | | | | |
| GAD | T | 1.4 | 0.9 | | | | 2.4 | | | |
| | M | 0.2 | 0.2 | | | | | | | |
| | F | 1.6 | 1.6 | | | | | | | |
| PAN | T | 2.1 | 1.6 | | | | 0.4 | | | |
| | M | 0.8 | 0.4 | | | | | | | |
| | F | 3.4 | 2.7 | | | | | | | |
| OCD | T | | | 2.1 | 1.3 | | | | | |
| | M | | | 1.0 | | | | | | |
| | F | | | 3.2 | | | | | | |
| ALC | T | 25.1 | 16.4 | 32.4 | 26.1 | 6.7 | 2.6 | | | |
| | M | 31.0 | 21.0 | 37.6 | | 10.1 | 3.6 | | | |
| | F | 19.4 | 11.8 | 26.8 | | 4.1 | 1.7 | | | |
| DRG | T | | | 9.8 | | | | | | |
| | M | | | 10.8 | | | | | | |
| | F | | | 8.9 | | | | | | |

NAP, non-affective psychosis; MDD, major depressive disorder; DYS, dysthymia; BIP, bipolar disorder; GAD, generalized anxiety disorder; PAN, panic disorder; OCD, obsessive–compulsive disorder; ALC, alcohol abuse/dependence; DRG, drug abuse/dependence; L, lifetime prevalence; Y, one-year prevalence; S, six-month prevalence; C, current prevalence; Cache, Cache County, Utah; VA, Virginia.

groups as there was methodological variance across studies.

Despite this limitation, the American Indian Service Utilization, Psychiatric Epidemiology, Risk and Protective Factors Project (AI-SUPERPFP) of the Southwest Indians and the Northern Plains Indians has provided the first comprehensive insight into the mental health of the American Indian population. Alcohol disorders and post-traumatic stress disorder were more common among these Indians than among other ethnic groups, but they were at lower risk for major depression. Studies of American Northern Plains and Southwest Indian Vietnam veterans also found very high rates of post-traumatic stress disorder: 31 per cent and 27 per cent for current prevalence and 57 per cent and 45 per cent for lifetime prevalence, respectively. This is significantly higher than

other ethnic groups including white, black and Japanese Americans. However, controlling for differential exposure to war-zone stress ethnicity was no longer a predictor. In addition, these veterans had higher rates of alcohol use disorders, over 70 per cent current and 80 per cent lifetime prevalence, in contrast to 11 per cent to 32 per cent current and 33 per cent to 50 per cent lifetime for the other ethnic groups examined (US Department of Health and Human Services, 2001; Beals *et al.*, 2002).

Direct comparisons between ethnic groups were made in the ECA, Florida, NCS, NCS-R, NLAES, NESARC, and NHANES-III studies, as well as an early study conducted in California using the Schedule for Affective Disorders and Schizophrenia (SADS) (Vernon and Roberts, 1982; see Tables 22.8–22.10). African Americans had lower rates of major depression and were found to be more likely

**Table 22.7**  *Prevalence rates (per cent) in USA surveys conducted in specific ethnic groups*

| | | AFA | MA | CHI | | PWI | | SCI | SWI | | NPI | |
|---|---|---|---|---|---|---|---|---|---|---|---|---|
| | | Y | L | L | Y | L | C | L | L | Y | L | Y |
| NAP | T | | | | | 2.1 | 2.1 | | | | | |
| | M | | | | | 4.4 | 4.4 | | | | | |
| | F | | | | | 0.0 | 0.0 | | | | | |
| MDD | T | 3.1 | 9.0 | 6.9 | 3.4 | 21.2 | 3.8 | 18.0 | 10.7 | 6.5 | 7.8 | 4.3 |
| | M | 2.8 | 6.1 | | | 17.0 | 2.2 | 14.0 | 8.5 | 5.6 | 6.6 | 2.9 |
| | F | 3.2 | 12.3 | | | 26.2 | 6.3 | 20.0 | 12.3 | 7.2 | 9.1 | 5.6 |
| DYS | T | | 3.3 | 5.2 | 0.9 | 4.0 | 1.9 | 2.0 | 3.5 | 2.1 | 22.3 | 0.9 |
| | M | | 3.1 | | | 1.5 | 1.5 | 3.0 | 3.0 | 2.2 | 1.7 | 0.5 |
| | F | | 3.7 | | | 6.2 | 2.3 | 2.0 | 3.9 | 2.0 | 3.0 | 1.3 |
| BIP | T | | 1.7 | | | 1.5 | | 0.0 | | | | |
| | M | | 0.9 | | | 0.0 | | 0.0 | | | | |
| | F | | 2.4 | | | 2.8 | | 1.0 | | | | |
| GAD | T | | | | | 0.4 | | | 3.3 | 1.8 | 1.7 | 1.0 |
| | M | | | | | 0.0 | | | 2.4 | 1.0 | 1.5 | 0.6 |
| | F | | | | | 0.8 | | | 4.1 | 2.3 | 1.8 | 1.3 |
| PAN | T | | 3.5 | | | 0.6 | 0.6 | 4.0 | 4.5 | 2.3 | 2.4 | 1.3 |
| | M | | 2.0 | | | 0.0 | 0.0 | 2.0 | 3.6 | 1.5 | 1.7 | 0.5 |
| | F | | 5.0 | | | 1.1 | 1.1 | 5.0 | 5.2 | 3.0 | 3.1 | 2.0 |
| OCD | T | | | | | | | 2.0 | | | | |
| | M | | | | | | | 3.0 | | | | |
| | F | | | | | | | 1.0 | | | | |
| ALC | T | | 14.4 | | | 56.9 | 20.9 | 58.0 | 23.9 | 8.6 | 34.7 | 16.4 |
| | M | | 21.3 | | | 76.5 | 36.4 | 66.0 | 38.7 | 16.3 | 41.0 | 20.9 |
| | F | | 6.7 | | | 39.4 | 7.0 | 53.0 | 12.1 | 2.6 | 18.7 | 12.1 |
| DRG | T | | 8.6 | | | | 1.0 | | 9.1 | 3.5 | 13.2 | 5.9 |
| | M | | 11.3 | | | | 2.2 | | 14.0 | 5.5 | 15.5 | 7.1 |
| | F | | 5.5 | | | | 0.0 | | 5.3 | 2.0 | 10.9 | 4.7 |

NAP, non-affective psychosis; MDD, major depressive disorder; DYS, dysthymia; BIP, bipolar disorder; GAD, generalized anxiety disorder; PAN, panic disorder; OCD, obsessive–compulsive disorder; ALC, alcohol abuse/dependence; DRG, drug abuse/dependence; L, lifetime prevalence; Y, one-year prevalence; C, current prevalence; AFA, African American; CHI, Chinese American; MA, MAPSS study, Mexican American; PWI, Pacific Northwest Indians; SCI, Southwest California Indians; SWI, AI-SUPERPFP study, Southwest Indian; NPI, AI-SUPERPFP study, Northern Plains Indian.

to suffer from phobia in the ECA study (Zhang and Snowden, 1999), although differences in overall rates in the ECA which were higher in African Americas were eliminated when adjusted for socio-economic status (US Department of Health and Human Services, 2001). The NCS, however, found lower lifetime rates of mental illness among African Americans than in white populations (Kessler *et al.*, 1994), and in particular with mood, anxiety and substance use disorders. Hispanics, and in particular Mexican Americans, were found to have lower risk for substance use and anxiety disorders than white populations.

Breslau and colleagues (2005) concluded that members of disadvantaged ethnic groups in the USA do not have an increased risk for psychiatric disorders; however, they do tend to have more persistent disorders. The NHANES-III study also found major depression to be significantly higher among white populations than African American or Mexican American populations (Riolo *et al.*, 2005). Similar results were found in the epidemiological study conducted in Florida (Turner and Gil, 2002); substantially lower rates were observed among African Americans for depressive disorders and substance abuse and dependence. The findings of

**Table 22.8**  *Prevalence rates (per cent) in USA surveys comparing rates across ethnic and racial groups*

| | | ECA | | | | | | NESARC | | | | | | |
|---|---|---|---|---|---|---|---|---|---|---|---|---|---|---|
| | | White | | Black | | Hispanic | | White | | Hispanic | | Black | Asian | Indian |
| | | L | Y | L | Y | L | Y | L | Y | L | Y | Y | Y | Y |
| NAP | T | 1.4 | 0.9 | 2.1 | 1.6 | 0.8 | 0.4 | | | | | | | |
| | M | 1.1 | 0.9 | 2.0 | 1.4 | 0.3 | 0.3 | | | | | | | |
| | F | 1.7 | 1.0 | 2.2 | 1.7 | 1.2 | 0.6 | | | | | | | |
| MDD | T | 5.1 | 2.8 | 3.1 | 2.2 | 4.4 | 3.3 | 17.8 | | 10.9 | | | | |
| DYS | T | 3.3 | | 2.5 | | 4 | | 4.5 | | 2.2 | | | | |
| BIP | T | 1.2 | 1.0 | 1.6 | 1.4 | 1.2 | 0.8 | 5.5 | | 5 | | | | |
| GAD | T | | 3.5 | | 6.1 | | 3.7 | 4.6 | | 2.3 | | | | |
| | M | | 2.1 | | 5.5 | | 1.8 | | | | | | | |
| | F | | 4.7 | | 6.6 | | 5.3 | | | | | | | |
| PAN | T | 1.6 | 0.9 | 1.3 | 1.0 | 0.9 | 0.7 | 5.5 | | 2.9 | | | | |
| | M | 1.0 | 0.6 | 0.6 | 0.6 | 0.4 | 0.3 | | | | | | | |
| | F | 2.2 | 1.2 | 1.9 | 1.4 | 1.3 | 1.0 | | | | | | | |
| OCD | T | 2.6 | 1.7 | 2.3 | 1.6 | 1.8 | 1.0 | | | | | | | |
| | M | 2.0 | 1.4 | 2.0 | 1.4 | 1.8 | 1.0 | | | | | | | |
| | F | 3.2 | 1.9 | 2.6 | 1.9 | 1.8 | 0.9 | | | | | | | |
| ALC | T | 13.6 | 6.7 | 13.8 | 6.6 | 16.7 | 9.1 | 33.9 | 8.9 | 21.9 | 8.9 | 6.9 | 4.5 | 12.2 |
| | M | 23.4 | 11.7 | 23.7 | 11.5 | 30.0 | 16.0 | | 12.9 | | 12.1 | 10.8 | 6.8 | 15.9 |
| | F | 4.5 | 2.1 | 5.5 | 2.5 | 3.9 | 2.5 | | 5.3 | | 3.6 | 3.8 | 2.4 | 8.7 |
| DRG | T | 6.4 | 2.7 | 5.5 | 2.7 | 4.4 | 2.0 | 11.2 | | 6.1 | | | | |
| | M | 7.8 | 4.1 | 7.2 | 4.2 | 6.3 | 3.3 | | | | | | | |
| | F | 5.0 | 1.3 | 4.0 | 2.3 | 2.5 | 0.7 | | | | | | | |

NAP, non-affective psychosis; MDD, major depressive disorder; DYS, dysthymia; BIP, bipolar disorder; GAD, generalized anxiety disorder; PAN, panic disorder; OCD, obsessive–compulsive disorder; ALC, alcohol abuse/dependence; DRG, drug abuse/dependence; L, lifetime prevalence; Y, one-year prevalence; ECA, Epidemiological Catchment Area Study; NESARC, National Epidemiologic Survey on Alcohol and Related Conditions.

**Table 22.9** Prevalence rates (per cent) in USA surveys comparing rates across ethnic and racial groups

| | | California SADS White | | California SADS Black | | California SADS Hispanic | | NLAES White | NLAES Hisp | NLAES Black | NLAES Asian | NLAES Indian | NHANES-III White | NHANES-III Black | NHANES-III Hisp |
|---|---|---|---|---|---|---|---|---|---|---|---|---|---|---|---|
| | | L | C | L | C | L | C | Y | Y | Y | Y | Y | L | L | L |
| MDD | T | 18.9 | 2.5 | 9.6 | 2.1 | 19.2 | 1.8 | | | | | | 9.6 | 6.8 | 6.7 |
| | M | 8.0 | | 6.0 | | 9.5 | | | | | | | | | |
| | F | 26.4 | | 18.9 | | 25.2 | | | | | | | | | |
| DYS | T | 2.3 | | 3.7 | | 4.1 | | | | | | | 5.7 | 7.8 | 7.5 |
| BIP | T | | | | | | | | | | | | 1.8 | 1.5 | 1.0 |
| ALC | T | | | | | | | 7.7 | 5.3 | 17.1 | 3.4 | 8.3 | | | |
| | M | | | | | | | 11.3 | 8.3 | 23.8 | 4.8 | 13.6 | | | |
| | F | | | | | | | 4.4 | 2.9 | 11.7 | 1.9 | 3.1 | | | |

MDD, major depressive disorder; DYS, dysthymia; BIP, bipolar disorder; ALC, alcohol abuse/dependence; L, lifetime prevalence; Y, one-year prevalence; C, current prevalence; Hisp, Hispanic; SADS, Schedule for Affective Disorders and Schizophrenia; NLAES, National Longitudinal Alcohol Epidemiologic Survey; NHANES-III, National Health and Nutrition Examination Survey III.

**Table 22.10** Prevalence rates (per cent) in USA surveys comparing rates across ethnic and racial groups

| | NCS White | | NCS Black | | NCS Hispanic | | Florida White | | Florida Black | | Florida Cuban | | Florida Other Hispanic | |
|---|---|---|---|---|---|---|---|---|---|---|---|---|---|---|
| | L | Y | L | Y | L | Y | L | Y | L | Y | L | Y | L | Y |
| Mood | 19.8 | 10.7 | 13.7 | 9.3 | 17.9 | 13.4 | 19.8 | 13.0 | 12.8 | 15.7 | 19.7 | 8.1 | 18.5 | 13.3 |
| Anxiety | 29.1 | 18.9 | 24.7 | 18.7 | 28.4 | 21.4 | 14.6 | 11.0 | 15.7 | 11.6 | 11.4 | 11.6 | 19.9 | 12.3 |
| Substance | 29.5 | 12.3 | 13.1 | 6.3 | 22.9 | 10.7 | 49.7 | 36.5 | 20.4 | 14.3 | 44.5 | 14.3 | 46.4 | 29.7 |

Mood, any mood disorder; anxiety, any anxiety disorder; substance, any substance disorder; L, lifetime; Y, one-year prevalence; NCS, National Comorbidity Study.

Indians having higher risk for alcohol use disorders, substance use disorders and affective disorders was also noted among Mexican Americans of Indian and non-Indian origin (Alderete *et al.*, 2000).

## STUDIES OF CHILD PSYCHIATRIC DISORDERS

For most psychiatric disorders, using data from the Great Smoky Mountains Study (Costello *et al.*, 1997), there were few differences found between American Indian and white children aged 9–13. The American Indian children had lower rates of tics and higher rates of substance use disorders. In a school-based sample, Beals *et al.* (1997) studied 109 North Plain Indians aged 13–17 years. They found that American Indians were less likely to receive a diagnosis of an anxiety disorder, but were more likely to receive diagnoses of attention deficit hyperactivity disorder (ADHD), conduct disorders, oppositional disorders and substance use disorders. African American children have been reported to have higher rates of functional enuresis than white children (Costello *et al.*, 1996), obsessive–compulsive disorder (Valleni-Basile *et al.*, 1996), symptoms of conduct disorders (Costello *et al.*, 1988), and symptoms of depression (Roberts *et al.*, 1977). However, Siegel *et al.* (1998) found no differences between African American and white populations.

## SUICIDE, HOMICIDE AND VIOLENCE

In 2002, the rate of suicide for the USA was 11 per 100 000. Among white populations this was 12.2 and black populations 5.2 per 100 000. The rate of African American and Hispanic suicide, however, has increased, in particular among the youth; although overall among all age groups, the rates among Hispanic people were low at 5.0 per 100 000 (Centers for Disease Control, 2004). Native Americans in the USA have 1.5 times higher suicide rates than the national average, and in particular for those aged 15–24 (US Department of Health and Human Services, 2001). Violent deaths account for

75 per cent of all mortality in young Indian American adults (Resnick *et al.*, 1997). A survey of adolescent Indians found that 22 per cent of females and 12 per cent of males had attempted suicide (Blum *et al.*, 1992). Those who have higher levels of cultural spiritual orientation have reduced prevalence of suicide ideations and attempts (Garroutte *et al.*, 2003).

In 1997, the overall rate for suicide in Canada was 12 per 100 000 and has steadily increased since the 1970s. Immigrants to Canada have a lower rate of suicide than non-immigrants, 7.9 compared to 13.3 per 100 000. The rate among Canada's indigenous population is extraordinarily high, twice the general population rate: 56.3 per 100 000 among males and 11.8 per 100 000 among females. For the 15–24 years age group among indigenous males the rate reaches 90 per 100 000.

Half of all incarcerated individuals in state and federal prisons in the USA are African Americans, and nearly 40 per cent of juveniles in legal custody are African Americans. Rates of mental illness among incarcerated African Americans have been noted to be somewhat less than those among white inmates (Jordan *et al.*, 1996; Teplin, 1990; Teplin *et al.*, 1996). Incarcerated African Americans with mental illness are less likely to receive mental health care than white inmates (Bureau of Justice Statistics, 1998). African Americans are more likely to be victims of violent crimes (Jenkins and Bell, 1997). Fifty per cent of all homicides are of African Americans. In 2002 black people were 5.7 times more likely than white people to die of homicide, and Hispanics were 2.6 times more likely to be victims of homicide than non-Hispanic white people. These findings are similar to the criminal justice experiences and mental health service experiences of black people, mainly Caribbean-origin black people, in the UK (see Chapter 30).

## REFUGEES AND IMMIGRANTS

In 2000, 93 000 refugees entered the USA. In the 1990s only 3 per cent of refugees came from Africa; however, by 2000 this was nearly one-quarter. The refugee population of the USA in 2004 was over

420 000 and in Canada over 141 000 (United Nations High Commission for Refugees, 2005). Only France and the UK accepted more asylum seekers than the USA in 2004 (84 000). Canada was fifth, taking in 25 800 asylum seekers. There are about 264 000 asylum seekers residing in the USA and 27 290 in Canada. Asylum seekers are a population at high risk for psychiatric disorders. A US study of 70 asylum seekers held in detention whilst pending their asylum claims used self-report questionnaires and reported that 77 per cent had significant symptoms of anxiety, 86 per cent depression and 50 per cent post-traumatic stress disorder. The rate of symptoms was related to the length of detention and decreased following release from detention (Keller et al., 2003; see Chapters 24 and 30 for comparison with other countries).

## Migration and psychological stress

Psychological stress associated with immigration has been examined in a number of ethnic groups. The greatest stress is associated with the first three years after arrival in the USA as noted in studies of Hispanics and the former Soviet Union (Vega and Rumbaut, 1991; Flaherty et al., 1986). Refugees from South-East Asia have been shown to have an initial euphoria followed by increased demoralization in the second year and a return to wellbeing beginning in the third year. Similar findings have been noted in Cubans (Portes and Rumbaut, 1990), Eastern Europeans and Chinese immigrants (Ying, 1988). Among Korean immigrants to the USA the highest levels of depressive symptoms are noted in the first two years, with symptom remission in the third (Hurh and Kim, 1988). Flaherty et al. (1988), comparing refugees from the former Soviet Union immigrating to both Israel and the USA, were able to demonstrate that the economic benefits of the USA were not sufficient to overcome increased marginality as a risk for psychological distress.

South-East Asian refugees have been noted to be at high risk for post-traumatic stress disorder (PTSD) due to pre-migratory trauma. The pre-migratory trauma was a significant factor in psychological distress even five years after immigration (Chung and Kagawa-Singer, 1993). Some studies

have suggested that up to 70 per cent of Laotian and Cambodian refugees have PTSD (Kinzie et al., 1990). A community survey among Cambodian refugees found that 45 per cent had PTSD and 51 per cent had depression (Blair, 2000). Cambodian adolescent refugees also have been found to have high rates of depression: 41 per cent had depression even 10 years after the traumatic exposure (Kinzie et al., 1989). Vietnamese adult refugees have been found to be at higher risk for depression compared with Chinese refugees (Hinton et al., 1997). More recently, a study examining Cambodian immigrants found even two decades after resettlement extremely high rates of PTSD (62 per cent) and major depression (51 per cent), with over 70 per cent having been exposed to violence in the USA (Marshall et al., 2005).

## Migration and mental illness

A number of epidemiological studies have found that foreign-born individuals are at lower risk for specific psychiatric disorders than US-born individuals. Psychiatric epidemiological studies in the USA began in the nineteenth century with Edward Jarvis' (1971) study that suggested that Irish immigrants had a higher prevalence of mental illness. A reanalysis of his data questions his conclusions (Vander Stoep and Link, 1998) Table 22.11 provides an overview of a number of the current studies. Grant et al. (2004) found that foreign-born Mexican Americans and foreign-born non-Hispanic white people were at significantly lower risk of DSM-IV substance use and mood and anxiety disorders compared with their US-born subjects. The risk of specific psychiatric disorders was noted to be similar between foreign-born Mexican Americans and foreign-born non-Hispanic white people; however, US-born Mexican Americans were at significantly lower risk of psychiatric morbidity than US-born non-Hispanic white people. The NCS also found higher rates in Hispanics born in the USA than those born in Mexico, in particular for diagnoses of phobia and depression (Burnam et al., 1987). Similar findings were noted when Mexican Americans born in the USA and Mexico were compared in the Los Angeles site of the ECA

**Table 22.11** *Lifetime prevalence rates (per cent) in USA surveys examining immigration*

| | NESARC | | | | MAPSS | | Florida | | | |
| | Hispanic | | White | | Mexican American | | Cuban American | | Other Hispanics | |
| | FRG | USA | FRG | USA | FRG | USA | FRG | USA | FRG | USA |
| --- | --- | --- | --- | --- | --- | --- | --- | --- | --- | --- |
| MDD | 7.7 | 15.2 | 12.0 | 18.2 | 5.2 | 14.8 | 17.8 | 19.0 | 18.0 | 18.3 |
| DYS | 1.7 | 2.8 | 3.1 | 4.6 | 1.9 | 5.2 | 0.0 | 1.7 | 0 | 0.5 |
| BIP | 3.5 | 7.0 | 4.5 | 5.5 | 1.1 | 2.8 | | | | |
| GAD | 1.5 | 3.3 | 3.2 | 4.7 | | | 0.8 | 1.0 | 1.2 | 2.6 |
| PAN | 1.3 | 5.0 | 3.4 | 5.7 | 2.0 | 1.4 | 1.0 | 3.0 | 2.1 | 3.6 |
| PTSD | | | | | | | 8.9 | 8.4 | 9.4 | 15.9 |
| AS | | | | | | | 6.8 | 6.4 | 8.7 | 12.8 |
| ALC | 15.3 | 30.5 | 16.2 | 35.0 | 9.3 | 22.2 | 28.1 | 29.0 | 24.8 | 31.2 |
| DRG | 1.7 | 12.0 | 4.8 | 11.6 | 3.9 | 16.2 | | | | |
| ANY | 28.5 | 47.6 | 32.3 | 52.5 | 24.9 | 46.2 | 59.3 | 60.9 | 56.5 | 71.3 |

MDD, major depressive disorder; DYS, dysthymia; BIP, bipolar disorder; GAD, generalized anxiety disorder; PAN, panic disorder; PTSD, post-traumatic stress disorder; AS, antisocial personality disorder; ALC, alcohol abuse/dependence; DRG, drug abuse/dependence; ANY, any psychiatric disorder; FRG, foreign born; USA, USA born; white, non-Hispanic white; NESARC, National Epidemiologic Survey on Alcohol and Related Conditions; MAPSS, Mexican American Prevalence and Services Survey.

(Escobar *et al.*, 1988), and when young adult Cuban and other Hispanic immigrants to Florida were compared (Turner and Gil, 2002).

Increasing acculturation is believed to increase the prevalence of psychiatric and substance use disorders in Hispanics examined in the NCS (Ortega *et al.*, 2000). Vega *et al.* (1998) found that immigrants who had lived in the USA for more than 13 years had higher rates than those who had lived in the USA for less than 13 years. They also found the rates for USA-born Mexican Americans to be 48 per cent overall, whereas those born in Mexico had rates of 25 per cent for mental and substance use disorders.

## SERVICE UTILIZATION AND INEQUALITIES IN MENTAL HEALTH CARE

The Canadians have attempted to develop specific cross-cultural services within their mental health care system (Ganesan and Janzé, 2005). Despite such programmes, minority groups in Canada, particularly the Chinese immigrant community (Chen and Kazanjian, 2005), remain underserved. A focus group study identified numerous barriers to care among the elderly Chinese community in Canada:

inadequate numbers of trained and acceptable mental health workers; limited awareness of mental disorders; and reliance on ethno-specific social agencies that are not designed to provide specialized mental health care. There was also inadequacy of interpreter services, lack of appropriate professional responses and inappropriate referral patterns (Sadavoy *et al.*, 2004). The rate of service utilization in Canada, at least for major depression, has changed little in the last decade, possibly due to the lack of national initiatives (Wang *et al.*, 2005).

Barriers to care for minorities have also been described in the USA. Mental illness has been found to have greater stigma among African Americans than white people (Sussman *et al.*, 1987; Cooper-Patrick *et al.*, 1997). In addition, African Americans were less likely to label their children with an ADHD diagnosis (Bussing *et al.*, 1998). Investigators have also found older African Americans to be less knowledgeable about depression than white people (Zylstra and Steitz, 1999). Minority patients receive differential treatment for depression and anxiety compared with white patients (Wang *et al.*, 2000; Young *et al.*, 2001).

Asian Americans have also been shown to have their mental health problems overlooked (Takeuchi and Uehara, 1996) and are less likely to use mental health services than are white people (Zhang *et al.*, 1998). Asian Americans seek care mainly when they have severe illness, in part because of discouragement by family members to use mental health services (Sue and Sue, 1999). One study suggested that primary care physicians were less likely to identify depression in Asian patients than in white patients (Borowsky *et al.*, 2000). Studies also suggest that Asian Americans may respond to lower dosages of psychotropic medications (Lin and Cheung, 1999). Asian Americans who are matched with an Asian American therapist are more likely to continue in treatment, in particular for those who were less acculturated (Sue *et al.*, 1991); in addition, those who attended culturally specific clinics had better outcomes (Yeh *et al.*, 1994).

Similarly Hispanics utilize mental health services less than white populations (Hough *et al.*, 1987). Mexican Americans born in Mexico with mental illness have even lower use of services than those born in the USA (Vega *et al.*, 1998). Hispanics, as well as African Americans, are less frequently prescribed new antipsychotic medications during the initial introduction of these drugs (Valenstein *et al.*, 2006), yet they were more likely to be diagnosed with schizophrenia (Blow *et al.*, 2004). Hispanic patients are less than half as likely as white patients to receive care for depression in the primary care setting (Lagomasino *et al.*, 2005).

One to two-thirds of American Indians in primary care settings utilize native healers (Kim and Kwok, 1998; Marbella *et al.*, 1998; Buchwald *et al.*, 2000), and also do so very commonly for mental health conditions (Gurley *et al.*, 2001; Beals *et al.*, 2005b). The Great Smoky Mountains Study found similar rates of mental health treatment among Cherokee Indian children and non-Indians, 1 in 7; however, the American Indian children were more likely to receive treatment though the juvenile justice system and inpatient facilities (Costello *et al.*, 1997). Among adults, Indians have higher rates of help-seeking for substance use problems, but less for depression and anxiety disorders than white people (Beals *et al.*, 2005a). Less than 30 per cent of those with a psychiatric disorder obtain help from specialty providers.

In the USA, African American youths were four times more likely than white youths to be physically restrained after acting in similar aggressive ways; behaviour among African Americans was interpreted as stereotypical of African Americans as violent, and this motivated the clinicians' judgement (Bond *et al.*, 1988). In addition, African Americans are more likely to be treated as inpatients (Snowden and Cheung, 1990; Braeux and Ryujin, 1999; Snowden, 1999) and involuntarily treated (Takeuchi and Cheung, 1988; Akutsu *et al.*, 1996). Similarly, African American children were less likely to receive inpatient psychiatric care, but more likely to be in residential treatment centres (Firestone, 1990; Chabra *et al.*, 1999), and to be in the public mental health service (Bui and Takeuchi, 1992; McCabe *et al.*, 1999). African American patients with depression are rated more negatively than white patients with identical symptoms (Jenkins-Hall and Sacco, 1991). African Americans have been shown to be overdiagnosed with schizophrenia (Trierweiler *et al.*, 2000; Blow *et al.*, 2004), and underdiagnosed with bipolar disorder (Bell and Mehta, 1980, 1981; Mukherjee *et al.*, 1983), depression and anxiety (Neal-Barnett and Smith, 1997; Baker and Bell, 1999; Borowsky *et al.*, 2000). Based on the ECA study African Americans have about half the mental health service utilization of white patients with similar needs (Swartz *et al.*, 1998). The NCS found that only 16 per cent of African Americans with a mood disorder saw a mental health specialist and less than one-third consulted a health care provider. For anxiety disorders, 13 per cent went to a mental health specialist and 26 per cent saw any provider (US Department of Health and Human Services, 2001). African American patients terminate treatment prematurely compared with white patients (Sue *et al.*, 1994), are more likely to be less adherent to medications (Valenstein *et al.*, 2004) and receive more emergency care (Hu *et al.*, 1991). The disparity in obtaining treatment, however, between African American and white populations appears to be closing (Cooper-Patrick *et al.*, 1999). However, African American patients when first diagnosed with depression are less likely to receive antidepressant treatment than white patients, and less likely to be started on selective serotonin reuptake inhibitors (SSRIs) (Melfi *et al.*, 2000). In the Veterans Hospital system African Americans with bipolar disorder were less likely to be given an outpatient appointment within 90 days of the initial diagnosis (Kilbourne *et al.*, 2005).

This chapter has set out the rates of mental disorders across ethnic groups and national groups in North America, as well as among asylum seeker and refugee populations. The rates of disorders among indigenous North Americans are also considered. Some causes of psychological distress among migrants and ethnic groups are considered. Inequalities of access to services and studies showing ethnic variations of the impact of racism and poorer access to services are considered. The limitations of these studies are not considered here (see Chapter 4 on epidemiology, and Chapter 9 on health service use). More details of indigenous systems of healing and local folk categories of illness are not presented, but a critique of these can be found in Chapters 2 and 11.

# REFERENCES

Akutsu, P.D., Snowden, L.R. and Organista, K.C. 1996: Referral patterns to ethnic-specific and mainstream mental health programs for Hispanic and non-Hispanic Whites. *Journal of Counseling Psychology* 43, 56–64.

Alderete, E., Vega, W. A., Kolody, B. and Aguilar-Gaxiola, S. 2000: Effects of time in the United States and Indian ethnicity on DSM-III-R psychiatric disorders among Mexican Americans in California. *Journal of Nervous and Mental Disease* 188, 90–100.

Baker, F.M. and Bell, C.C. 1999: Issues in the psychiatric treatment of African Americans. *Psychiatric Services* 50, 362–68.

Beals, J., Piasecki, J., Nelson, S., Jones, M., Keane, E., Dauphinais, P., Shirt, R.R., Sack, W.H. and Manson, S.M. 1997: Psychiatric disorder among American Indian adolescents: prevalence in Northern Plains youth. *Journal of the American Academy of Child and Adolescent Psychiatry* 36, 1252–59.

Beals, J., Manson, S.M., Shore, J.H., Friedman, M., Ashcraft, M., Fairbank, J.A. and Schlenger, W.E. 2002: The prevalence of posttraumatic stress disorder among American Indian Vietnam veterans: disparities and context. *Journal of Traumatic Stress* 15, 89–97.

Beals, J., Manson, S.M., Whitesell, N.R., Spicer, P., Novins, D.K. and Mitchell, C.M. 2005a: Prevalence of DSM-IV disorders and attendant help-seeking in 2 American Indian reservation populations. *Archives of General Psychiatry* 62, 99–108.

Beals, J., Novins, D.K., Whitesell, N.R., Spicer, P.P., Mitchell, C.M. and Manson, S.M. 2005b: American Indian Service Utilization, Psychiatric Epidemiology, Risk and Protective Factors Project Team. Prevalence of mental disorders and utilization of mental health services in two American Indian reservation populations: mental health disparities in a national context. *American Journal of Psychiatry* 162, 1723–32.

Bell, C.C. and Mehta, H. 1980: The misdiagnosis of black patients with manic depressive illness. *Journal of the National Medical Association* 72, 141–45.

Bell, C.C. and Mehta, H. 1981: The misdiagnosis of black patients with manic depressive illness: Second in a series. *Journal of National Medical Association* 73, 101–107.

Blair, R.G. 2000: Risk factors associated with PTSD and major depression among Cambodian refugees. *Health and Social Work* 25, 23–30.

Bland, R.C., Orn, H. and Newman, S.C. 1988a: Lifetime prevalence of psychiatric disorders in Edmonton. *Acta Psychiatrica Scandinavica* 338, 24–32.

Bland, R.C., Newman, S.C. and Orn, H. 1988b: Period prevalence of psychiatric disorders in Edmonton. *Acta Psychiatrica Scandinavica* 338, S33–42.

Blow, F.C., Zeber, J.E., McCarthy, J.F., Valenstein, M., Gillon, L. and Bingham, C.R. 2004: Ethnicity and diagnostic patterns in veterans with psychoses. *Social Psychiatry and Psychiatric Epidemiology* 39, 841–51.

Blum, R.W., Harmon, B., Harris, L., Bergeisen, L. and Resnick, M.D. 1992: American Indian-Alaska Native youth health. *Journal of the American Medical Association* 267, 1637–44.

Bond, C.F., DiCandia, C.G. and MacKinnon, J.R. 1988: Responses to violence in a psychiatric setting: The role of patient's race. *Personality and Social Psychology Bulletin* 14, 448–58.

Borowsky, S.J., Rubenstein, L.V., Meredith, L.S., Camp, P., Jackson-Triche, M. and Wells, K.B. 2000: Who is at risk of nondetection of mental health problems in primary care? *Journal of General Internal Medicine* 15, 381–88.

Braeux, C. and Ryujin, D.H. 1999: Use of mental health services by ethnically diverse groups within the United States. *The Clinical Psychologist* 52, 4–14.

Breslau, J., Kendler, K.S., Su, M., Gaxiola-Aguilar, S. and Kessler, R.C. 2005: Lifetime risk and persistence of psychiatric disorders across ethnic groups in the United States. *Psychological Medicine* 35, 317–27.

Brown, D.R., Ahmed, F., Gary, L.E. and Milburn, N.G. 1995: Major depression in a community sample of African Americans. *American Journal of Psychiatry* 152, 373–78.

Brown, E.R., Ojeda, V.D., Wyn, R. and Levan, R. 2000: *Racial and Ethnic Disparities in Access to Health Insurance and Health care*. Los Angeles: UCLA Center for Health Policy Research and the Henry J. Kaiser Family Foundation.

Bui, K.V. and Takeuchi, D.L. 1992: Ethnic minority adolescents and the use of community mental health care services. *American Journal of Community Psychology* 20, 403–17.

Bureau of Justice Statistics 1998: *Probation and Parole Populations 1997*. Washington, DC: Bureau of Justice.

Burnam, M., Hough, R., Escobar, J., Karno, M., Timbers, D.M., Telles, C.A. and Locke, B.Z. 1987: Six-month prevalence of specific psychiatric disorders among Mexican American and non-Hispanic whites in Los Angeles. *Archives of General Psychiatry* 44, 687–94.

Buchwald, D.S., Beals, J. and Manson, S.M. 2000: Use of traditional healing among Native Americans in primary care setting. *Medical Care* 38, 1191–99.

Bussing, R., Schoenberg, N.E., Rogers, K.M., Zima, B.T. and Angus, S. 1998: Explanatory models of ADHD: do they differ by ethnicity, child gender, or treatment status? *Journal of Emotional and Behavioral Disorders* 6, 233–42.

Centers for Disease Control 2004: *Deaths: Final Data for 2002*. Atlanta, GA: National Vital Statistics Reports 53, No. 5.

Chabra, A., Chavez, G.F., Harris, E.S. and Shah, R. 1999: Hospitalization for mental illness in adolescents: risk groups and impact on the health care system. *Journal of Adolescent Health* 24, 349–56.

Chen, A.W. and Kazanjian, A. 2005: Rate of mental health service utilization by Chinese immigrants in British Columbia. *Canadian Journal of Public Health* 96, 49–51.

Chung, R.C. and Kagawa-Singer, M. 1993: Predictors of psychological distress among Southeast Asian refugees. *Social Science and Medicine* 36, 631–39.

Cooper-Patrick, L., Powe, N., Jenekes, M.W., Gonzales, J.J., Levine, D.M. and Ford, D.E. 1997: Identification of patient attitudes and preferences regarding treatment of depression. *Journal of General Internal Medicine* 12, 431–38.

Cooper-Patrick, L., Gallo, J.J., Gonzales, J.J., Vu, H.T., Powe, N.R., Nelson, C. and Ford, D.E. 1999: Race, gender, and partnership in the patient–physician relationship. *Journal of the American Medical Association* 37, 1034–45.

Costello, E.J., Costello, A.J., Edelbrock, C., Burns, B.J., Dulcan, M.K., Brent, D. and Janiszewski, S. 1988: Psychiatric disorders in pediatric primary care. Prevalence and risk factors. *Archives of General Psychiatry* 45, 1107–16.

Costello, E.J., Angold, A., Burns, B.J., Erkanli, A., Stangl, D.K. and Tweed, D.L. 1996: The Great Smoky Mountains Study of Youth. Functional impairment and serious emotional disturbance. *Archives of General Psychiatry* 53, 1137–43.

Costello, E.J., Famer, E.M., Angold, A., Burns, B.J. and Erkanli, A. 1997: Psychiatric disorders among American Indian and white youth in Appalachia: the Great Smoky Mountains Study. *American Journal of Public Health* 87, 827–32.

De Marco, R.R. 2000: The epidemiology of major depression: implications of occurrence, recurrence, and stress in a Canadian community sample. *Canadian Journal of Psychiatry* 45, 67–74.

Escobar, J.I., Karno, M., Burnam, A., Hough, R.L. and Golding, J. 1988: Distribution of major mental disorders in a US metropolis. *Acta Psychiatrica Scandinavica Supplementum* 344, 45–53.

Finch, B.K., Kolody, B. and Vega, W.A. 2000: Perceived discrimination and depression among Mexican origin adults in California. *Journal of Health and Social Behavior* 41, 295–313.

Firestone, B. 1990: *Information Packet on Use of Mental Health Services by Children and Adolescents*. Rockville, MD: Center for Mental Health Services Survey and Analysis Branch.

Flaherty, J.A., Kohn, R., Golbin, A., Gaviria, M. and Birz, S. 1986: Demoralization and social support in Soviet-Jewish immigrants to the United States. *Comprehensive Psychiatry* 27, 149–58.

Flaherty, J.A., Kohn, R., Levav, I. and Birz, S. 1988: Demoralization in Soviet-Jewish immigrants to the United States and Israel. *Comprehensive Psychiatry* 29, 588–97.

Fournier, L., Lesage, A.D., Toupin, J. and Cyr, M. 1997: Telephone surveys as an alternative for estimating prevalence of mental disorders and service utilization: a Montreal catchment area study. *Canadian Journal of Psychiatry* 42, 737–43.

Ganesan, S. and Janzé, T. 2005: Overview of culturally-based mental health care in Vancouver. *Transcultural Psychiatry* 42, 478–90.

Garroutte, E.M., Goldberg, J., Beals, J., Herrell, R. and Manson, S.M. and the AI-SUPERPFP Team. 2003: Spirituality and attempted suicide among American Indians. *Social Science and Medicine* 56, 1571–79.

Gilder, D.A., Wall, T.L. and Ehlers, C.L. 2004: Comorbidity of select anxiety and affective disorders with alcohol dependence in southwest California Indians. *Alcohol and Clinical Experimental Research* 28, 1805–13.

Grant, B. 1995: Comorbidity between DSM-IV drug use disorders and major depression: results of a national survey of adults. *Journal of Substance Abuse* 7, 481–97.

Grant, B.F., Stinson, F.S., Hasin, D.S., Dawson, D.A., Chou, S.P. and Anderson, K. 2004: Immigration and lifetime prevalence of DSM-IV psychiatric disorders among Mexican Americans and non-Hispanic whites in the United States: results from the National Epidemiologic Survey on Alcohol and Related Conditions. *Archives of General Psychiatry* 61, 1226–33.

Gurley, D., Novins, D.K., Jones, M.C., Beals, J., Shore, J.H. and Manson, S.M. 2001: Comparative use of biomedical services and traditional health options by American Indian veterans. *Psychiatric Services* 52, 68–74.

Hinton, W.L., Tiet, Q., Tran, C.G. and Chesney, M. 1997: Predictors of depression among refugees from Vietnam: a longitudinal study. *Journal of Nervous and Mental Disease* 185, 39–45.

Hough, R.L., Landsverk, J.A., Karno, M., Burnam, M.A., Timbers, D.M., Escobar, J.I. and Regier, D.A. 1987: Utilization of health and mental health services by Los Angeles Mexican Americans and non-Hispanic whites. *Archives of General Psychiatry* 44, 702–709.

Hu, T.W., Snowden, L.R., Jerrell, J.M. and Nguyen, T.D. 1991: Ethnic populations in public mental health: services choice and level of use. *American Journal of Public Health* 81, 1429–34.

Hurh, W.M. and Kim, K.C. 1988: *Uprooting and Adjustment. A Sociological Study of Korean Immigrants' Mental Health*. Final report to the National Institute of Mental Health. Macomb, IL: Western Illinois University, Department of Sociology and Anthropology.

Jarvis, E. 1971: *Insanity and Idiocy in Massachusetts: Report of the Commission of Lunacy (1855)*. Cambridge, MA: Harvard University Press.

Jencks, C. 1994: *The Homeless*. Cambridge, MA: Harvard University Press.

Jenkins-Hall, K.D. and Sacco, W.P. 1991: Effect of client race and depression on evaluation by white therapists. *Journal of Social and Clinical Psychology* 10, 322–33.

Jenkins, E.J. and Bell, C.C. 1997: Exposure and response to community violence among children and adolescents. In Osofsy, J. (ed.) *Children in a Violent Society*. New York: Guilford Press, 9–31.

Jonas, B.S., Brody, D., Roper, M. and Narrow, W.E. 2003: Prevalence of mood disorders in a national sample of young American adults. *Social Psychiatry and Psychiatric Epidemiology* 38, 618–24.

Jordan, B.K., Schenger, W.E., Fairbank, J. and Caddell, J.M. 1996: Prevalence of psychiatric disorders among incarcerated women II: convicted felons entering prison. *Archives of General Psychiatry* 53, 514–19.

Keller, A.S., Rosenfeld, B., Trinh-Shevrin, C., Meserve, C., Sachs, E., Leviss, J.A., Singer, E., Smith, H., Wilkinson, J., Kim, G., Allden, K. and Ford, D. 2003: Mental health of detained asylum seekers. *Lancet* 362, 1721–23.

Kessler, R.C., McGonagle, K.A., Zhao, S., Nelson, C.B., Hughes, M., Eshleman, S., Wittchen, H.U. and Kendler, K.S. 1994: Lifetime and 12-month prevalence of DSM-III-R psychiatric disorders in the United States. *Archives of General Psychiatry* 51, 8–19.

Kessler, R.C., Mickelson, K.D. and Williams, D.R. 1999: The prevalence, distribution, and mental health correlates of perceived discrimination in the United States. *Journal of Health and Social Behavior* 40, 208–30.

Kessler, R.C., Chiu, W.T., Demler, O., Merikangas, K.R. and Walters, E.E. 2005: Prevalence, severity, and comorbidity of 12-month DSM-IV disorders in the National Comorbidity Survey Replication. *Archives of General Psychiatry* 62, 617–27.

Kilbourne, A.M., Bauer, M.S., Han, X., Haas, G.L., Elder, P., Good, C.B., Shad, M., Conigliaro, J. and Pincus, H. 2005: Racial differences in the treatment of veterans with bipolar disorder. *Psychiatric Services* 56, 1549–555.

Kim, C. and Kwok, Y.S. 1998: Navajo use of native healers. *Archives of Internal Medicine* 158, 2245–49.

Kinzie, J.D., Sack, W., Angell, R., Clarke, G. and Ben, R. 1989: A three-year follow-up of Cambodian young people traumatized as children. *Journal of the American Academy of Child and Adolescent Psychiatry* 45, 923–26.

Kinzie, J.D., Boehnlein, J.K., Leung, P.K., Moore, L.J., Riley, C. and Smith, D. 1990: The prevalence of post-traumatic stress disorder and its clinical significance among Southeast Asian refugees. *American Journal of Psychiatry* 147, 913–17.

Kinzie, J.D., Leung, P.K., Boehnlein, J., Matsunaga, D., Johnson, R., Manson, S., Shore, J.H., Heinz, J. and Williams, M. 1992: Psychiatric epidemiology of an Indian village. A 19-year replication study. *Journal of Nervous and Mental Disease* 180, 33–39.

Lagomasino, I.T., Dwight-Johnson, M., Miranda, J., Zhang, L., Liao, D., Duan, N. and Wells, K.B. 2005: Disparities in depression treatment for Latinos and site of care. *Psychiatric Services* 56, 1517–23.

Lin, K.M. and Cheung, F. 1999: Mental health issues for Asian Americans. *Psychiatric Services* 50, 774–80.

Manson, S.M., Shore, J.H. and Bloom, J.D. 1985: The depressive experience in American Indian communities: A challenge for psychiatric theory and diagnosis. In Kleinman, A. and Good, B. (eds) *Culture and Depression*. Berkley, CA: University of California Press, 331–68.

Marbella, A.M., Harris, M.C., Diehr, S., Ignace, G. and Ignace, G. 1998: Use of Native American healers among Native American patients in an urban Native American health center. *Archives of Family Medicine* 7, 182–85.

Marshall, G.N., Schell, T.L., Elliott, M.N., Berthold, S.M. and Chun, C.A. 2005: Mental health of Cambodian refugees 2 decades after resettlement in the United States. *Journal of the American Medical Association* 294, 571–79.

McCabe, K.M., Clark, R. and Barnett, D. 1999: Family protective factors among urban African American youth. *Journal of Clinical and Child Psychology* 28, 137–50.

Melfi, C., Croghan, T., Hanna, M. and Robinson, R. 2000: Racial variation in antidepressant treatment in a Medicaid population. *Journal of Clinical Psychiatry* 61, 16–21.

Mukherjee, S., Shulka, S., Woodle, J., Rosen, A.M. and Olarte, S. 1983: Misdiagnosis of schizophrenia in bipolar patients: A multiethnic comparison. *American Journal of Psychiatry* 140, 1571–74.

Murphy, J.M., Laird, N.M., Monson, R.R., Sobol, A.M. and Leighton, A.H. 2000: A 40-year perspective on the prevalence of depression. The Stirling County Study. *Archives of General Psychiatry* 57, 209–15.

Narrow, W.E., Rae, D.S., Mościcki, E.K., Locke, B.Z. and Regier, D.A. 1990: Depression among Cuban Americans. The Hispanic Health and Nutrition Examination Survey. *Social Psychiatry and Psychiatric Epidemiology* 25, 260–68.

Neal-Barnett, A.M. and Smith, J. 1997: African Americans. In Friedman, S. (ed.) *Cultural Issues in the Treatment of Anxiety*. New York: Guilford Press, 154–74.

Noh, S., Beiser, M., Kaspar, V., Hou, F. and Rummens, J. 1999: Perceived racial discrimination, depression and coping: A study of Southeast Asian refugees in Canada. *Journal of Health and Social Behavior* 40, 193–207.

Offord, D.R., Boyle, M.H., Campbell, D., Goering, P., Lin, E., Wong, M. and Racine, Y.A. 1996: One-year prevalence of psychiatric disorder in Ontarians 15 to 64 years of age. *Canadian Journal of Psychiatry* 41, 559–63.

Ortega, A. N., Rosenheck, R., Alegría, M. and Desai, R.A. 2000: Acculturation and the lifetime risk of psychiatric and substance use disorders among Hispanics. *Journal of Nervous and Mental Disease* 188, 728–35.

Pan American Health Organization 2002: *Health in the Americas 2002*. Washington, DC: PAHO.

Patten, S.B. 2000: Major depression prevalence in Calgary. *Canadian Journal of Psychiatry* 45, 923–26.

Patten, S.B. and Charney, D.A. 1998: Alcohol consumption and major depression in the Canadian population. *Canadian Journal of Psychiatry* 43, 502–506.

Patten, S.B., Wang, J.L., Williams, J.V.A., Currie, S., Beck, C.A., Maxwell, C.J. and el-Guebaly, N. 2006: Descriptive epidemiology of major depression in Canada. *Canadian Journal of Psychiatry* 51, 84–90.

Portes, A. and Rumbaut, R.G. 1990: *Immigrant America: A Portrait*. Berkeley, CA: University of California Press.

Reinherz, H.Z., Giaconia, R.M., Lefkowitz, E.S., Pakiz, B. and Frost, A.K. 1993: Prevalence of psychiatric disorders in a community population of older adolescents. *Journal of the American Academy of Child and Adolescent Psychiatry* 32, 369–77.

Ren, X.S., Amick, B. and Williams, D.R. 1999: Racial/ethnic disparities in health: the interplay between discrimination and socioeconomic status. *Ethnicity and Disease* 9, 151–65.

Resnick, M.D., Bearman, P.S., Blum, R.W., Bauman, K.E., Harris, K.M., Jones, J., Tabor, J., Beuhring, T., Sieving, R.E., Shew, M., Ireland, M., Bearinger, L.H. and Udry, J.R. 1997: Protecting adolescents from harm. Findings from the National Longitudinal Study on Adolescent Health. *Journal of the American Medical Association* 278, 823–32.

Riolo, S.A., Nguyen, T.A., Greden, J.F. and King, C.A. 2005: Prevalence of depression by race/ethnicity: findings from the National Health and Nutrition Examination Survey III. *American Journal of Public Health* 95, 998–1000.

Roberts, R.E., Roberts, C. and Chen, Y.R. 1977: Ethnocultural differences in prevalence of adolescent depression. *American Journal of Community Psychology* 25, 95–110.

Robins, L.N. and Regier, D.A. 1991: *Psychiatric Disorders in America: the Epidemiological Catchment Area Study*. New York: Free Press.

Robins, L.N., Helzer, J.E., Croughan, J. and Ratcliff, K.S. 1981: National Institute of Mental Health Diagnostic Interview Schedule: its history, characteristics, and validity. *Archives of General Psychiatry* 38, 381–89.

Robins, L.N., Wing, J., Wittchen, H.U., Helzer, J.E., Babor, T.F., Burke, J., Farmer, A., Jablenski, A., Pickens, R., Regier, D.A., Sartorius, N. and Towle, L.H. 1988: The Composite International Diagnostic Interview: an epidemiologic instrument suitable for use in conjunction with different diagnostic systems and in different cultures. *Archives of General Psychiatry* 45, 1069–77.

Rumbaut, R.G. 1994: The crucible within: ethnic identity, self-esteem and segmented assimilation among children of immigrants. *International Migration Review* 28, 748–94.

Sadavoy, J., Meier, R. and Ong, A.Y. 2004: Barriers to access to mental health services for ethnic seniors: the Toronto study. *Canadian Journal of Psychiatry* 49, 192–299.

Siegel, J.M., Aneshensel, C.S., Taub, B., Cantwell, D.P. and Driscoll, A.K. 1998: Adolescent depressed mood in a multiethnic sample. *Journal of Youth and Adolescence* 27, 413–27.

Snowden, L.R. 1999: African American service use for mental health problems. *Journal of Community Psychology* 27, 303–13.

Snowden, L.R. and Cheung, F.K. 1990: Use of inpatient mental health services by members of ethnic minority groups. *American Psychologist* 45, 347–55.

Steffens, D.C., Skoog, I., Norton, M.C., Hart, A.D., Tschanz, J.T., Plassman, B.L., Wyse, B.W., Welsh-Bohmer, K.A. and Breitner, J.C. 2000: Prevalence of depression and its treatment in an elderly population: the Cache County study. *Archives of General Psychiatry* 57, 601–607.

Sue, D.W. and Sue, D. 1999: *Counseling the Culturally Different: Theory and Practice,* 3rd edn. New York: Wiley.

Sue, S., Fujino, D., Hu, L.T., Takeuchi, D.T. and Zane, N.W. 1991: Community mental health services for ethnic minority groups: a test of the cultural responsiveness hypothesis. *Journal of Consulting and Clinical Psychology* 59, 533–40.

Sue, S., Zane, N. and Young, K. 1994: Research on psychotherapy on culturally diverse populations. In Bergin, A. and Garfield, S. (eds) *Handbook of Psychotherapy and Behavior Change*, 4th edn. New York: Wiley, 783–817.

Sussman, L.K., Robins, L.N. and Earls, K. 1987: Treatment-seeking for depression by black and white Americans. *Social Science and Medicine* 24, 187–96.

Swartz, M.S., Wagner, H.R., Swanson, J.W., Burns, B.J., George, L.K. and Padgett, D.K. 1998: Administrative update: utilization of services. 1. Comparing use of public and private mental health services. The enduring barriers of race and age. *Community Mental Health Journal* 34, 133–44.

Takeuchi, D.T. and Uehara, E.S. 1996: Ethnic minority mental health services: current research and future conceptual directions. In Levin, B.L. and Petrila, J. (eds) *Mental Health Services: A Public Health Perspective*. New York: Oxford University Press, 63–80.

Takeuchi, D.T. and Cheung, M.K. 1998: Coercive and voluntary referrals: how ethnic minority adults get into mental health treatment. *Ethnicity and Health* 3, 149–58.

Takeuchi, D.T., Chung, R.C., Lin, K.M., Shen, H., Kurasaki, K., Chun, C.A. and Sue, S. 1998: Lifetime and twelve-month prevalence rates of major depressive episodes and dysthymia among Chinese Americans in Los Angeles. *American Journal of Psychiatry* 155, 1407–14.

Teplin, L.A. 1990: The prevalence of severe mental disorders among male urban jail detainees: comparison with the Epidemiologic Catchment Area Program. *American Journal of Public Health* 80, 663–69.

Teplin, L.A., Abram, K.M. and McClelland, G.M. 1996: Prevalence of psychiatric disorders among incarcerated women. *Archives of General Psychiatry* 53, 505–12.

Trierweiler, S.J., Neighbors, H.W., Munday, C., Thompson, S.E., Binion, V.J. and Gomez, J.P. 2000: Clinician attributions associated with diagnosis of schizophrenia in African American and non-African American patients. *Journal of Consulting and Clinical Psychology* 68, 171–75.

Turner, R.J. and Gil, A.G. 2002: Psychiatric and substance use disorders in South Florida: racial/ethnic and gender contrasts in a young adult cohort. *Archives of General Psychiatry* 59, 43–50.

Turvey, C.L., Wallace, R.B. and Herzog, R. 1999: A revised CES-D measure of depressive symptoms and a DSM-based measure of major depressive episodes in the elderly. *International Psychogeriatrics* 11, 139–48.

US Department of Health and Human Services. Mental Health 2001: *Culture, Race, and Ethnicity – A Supplement to Mental Health: A Report of the Surgeon General*. Rockville, MD: US Department of Health and Human Services, Substance Abuse and Mental Health Services Administration, Center for Mental Health Services.

United Nations High Commission for Refugees 2005: *2004 Global Refugee Trends*. Geneva: UNHCR.

Valenstein, M., Blow, F.C., Copeland, L.A., McCarthy, J.F., Zeber, J.E., Gillon, L., Bingham, C.R. and Stavenger, T. 2004: Poor antipsychotic adherence among patients with schizophrenia: medication and patient factors. *Schizophrenia Bulletin* 30, 255–64.

Valenstein, M., McCarthy, J.F., Ignacio, R.V., Dalack, G.W., Stavenger, T. and Blow, F.C. 2006: Patient- and facility-level factors associated with diffusion of a new antipsychotic in the VA health system. *Psychiatric Services* 57, 70–76.

Valleni-Basile, L.A., Garrison, C.Z., Waller, J.L., Addy, C.L., McKeown, R.E., Jackson, K.L. and Cuffe, S.P. 1996: Incidence of obsessive-compulsive disorder in a community sample of young adolescents. *Journal of the American Academy of Child and Adolescent Psychiatry* 35, 898–906.

Vander Stoep A. and Link, B. 1998: Social class, ethnicity, and mental illness: the importance of being more than earnest. *American Journal of Public Health* 88, 1396–402.

Vega, W.A. and Rumbaut, R.G. 1991: Ethnic minorities and mental health. *Annual Review of Sociology* 17, 351–83.

Vega, W.A., Kolody, B., Aguilar-Gaxiola, S., Alderate, E., Catalano, R. and Carveo-Anduaga, J. 1998: Lifetime prevalence of DSM-III-R psychiatric disorders among urban and rural Mexican Americans in California. *Archives of General Psychiatry* 55, 771–78.

Vernon, S.W. and Roberts, R.E. 1982: Use of the SADS-RDC in a tri-ethnic community survey. *Archives of General Psychiatry* 39, 47–52.

Wang, J., Patten, S.B., Williams, J.V., Currie, S., Beck, C.A., Maxwell, C.J. and El-Guebaly, N. 2005: Help-seeking behaviours of individuals with mood disorders. *Canadian Journal of Psychiatry* 50, 652–59.

Wang, P.S., Berglund, P. and Kessler, R.C. 2000: Recent care of common mental disorders in the United States. *Journal of General Internal Medicine* 15, 284–92.

Weissman, M.M., Myers, J.K. and Harding, P.S. 1978: Psychiatric disorders in a U.S. urban community: 1975–1976. *American Journal of Psychiatry* 35, 459–62.

Williams, D.R., Yu, Y., Jackson, J.S. and Anderson, N.B. 1997: Racial differences in physical and mental health socio-economic status, stress and discrimination. *Journal of Health Psychology* 2, 335–51.

World Health Organization 2002: *Global Burden of Disease Project*. http://www.who.int/healthinfo/bodabout/en/index.html (accessed 26 November 2005).

Yeh, M., Takeuchi, D.T. and Sue, S. 1994: Asian-American children treated in the mental health system: a comparison of parallel and mainstream outpatient service centers. *Journal of Clinical Child Psychology* 23, 5–12.

Ying, Y. 1988: Depressive symptomatology among Chinese-Americans as measured by the CES-D. *Journal of Clinical Psychology*, 44, 739–46.

Young, A.S., Klap, R., Shebourne, C.D. and Wells, K.B. 2001: The quality of care for depressive and anxiety disorders in the United States. *Archives of General Psychiatry* 58, 55–61.

Zhang, A.Y. and Snowden, L.R. 1999: Ethnic characteristics of mental disorders in five US communities. *Cultural Diversity and Ethnic Minority Psychology* 5, 134–46.

Zhang, A.Y., Snowden, L.R. and Sue, S. 1998: Differences between Asian- and White-Americans' help-seeking and utilization patterns in the Los Angeles area. *Journal of Community Psychology* 26, 317–26.

Zylstra, R.G. and Steitz, J.A. 1999: Public knowledge of late-life depression and aging. *Journal of Applied Gerontology* 18, 63–76.

# 23

# Culture and mental health care in New Zealand: indigenous and non-indigenous people

Rajendra Pavagada and Ruth DeSouza

## INTRODUCTION

*A distant land, cloud capped, with plenty of moisture and sweet scented soil.*
**Kupe (cited in Te Matorohanga, 1913)**

This chapter sets out to provide an overview of mental health services in New Zealand, with specific attention to the cultural aspect of these services for both indigenous people (*Mäori*) and migrants. We are ourselves both migrants to New Zealand and approach this chapter as insiders and outsiders to the system, giving us a unique perspective. There are a number of limitations we would like to highlight: We do not claim to speak for all New Zealanders and acknowledge that this chapter is a beginning reference point, not a comprehensive review of all mental health issues. This chapter focuses on adult mental health and excludes in-depth discussion of child and youth mental health issues, problem gambling and alcohol and other drugs. We do not claim to be experts in issues related to *Mäori*, since we are not ourselves *Mäori*.

Throughout the chapter we use the term '*tangata whai ora*' rather than 'patient'. We do this to recognize and acknowledge the unique context of the New Zealand consumer's reality but in doing so also acknowledge that all terms have their politics and limitations. *Mäori* words and terms used in this chapter are italicized for the benefit of the non-New Zealand reader and a glossary is provided at the end.

The chapter begins with an overview of the unique background and contextual issues that have shaped the New Zealand mental health system. It presents demographic information, discusses the significance of the Treaty of Waitangi and the structure of the health system, with particular reference to the health reforms of the 1980s and 1990s. It emphasizes the importance of the recovery model and the role of consumers in the delivery and development of mental health services. The first section concludes with a summary of the role of the Mental

Health Commission. The chapter then continues with a discussion of the unique bicultural nature of New Zealand, with particular reference to *Mäori* and the role of the Treaty of Waitangi. There follows a discussion of key aspects of psychiatric practice in New Zealand and a separate section describing the mental health services that are provided for *Mäori*. Issues of workforce development are discussed and the chapter concludes with a discussion on migrant and refugee communities and their mental health requirements and service provision.

## BACKGROUND AND CONTEXT

New Zealand achieved independent dominion from Britain in 1907 and today has a population of four million people. Three-quarters of the population live in the North Island and 85 per cent live in urban areas. Like other Western countries, the population is ageing and the median age is 35. Twenty-nine per cent of New Zealanders live in its largest city, Auckland. Changes heralded in the Immigration Act 1987 have led to an increasingly diverse population. Whilst European New Zealanders make up 75 per cent of the population and *Mäori* account for 14.7 per cent, Pacific people make up 6.5 per cent and Asians now account for 9 per cent (and 12 per cent in Auckland). Asians are also the fastest-growing ethnic group, increasing by around 140 per cent over the last ten years. The predominant language spoken in New Zealand is English (96.1 per cent) followed by *Mäori* (4.5 per cent), which is an official language. Sixteen per cent of people are bilingual or multilingual speakers. The median income for the population is US$21 000 (Statistics New Zealand, 2005).

## THE TREATY OF WAITANGI AND CULTURAL SAFETY

When Britain assumed governance of its new colony in 1840, it signed a treaty with *Mäori* tribes. *Te Tiriti O Waitangi*/The Treaty of Waitangi is today recognized as New Zealand's founding document and its importance is strongly evident in health care and social policy. As a historical accord between the Crown and *Mäori*, the treaty defines the relationship between *Mäori* and *Pakeha* (non-*Mäori*) and forms the basis for biculturalism, which Sullivan (1994) defined as:

- Equal partnership between two groups.
- *Mäori* are acknowledged as *tangata whenua* ('people of the land').
- The *Mäori* translation of *Te Tiriti O Waitangi* is acknowledged as the founding document of *Aotearoa*/New Zealand.
- Biculturalism is concerned with addressing past injustices and re-empowering indigenous people.

Durie (1994) suggests that the contemporary application of the Treaty of Waitangi involves the concepts of biculturalism and cultural safety, which are at the forefront of delivery of mental health services. This means incorporating 'principles of partnership, participation, protection and equity' (Cooney, 1994, p. 9) into the care that is delivered. There is an expectation that mental health staff in New Zealand ensure care is culturally safe for *Mäori* (Mental Health Commission, 2001). Simply put, 'unsafe practitioners diminish, demean or disempower those of other cultures, whilst safe practitioners recognize, respect and acknowledge the rights of others' (Cooney, 1994, p. 6). The support and strengthening of identity are seen as crucial for recovery for *Mäori* along with ensuring services meet *Mäori* needs and expectations (Mental Health Commission, 2001). Cultural safety goes beyond learning about such things as the dietary or religious needs of different ethnic groups; it also involves engaging with the socio-political context (McPherson *et al.*, 2003; DeSouza, 2004).

## THE PUBLIC HEALTH SYSTEM

The health system is predominantly a public-based system. The country is divided into 21 District Health Boards (DHBs), which provide services with the objective of improving, promoting and protecting the health of people and communities. There is a strong emphasis in psychiatric practice on community-based services. Recently, primary mental health care has been strengthened with the development of the Primary Health Care strategy and establishment of primary health organizations (PHOs) whose focus includes addressing the mental health needs of their populations who present with mild to moderately severe mental health problems or disorders as well as working in partnership with mental health services to provide care for moderate to severe disorders. Building up the capacity and responsivity of PHOs in primary care is a priority as they are seen as having a pivotal role in the overall provision of mental health care.

New Zealand's first psychiatric hospital was opened in Dunedin in 1863 (Bloomfield, 2001). It accommodated 21 *tangata whai ora*. By 1938, New Zealand had become the first country in the world to introduce universal health care, as part of a post-depression welfare state. The modern health system has been shaped by the shift to neo-liberal ideologies from the mid-1980s (Crowe *et al.*, 2001). No other country embraced the market-driven model and corporatization of public assets to the extent New Zealand did. Underpinned by free trade, market liberalization, limited government involvement and a deregulated labour market, New Zealand's public service underwent dramatic reforms between 1987 and 1999 (Crowe, 1997). Unsurprisingly, this has profoundly influenced the provision of mental health care. Since the election of a Labour-led coalition government in 1999, there has been a gradual winding back of neo-liberalism and a return to more socially oriented measures with greater state involvement in public service delivery (Saul, 2005).

The legacy of the reforms is seen in the transition from large mental hospitals to psychiatric inpatient units within general hospitals, which also began in the 1980s. Law and policy changes throughout the 1990s encouraged the process of deinstitutionalization and hospital beds were reduced from over 10 000 in 1973 to less than 2000 by 1996 (Currier, 1997). The Mental Health (Community Assessment and Treatment) Act 1992 allows for the compulsory treatment of people with serious mental illness in the community while the Looking Forward strategy (Ministry of Health, 1994) advocated for more community-based mental health services to be provided by publicly funded non-governmental organizations (NGOs) as well as by DHBs and for the continued reduction of hospital admissions.

Dew and Kirkman (2002) suggest that the process of deinstitutionalization was flawed in that it was not government-led and occurred erratically. The result has been fragmentation and underfunding of community mental health services. They argue that the workforce was ill-prepared and the result has been a dearth of recovery/rehabilitation-orientated professionals and a paucity of services and resources, such as accommodation, which has seriously impeded service delivery. These issues are addressed by the national mental health strategy, 'the Blueprint' (Mental Health Commission, 1998), which promotes a recovery approach for mental health service providers and incorporates notions of consumer empowerment, self-determination, awareness, maintenance of rights and full participation in society (Ministry of Health, 2003). Hospital-based mental health services now provide short-term care for people while they are acutely unwell, but bed shortages remain a concern.

A recent policy is *Te Tāhuhu – Improving Mental Health 2005–2015* (Ministry of Health, 2005b). This develops plans for a comprehensive integrated mental health and addiction system. It emphasizes early access to effective primary care services, and an improved range and quality of specialist community mental health and addiction services. It covers the spectrum of interventions from prevention/promotion to primary care to specialist services. Another new document was published in August 2006. *Te Kōkiri: The Mental Health and Addiction Action Plan 2006–2015* sets out the next steps for progressing the 10 leading challenges indentified in *Te Tāhuhu* for improving mental health and addiction over the next 10 years.

## RECOVERY AND THE CONSUMER MOVEMENT

In parallel to the economic reforms, the consumer movement has influenced a movement in mental health service delivery from a medical to a recovery model. New opportunities have arisen for consumers to interact with policy-makers, professionals and others from a position of strength. Consumer-operated programmes and initiatives have emerged from dissatisfaction with clinical mental health services and consumers now report finding consumer-staffed organizations more empathetic, tolerant and understanding because of their own struggles with psychiatric disability (Worley, 1997). Guidelines have been developed as a result of increased consumer participation in professionally run mental health agencies (Ministry of Health, 1995) and this led to changes in the relationship between consumers and professionals. There is a growing recognition on the part of professionals of the value of experiential knowledge and what consumers have to offer other consumers.

## MENTAL HEALTH COMMISSION

Established in 1997 to ensure the implementation of the National Mental Health Strategy, the Mental Health Commission's role is to improve services and outcomes for people with mental illness and their families/*whänau*. It evolved from the Mason Committee, set up to inquire into mental health services and the findings of which revealed strengths and significant weaknesses in New Zealand mental health services (Mason *et al.*, 1996). Initially, the Commission was involved in reviewing the standards for mental health services and strategic planning for implementing better services over a five-year period. The Commission formulated a blueprint for mental health services and proposed that the recovery approach become standard practice in all services. This document is now government policy, setting out expectations around what levels of service need to be present to meet the needs of different groups. It defines guidelines for delivering services to *Mäori*, so that they have a choice of accessing high-quality, culturally effective mainstream services. It has also responded to the growing populations of Pacific and Asian communities through the development of resources.

The Commission defines recovery as something that:

*happens when people can live well in the presence or absence of their mental illness and the loss that may come in its wake, such*

*as isolation, poverty, unemployment and discrimination. Recovery does not always mean that people will return to full health or retrieve all their losses, but it does mean that people can live well in spite of losses.*

**(Mental Health Commission, 1998, p. 1)**

The concept of recovery originates in the USA and is derived from the self-help movement, users of mental health services and psychiatric rehabilitation principles.

It is noted that stigma and discrimination associated with mental illness are major barriers to recovery. In New Zealand, the 'Like Minds Like Mine' Project, a public health-funded project, began in 1997 to reduce stigma associated with mental illness and the discrimination that people with mental illness face in the community. Nationwide and community-based programmes are making significant progress through advertising campaigns, policy initiatives and so forth. A co-ordinated cross-sectoral approach with the Mental Health Commission, the Human Rights Commission and the Office for Disability Issues is also under development.

The Mental Health Commission (2001) suggests that understanding, supporting and strengthening identity are important components of recovery. Cultural assessment, or the process through which the relevance of culture to mental health is ascertained, in the treatment and support of *tangata whai ora* is strongly advocated. While undertaking a cultural assessment helps to identify a person's cultural needs, cultural supports or healing practices are also needed to strengthen identity and enhance wellness. Cultural assessment can be used to assess mental status and it is also important as a tool for planning treatment and rehabilitation (Mental Health Commission, 2001).

## *MÄORI/TANGATA WHENUA*

Durie (1999) suggests that the greatest threat to good health for *Mäori* is poor mental health. Prior to Western systems of health *Mäori* followed indigenous practices where illnesses were generally attributed to the violation of *tapu* (supernatural influence or restriction) or the presence of *makutu* (curse).

The *tohunga* acted as an intermediary between humans and *atua* (gods) and performed atonement or addressed imbalances of supernatural power (Sachdev, 1998). As Durie (1985) explains, *Māori* concepts of health are broader than Western concepts, encompassing spiritual and family components in addition to the physical and psychological aspects. Furthermore, *whenua* (land), *whānau* (family) and *reo* (language) are crucial determinants of good mental health for *Māori*.

There remain significant disparities between *Māori* and non-*Māori* in mental health. Mental health services have a responsibility to respond to *Māori* health issues by improving care through understanding the socio-political issues and historical processes that impact on the status of *Māori*. Furthermore, *Māori* are underrepresented in the health workforce despite the proliferation of *Māori* mental health service providers (Mental Health Commission and Ministry of Health, 1999).

Whilst the health status of *Māori* has improved significantly over the last four decades, their indices of health still lag behind non-*Māori*, with higher rates of common disorders. *Māori* are overrepresented in crisis, acute inpatient and forensic services and have substantially higher rates of readmission than non-*Māori* (Pomare, 1986; Pomare and deBoer, 1988). Hyslop *et al.* (1983) suggest that this is due to poor delivery of health care services to *Māori* or an ineffective use of these services by *Māori*.

The leading causes of first admission for *Māori* are alcohol dependence or abuse and, for readmission, schizophrenia (men) and affective psychosis (women). *Māori* are more likely to be admitted through involuntary and committal procedures (36 per cent versus 24 per cent). *Māori*, and in particular *Māori* youth, have higher than average rates of suicide. In 1997 the suicide rate for *Māori* was 33.9/100 000 and for non-*Māori* was only 24.2/100 000.

*Māori* communities have experienced considerable change since 1945, with a significant population drift from rural to urban areas, a related dislocation from tribal affiliations and inter-marriage with Europeans (Harre, 1968). Westernization and urbanization have altered the traditional fabric of society and the role of extended family and tribal structure (*whānau*, *hapu* and *iwi*) as a fundamental unit has been broken with no suitable substitute (McCreary, 1968). Traditional supports and controls on behaviour have consequently been lost (Sachdev, 1989) and other risk factors such as cultural alienation, the impact of history through intergenerational modelling, behavioural transfer and confusion over identity remain for many.

## PSYCHIATRIC PRACTICE IN NEW ZEALAND

In 2002, 1.7 per cent of the New Zealand population were users of mental health services. In the first six months of 2002, 0.14 per cent of the population received inpatient care and 0.3 per cent of the population was treated by alcohol and drug services (Gaudin, 2004). At this time, the total number of general adult inpatient beds was 1375. Forty-seven per cent of *tangata whai ora* were being assessed and treated under the Mental Health Act 1992.

More than 90 per cent of mental health services are provided free of charge to *tangata whai ora* through government subsidy and this funding is allocated through local DHBs. In 2001/2002, funding totalled NZ$725 million, the equivalent of NZ$184 per capita. Approximately 69 per cent of this funding went to community mental health services and 31 per cent to inpatient services. *Māori* services received 9.5 per cent of the total mental health budget and services for Pacific people received 1.4 per cent (Gaudin, 2004).

Benchmarking for various service components such as the number of inpatient beds is set by the National Mental Health Strategy. However, it does not discuss the gradient required in those benchmarks in order to effectively address deprivation. There is a strong association between areas of deprivation and psychiatric bed utilization (Abas *et al.*, 2003). People living in deprived areas, such as south of Auckland, have approximately three times the admission prevalence of those living in the least deprived areas. It is suggested that the higher admission rates in the most deprived areas are the result of poor access to primary care, poorer quality of primary care or poorer access to outpatient mental health care (Stuart *et al.*, 1996; Jacobson, 1999).

## Public services

The New Zealand Government provides the vast majority of funding made available to mental health services and 70 per cent of all funding is spent by public providers through DHBs and GPs, including PHOs. The government identifies five key outcome perspectives for service delivery (Krieble, 2003): Consumer, Cultural, Family, Care, and Public.

## Non-government organizations (NGOs)

NGOs have become an integral part of mental health service delivery. Services provided by NGOs include residential care, community support, employment services and consumer and family support services. NGOs receive one-third of the funding allocated to mental health and are co-ordinated through their own national network, Platform, the New Zealand Association of Support Services and Community Development in Mental Health.

## Accident compensation scheme

New Zealand has a publicly funded model of no-fault accident insurance. Whilst this relates primarily to physical (and particularly sporting) injuries, the Accident Compensation Corporation (ACC), which administers the scheme and provides personal injury cover for all New Zealand citizens, residents and temporary visitors to New Zealand, also deals with the mental health effects of sexual abuse or sexual assault. These 'sensitive claims' include depression and post-traumatic stress disorder (PTSD). The ACC provides cover for a mental injury resulting from a physical injury, such as PTSD or depression resulting from a motor vehicle accident.

## Housing

According to the Mental Health Commission (1999), recovery from mental illness often requires specific housing arrangements combining support, a quality physical environment and suitable local environment. With the shift to community-based care, housing difficulties now affect 17 per cent of *tangata whai ora*, with a similar number living in circumstances that could involve a heightened risk of future homelessness. About 4 per cent of *tangata whai ora* are homeless or living in temporary or emergency accommodation. One-third of *tangata whai ora* have problems affording housing and another third face a lack of choice (Peace and Kell, 2001). Peace and Kell note that discrimination, unsuitable locations, loss of accommodation during acute illness or hospitalization can affect between 10 and 20 per cent of *tangata whai ora*. Problems with accommodation can lead to deterioration in mental health, particularly during the transition from clinical care to independent housing. Peace and Kell contend that an additional factor affecting Pacific consumers is overcrowding and many mental health providers identify housing difficulties as being a serious issue for *Māori*.

## Compulsory treatment

With the introduction of the Mental Health (Compulsory Assessment and Treatment) Act 1992 (MHA) there occurred a major revision in the law regulating the involuntary admission of psychiatric *tangata whai ora*. The MHA defines the circumstances and conditions under which a person can be subjected to compulsory psychiatric assessment and treatment. The Act reformed and consolidated the law relating to the assessment and treatment of persons suffering from mental disorder. It defines the rights of such persons and provides protection for those rights. The MHA placed greater emphasis on the protection of civil rights through regular judicial review and, under this legislation the initiation of involuntary hospitalisation is carried out by a Duly Authorised Officer (DAO) appointed by the Director of Area Mental Health Services. The Act defines the rights of *tangata whai ora*, recognizes cultural safety and provides a multi-tiered system of advocacy. *Tangata whai ora* can challenge their compulsory status, including requesting a second opinion, a judicial review or making a request to the Mental Health Review Tribunal for a review of their compulsory status. Contrary to previous legislation but in line with current practice, the Act emphasizes community treatment over institutional treatment (Currier, 1997). Further refinements have been made in the Amendments to the MHA, which came into force in 1999.

*Tangata whai ora* committed to community care have the right to refuse medication after the first month of treatment and a process of second opinion must be initiated to enforce medication compliance. The MHA defines grounds for involuntary hospitalization as the person must be suffering from an 'abnormal state of mind', including delusion or impairment of cognition, volition or perception and the mental disorder results in significant risk to danger to self or others or in a substantial impairment of ability to care for self. The MHA does not recognize cultural beliefs, sexual preferences, criminal or delinquent behaviour, substance abuse or an intellectual handicap as mental disorder.

## Forensic psychiatry

Forensic psychiatric services provide care for prison inmates, mentally ill persons proceeding through the courts and those found to be not guilty through disability and insanity. Decisions regarding violent inmates with mental health concerns are made on a clinical basis and not through reference to legal status. A dilemma exists regarding the forensic status of personality-disordered or intellectually disabled prisoners, since there is no equivalent psychopathic disorder defined. Inpatient forensic services work almost exclusively with patients subject to compulsory inpatient treatment orders either through civil commitments or by the criminal justice legislation.

The Mason Report (Mason *et al.*, 1996) shaped the future of forensic psychiatry in New Zealand. Following this report, four new types of forensic service were established:

1. Medium and a minimum security psychiatric units
2. A prison liaison service
3. A court liaison service
4. A community forensic psychiatric service.

In addition, a consultation and liaison service for general psychiatric services was established. Regional forensic psychiatric services were created as a part of the regional mental health services and

established to cater for *tangata whai ora* for a period of up to three years in secure rehabilitation. However, as some *tangata whai ora* have required significant longer rehabilitation periods, long-term rehabilitation units have also been built.

Clinical practice in this area is largely influenced by the Mental Health Act 1992, which provides for compulsory care of the mentally ill both within an inpatient unit and also in the community. Criminal law deals with concerns of criminal responsibility, fitness to plead and the legal definition of mental disorder. The person found to be mentally disordered before the court in a criminal matter can be dealt with through provisions in MHA, the Summary Proceedings Act 1957 and the Criminal Justice Act 1985. Insanity provisions are contained in section 23 of the Crimes Act 1961 (see Chapter 7, section on New Zealand mental health law).

A psychiatric report can be requested by the Court for a person either charged (before or during their trial) or convicted of an offence under section 121 of the Criminal Justice Act 1985. This allows a person to be remanded to prison or psychiatric care pending such report or for the report to be prepared as a condition of bail. Such reports address fitness to plead, insanity or other pre-sentence issues that might assist the presiding Judge in arriving at an appropriate disposition. The assessment of 'fitness to plead' under New Zealand law is similar to that of other Commonwealth jurisdictions but New Zealand law lacks a provision for claiming 'diminished capacity' through mental disorder at the time of offending (Brinded, 2000). The disposition available to the court for an individual found to be not guilty by virtue of insanity is similar to that for a person unfit to plead under section 115 of the Criminal Justice Act 1985. The experienced member of the multidisciplinary team provides the court liaison service based in the court. Following a reference from the judge, police, lawyers or the family of the accused person the health professionals perform the initial assessment. This service is available in almost all high courts of New Zealand.

Outpatient forensic psychiatry services work closely with inpatient services and also with community mental health centres. This facilitates the smooth transfer of the *Tangata whai ora* and tends to avoid the artificial barriers between inpatient care and the community. The treatment for sex and violent offenders remains largely based in correctional facilities.

## Suicide

Suicide is one of the indicators of mental health in the population. New Zealand has the highest reported male youth (15–24 years) suicide rate and the second highest female youth suicide rate amongst OECD (Organization for Economic Co-operation and Development) countries. For all ages suicide rates for males in New Zealand ranks fifth amongst OECD countries and for females, sixth. Local research suggests that almost 90 per cent of people who die by suicide or make serious suicide attempts will have one or more mental disorders at the time of their attempt, with these disorders typically being accompanied by other sources of stress and difficulty (Beautrais *et al.*, 2005). The government's youth suicide prevention strategy provides a framework for understanding what suicide prevention is and signals the steps a range of government agencies, communities, service providers, *iwi* and *whänau* must take to reduce the incidence of suicide. Since 2001 the Ministry of Youth Development (2004) has led the promotion and co-ordination of this strategy. *Mäori* have higher rates of suicide than non-*Mäori* for both men and women. Additional risk factors appear to be related to cultural alienation and confusion over identity. Official statistics indicate that suicide among *Mäori* aged over 45 years is virtually non-existent, suggesting that there may be culturally specific factors that may be protecting this group against suicide.

## Rural services

New Zealand has significant rural populations and this provides challenges for the delivery of mental health services. These include staff retention, a shortage of skilled mental health staff, limited access to hospital-based services, lack of funding for psychiatric services, frequently being on call and effective management of risk is challenging in rural psychiatry. Risk exists in the limited opportunities to obtain a second opinion and the lack of collegiate

support. There are few opportunities for rural mental health staff to participate in continuing medical education (CME) and quality assurance issues can arise due to professional isolation. The lack of trainees is also a significant problem for those working in rural areas.

## *MÄORI* MENTAL HEALTH SERVICES

Durie (1985) reported that communication problems between professionals and *Mäori tangata whai ora* and the inflexibility of the health system to accommodate cultural differences presented by *Mäori* caused under-utilization of mental health services by *Mäori*. The health system has traditionally been dominated by the Western medical model and *Mäori* have been an underrepresented minority as well as a socio-economically disadvantaged minority.

Since the early 1990s, mental health services have increasingly recognized the need to develop a *Mäori* mental health workforce. New Zealand has developed parallel services that are 'for *Mäori* by *Mäori*' and 'For Pacific people by Pacific people'. One aim of the national strategic framework for *Mäori* mental health, *Te Puawaitanga* (Ministry of Health, 2002a) is to increase the number of *Mäori* mental health workers, resulting in new research, tertiary training and workforce development initiatives. *Te Rau Matatini* was established to ensure that *Mäori tangata whai ora* have access to a well-prepared and well-qualified *Mäori* mental health workforce. The goal was to increase recruitment and retention of *Mäori* staff through increasing *Mäori* participation, to increase the expertise of the broader *Mäori* workforce and of *Mäori* staff in related sectors. This model promotes excellence in the workforce through the development of clinical and cultural expertise (Te Rau Matatini, 2004).

Awareness of cultural differences is needed not only in culturally specific services but also in the mainstream services, since not all *Mäori* or members of other ethnic or cultural groups have access to or choose to use culturally specific services. Fears regarding treatment can arise from concepts that are generally disregarded in the Western construction of mental health. As Durie (1977) observes, *Māori tangata whai ora* can present with an 'unspoken and unconscious fear' (p. 484) of some infringement of *tapu* and families might seek the services of a traditional healer in *tohunga* in order to identify and 'treat' such an infringement. The traditional role of the *tohunga* does not replace the doctor, rather it may be complementary, with some *Māori* leaders arguing for a greater degree of co-operation between the two systems. They suggest that the two roles could be seen as serving different but complementary functions for *tangata whai ora*. There is evidence of improved health outcomes within *Māori* communities when culturally appropriate responses emerge from the community itself and such that Western medical practices are re-conceptualized within a *Māori kaupapa* (Department of Health, 1984).

Localized attempts to provide culturally based care in the community include GP services based within *Marae*, specialist outreach clinics, culturally specific health education programmes and *Māori* mental health teams. However, research shows that health professionals can feel ill-prepared to deal with such services: Johnstone and Read (2000) found that whilst 70 per cent of psychiatrists responding to their survey believed there was a need to consult with *Māori* when working with *Māori tangata whai ora*, only 40 per cent felt that their training had prepared them to work effectively with *Māori*.

## *Kaupapa Māori* services and strategies for managing overrepresentation

The establishment of *kaupapa Māori* mental health services appears to be an effective strategy in that they deliver a culturally safe, specific and responsive service to *Māori tangata whai ora*. In addition to educating health care professionals, and training and employing more *Māori* in the health professions, the use of bicultural intermediaries has been adopted as a strategy for increasing *Māori* utilization of mental health services. *Marae*-based health programmes have been developed and *kaumatua* have been used as cultural interpreters by health professionals. Psychiatric hospitals

can now be expected to have the services of a *kaumatua* available to act as a counsellor for *Māori tangata whai ora* and to assist and advise the staff with regard to providing culturally appropriate care.

Since the *marae* is central to many aspects of *Māori* culture and a place of both belonging and contact, *marae*-based services offer the potential for addressing poor access to mainstream services and for providing culturally appropriate services in a safe and familiar setting. Their purpose is to complement community health services already in place, rather than to replace them, and many *marae*-based programmes are attempts to educate and enrich *tangata whai ora* and their *whānau*.

Durie (1997) suggests five strategies that can lead to improved mental health outcomes for *Māori*:

1. Development of a secure identity. Identity is a prerequisite for good mental health and *Māori* identity requires more than a superficial knowledge of tribal affiliation or ancestry, depending as it does on access to the cultural, social and economic resources of *te ao Māori* (the *Māori* world).

2. Active participation of *Māori* in society and in the economy. Unemployment, unrewarding work, negative experiences at school and powerlessness and marginalization within society is not compatible with good mental health and can lead to drug and alcohol abuse, violence and parental abandonment.

3. Improving the quality and quantity of mental health services so that *Māori* can access them and *Māori* outcomes are enhanced. This can be done through *kaupapa Māori* services focused on both cultural and clinical goals and when *kaumatua* guide and work alongside clinicians to bring a more comprehensive approach to treatment than possible in usual services.

4. Accelerated *Māori* workforce development as *Māori* are underrepresented in the mental health discipline.

5. Autonomy and control for *Māori* for service delivery and for policy formulation, planning and key decision-making.

## Transferability

*Māori* initiatives to address mental health disparities have been innovative and offer potential for others. Sachdev (1998) sees the *Māori* experience in New Zealand as being relevant for other minority ethnic communities. The major lesson, he suggests, is that primary initiatives must come from communities themselves and for this change to occur the appropriate socio-political conditions must be created. Disadvantaged communities must be empowered to bring about change and the mainstream health system must recognize such change as adaptive, rational and even cost-effective (see the approach in the UK described in Chapter 5, in Australia in Chapter 25 and in Europe in Chapter 30).

## WORKFORCE DEVELOPMENT

The quality and further development of New Zealand's mental health services have been constrained by a shortage of appropriately trained staff (Health Funding Authority, 2000). More precisely issues such as the poor co-ordination of development, lack of skilled staff, problems with recruitment and retention and unsatisfactory and inappropriate skill mixes have been identified as important issues. It has been suggested by the Health Funding Authority that too little staff training has been available to assist with the transition into the changed health environment. The areas of most concern have been *Māori*, Pacific and child and youth mental health services. The mental health sector faces particular challenges in recruiting and retaining skilled and experienced staff, which also reflect global factors, such as an international shortage of doctors and mental health nurses. New Zealand trained staff often move overseas and New Zealand must compete with other countries (most notably Australia, Canada and the UK) for new staff. In 2003 there were 5293 FTE mental health positions in the public mental health system and 523 vacancies (Mental Health Commission, 2004). Staff shortages directly impact on service delivery and negatively impact on the ability to achieve previously agreed strategic targets for mental health.

Reflecting a systemic approach, the Workforce Development Framework (Ministry of Health, 2002b) shown in Figure 23.1 identifies five areas that aim to broaden the focus from training to

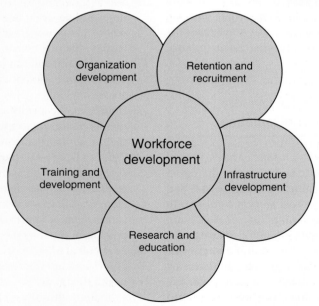

Figure 23.1 *Workforce development framework (Ministry of Health, 2002, p. 21).*

include a more comprehensive approach to the development of the mental health workforce.

# MIGRANTS AND REFUGEES

Almost one in five New Zealanders was born overseas. This rises to one in three in Auckland, where half of the migrant population resides. The highest proportion of Pacific and Asian migrants live in Auckland. The great Tahitian Chief, Kupe, first discovered *Aotearoa* in AD 950. Europeans began arriving after 1769, with organized settlement occurring from 1840 (King, 2003). Visibly different migrants, such as Indians, Chinese and Samoans, became 'others' because of their different physical appearance, religion or culture. Though the first Indians and Chinese came to New Zealand in 1850s and 1860s, fear of the impact of foreigners led to restrictive Acts of Parliament being introduced between 1870 and 1899, such as the Asiatic Restriction Bill 1879 and the Chinese Immigrants Act 1881. These were repealed only when labour market demands increased (Thakur, 1995).

In the last three decades different trends have impacted on migration. The first was an initial increase in migration from the Pacific Islands during the late 1970s and again following the Fiji coup of 1987. Pacific Island migration decreased in the 1990s due to the shrinkage in manufacturing and the closure of factories as trade tariffs were removed. The second trend saw an increase in Asian migration through the encouragement of foreign investment. Refugees arrived from Cambodia and Vietnam and migration from Hong Kong increased as the colony was returned to China. The third trend saw an increase in migration from South Africa and the Middle East. These trends have led to an increase in the number of migrants from non-traditional source areas. Critics such as Thakur (1995) argue that the official rhetoric recognizes the legitimacy of *Māori* and *Pakeha* but excludes migrant cultures that are non-white and non-indigenous, excluding them from the debate on identity and the future of the country in which they live. As Mohanram (1998, p. 21) asks, 'what place does the visibly different coloured immigrant occupy within the discourse of biculturalism?' This tension around inclusion and belonging exists for many other groups as well, for example Wittman (1998, p. 39) has commented 'on the exclusionary effect of any others by the ideology of biculturalism' for Jewish people in New Zealand.

The post-1945 notion of assimilation positioned the ideal migrant as 'invisible'. Migrants were expected to fit in, not change the society they had entered, and so change was one-way. Whilst Canada and Australia embraced multiculturalism during the 1960s, transforming the notion of settlement into a two-way process whereby change was required by both migrants and the host society, New Zealand policy made this strategic move only as recently as 1986. The Immigration Act 1987 eased access into New Zealand from non-traditional source countries and replaced entry criteria based on nationality and culture with ones initially based on skills. This changed in 1991 to a points-based system that saw migrants with experience, skills, qualifications and money being selected for business investment in New Zealand.

Today Asians make up the fastest-growing ethnic population; between 1991 and 2001 the number of people identifying as Asians more than doubled to almost 6.4 per cent of the population. Chinese are the largest ethnic group within the Asian population, followed by Indian and Korean.

Research has identified factors such as unemployment, communication and lack of English proficiency as significant in adjustment. Several studies have found that unemployment or under-employment, having experienced discrimination in New Zealand, not having close friends, being unemployed and spending most of one's time with one's own ethnic group are predictors for poor adjustment among migrant groups (Pernice *et al.*, 2000).

## Pacific people

People from the Pacific Islands began migrating to New Zealand in the 1950s and continued through to a peak in the late 1970s. According to the Mental Health Commission and Ministry of

Health (1999), unemployment, low income, poor housing, the breakdown in family networks, cultural fragmentation and rising alcohol and drug problems have led to increasing concerns about the mental health of Pacific people. An identified priority is to develop a skilled Pacific Island mental health workforce and this initiative has been successful in bringing mature, culturally knowledgeable and bilingual staff into the workforce. These services have facilitated improvements in the delivery of mental health services to Pacific *tangata whai ora*. Recently, *Te Orau Ora: Pacific Mental Health Profile* was published, which is the first document targeted specifically at Pacific people's mental health to be published by the Ministry of Health (2005). It provides demographic and mental health-related information to assist in the planning of cultural specific services.

## Refugees

Refugees who have resettled in New Zealand mostly originate from Africa, the Middle East, South-East Asia and Eastern Europe. A United Nations-mandated quota of 750 refugees per year is accepted, along with approximately the same number of asylum seekers. Increased numbers of immigrants and refugees have led to the formation of specialized mental health services, for example the Refugees as Survivors (RAS) centre. A study of Somali communities in Hamilton found that GPs played a significant role in terms of the mental health of the research sample and were key gatekeepers of health (Guerin *et al.*, 2003).

## Asians

There are no official data available on the mental health of Asians (the use of the term in New Zealand is broader than in the UK and includes people from China and South-East Asia). However, an outcome of a report on the mental health of Asians in New Zealand has been an increase in responsivity to the needs of those communities (Yee, 2003). Research activity, information provision, collaboration and Asian-focused operational activities and policy are some of the strategies that are being used by government agencies (Yee, 2003).

A study among recent Chinese migrants using the General Health Questionnaire found that 19 per cent reported psychiatric morbidity (Abbott *et al.*, 1999). A study of older Chinese migrants aged 55 found that 26 per cent showed depressive symptoms (Abbott *et al.*, 2003). Lower emotional supports, greater number of visits to doctor, difficulties in accessing health services and low New Zealand cultural orientation increased the risk of developing depression. Research with Asian immigrants, refugees and student sojourners in New Zealand shows that social supports can assist newcomers to cope with the stresses of migration and reduce the risk of emotional disorder (Abbott *et al.*, 1999). Conversely, research shows that language and cultural barriers can limit access to health services (Abbott *et al.*, 1999; Ngai *et al.*, 2001).

Asians underutilize mental health services, making up only 1.9 per cent of *tangata whai ora* seen by DHBs in 2002; yet they are more than 6.5% of the population (New Zealand Health Information Service, 2005). The new policy *Te Tāhuhu* acknowledges the need for responsiveness to Asian peoples, other ethnic communities and refugee and migrant communities (De Souza, 2006). There is also an emphasis on developing a culturally capable workforce and developing a research agenda that informs service planning, delivery and training. The Mental Health Commission's Recovery Competencies for Mental Health Workers (O'Hagan, 2001) suggests that competent mental health workers need to demonstrate knowledge of Asian cultures, an understanding of their diversity and the ability to involve Asian families, communities and service users in care. Other initiatives include: the New Zealand Mental Health Foundation's information sheets on the mental health needs of Chinese adults and older Korean people; and there is a project for training Asian interpreters and mental health practitioners serving the diverse Asian immigrant population in the Auckland region (Lim and Walker, 2006). An emergent Asian research agenda will lead to a profile of Asian health needs; for example, the *Asian Health Chart Book* (Ministry of Health, 2006a) suggests a need to focus on longer-term settled migrant Asian communities. Regionally specialized mental health services are being established with unique configurations of 'transcultural' teams or Asian mental health workers. NGOs are at the forefront of responding to the needs of Asian *tangata whai ora*.

## CONCLUSION

Mental health services in New Zealand have many similarities with services elsewhere; however, New Zealand also offers a unique insight into the value of delivering culturally specific services alongside mainstream mental health services. The New Zealand experience also offers a useful case study into the dramatic effects of neo-liberalism, their failure and a subsequent attempt to refocus health care on a more socially constructed basis. Structural and systemic problems clearly exist in New Zealand, as elsewhere. Financial constraints and a shortage of appropriately trained staff continue to impinge on service delivery.

Mental health practice in New Zealand has been significantly influenced and enhanced by consumer participation, ranging from self-help groups and NGO-based service delivery to providing policy input. New Zealand today is a multicultural country with varied ethnic groups but one which is grounded in biculturalism, the relationship between *Māori* and *Pakeha* inherent in the principles of the Treaty of Waitangi. This results in a general acceptance that the incorporation of cultural perspectives in psychiatric services is crucial.

## REFERENCES

Abas, M., Vanderpyl, J., Proux, T.L., Kydd, R., Emery, B. and Foliaki, S.A. 2003: Psychiatric hospitalisation: reason for admission and alternatives to admission in South Auckland, New Zealand. *Australian and New Zealand Journal of Psychiatry* 37, 620–25.

Abbott, M.W., Wong, S., Williams, M., Au, M.K. and Young, W. 1999: Chinese migrants' mental health and adjustment to life in New Zealand. *Australian and New Zealand Journal of Psychiatry* 33, 13–21.

Abbott, M.W., Wong, S., Giles, L.C., Wong, S., Young, W. and Au, M. 2003: Depression in older Chinese migrants to Auckland. *Australian and New Zealand Journal of Psychiatry* 37, 445–51.

Beautrais, A.L., Collings, S.C.D., Ehrhardt, P. and Henare, K. 2005: *Suicide Prevention: A Review of Evidence of Risk and Protective Factors, and Points of Effective Intervention.* Wellington: Ministry of Health.

Bloomfield, J.H. 2001: Dunedin Lunatic Asylum 1863–1873. In Brookes, B. and Thompson, J. (eds) *Unfortunate Folk – Essays on Mental Health Treatment 1863–1992.* Dunedin: University of Otago Press.

Brinded, P.M.J. 2000: Forensic psychiatry in New Zealand. A review. *International Journal of Law and Psychiatry* 23, 453–65.

Cooney, C. 1994: A comparative analysis of transcultural nursing and cultural safety. *Nursing Praxis in New Zealand* 9, 6–12.

Crowe, M. 1997: An analysis of the sociopolitical context of mental health nursing practice. *Australian and New Zealand Journal of Mental Health Nursing* 6, 59–65.

Crowe, M., O'Malley, J. and Gordon, S. 2001: Meeting the needs of consumers in the community: A working partnership in mental health in New Zealand. *Journal of Advanced Nursing* 35, 88–96.

Currier, G.W. 1997: A survey of New Zealand psychiatrists' clinical experience with the Mental Health Act of 1992. *New Zealand Medical Journal* 10, 6–9.

DeSouza, R. 2004: Working with refugees and migrants. In Wepa, D. (ed.) *Cultural Safety.* Auckland: Pearson Education New Zealand, 122–33.

DeSouza, R. 2006: Sailing in a new direction: multicultural mental health in New Zealand. Australian e-Journal for the Advancement of Mental Health 5(2) www.auseinet.com/journal/vol15iss2/desouza.pdf.

Department of Health 1984: Paper presented at the Hui Whakaoranga: Māori health planning workshop. Wellington.

Dew, K. and Kirkman, A. 2002: *Sociology of Health in New Zealand.* Melbourne: Oxford University Press.

Durie, M. 1977: Māori attitudes to sickness, doctors and hospitals. *New Zealand Medical Journal* 86, 483–85.

Durie, M. 1985: Māori health institutions. *Community Mental Health in New Zealand* 2, 63–69.

Durie, M. 1994: *Whaiora: Māori health development.* Auckland: Oxford University Press.

Durie, M. 1997: *Puahou: A Five Point Plan for Improving Māori Mental Health.* Wellington: Māori Mental Health Summit.

Durie, M. 1999: Mental health and Māori development. *Australian and New Zealand Journal of Psychiatry* 33, 5–12.

Gaudin, A. 2004: *Report to the Mental Health Commission: Review of Mental Health Services Expenditure for the Year Ended 30 June 2003.* Wellington: Mental Health Commission.

Guerin, B., Abdi, A. and Guerin, P. 2003: Experiences with the medical and health systems for Somali refugees living in Hamilton. *New Zealand Journal of Psychology* 32, 27–32.

Harre, J. 1968: Mäori-Pakeha intermarriage. In Schwimmer, E. (ed.) *The Mäori People in the Nineteen-Sixties*. Auckland: Longman Paul, 118–31.

Health Funding Authority 2000: *Tuutahitia te wero: Meeting the Challenges – Mental Health Workforce Development Plan 2000–2005*. Christchurch: Health Funding Authority.

Hyslop, J., Downland, J. and Hickling, J. 1983: *Health Facts: New Zealand*. Wellington: Department of Health.

Jacobson, B. 1999: Tackling inequalities in health and health care – the role of NHS. In Gordon, D., Shaw, M., Dorling, D. and Smith, G.D. (eds) *Inequalities in Health. The Evidence*. Bristol: Policy Press, 110–17.

Johnstone, K. and Read, J. 2000: Psychiatrists' recommendations for improving bicultural training and Maori mental health services: A New Zealand Survey. *Australian and New Zealand Journal of Psychiatry* 34, 135–45.

King, M. 2003: *The Penguin History of New Zealand*. Auckland: Penguin Books.

Krieble, T. 2003: Towards an outcome-based mental health policy for New Zealand. *Australasian Psychiatry* 11, S78.

Lim, S. and Walker, R. 2006: *Asian Mental Health Interpreter Workforce Development Project: Report on Curricula & Guidelines Development for Asian Interpreters and Mental Health Practitioners to Work Effectively Together*. Auckland: Northern DHB Support Agency.

Mason, K., Johnston, J. and Crowe, J. 1996: *Inquiry under Section 47 of the Health and Disability Services Act 1993 in Respect of Certain Mental Health Services: Report of the Ministerial Inquiry to the Minister of Health*. Wellington: Ministry of Health.

McCreary, J.R. 1968: Population growth and urbanisation. In Schwimmer, E. (ed.) *The Mäori People in the Nineteen-Sixties*. Auckland: Longman Paul, 187–204.

McPherson, K.M.M., Harwood, M. and McNaughton, H.K. 2003: Ethnicity, equity, and quality: lessons from New Zealand. *British Medical Journal* 327, 443–44.

Mental Health Commission 1998: *Blueprint for Mental Health Services in New Zealand: How Things Need to Be*. Wellington: Mental Health Commission.

Mental Health Commission 1999: *Housing and Mental Health: Reducing Housing Difficulties for People with Mental Illness. Discussion Paper*. Wellington: Mental Health Commission.

Mental Health Commission 2001: *Cultural Assessment Processes for Mäori – Guidance for Mainstream Health Services*. Wellington: Mental Health Commission.

Mental Health Commission 2004: *Annual Report of the Mental Health Commission for the Year Ended 30 June 2004*. Wellington: Mental Health Commission.

Mental Health Commission and Ministry of Health 1999: *Developing the Mental Health Workforce: The Report of the National Mental Health Workforce Development Coordinating Committee*. Wellington: Mental Health Commission and Ministry of Health.

Ministry of Health 1994: *Looking Forward: Strategic Directions for Mental Health Services*. Wellington: Ministry of Health.

Ministry of Health 1995: *A Guide to Effective Consumer Participation in Mental Health Services*. Wellington: Ministry of Health.

Ministry of Health 2002a: *Te puawaitanga: Mäori Mental Health National Strategic Framework*. Wellington: Ministry of Health.

Ministry of Health 2002b: *Mental Health (Alcohol and Other Drugs) Workforce Development Framework*. Wellington: Ministry of Health.

Ministry of Health 2003: *New Zealand Health Strategy: District Health Board Toolkit, Mental Health*. Wellington: Ministry of Health.

Ministry of Health 2005a: *Te Orau Ora: Pacific Mental Health Profile*. Wellington: Ministry of Health.

Ministry of Health 2005b: *Draft Action Plan Te Tähuhu – Improving Mental Health 2005–2015: The Second New Zealand Mental Health and Addiction Plan*. Wellington: Ministry of Health.

Ministry of Health 2006a: *Asian Health Chart Book 2006*. Wellington: Ministry of Health.

Ministry of Health 2006b: *Te Kökiri: The Mental Health and Addiction Action Plan 2006–2015*. Wellington: Ministry of Health.

Ministry of Youth Development 2004: *Guidelines for Primary Care Providers: Detection and Management of Young People at Risk of Suicide*. Wellington: Ministry of Youth Development.

Mohanram, R. 1998: (In)visible bodies? Immigrant bodies and constructions of nationhood in Aotearoa/New Zealand. In Plessis, R.D. and Alice, L. (eds) *Feminist Thought in Aotearoa, New Zealand*. Auckland: Oxford University Press, 21–29.

New Zealand Health Information Service 2005: *Mental Health: Service Use in New Zealand 2002*. Wellington: Ministry of Health.

Ngai, M.M.Y., Latimer, S. and Cheung, V.Y.M. 2001: *Healthcare Needs of Asian People: Surveys of Asian People and Health Professionals in the North and West Auckland*. Takapuna: Asian Health Support Service, Waitemata District Health Board.

O'Hagan, K. 2001: *Cultural Competence in the Caring Professions*. London: Jessica Kingsley.

Peace, R. and Kell, S. 2001: Mental health and housing research: Housing needs and sustainable independent living. *Social Policy Journal of New Zealand* 17, 101–23.

Pernice, R., Trlin, A., Henderson, A. and North, N. 2000: Employment and mental health of three groups of immigrants to New Zealand. *New Zealand Journal of Psychology* 29, 24–29.

Pomare, E.W. 1986: Mäori health: New concepts and initiatives. *New Zealand Medical Journal* 99, 410–11.

Pomare, E.W. and deBoer, G. 1988: *Hauroa: Mäori Standards of Health: A Study of the Years 1970–1984*. Wellington: Department of Health.

Sachdev, P. 1989: Psychiatric illness in the New Zealand Mäori. *Australian and New Zealand Journal of Psychiatry* 23, 529–41.

Sachdev, P. 1998: The New Zealand Mäori and the contemporary health system. Response of an indigenous people to mainstream medicine. In Okpaku, S.O. (ed.) *Clinical Methods in Transcultural Psychiatry*. Washington, DC: American Psychiatric Press, 111–36.

Saul, J.R. 2005: *The Collapse of Globalism and the Reinvention of the World*. London: Penguin.

Statistics New Zealand 2005: *National Population Estimates (December 2004 quarter) – Hot Off The Press*. Available online: www2.stats.govt.nz/domino/external/pasfull/pasfull.nsf/web/Hot+Off+The+Press+National+Population+Estimates+December+2004+quarter?open (accessed 9 September 2005).

Stuart, G., Minas, I.H., Klimidis, S. and Connell, S.O. 1996: English language ability and mental health service utilization: a census. *Australian and New Zealand Journal of Psychiatry* 30, 270–77.

Sullivan, K. 1994: Bicultural education in Aotearoa/New Zealand. In Manson, H. (ed.) *New Zealand Annual Review of Education/Te arotake a tau o te ao o te mataurangi i Aotearoa*. Wellington: Victoria University.

Te Matorohanga, M. 1913: Te kauae raro. *Journal of the Polynesian Society* 4, 118–33.

Te Rau Matatini 2004: *About Te Rau Matatini*. Available online: www.matatini.co.nz/aboutTRM/aboutTRM.htm (accessed 6 June 2004).

Thakur, R. 1995: In defence of multiculturalism. In Greif, S.W. (ed.) *Immigration and National Identity in New Zealand: One People, Two Peoples, Many Peoples*. Palmerston North: Dunmore Press, 255–81.

Wittman, L.K. 1998: *Interactive Identities; Jewish Women in New Zealand*. Palmerston North: Dunmore Press.

Worley, N. 1997: *Mental Health Nursing in the Community*. St Louis: Mosby.

Yee, B. 2003: *Asian Mental Health Recovery – Follow Up to the Asian Report*. Wellington: Mental Health Commission.

# GLOSSARY

| | |
|---|---|
| *Aotearoa* | Lit. 'Land of the long white cloud'. The *Mäori* term for New Zealand |
| *Hapu* | Subtribe |
| *Iwi* | Tribe |
| *Kaupapa [Mäori]* | The philosophy of *Mäori* knowledge and learning |
| *Mäori* | The indigenous people of *Aotearoa*/New Zealand |
| *Marae* | Communal meeting house (for *iwi* or *hapu*) |
| *Pakeha* | Europeans and other non-*Mäori* |
| *Tangata whenua* | *Mäori*, literally, the people of the land |
| *Tapu* | Sacred, to be treated with respect, a restriction, being with potentiality for power, integrity |
| *Te reo [Mäori]* | The *Mäori* language |
| *Tohunga* | A spiritual adviser and traditional healer |
| *Whänau* | Extended family |
| *Whenua* | The land |

# 24

# The culture of deterrence: the mental health impact of Australia's asylum policies

Derrick Silove and Zachary Steel

## INTRODUCTION

Since World War II, psychiatry has taken a strong interest in the mental health of refugees displaced by persecution, war and other forms of conflict (Eitinger and Grunfeld, 1966; Krupinski et al., 1973). The field is complex, drawing on concepts from diverse disciplines, including transcultural and disaster psychiatry, human rights, traumatology and models of international development (Silove, 1999).

Australia has played a pivotal role as a recipient country of refugees, admitting more displaced persons per capita since World War II than most other Western countries (Department of Immigration and Multicultural Affairs, 2001). Australia's shift in the 1990s towards a policy of deterring asylum seekers (Silove et al., 2000) therefore represents a radical change in direction, with the psycho-social consequences offering lessons to other countries considering adopting such approaches. Here, we consider how these policy changes have affected the mental health and psycho-social adjustment of refugees and the consequent impact this shift has had on the roles and modes of operation of mental health professionals working in the field (Silove, 2002; Steel et al., 2004a).

## HISTORY SINCE WORLD WAR II

In the wake of World War II, Australia accepted a large number of displaced persons from Europe, as did other Western countries (Department of Immigration and Multicultural Affairs, 2001). The influx profoundly altered the ethnic composition of the settler population, which previously was almost entirely of Anglo-Celtic background. There was some prejudice against the non-English-speaking newcomers (referred to colloquially as 'reffos') but most of the displaced persons and their offspring became well-integrated into the host community, thereby laying the foundations for the future policy of multiculturalism. Nevertheless, in parallel, a 'White Australian' policy remained in place until the 1970s (in spite of the indigenous population being black), with successive waves of refugees and migrants being from Caucasian backgrounds.

A key historical shift occurred with the influx of South-East Asian refugees after the fall of Saigon in 1975. Although their arrival triggered some initial communal unease in Australia, the administration of the time adopted a receptive policy, offering the Vietnamese, Cambodian and Lao refugees permanent residency, family reunion, and access to the full array of educational, welfare, health and occupational services (Lee, 1997; Lewins and Ly, 1985).

A recent epidemiological study (Steel *et al.*, 2005) has demonstrated how well the Vietnamese have adapted to their new country. Vietnamese refugees reported a stepwise reduction in symptoms the longer they had been resettled in Australia, with that pattern of improvement applying even to those who suffered the most severe war trauma (Steel *et al.*, 2002). At the time of the study in 2001, the prevalence of post-traumatic stress disorder (PTSD) (1.5 per cent) was no higher than amongst the Australian-born population. These results suggest, albeit indirectly, that the policy of receptiveness applied to Vietnamese refugees may have contributed substantially to their post-settlement trajectory of improved mental health.

## DEVELOPMENT OF SPECIALIST MENTAL HEALTH SERVICES

It was during that epoch of receptiveness to refugees that torture and trauma services were established in all the states of Australia. The country is one of only a few worldwide that maintains an active offshore refugee programme, accepting for permanent settlement an annual quota of 13 000 refugees screened overseas. In the 1980s, it became apparent that there were no specialist mental health services to deal with the traumatic stress reactions that some of these refugees suffered. It was in the spirit of optimism about the potential to assist these traumatized refugees (Somnier and Genefke,

1986) that Australian mental health professionals joined the international movement to develop specialist torture and trauma rehabilitation services to fill that gap (Reid *et al.*, 1990; Silove *et al.*, 1991). The two largest centres are based in Sydney (Service for the Treatment and Rehabilitation of Torture and Trauma Survivors – STARTTS) and Melbourne (Victorian Service for Torture Survivors), with a network of smaller services operating in other states and territories of the country. Throughout its period of operation, STARTTS (the service with which the present authors are affiliated) has received funding from the state government of New South Wales, with the federal government contributing to special programmes, most recently to an innovative Early Intervention Program which offers screening, referral, resettlement and acculturation programmes, and short-term counselling to newly arrived refugees.

From the outset, STARTTS adopted a model that offered both direct clinical interventions (various forms of psychotherapy, psychiatric services, family therapy, somatotherapy) as well as targeted community development activities. The cultural focus has been a key element (Aroche and Coello, 2004; Silove and Kinzie, 2001), with the early adoption of a bicultural counsellor model first pioneered at the Indochinese Psychiatric Clinic in Boston (Mollica, 1988). Until the early 1990s, there was a strong sense of common purpose and intersectoral collaboration between the torture and trauma services and state and federal government departments. Overall, there was a national consensus that refugees should be treated with compassion and respect, a principle based on two decades of political developments during which Australia's foundations of multiculturalism and promotion of human rights had been consolidated.

## SHIFT IN ASYLUM POLICY

The early 1990s marked a watershed with a fundamental shift in Australia's approach to dealing with refugees. At the time, there was an increase in the number of asylum seekers entering Australia and other Western nations (United Nations High

Commissioner for Refugees, 2000). Unlike quota or 'offshore' refugees, asylum seekers ('onshore' refugees) applied for protection once they entered the country. Recipient countries of the West began instituting 'policies of humane deterrence', aimed at discouraging asylum arrivals (Silove *et al.*, 2000). In Australia, legislation was adopted to limit the rights of asylum seekers living in the community, by restricting their access to health services, work opportunities, education, government-funded welfare support and ability to reunite with their families.

In addition, Australia stood alone in introducing mandatory detention based solely on the mode of entry (unauthorized arrival by boat or without valid entry documents) rather than on the strength of refugee claims or degree of persecution experienced. That policy disadvantaged those who had to flee under extreme duress, since they were more likely to leave their homelands without passports or temporary entry visas and hence be detained at the border (Steel and Silove, 2001).

Until recently, detention was indefinite, non-reviewable by courts of law and applied equally to adults and children. Provisions for releasing certain categories of detainees, such as those who had been severely tortured, have been applied in only a few exceptional circumstances. Newcomers to the country, many of whom do not speak English or understand the culture, are bewildered and disorientated by being immediately confined in remote detention compounds with restricted contact with family, and no access to meaningful cultural, leisure or occupational activities to help pass the time. As the 1990s progressed, Immigration Reception and Processing Centers (IRPCs) were expanded, often being located in remote semi-desert areas, far from services and compatriot communities who live in the larger coastal cities. The IRPCs are run by a multinational private prison corporation and have been built as prisons, surrounded by double layers of razor wire and palisade fencing. Inmates are regimented, commonly being identified by numbers rather than by names, and subjected to multiple daily headcounts, and night musters and searches. Strict behavioural management regimes to control dissent and to manage suicidal tendencies were implemented using physical constraint

and solitary confinement in 'management units', where detainees could be held in isolation for weeks or months. Rapid response units were staffed by officers equipped with full riot gear to physically subdue and apprehend 'trouble makers'. Successive commissions of inquiry have detailed inadequacies and neglect in the provision of basic services within IRPCs including general and mental health care (Commonwealth Ombudsman, 2001; Human Rights and Equal Opportunity Commmission, 1998, 2004; Koutroulis, 2003; Silove, 2002; Silove *et al.*, 2001). Multiple ethnic groups are held together even where there are known historical tensions amongst them. Until recently, women and children have been housed in general compounds along with adult male detainees.

In 1999, the tradition of offering permanent protection to asylum seekers found to be genuine refugees was overturned, with new legislation creating a category of temporary protection visas (TPVs). This meant that many asylum seekers who had spent years in detention found that, in spite of the refugee claims finally being successful, they were only offered three-year visas with the likelihood of their being forcibly repatriated after that time. People given a TPV are prohibited from family reunion, provisions that are available to permanent refugees. They are restricted in their access to resettlement assistance services and they are refused the right of return to Australia if they travel overseas; for example, to attend to a sick family member. The most serious consequence of the new policy, however, is that people given a TPV live in constant fear that they will be forcibly repatriated and hence lack the security to create a new life in Australia for themselves and their children.

## IMPACT ON MENTAL HEALTH

### Theoretical underpinnings

Soon after the introduction of detention, cases came to light of asylum seekers exhibiting marked deterioration in their mental state after being confined (Becker and Silove, 1993; Silove *et al.*, 1993), raising concerns that the conditions in detention were leading to the re-traumatization of survivors who had experienced past abuses. Those living in the community also were noted to manifest severe stress reactions related to their insecure status. These observations led our group to initiate a decade of research which has had theoretical, policy-related and direct service implications. Our initial clinical observations recast our perspectives on the avoidance and arousal symptoms typical of PTSD, since these responses appeared to be normative and potentially adaptive in asylum seekers, manifesting universally across cultural groups and fluctuating according to the immediacy of the threat. For example, if an asylum seeker received news of a further legal setback in pursuing a refugee claim, symptoms invariably worsened.

We also considered the possibility that the third domain of PTSD symptoms, the intrusive imagery (flashbacks, nightmares), may represent primitive survival-learning mechanisms that were functionally important (Silove, 1998). Rehearsing memories of the threat and thereby triggering flight and fight survival mechanisms would ensure a rapid response to re-exposure, either to the real threat or to analogous environments. In that sense, the post-traumatic stress reaction may be conceptualized as having its roots in a teleologically meaningful and future-oriented survival response, preparing the human – albeit in a rigid and stereotypic way – to deal with later danger by encoding a catalogue of readily retrievable threat memories. The corollary of this general theory is that if asylum seekers exposed to past trauma such as torture and incarceration are re-exposed to conditions such as detention that constantly trigger these memories in a threatening environment, then there is little potential for therapeutic interventions to resolve the consequent primitive survival reaction, the clinical correlate being that PTSD symptoms are resistant to change.

## Empirical studies

Commencing in the mid-1990s, our group initiated a series of studies of asylum seekers living in the community (Silove et al., 1997, 1998, 2002, 2006), and two amongst detainees (Thompson et al., 1998;

Steel et al., 2004b). More recently, we have conducted two studies examining the psycho-social impact of temporary protection (Momartin et al., 2006; Steel et al., 2005).

### Asylum seekers in the community

Asylum seekers are a hidden minority often alienated from mainstream society, making studies in the field a particular challenge to researchers who aim to apply rigorous sampling methods. As a consequence, we have used targeted sampling strategies, recruiting asylum seekers from a support centre (Silove et al., 1997), by snowball sampling (Silove et al., 1998), and through an outreach service linked to STARTTS (Silove et al., 2002). To achieve greater representativeness, our recently completed study (Silove et al., 2006) recruited a random sample of immigration agents as the source of our asylum sample, since almost all refugee applicants consult these people in Australia.

In all studies, we applied a purpose-designed post-migration life difficulties checklist in addition to standard measures of past trauma, PTSD, depression and anxiety. In keeping with research in the general refugee field (Chung and Kagawa-Singer, 1993; Mollica et al., 1998; de Jong et al., 2001; Steel et al., 2002), we found a consistent and predictable relationship between pre-migration trauma and psychiatric ill-health, particularly ongoing PTSD. In addition, however, in all studies, post-migration stresses contributed substantially to adverse psychiatric outcomes. The longer asylum seekers lived in Australia, the more severe their symptoms, a finding corroborated by a study in the Netherlands (Laban et al., 2004). In a path analysis (Steel et al., 1999), we showed that key post-migration stresses (insecure residency/fear of repatriation; acculturation stress; and socio-economic deprivation/poor access to services) all contributed independently to ongoing PTSD symptoms, even when exposure to past trauma was taken into account.

In a study amongst Tamils from Sri Lanka, we were able to compare asylum seekers with compatriot refugees and immigrants who were permanently resettled. Asylum seekers manifested much higher levels of PTSD, depression and anxiety, even when past trauma was taken into account.

## Detention

Administrative obstacles have limited the capacity of researchers to gain access to detention centres in spite of calls by national bodies such as the Australian Medical Association (Australian Medical Association, 2001) to allow the health status of detainees to be investigated. Nevertheless, in the early years of the detention policy, torture and trauma experts were able to document the clinical status of two detainee groups from East Timor (Victorian Foundation for Survivors of Torture, 1998) and Sri Lanka (Thompson *et al.*, 1998). Both studies showed unusually high levels of post-traumatic stress, depression, anxiety and, in particular, suicidality (suicidal thinking and behaviour). In the Tamil study, the rates of psychiatric morbidity amongst detainees were much higher than those reported by compatriot asylum seekers living in the community.

Subsequently, an Iraqi doctor, a long-term detainee, undertook a participant-observer study of inmates held for over two years in a detention centre in Sydney (Sultan and O'Sullivan, 2001). He documented a progressive and universal deterioration in mental health, the longer asylum seekers were held in detention. All eventually lost hope and descended into a state of severe, vegetative depression.

In a more recent study, all family members of one ethnic group held for a prolonged period in a remote detention centre were interviewed by phone by same-language psychologists using structured interviews (Steel *et al.*, 2004b). Lifetime histories indicated moderate levels of PTSD and depression in adults and their children prior to detention, rates that were equivalent to those expected of refugee populations. The rates in detention, however, had increased substantially, with 100 per cent of adults and children receiving at least one psychiatric diagnosis and with co-morbidity being common. Both age groups reported experiences in detention that coincided with media reports, namely, exposure to prison-like conditions with head counts and daily musters, being called by number rather than name, lack of respect for culture and religion, and exposure to violence, riots, public displays of self-mutilation and suicidal behaviour, hunger strikes, and intimidation by guards.

A parallel study (Mares and Jureidini, 2004) undertaken by mental health clinicians providing care to ten family groups held in detention documented similarly high levels of psychiatric morbidity. All children aged 6–16 were diagnosed with PTSD attributable to experiences in detention while the majority (80 per cent) of pre-school age children displayed marked developmental delays and various forms of emotional disturbance.

## Temporary protection

Our group has also completed two studies of asylum seekers who were found to be *bona fide* refugees and who were then offered temporary protection status. The first study applied a multilevel statistical method to data obtained from refugees on a TPV and those on permanent visas who were members of an ethnic minority, the Mandaeans, originating from Iran (Steel *et al.*, in press). The key determinants of ongoing PTSD that emerged were past detention and ongoing TPV status, predictors that remained robust even when other correlates such as family composition and past trauma were taken into account. A second, clinic-based study supports these findings, indicating that the combination of TPV status and past detention is a powerful determinant of ongoing PTSD and related psychiatric disabilities (Momartin *et al.*, 2006).

## IMPLICATIONS FOR MENTAL HEALTH PROFESSIONALS AND SERVICES

As indicated, the recent history of refugee mental health in Australia as in other countries such as the UK has been strongly influenced by asylum policy. In the 1980s, the pioneering period in establishing torture and trauma rehabilitation services for refugees was marked by consensus and collaboration with government. Co-operation continues in providing services for permanent refugees accepted according to Australia's offshore quota programme. At the same time, once policies of deterrence were introduced in the early 1990s, the culture of co-operation changed, with mental health professionals feeling compelled to take a public stand on human rights grounds about the treatment of onshore asylum applicants (Silove *et al.*, 1993; Professional Alliance for the Health of Asylum Seekers and their Children, 2003).

The consequences for service interventions have been profound. For permanently resettled refugees, torture and trauma services continue to offer an array of services, focusing not only on treating PTSD and related psychiatric disorders, but also on acculturation and resettlement issues. STARTTS has initiated a range of innovative programmes including a manualized Family in Cultural Transition group programme (Silove *et al.*, 2005) that assists whole families to gain skills in a range of areas, including dealing with services, changes in cultural expectations, gender and childhood development, and understanding local customs. The overriding philosophy of the community development programme is to support emerging refugee communities in maintaining their culture and traditions while achieving competence in living in the wider, mainstream society.

The contrast in working with asylum seekers is stark. Even though many asylum seekers are from the same backgrounds as their permanently resettled compatriots in terms of culture and traumatic histories, the approach to interventions for the former group, of necessity, is different. For example, the major challenge in working with East Timorese asylum seekers was to overcome their profound distrust of and alienation from the mainstream society, based on years of conflict with the Australian government about their refugee status (Silove *et al.*, 2002). To engage the community, we developed a researcher-advocacy model which aimed to achieve several outcomes: to win the trust of the community; to document their past persecution so that their leaders were better placed to advocate on their community's behalf for a more sympathetic understanding of their plight; to support the documentation needed in advancing refugee claims; to develop networks of voluntary services in health and social support for a group that was restricted in its access to government services; and to provide immediate mental health care for those who reached crisis point because of their insecure residency status. In direct work with individual asylum seekers, the relevance of the re-traumatization hypothesis is often clear: each legal

setback in the prolonged and complex process of seeking asylum leads predictably to a recurrence of PTSD and depressive symptoms, at times resulting in a psychiatric emergency often associated with suicidal urges. Psychiatric interventions often involve supporting traumatized asylum seekers through successive crises without the expectation of a durable remission from PTSD symptoms until their legal status is clarified, a process that can take many years (Silove, 2002; Steel *et al.*, 2004a).

## POLICY OUTCOMES AND LESSONS

After years of advocacy by key sectors of society, including the medical profession, and recent public outcry triggered by the mistaken confinement of an Australian citizen with mental illness in an IRPC, the Australian government tempered its detention policy in mid-2005, releasing all children and their families and implementing a review process for long-term detainees. While the reforms failed to address a number of key concerns about the management of the centres or to abolish the practice of detention, the changes nevertheless represent a major shift in policy in a setting that appeared entirely intransigent. It is noteworthy that the documentation and advocacy by mental health professionals played a pivotal role in prompting this policy change.

At a theoretical level, the social experiment applied to asylum seekers in Australia has the potential to cast theoretical light on the ecosocial factors that can perpetuate traumatic stress reactions, potentially revealing the functional if primitive underpinnings of the symptoms we refer to as PTSD. In particular, PTSD may have its roots in survival-learning substrates in the brain, a memory bank that can be repeatedly rekindled by threats that are analogous to the initial exposure. Hence, the consequent state of avoidance and arousal can become chronic and dysfunctional, in settings where threat is prolonged and uncontrollable.

More specifically, the overall lessons that can be derived from the Australian experience is that asylum seekers and refugees can adapt well to their adopted societies if offered conditions of security

(Silove, 1999, 2004; Steel *et al.*, 2002): to live in safety, to reunite with families, to be treated with justice; to have the opportunity to preserve cultural identities while establishing new roles in the host society; and to pursue their chosen traditions, cultural rituals and religious practices. Where conditions of insecurity are imposed on asylum seekers, the consequences are the perpetuation of psychiatric disability and alienation, a wastage of the human potential that displaced populations have to offer host societies. The impact on the fabric of host countries in the developed world is also of concern, with contemporary asylum policies potentially undermining the foundations of multiculturalism and human rights on which modern, pluralistic societies are built.

## REFERENCES

Aroche, J. and Coello, M. 2004: Ethnocultural considerations in the treatment of refugees and asylum seekers. In Wilson, J.P. and Drozdek, B. (eds) *Broken Spirits: The Treatment of Traumatised Asylum Seekers, Refugees, War and Torture Survivors*. New York: Brunner-Routledge, 53–80.

Australian Medical Association 2001: Media release, 8 August: *Asylum Seekers Should have Access to Quality Health Services Under Medicare*. http://www.ama.com.au/web.nsf/doc/WEEN-5GB46R (accessed 8 January 2007).

Becker, R. and Silove, D. 1993: Psychiatric and psycho-social effects of prolonged detention on asylum-seekers. In Crock, M. (ed.) *Protection or Punishment: the Detention of Asylum-Seekers in Australia*. Sydney: The Federation Press, 46–63.

Chung, R.C. and Kagawa-Singer, M. 1993: Predictors of psychological distress among southeast Asian refugees. *Social Science and Medicine* 36, 631–39.

Commonwealth Ombudsman 2001: *Report of an Own Motion Investigation into The Department of Immigration and Multicultural Affairs' Immigration Detention Centres*. Canberra: Commonwealth of Australia.

de Jong, J.T., Komproe, I.H., van Ommeren, M., El Masri, M., Araya, M., Khaled, N., van De Put, W. and Somasundaram, D. 2001: Lifetime events and posttraumatic stress disorder in 4 postconflict settings. *Journal of the American Medical Association* 286, 555–62.

Department of Immigration and Multicultural Affairs 2001: *Immigration Federation to Century's End 1901–2000*. Canberra: Commonwealth of Australia.

Eitinger, L. and Grunfeld, B. 1966: Psychoses among refugees in Norway. *Acta Psychiatrica Scandinavica* 42, 315–28.

Human Rights and Equal Opportunity Commission 1998: *Those Who've Come Across the Seas: The Report of the Commission's Inquiry into the Detention of Unauthorised Arrivals*. Canberra: Commonwealth of Australia.

Human Rights and Equal Opportunity Commission 2004: *A Last Resort? National Inquiry into Children in Immigration Detention*. Sydney: Human Rights and Equal Opportunity Commission.

Koutroulis, G. 2003: Detained asylum seekers, health care, and questions of human(e)ness. *Australian and New Zealand Journal of Public Health* 27, 381–84.

Krupinski, J., Stoller, A. and Wallace, L. 1973: Psychiatric disorders in East European refugees now in Australia. *Social Science and Medicine* 7, 31–49.

Laban, C.J., Gernaat, H.B., Komproe, I.H., Schreuders, B.A. and de Jong, J.T. 2004: Impact of a long asylum procedure on the prevalence of psychiatric disorders in Iraqi asylum seekers in the Netherlands. *Journal of Nervous and Mental Disease* 192, 843–51.

Lee, G.Y. 1997: *Indochinese Refugee Families in Australia: A Multicultural Perspective*. Sydney: Ethnic Affairs Commission of NSW.

Lewins, F. and Ly, J. 1985: *The First Wave: The Settlement of Australia's First Vietnamese Refugees*. Sydney: Allen and Unwin.

Mares, S. and Jureidini, J. 2004: Psychiatric assessment of children and families in immigration detention: clinical, administrative and ethical issues. *Australian and New Zealand Journal of Public Health* 28.

Mollica, R.F. 1988: The trauma story: The psychiatric care of refugee survivors of violence and torture. In Ochberg, F.M. (ed.) *Post-traumatic Therapy and Victims of Violence Brunner/Mazel Psychosocial Stress Series, No. 11*. Philadelphia, PA: Brunner/Mazel, 295–314.

Mollica, R.F., McInnes, K., Poole, C. and Tor, S. 1998: Dose-effect relationships of trauma to symptoms of depression and post-traumatic stress disorder among Cambodian survivors of mass violence. *British Journal of Psychiatry* 173, 482–88.

Momartin, S., Steel, Z., Coello, M., Aroche, J., Silove, D. and Brooks, R. 2006: A comparison of mental health of refugees with temporary versus permanent protection visas. *Medical Journal of Australia* 185(7), 357–61.

Professional Alliance for the Health of Asylum Seekers and their Children 2003: Summary and Recommendations from A National Summit 'Forgotten Rights – Responding to the Crisis in Asylum Seeker Health Care', 12 November, 2003. http://www.nswiop.nsw.edu.au/asylum_seekers.htm (accessed 2 February 2004).

Reid, J., Silove, D. and Tarn, R. 1990: The development of a NSW Service for the Treatment and Rehabilitation of Torture and Trauma Survivors (STARTTS): experience of the first year.

*Australian and New Zealand Journal of Psychiatry* 24, 486–95.

Silove, D. 1998: Is posttraumatic stress disorder an overlearnt survival response? An evolutionary-learning hypothesis. *Psychiatry* 61, 181–90.

Silove, D. 1999: The psychosocial effects of torture, mass human rights violations, and refugee trauma: toward an integrated conceptual framework. *Journal of Nervous and Mental Disease* 187, 200–207.

Silove, D. 2002: The asylum debacle in Australia: a challenge for psychiatry. *Australian and New Zealand Journal of Psychiatry* 36, 290–96.

Silove, D. 2004: The challenges facing mental health programs for post-conflict and refugee communities. *Prehospital and Disaster Medicine* 19, 90–96.

Silove, D. and Kinzie, J.D. 2001: Survivors of war trauma, mass violence, and civilian terror. In Gerrity, E., Keane, T.M. and Tuma, F. (eds) *The Mental Health Consequences of Torture.* New York: Kluwer Academic/Plenum, 159–74.

Silove, D., Tarn, R., Bowles, R. and Reid, J. 1991: Psychosocial needs of torture survivors. *Australian and New Zealand Journal of Psychiatry* 25, 481–90.

Silove, D., McIntosh, P. and Becker, R. 1993: Risk of retraumatisation of asylum-seekers in Australia. *Australian and New Zealand Journal of Psychiatry* 27, 606–12.

Silove, D., Sinnerbrink, I., Field, A., Manicavasagar, V. and Steel, Z. 1997: Anxiety, depression and PTSD in asylum seekers: associations with pre-migration trauma and post-migration stressors. *British Journal of Psychiatry* 170, 351–57.

Silove, D., Steel, Z., McGorry, P. and Mohan, P. 1998: Psychiatric symptoms and living difficulties in Tamil asylum seekers: comparisons with refugees and immigrants. *Acta Psychiatrica Scandinavica* 97, 175–81.

Silove, D., Steel, Z. and Watters, C. 2000: Policies of deterrence and the mental health of asylum seekers in western countries. *Journal of the American Medical Association* 284, 604–11.

Silove, D., Steel, Z. and Mollica, R. 2001: Detention of asylum seekers: assault on health, human rights, and social development. *Lancet* 357, 1436–37.

Silove, D., Coello, M., Tang, K., Aroche, J., Soares, M., Lingam, R., Chaussivert, M., Manicavasagar, V. and Steel, Z. 2002: Towards a researcher-advocacy model for asylum seekers: A pilot study amongst East Timorese living in Australia. *Transcultural Psychiatry* 39, 452–68.

Silove, D., Manicavagasgar, V., Coello, M. and Aroche, J. 2005: PTSD and acculturation. *Interventions: International Journal of Mental Health, Psychosocial Work and Counselling in Areas of Armed Conflict* 3(1), 46–50.

Silove, D., Steel, Z., Susljik, I., Frommer, N., Loneragan, C., Brooks, R. *et al.* 2006: Torture, mental health status and the outcomes of refugee applications amongst recently arrived asylum seekers in Australia. *International Journal of Migration, Health and Social Care* 2(1), 4–14.

Somnier, F.E. and Genefke, I.K. (1986): Psychotherapy for victims of torture. *British Journal of Psychiatry* 149, 323–29.

Steel, Z. and Silove, D.M. 2001: The mental health implications of detaining asylum seekers. *Medical Journal of Australia* 175, 596–99.

Steel, Z., Silove, D., Bird, K., McGorry, P. and Mohan, P. 1999: Pathways from war trauma to posttraumatic stress symptoms among Tamil asylum seekers, refugees and immigrants. *Journal of Traumatic Stress* 12, 421–35.

Steel, Z., Silove, D., Phan, T. and Bauman, A. 2002: Long-term effect of psychological trauma on the mental health of Vietnamese refugees resettled in Australia: a population-based study. *Lancet* 360, 1056–62.

Steel, Z., Mares, S., Newman, L., Blick, B. and Dudley, M. 2004a: The politics of asylum and immigration detention: advocacy, ethics and the professional role of the therapist. In Wilson, J.P. and Drozdek, B. (eds) *Broken Spirits: The Treatment of Traumatised Asylum Seekers, Refugees, War and Torture Survivors.* New York: Brunner-Routledge, 659–87.

Steel, Z., Momartin, S., Bateman, C., Hafshejani, A., Silove, D., Everson, N., Roy. K., Dudley, M., Newman, L., Blick, B. and Mares, S. 2004b: Psychiatric status of asylum seeker families held for a protracted period in a remote detention centre in Australia. *Australian and New Zealand Journal of Public Health* 28, 23–32.

Steel, Z., Silove, D.M., Chey, T., Bauman, A., Phan, T. and Phan, T. 2005: Mental disorders, disability and health service use amongst Vietnamese refugees and the host Australian population. *Acta Psychiatrica Scandinavica* 111(4), 300–309.

Steel, Z., Silove, D., Brooks, R., Momartin, S., Alzuhairi, B. and Susljik, I. 2006: The impact of immigration detention and temporary protection on the mental health of refugees. *British Journal of Psychiatry* 188(1), 58–64.

Sultan, A. and O'Sullivan, K. 2001: Psychological disturbances in asylum seekers held in long term detention: a participant-observer account. *Medical Journal of Australia* 175, 593–96.

Thompson, M., McGorry, P., Silove, D. and Steel, Z. 1998: Maribyrnong Detention Centre Tamil survey. In Silove, D.M. and Steel, Z. (eds) *The Mental Health and Well-Being of On-Shore Asylum Seekers in Australia.* Sydney, Australia: Psychiatry Research and Teaching Unit, 27–31.

United Nations High Commissioner for Refugees 2000: *State of the World's Refugees: Fifty years of Humanitarian Intervention.* Oxford, UK: Oxford University Press.

Victorian Foundation for Survivors of Torture 1998: The East Timorese: clinical and social assessments of applicants for asylum. In Silove, D.M. and Steel, Z. (eds) *The Mental Health and Well-Being of On-Shore Asylum Seekers in Australia.* Sydney, Australia: Psychiatry Research and Teaching Unit, 23–27.

# 25

# Multicultural mental health in Australia

## Beverley Raphael

## INTRODUCTION

This chapter explores culture and mental health in Australian peoples, and progresses a global understanding of the relationship between culture and mental health based on these regional peoples and contexts. The understanding of culture and its relationship to mental health can be viewed from many different perspectives. These range from its representation as patterns of values, beliefs, personal behaviours and social ritual, to considerations of phenomena identified as characteristic of particular nationalities, or ethnic, racial or religious groupings. Culture may also be applied to certain stages of development, for instance 'youth culture' or geographical areas, for instance rural or 'bush' cultures in Australia. Language has constituted one variable that can preserve and transmit cultural meanings, separateness and uniqueness. Distance, isolation and restrictive borders may also contain cultures or preserve them in certain forms. Therefore, definitions of culture need to be closely tied to the regions and the peoples to whom these definitions apply.

While definitions of culture frequently include the concept of vertical transmission of values,

beliefs and expectations of behaviour from one generation to the next, values, beliefs, personal behaviour and social rituals will also be shaped by horizontal forces such as developmental demand at stages of the life cycle, and in response to major social forces such as war-time, baby boomer generations, mass communication developments such as the internet and so forth. It is important to recognize that there are many cultural interfaces, diverse multiculturalisms and significant global forces which may shape the cultural mix, and may have psychological and social impacts. These can lead to particular developments in the personal spheres of social and emotional wellbeing and mental health, and enhanced social capital; or alternatively, can impact negatively, bringing psychological trauma, loss and dislocation to individuals, or conflict, social disruption and even destruction to communities, for instance through tragedies of 'ethnic cleansing' or even genocide.

Australia could be said to be one of the most multicultural countries with 30 per cent of the population identifying themselves as being of culturally and linguistically diverse backgrounds. Languages other than English are the primary language spoken at home by at least 15 per cent of the population, and more than two and a half million residents were born in countries where English was not the first language. Most of the world's religions are practised in Australia and over 200 languages are spoken by Australians of culturally and linguistically diverse backgrounds. Many different government, non-government, academic and community agencies and structures support these directions. One of the most notable is the public broadcasting and television network SBS, as well as bodies such as the Federation of Ethnic Community Councils of Australia (FECCA), and anti-discrimination legislation (Commonwealth of Australia, 1999, 2003, 2004). The mental health of peoples of culturally and linguistically diverse backgrounds is recognized in all relevant policy documents including the *National Statement of Mental Health Rights and Responsibilities* (Commonwealth of Australia, 2000).

Australia has made a strong political commitment to multiculturalism and, in line with this, health services delivery, and specifically mental health care, has been shaped to respond appropriately, through national and state and territory initiatives. Before describing these initiatives and systems, however, it is vital to examine the challenges that must be dealt with if the mental health needs of those of culturally and linguistically diverse backgrounds are to be met. This has also to be viewed in terms of the multiple layers of culture that must be understood and addressed. This approach is even more important than usual as health and mental health policies, and their related programmes, are mostly developed and shaped within the dominant and usually Western cultural view of mental health needs and how these may best be addressed. The culture of a dominant community will be more influential than might be useful to address the needs of diverse groups. Similarly the culture of health care provision will also be very relevant in terms of systems of care, as well as the culture of health and mental health care carried by the individual providers.

Health care cultures are more clearly delineated in terms of clinical processes where appointed physicians or healers have socially sanctioned roles for the diagnosis of the problem or disease, communication about it to the affected person, and provision of agreed treatment. Public health and prevention are understood in general terms, for example in terms of issues such as clean water, good nutrition, protection from toxic exposures, immunization against disease and to a lesser degree healthy lifestyles and behaviours and risky lifestyles and behaviours. The cultural issues are more complex in terms of these strategies, their acceptability and purpose.

## CHALLENGES TO THE DEVELOPMENT OF MULTICULTURAL MENTAL HEALTH POLICY AND PROGRAMMES

### Evidence base for care

In the context of a population mental health framework (Raphael, 2000) it is critical to understand the epidemiology of disorders in different population groups. However, population-based studies such as the 1997 Australian National Survey of Mental Health and Wellbeing (Australian Bureau of Statistics, 1998) did not have sufficient power to provide any detailed analysis at the level of different ethnic or language groups. Nevertheless, a more generic evaluation of these data suggests that over a quarter of a million first-generation Australian adults of culturally and linguistically diverse backgrounds experience a mental health disorder in a 12-month period.

An excellent report called *Immigrants and Mental Health* (McDonald and Steel, 1997) drew together the information at that time, in terms of utilization data in the state of New South Wales (NSW) and other available data. It highlighted patterns of utilization but could not provide data on levels of problems in the different populations. Never has information been available in terms of children and adolescents from culturally diverse backgrounds. More recently it has been suggested that there are high levels of disability and psychological distress and lower rates of service use by people of culturally diverse backgrounds (Boufous *et al.*, 2005).

Evidence is not readily available for culturally and linguistically diverse populations either about the most effective individual interventions, apart from those related to medication regimes. The psycho-social aspects of care across cultural boundaries have not been adequately researched, nor have interventions for children in such contexts. The different pharmacokinetics of some psychotropic medications in different racial groups adds to the complexity of defining any single set of guidelines for care across cultural boundaries.

Such issues are also relevant for indigenous populations. Data at population-based levels demonstrate a significantly higher level of psychological distress than for the non-indigenous population. Here also there is a need for a stronger evidence base to support strategies for care (Chief Health Officer's Report, 2000).

## Capacity for programme delivery

Effective service delivery, care that is equitable, requires a system of care and individual providers who can assess and treat people from diverse cultural backgrounds. Such systems should be based on a population mental health service model (Raphael, 2000; see Chapter 9). This requires a number of elements to be in place:

- Mental health and health workforce providers who understand, who are educated and trained to assess and provide care to peoples of culturally and linguistically diverse backgrounds.
- Resources in community languages to provide information to clients including children, adolescents adults and older people. Such information would cover the nature of any mental health problems, what can be done for them and where to get help.
- Health and mental health care interpreter services to facilitate assessment and care for those whose first language is not English.
- Bilingual health care workers.
- Cultural consultants.
- Resources to provide for infrastructure and funding to sustain effective health care systems.
- Health care systems and programmes that are accessible and acceptable, for all populations and all age groups.

Evidence is not readily available for the most effective models of service delivery, but special programmes incorporating the above elements into the provision of mental health care for people from such diverse backgrounds generally are perceived as more helpful. A special model of Cultural Consultation for mental health programmes has demonstrated benefit in such circumstances and is being trialled currently for its utility in the Australian multicultural mental health service provision context (Kirmayer *et al.*, 2003). Developing an appropriately skilled and representative workforce is a major challenge in mental health services and public services generally (Commonwealth of Australia, 2002).

## Special issues

Many factors need to be specifically recognized due to their contribution to positive mental health or because of negative impacts. These include past or present experiences of psychological trauma, abuse, violence; multiple and major losses; disruption and dislocation of families and communities through conflict, refugee and disaster status; nostalgia, grief and longing for what has been left behind. Difficulties during or after migration, such as not having qualifications recognized, finding a place in the new society, disadvantage, discrimination and other adversities may all impact. While such issues need to be taken into account for all populations in clinical assessment and care provision, they have special significance for those of culturally and linguistically diverse backgrounds. These issues have been well highlighted by Bhugra and Becker (2005) in their discussions on migration, cultural bereavement, cultural identity (Chen, 2000) and cultural congruity as key elements for mental health in culturally and linguistically diverse populations. Such factors and others have also been recognized in Australia's multicultural mental health strategic framework with identification of populations who may have special needs: refugees and those displaced; those who have experienced torture and trauma; people from diverse backgrounds settling in rural and remote areas; women from culturally and linguistically diverse backgrounds in terms of gender values; adolescents and young adults; older people. Significant research and service delivery initiatives have progressed understanding and mental health care in all of these areas in the Australian context (e.g. Minas *et al.*, 1996; Jacques and Abbott, 1997; Fitzgerald *et al.*, 1998; Silove, 1999; Mihalopoulos *et al.*, 1999).

## Cultural competency in service delivery

This is highly relevant both for service systems and for individual providers. 'Cultural competency' and 'cultural safety' have become metaphors to cover ambiguous behaviour sets that are perceived as better addressing the needs of clients of diverse cultural backgrounds. Operationalizing cultural competence for individuals or service systems is difficult, but inherent in this concept is knowledge about cultures, the cultures of those presenting for care, respect for the person's beliefs, values and behaviours as far as is possible in terms of caring for them and their illness and practising in ways which reflect this. For instance, Long *et al.* (1999) developed a template for 'best practice' in the provision of access to public mental health services for people of culturally and linguistically diverse backgrounds using as a basis the National Standards for Mental Health Services for Australia (Commonwealth of Australia, 1997). These standards also include requirements for culturally competent provision of services to people of such backgrounds. Other endeavours have focused on guidelines for cultural competence. Cultural competence also requires awareness of providers' own culture.

Numerous tools and resources have been developed to support programmes in this area. These included: *Cultural Awareness Tool: Understanding Cultural Diversity in Mental Health* (Multicultural Mental Health Australia, 2002) for providers; and tools for consumers (Multicultural Mental Health Australia, 2004a) and carers (Multicultural Mental Health Australia, 2004b).

## Information systems

Information systems are critical both to guide service planning and to evaluate outcomes and effectiveness of service delivery. The information needs to be culturally appropriate and to be based on tools that are reliable and valid. *National Mental Health Information Priorities* (Commonwealth of Australia, 2005) and *Information Strategies under the National Mental Health Plan* (Australian Government, 2005) fulfil generic mental health information requirements, but the specifics of information requirements in terms of diverse populations have yet to be better delineated both generally and in terms of the *National Performance Indicators* (Australian Government, 2005).

## STRUCTURES, POLICIES AND PROGRAMMES

There have been a number of important national initiatives to progress multicultural mental health in Australia, and in each of the states and territories of this country. These include policy recommendations, a multicultural mental health steering committee and ultimately a *National Multicultural Mental Health Policy Framework* (Commonwealth of Australia, 2004), and importantly the overseeing, management and representative body Multicultural Mental Health Australia. National conferences have contributed, as have international partnerships.

Transcultural or multicultural mental health programmes exist in states and territories and have contributed excellent initiatives at both an individual jurisdiction level, as well as towards the national programme focus. In addition there have been torture and trauma services as well as specific programmes for refugees, and more recently, advice and support for the mental health needs of those in immigration detention centres.

The Transcultural Mental Health Centre in NSW is one example of a state-based initiative. It has been a focus for the development of resources in multiple community languages; the development of bilingual counselling programmes; special developments for children and young people of culturally and linguistically diverse backgrounds; education; service provision; specialized projects including promotion and prevention, consumer development and advocacy; monograph publication services;

newsletter; provision of call-centre assistance to communities affected following terrorist incidents (Raphael and Malak, 2001).

## MULTICULTURAL MENTAL HEALTH AUSTRALIA

Multicultural Mental Health Australia is the strong central organization representing both states and territories but also relevant non-government organizations and other stakeholders. It promotes and contributes to broader diversity initiatives in the population, and is a national and international focus in Australia for multicultural mental health. It has been responsible for the development of a national mental health policy framework for multicultural mental health directions at a national level.

### Framework – for the implementation of the National Mental Health Plan 2003–2008 in Multicultural Australia (2004)

This framework is the national policy direction and encourages states and territories to fulfil their responsibilities to their diverse populations in terms of the directions set, and also provides for Australia-wide initiatives. The main action areas reflect the overarching mental health policy and strategies for Australia:

- A population mental health approach to mental health for people from culturally and linguistically diverse (CALD) backgrounds: This aims to promote mental health and wellbeing, and the full spectrum of culturally appropriate interventions from prevention, early intervention through to relapse prevention and recovery. The policy also aims to improve service responsiveness for culturally diverse populations with services that are accessible and responsive to the needs of such populations across the lifespan. This includes services for children and adolescents, adults and older people and both community and inpatient programmes in mainstream settings.

- Strengthening quality: This involves the enhancement of the cultural competency of the workforce, appropriate monitoring of performance against quality indicators reflecting culturally and linguistically diverse populations, and through the active engagement and participation of consumers, families and carers from such backgrounds.
- Fostering culturally inclusive research, innovation and sustainability: This aims to develop a culturally competent and inclusive research agenda for mental health in this field.

This strategic framework builds on the established commitments of Australia's heath and mental health policies, and its commitment to multiculturalism. The following represent some of the many structural and policy processes that provide such support.

- Multicultural policy: Multicultural Australia United in Diversity (Commonwealth of Australia, 2003) emphasizes earlier commitment to valuing cultural diversity, promoting it as a unifying force with substantial benefits, inclusiveness, equity in public sector service provision and cultural responsiveness in mainstream services.
- Australian mental health policy (currently being updated) makes specific commitment to the mental health needs of culturally and linguistically diverse populations, both directly and through its instruments. These include the Mental Health Statement of Rights and Responsibilities (Commonwealth of Australia, 2000), First National Mental Health Plan (Australian Health Ministers, 1992), Second National Mental Health Plan (Australian Health Ministers, 1998), and the current National Mental Health Plan (Australian Health Ministers, 2003), National Standards for Mental Health Services (Commonwealth of Australia, 1997) and the National Practice Standards for the Mental Health Workforce (Commonwealth of Australia, 2002).

The implementation of the framework above will be overseen through the National Mental Health Standing Committee which reports to the Australian Health Ministers Advisory Council. Achieving the aims of equity in such a culturally diverse society will take progressive and ongoing commitment, as well as building the research and knowledge base for this evolving social field.

## THE FUTURE OF MULTICULTURALISM AND IMPLICATIONS FOR MENTAL HEALTH

Multiculturalism as a policy is strongly incorporated in Australian life, perhaps symbolized by the song with the line 'we are one, but we are many'. Nevertheless there is a set of important issues that need to be recognized and shaped into the future.

Culture is a two-way process. The dominant cultural group propagates its values. It may be challenged by those who are different. It may need to be open to incorporating and valuing the diversities of the other. There has been a change in many countries suggesting a return to more conservative approaches, a retreat from some diversities. This has the potential to create conflict or to lead individuals or groups to experience themselves negatively against the dominant and sanctioned values, beliefs and behaviours of the broader society. This is particularly challenging for minorities when it touches on and threatens to erode core values: these include roles within family; the status of women; and cherished religious and secular beliefs.

Research to influence mental health care has been driven by a number of leaders in this field in Australia, for instance Minas, Silove and Steele. Nevertheless, there is a need for a nationally co-ordinated approach to research in this field to identify the significance of the core concepts underlying different cultures and their contribution or otherwise to mental health. This needs to encompass recognition of risk and resilience; how research dealing with different populations can contribute; the need for longitudinal studies to identify positive processes at societal and individual levels as well as trajectories of vulnerability over time. The needs of children, young people and families are particularly relevant in this context. The Western Australian Aboriginal Child Health Survey (Zubrick *et al.*, 2005) has shown how such

research is not only possible but can provide high-quality information to inform care.

Pooling of data, common instruments and shared methodologies can all progress this field. However, a more co-ordinated and networked approach is essential to answer relevant questions that will inform effective policy and programme implementation. This could also identify the ways in which information systems in public health and clinical service delivery could contribute; and how performance indicators such as those in the national multicultural mental health strategic framework can be met.

In a more global community there are opportunities and threats. Opportunities arise from increased travel, population movement, mass communication and technologies for information transfer. Risks arise from losses of culture, language and potentially identity. A particular threat currently arises with terrorism, which aims to, and does, make populations feel more fearful, feel more threatened and potentially be more likely to see the other as alien and dangerous. This has the potential to impact negatively on the mental health and wellbeing of those populations perceived as strangers and as different from the majority; these populations may be perceived to be associated with political movements that threaten society and democracy. If established, local cycles of vengeance, violence and hatred will impact negatively on everyone's mental health.

Improving services to meet greater expectations of health and mental health care requires strategies, tools, education and training to address the needs of all ages and segments of the population. The magnitude of need, and economic costs, and the complexity of needs among minorities are further challenges.

## CONCLUSION

Cultural diversity is inevitable and almost certainly a positive and powerful force for the future. But what has been discussed here touches on only the beginning of understanding the relevance for mental health and what we can do best to make this positive, to bring inclusiveness, human rights and human values to a hopeful way forward (see

Chapters 2, 3, 7 and 9). The oldest of cultural understandings come from first nations' peoples, in Australia from our Aboriginal peoples and Torres Strait Islanders. Their culture has endured for more than 40 000 years, and they have much wisdom to share. Research has shown how the disruption and loss of culture can contribute to adverse mental health and social outcomes. Nevertheless cultural adaptations are often critical both to survival and wellbeing. While major strategies are in place in Australia to address these issues, for instance in the National Strategic Framework for Aboriginal Mental Health, there is a need to learn from this first nations' platform. For as so powerfully stated:

> Our strength is that we have survived. We are strong, or we would not have survived. Our culture is alive, and is central to our strength. The colonisation process of dispossession made us strong. We depend on each other, we understand and support each other.
>
> (Human Rights and Equal Opportunity Commission, 1993)

## REFERENCES

Australian Bureau of Statistics 1998: *Mental Health and Wellbeing: Profile of Adults, Australia, 1997*. ABS Catalogue No. 4326.0. Canberra: ABS.

Australian Government National Mental Health Working Group Information Strategy Committee Performance Indicator Drafting Group 2005: Key Performance Indicators for Australian Public Mental Health Services. ISC Discussion Paper No. 6. Canberra: Australian Government Department of Health and Ageing.

Australian Health Ministers 1992: *National Mental Health Plan*. National Mental Health Strategy, Commonwealth of Australia.

Australian Health Ministers 1998: *Second National Mental Health Plan*. Mental Health Branch, Commonwealth Department of Health and Family Services, Commonwealth of Australia (July).

Australian Health Ministers 2003: *National Mental Health Plan 2003–2008*. Canberra: Australian Government, July.

Boufous, S., Silove, D., Bauman, A. and Steel, Z. 2005: Disability and health service utilization associated with psychological distress: the influence of ethnicity. *Mental Health Services Research* 7, 171–79.

Bhugra, D. and Becker, M. 2005: Migration, cultural bereavement and cultural identity. *World Psychiatry* 4(1), 18–24.

Chen, L. 2000: Ethnic identity and mental health of young Chinese immigrants. A thesis submitted to the Department of Psychiatry, the University of Queensland in candidacy for the degree of Doctor of Philosophy.

Chief Health Officer's Report 2000: *The Health of the People of New South Wales – Report of the Chief Health Officer*. Sydney: NSW Department of Health Population Health Division. Available at http://www.health.nsw.gov.au/public-health/chorep/toc/pre_foreword.htm (accessed 2000).

Commonwealth of Australia 1997: *National Standards for Mental Health Services*. Canberra: Australian Government Publishing Service.

Commonwealth of Australia 1999: *Australian Multiculturalism for a New Century: Towards Inclusiveness. A Report by the National Multicultural Advisory Council*. Canberra: Australian Government Publishing Service.

Commonwealth of Australia 2000: *Mental Health Statement of Rights and Responsibilities. Report of the Mental Health Consumer Outcomes Task Force Adopted by the Australian Health Ministers March 1991*. Canberra: Australian Government Publishing Service.

Commonwealth of Australia 2002: *National Practice Standards for the Mental Health Workforce*. Canberra: Commonwealth Department of Health and Ageing.

Commonwealth of Australia 2003: *Multicultural Australia, United in Diversity: Updating the 1999 Agenda for Multicultural Australia: Strategic Directions for 2003–2006*. Canberra: Australian Government Publishing Service.

Commonwealth of Australia 2004: *Framework for the Implementation of the National Mental Health Plan 2003–2008 in Multicultural Australia*. Canberra: Australian Government Publishing Service.

Commonwealth of Australia, 2005: *National Mental Health Information Priorities* (2nd Edition). Publications Approval Number 3676. Canberra: Department of Health and Ageing.

Fitzgerald, M., Barnett, B., Inv, V., Matthey, S., Ya, T.H., Silove, D., Hay, S.H., Mitchell, P., Yang, T., McNamara, J. and Duong, H.L. 1998: *Hear Our Voices: Trauma, Birthing and Mental Health among Cambodian Women*. Cultural and Mental Health current issues in transcultural mental health. Sydney: Transcultural Mental Health Centre.

Human Rights and Equal Opportunity Commission 1993: *Human Rights and Mental Illness Report of the National Inquiry into the Human Rights of People with Mental Illness*, Vol 2. Canberra: Australian Government Publishing Service.

Jacques, L. and Abbott, L. 1997: Resettlement disrupted: effects of having a family member in a conflict zone. In Ferguson, B. and Barnes, D. (eds) *Perspectives on Transcultural Mental Health*. Parramatta: NSW Transcultural Mental Health Centre, 68–76.

Kirmayer, L.J., Groleau, D., Gudzer, J., Caminee, B. and Jarvis, E. 2003: Cultural consultation: a model of mental health service for multicultural societies. *Canadian Journal of Psychiatry* 48(3), 145–53.

Long, H., Pirkis, J., Mihalopoulos, C., Naccarella, L., Summers, M. and Dunt, D. 1999: *Evaluating Mental Health Services for Non-English Speaking Background Communities.* Melbourne: Australian Transcultural Mental Health Network.

McDonald, R. and Steel, Z. 1997: *Immigrants and Mental Health: An Epidemiological Analysis.* Sydney: NSW Transcultural Mental Health Centre.

Mihalopoulos, C., Pirkis, J., Naccarella, L. and Dunt, D. 1999: *The Role of General Practitioners and other Primary Care Agencies in Transcultural Mental Health Care.* Melbourne: Australian Transcultural Mental Health Network.

Minas, I.H., Lambert, T.J.R., Kostov, S. and Boranga, G. 1996: *Mental Health Services for NESB Immigrants.* Canberra: Commonwealth of Australia.

Multicultural Mental Health Australia 2002: *Cultural Awareness Tool: Understanding Cultural Diversity in Mental Health.* Sydney: Multicultural Mental Health Australia.

Multicultural Mental Health Australia 2004a: *Reality Check: Culturally Diverse Mental Health Consumers Speak Out.* Sydney: Multicultural Mental Health Australia.

Multicultural Mental Health Australia 2004b: *In their Own Right: Assessing the Needs of Carers from Culturally and Linguistically Diverse Backgrounds.* Sydney: Multicultural Mental Health Australia.

Raphael, B. 2000: *A Population Health Model for the Provision of Mental Health Care.* Canberra: Commonwealth of Australia.

Raphael, B. and Malak, A. (eds) 2001: *Diversity and Mental Health in Challenging Times.* Sydney: Transcultural Mental Health Centre.

Silove, D. 1999: The psychological effects of torture, mass human rights violation, and refugee trauma. *Journal of Nervous and Mental Disease* 187, 200–207.

Zubrick, S.R., Silburn, S.R., Lawrence, D.M., Mitrou, F.G., Dalby, R.B., Blair, E.M., Griffin, J., Milroy, H., De Maio, J.A., Cox, A. and Li, J. 2005: *The Western Australian Aboriginal Child Health Survey: The Social and Emotional Wellbeing of Aboriginal Children and Young People.* Perth: Curtin University of Technology and Telethon Institute for Child Health Research.

# 26

# Aboriginal and Torres Strait Islander mental health

Ernest Hunter

## TIME AND HISTORY

While permanent European settlement in Australia dates from 1788, indigenous experiences of first contact spanned the seventeenth century to the 1970s. Despite significant variability in the timing and nature of European occupation, a number of phases can, generally, be defined. Although exploratory contact was not necessarily violent, the appropriation of land and resources that followed usually was, with frontier conflict ('pacification') lasting in remote settings through the nineteenth century. This was followed by institutional control as indigenous Australians were concentrated and contained in government, pastoral and mission settlements, disappearing from the gaze and awareness of mainstream Australia – a 'great Australian silence' lasting until the 1960s, this being Stanner's term for the 'cult of disremembering' regarding Aboriginal Australians in the wider Australian consciousness (Stanner, 1979).

This all changed through the 1970s, a decade separating a 'regulated' world of discrimination and foreshortened horizons for indigenous Australians,

and the quarter-century since, during which freedoms and 'opportunities' have, more often than not, delivered far less than anticipated. The 1960s began with a national policy to assimilate immigrants, requiring them to give up their own cultures and adopt those of the host society. In contrast, policies in support of Aboriginal affairs were almost exclusively devolved to local states. Significant political activism across the nation culminated in the 1967 Commonwealth Referendum which, passed by 90 per cent of the Australian electorate, included indigenous Australians in the national census and provided for the Commonwealth to legislate in indigenous affairs.

In the following decade funding and services were increased, and access facilitated to the social security system as missions and government settlements were transformed into 'communities' with variable (but illusory) degrees of self-government. However, there was little preparation or planning in this process of 'deregulation', with inevitable confusion and tension. Predictably, there were forces resisting social change and its pace varied. Regardless, momentum built through the 1970s with the expansion of community-controlled organizations (including health), the land rights movement and the first significant cohort of indigenous students progressing to tertiary education. Fundamentally, through the 1970s a paradigm shift occurred from a colonial mindset in which indigenous people were the objects of regulation, to indigenous leadership and participation in policy through the 1980s.

However, participation has not meant control. Investigations, commissions and reports have recommended that indigenous communities and organizations be empowered with greater control over their affairs. Despite this, in 2005 the peak national representative body, the Aboriginal and Torres Strait Islander Commission, was replaced by a government-nominated committee, the Office of Indigenous Policy Coordination. Used and abused, terms such as 'self-determination' and 'self-management' have been replaced by discussion of 'shared responsibility' and 'mutual obligation' in relationships with government, and 'social entrepreneurial' corporate partnerships. The certainties of discrimination have been replaced by ambiguities, with increasing divisions between indigenous leaders.

## CIRCUMSTANCES

The 460 140 Aboriginal and Torres Strait Islander Australians counted in the 2001 national census constitute only 2.4 per cent of the Australian population. The proportion aged less than 15 years is twice as great (40 per cent versus 21 per cent) and the proportion of those surviving to 65 years is one-fifth that of the wider society (2.6 per cent versus 12 per cent) (Australian Bureau of Statistics, 2002). Mortality rates for almost all conditions are higher for indigenous compared with non-indigenous Australians, with the standardized mortality rate ratios being 2.9 for males and 2.6 for females. Not surprisingly, the broader impact of ill-health is greater, with data from the Northern Territory indicating that the indigenous burden of disease is some 2.5 times that of non-indigenous Territorians, and in the 35–54-year age group being 4.1 times higher (Zhao et al., 2004).

While pervasive and persistent social disadvantage is clearly important, it is not sufficient to explain the appalling status of indigenous health. Examination of census data for 2001 according to location in Queensland (Socio-Economic Indexes for Areas – SEIFA) shows that indigenous residents are concentrated in lower socio-economic areas (Rawnsley and Baker, 2004). However, while the mortality rate ratio by SEIFA quintile for the state as a whole increases in a linear fashion from 0.80 to 1.23 for those living in least to most disadvantaged areas, the indigenous mortality rate ratio is 3.8 – some three times greater than for residents in those areas constituting the most disadvantaged quintile for Queensland (Kennedy, 2003).

Associated with social disadvantage is what Leonard Syme has called 'control of destiny' (Syme, 1998), the capacity for people to: 'influence the events that impinge their lives', being related to concepts such as 'mastery, self-efficacy, locus of control, sense of control, powerlessness, competence, and hardiness' (p. 494). The broader social and political context of 'control' has emerged as a critical determinant in Canadian First Nations' suicide research (Chandler et al., 2003). Cross-population comparisons are telling – Aboriginal and Islander health disadvantage relative to the wider national population is greater than that of indigenous populations in other areas of 'Anglo-settler colonialism' (Kunitz, 1994) and, further, by comparison to those other societies the situation in Australia is not improving (Ring and Brown, 2003).

## ENGAGEMENT

Systematic professional involvement in indigenous mental health spans barely four decades but has involved dramatic shifts in understanding processes (of inquiry and practice) (Hunter, 1997) and development of indigenous capacity. To put this in context, there is only one indigenous psychiatrist in Australia and similar underrepresentation in other mental health disciplines. There is now a national framework for indigenous social and emotional wellbeing (Social Health Reference Group, 2004) informed by nine 'guiding principles', being: a holistic understanding of health; self-determination; underpinning culturally valid understandings; recognition of historical trauma; respect for human rights; recognition and response to racism, stigma and environmental adversity; the centrality of family and kinship; recognition of indigenous diversity; and recognition of indigenous strengths.

## DATA

There are major deficiencies in terms of data. Sadly, an exception is suicide. In the State of Queensland the indigenous suicide rate (1999–2001) was 56 per cent higher than for the total population, with the rate for young males aged 15–24 years 3.5 times higher. Some 83 per cent of indigenous suicides were less than 35 years of age (42 per cent for Queensland as a whole) with 95 per cent of these deaths by highly lethal means (90 per cent hanging; 5 per cent firearms) (De Leo and Heller, 2004). However, indigenous suicide is changing. From very low rates in the early 1980s suicide began among heavy drinking, town-based males in their thirties and forties, often men experiencing frightening alcohol-related psychotic experiences or recent relationship crises (Hunter, 1993). In the late 1980s there was a dramatic increase among men in their teens and twenties, often intoxicated and in impulsive response to seemingly 'minor' precipitants. These deaths, increasingly in remote settings, clustered in particular communities suggesting a condition of 'community risk' associated with wider 'lifestyles of risk' (Hunter et al., 2001). In the last years there has been a number of deaths of children and young teens of both sexes who have been raised in families and communities in which 'lifestyles of risk', including self-harm, which is far more 'visible' in indigenous settings (Hunter, in press).

The Western Australian Aboriginal Child Health Survey report on social and emotional wellbeing, based on data for 3993 children aged 4–17 years (Zubrick et al., 2005) demonstrated an elevated risk for clinically significant emotional and behavioural disorders for Aboriginal children aged 4–11

(26 per cent) and 12–17 (21 per cent) compared with non-indigenous peers (17 per cent and 13 per cent respectively), with Aboriginal levels lower in areas of extreme isolation. Among associated social factors were the number of life stress events in the prior 12 months (22 per cent of children were living in families with seven or more life stresses), poor quality of parenting (25 per cent of those surveyed were so classified and were four times as likely to be at risk of emotional and behavioural difficulties), poor family functioning (21 per cent, twice as likely to be at risk), being raised by a sole parent or a non-parental carer (twice as likely to be at risk) and a history of parental forcible separation from their natural families (2.3 times as likely to be at risk).

Similar findings in relation to remoteness as a protective factor were found in the indigenous household sampling survey within the 2001 National Health Survey (Booth and Carroll, 2005), which showed:

> that non-remote Aborigines are more likely to report the following conditions compared to non-Aborigines: depression (9.2 per cent compared to 5.9 per cent), drug and alcohol dependency (3.3 per cent compared to 0.9 per cent) and anxiety (6.9 per cent compared to 5.4 per cent). It is striking that Aborigines living in remote areas are less likely to report these conditions than non-Aborigines.
>
> (p. 10)

These authors note that in relation to self-assessed health status, socio-economic variables explain only between one-third and one-half of the gap compared with non-indigenous Australians. Unfortunately, reliable population level mental health data are limited. However, information from the Australian Institute of Health and Welfare for 1998 and 1999 reveals indigenous:non-indigenous standardized morbidity ratios of 2.0 and 1.5 for indigenous males and females respectively for all mental and behavioural disorders, 4.1 and 3.5 for mental disorders due to psychoactive substances, and 1.8 and 2.0 for schizophrenia and delusional disorders. Given issues of access to services, these figures underrepresent the excess burden of mental health disorder in indigenous Australia.

## RESEARCH

Research has also changed, from indigenous people as the objects of descriptive research, to an expectation that the research agenda will be informed by indigenous priorities, increase Aboriginal and Torres Strait Islander research capacity and be solution-focused (Hunter, 2001). This has resulted in increasing attention to 'participatory action research' and to exploring the underlying values and power relationships of research. Systematic service and policy evaluation has demonstrated that, contrary to popular views of high expenditure on indigenous health, the situation is quite different. Most indigenous health services are provided through primary care and, as Dwyer and colleagues have identified (Dwyer *et al.*, 2004): 'the total Australian Government spending on primary health care services for Indigenous Australians was only about 70 per cent of that for other Australians' (p. xiii).

## TENSIONS

However, while there clearly is a need to acknowledge indigenous difference, there is cause for caution. Maggie Brady (2004) has pointed out that the appropriation of the definition of health promulgated by the World Health Organization in the 1970s introduced a: 'stress on fundamental differences [which] meant that "Western" and "Indigenous" approaches to health were often depicted as polarised, separate domains' (p. 125). In its extreme form this can include rejection of mental health nosology and practice. It is thus critical to be aware of the social, political and institutional currents that inform these ongoing debates.

This may demand confronting some cherished ideological positions. For instance, that because certain policies and initiatives in indigenous affairs were informed by concerns for equity and social justice they could not have harmful consequences (Hunter, 2002); or that 'culture' and 'tradition' are necessarily unproblematic. As Sutton (2001) has pointed out: 'a number of the serious

problems indigenous people in Australia face today arise from a complex joining together of recent, that is post-conquest, historical factors of external impact, with a substantial number of ancient, pre-existing social and cultural factors' (p. 127). Sutton challenges unquestioning acceptance of some manifestly harmful practices on the basis that they represent 'cultural' practice:

*What about the socialisation of children, or 'demand sharing' of resources, the pervasive importance of kinship, a high stress on personal autonomy, long patterns of internecine feuding, resistance to delegating authority, the blaming of deaths on out-group sorcerers rather than on those involved in episodes of drink driving or wife bashing, for example? While these and many other practices may contain powerful elements of classic traditions, they now exist under conditions that differ significantly from those of the pre-colonial era.*
**(p. 140)**

Another commentator with similar tenure in remote Aboriginal Australia, Richard Trudgen, agrees on the broad spectrum of problems, the effects of failed programmes, and pervasive social and economic dependence (Trudgen, 2000). Reflecting on issues such as suicide, petrol sniffing and the breakdown of authority structures, he comments: 'The people have suffered an almost total loss of control over their lives and living environment' (p. 218). However, in his analysis the fundamental problem relates to communication, the critical element in any solution demanding cultural and linguistic competence on the part of non-indigenous practitioners.

While these authors present different readings of how traditional practices and beliefs influence responses to contemporary social problems, there is agreement in relation to how instability impacts child development, and on exposure to 'trauma'. The literature and debate around trauma, particularly 'transgenerational trauma', captures tensions and ambiguities typical of the broader arena of indigenous mental health. As McCoy (2004) notes:

*From the 1990s the term trauma has been used to describe a wide range of Aboriginal*

*experience; the trauma of colonised history,
the trauma of separation of a person from
their family, trauma related to loss and grief,
ongoing events which add to trauma that has
already being experienced, and trauma that
is passed from one generation to the next.
Trauma has been used to cover not just a
wide field of human suffering but also personal and community experiences.*

(p. 12)

For McCoy 'intergenerational trauma' is the
'wounding' of culturally informed socializing
processes critical for personal development and
social/cultural integrity. However, trauma has also
come to represent the violation of rights experienced by past and present generations. It is a poly-
semous term, the ambiguities of which have
significant response implications as noted by Noel
Pearson (Pearson, 2000):

*I would however urge a distinction to be
drawn between that trauma which is
personal and immediate and may incapaci-
tate individuals or families, and that trauma
which is inherited and more remote – which
renders people susceptible to problems, but
does not leave them incapacitated. Prevailing
discussions of trauma in Aboriginal society
unhelpfully conflate these two kinds of
trauma.*

(p. 35)

## SERVICES

Ultimately, major and broad-ranging social change
will be necessary to eliminate the excess burden
of health and mental health disadvantage in
Aboriginal and Torres Strait Islander Australia –
this will not be brought about by mental health
interventions alone. Regardless, indigenous functional access to effective services is a right and
should be ensured. Manifest excess need is compounded by problems of availability of specialist
services in rural and remote Australia and limited
access to the resources of the private sector. Consequently, primary care is and will remain the major

conduit for the provision of indigenous mental
health services and there is a pressing need for effective integration of mental health into the broader
primary care agenda (Haswell-Elkins *et al.*, 2005).
Realistic, needs-based resourcing is critical (O'Kane
and Tsey, 2004), with a shift from project-based to
recurrent funding that will allow sensible forward
planning. Given the complexities of developing a
reliable evidence base for interventions in small
populations exposed to high levels of stress and
social adversity, supporting flexibility and innovation in terms of intervention and evaluation is
critical. A precondition of real improvement will
be enhancing the indigenous workforce capacity
across the range of disciplines including Aboriginal
mental health workers (Parker, 2003) in both mainstream and community controlled services. There
must also be a shift from tokenistic mantras regarding 'cultural sensitivity' towards carefully researched
culturally informed approaches to assessment and
intervention (Westerman, 2004).

## CONCLUSION

As with trauma, indigenous mental health is a con-
tested arena between artificially polarized 'holistic'
and 'biomedical' models. Pragmatically, comprehensively addressing indigenous social and mental
health challenges will demand conceptual flexibility with attention to historical and social factors,
equitable access to appropriate resources and services, and intensive investment in the environments
of childhood – that is, in childhood socialization.
As Pat Dodson and Noel Pearson (Dodson and
Pearson, 2004) have articulated in discussing
'mutual obligation': 'The aim must be to normalise
obligations between Aboriginal parents and their
children, between family members, and between
individuals and their communities' (p. 17).

Dodson and Pearson warn against the 'collapse
in expectations' of indigenous responsibilities. This
is particularly relevant in relation to indigenous
mental health where, for practitioners, it is important to understand history without being paralysed
by it. Paralysis is supported by the politicization of
indigenous health which may further diminish or

deny indigenous agency. There is a long history of indigenous agency being denied in Australia through processes of institutionalization and infantilization, particularly in what Peggy Brock has called 'outback ghettos' (Brock, 1993). Peter Sutton has invoked this image and points out that it is (Sutton, 2001): 'the complex combination of these forms of cultural persistence with the after-effects of colonisation, including ghettoisation, that makes Indigenous conditions such a challenge to reformers' (p. 149). One might ask – Reform what? By whom? For whom?

While history, social disadvantage, racism and disempowerment are all, clearly, influential factors, ultimately they are mediated through the processes by which identity is formed and transmitted by individuals and groups. On the one hand this may result in stereotypes and internalizations that reinforce vulnerability. On the other it may lead to growth, resilience and solutions. This is captured in the comments of an Aboriginal health professional (Bond, 2005) reflecting on public health constructions of 'Aboriginality' and on her own journey of awareness and engagement:

*Through my journey so far, I have found the strength in my identity as an Aboriginal person, in all of its 'inauthenticity', and the strength in my community, in all its unhealthiness, to see a way forward to improving the health of our people. For me, inherent in the task of improving Indigenous health and in achieving wellbeing as an Indigenous person is providing a space within public health practice and in our own minds that allows us, the 'public', to define and redefine our experiences of identity.*

(p. 40)

## REFERENCES

Australian Bureau of Statistics 2002: *Population Distribution, Aboriginal and Torres Strait Islander Australians, 2001*. Cat No. 4705.0. Canberra: Australian Bureau of Statistics.

Bond, C.J. 2005: A culture of ill health: public health or Aboriginality? *Medical Journal of Australia* 183, 39–41.

Booth, A. and Carroll, N. 2005: *The Health Status of Indigenous and Non-Indigenous Australians*. Bonn: Forschingsinstitut zur Zunkunft der Arbeit (Institute for the Study of Labor).

Brady, M. 2004: *Indigenous Australia and Alcohol Policy: Meeting Difference with Indifference*. Sydney: University of New South Wales Press.

Brock, P. 1993: *Outback Ghettos: A History of Aboriginal Institutionalisation and Survival*. Melbourne: Cambridge University Press.

Chandler, M.J., Lalonde, C.E., Sokol, B.W. and Hallett, D. 2003: Personal persistence, identity development, and suicide: a study of Native and Non-native North American adolescents. *Monographs of the Society for Research in Child Development* 68, vii–viii, 1–130; discussion 131–38.

De Leo, D. and Heller, T. 2004: *Suicide in Queensland 1999–2001: Mortality Rates and Related Data*. Brisbane: Australian Institute for Suicide Research and Prevention.

Dodson, P. and Pearson, N. 2004: The dangers of mutual obligation. *The Age* 15 December, 17.

Dwyer, J., Silburn, K. and Wilson, G. 2004: *National Strategies for Improving Indigenous Health and Health Care*. Canberra: Commonwealth of Australia.

Haswell-Elkins, M., Hunter, E., Nagel, T., Thompson, C., Hall, B., Mills, R., Wargent, R., Tsey, K., Knowles, L. and Wilkinson, Y. 2005: Reflections on integrating mental health into primary health care services in remote Indigenous communities in Far North Queensland and the Northern Territory. *Australian Journal of Primary Health* 11(2), 62–69.

Hunter, E. 1993: *Aboriginal Health and History: Power and Prejudice in Remote Australia*. Melbourne: Cambridge University Press.

Hunter, E. 1997: Double talk: changing and conflicting constructions of indigenous mental health. *Australian and New Zealand Journal of Psychiatry* 31, 820–27.

Hunter, E. 2001: A brief historical background to health research in Indigenous communities. *Aboriginal and Islander Health Worker Journal* 25, 6–8.

Hunter, E. 2002: 'Best intentions' lives on: untoward health outcomes of some contemporary initiatives in Indigenous affairs. *Australian and New Zealand Journal of Psychiatry* 36, 575–84.

Hunter, E. in press: The protracted dawning of the 'Bran Nue Dae': Aboriginal suicide in social context. In Chandler, M.J., Lalonde, C.E. and Lightfoot, C. (eds) *A Global Perspective on Problems of Identity and Suicide in Indigenous Minority Youth*. Mahwah, NJ: Lawrence Erlbaum Associates.

Hunter, E., Reser, J., Baird, M. and Reser, P. 2001: *An Analysis of Suicide in Indigenous Communities of North Queensland: the Historical, Cultural and Symbolic Landscape*. Canberra: Commonwealth Department of Health and Aged Care.

Kennedy, B. 2003: *Indigenous SEIFA scores*. Brisbane: Strategic Partnerships Office, Department of Aboriginal and Torres Strait Islander Policy.

Kunitz, S. 1994: *Disease and Social Diversity: The European Impact on the Health of Non-Europeans*. New York: Oxford University Press.

McCoy, B.F. 2004: Kanyirninpa: health, masculinity and wellbeing of desert Aboriginal men. PhD dissertation, University of Melbourne.

O'Kane, A. and Tsey, K. 2004: Towards a needs based mental health resource allocation and service development in rural and remote Australia. *Australasian Psychiatry* 12, 1–6.

Parker, R. 2003: The indigenous mental health worker. *Australasian Psychiatry* 11, 295–97.

Pearson, N. 2000: *Our Right to Take Responsibility*. Cairns: Noel Pearson and Associates.

Rawnsley, T. and Baker, J. 2004: *Indigenous SEIFA for Queensland. Report prepared for: Office of Economic and Statistical Research*. Canberra: Analysis Branch, Methodology Division, Australian Bureau of Statistics.

Ring, I. and Brown, N. 2003: The health status of indigenous peoples and others. *British Medical Journal* 327, 404–405.

Social Health Reference Group 2004: *Social and Emotional Well Being Framework: A National Strategic Framework for Aboriginal and Torres Strait Islander Mental Health and Social and Emotional Well Being (2004–2008)*. Canberra: Department of Health and Ageing.

Stanner, W.E.H. 1979: *White Man got no Dreaming: Essays 1938–1973*. Canberra: Australian National University Press.

Sutton, P. 2001: The politics of suffering: Indigenous policy in Australia since the 1970s. *Anthropological Forum* 11, 125–71.

Syme, S.L. 1998: Social and economic disparities in health: Thoughts about intervention. *The Milbank Quarterly* 76, 493–505.

Trudgen, R. 2000: *Why Warriors Lie Down and Die: Towards an understanding of why Aboriginal people of Arnhem Land face the greatest crisis in health and education since European contact*. Darwin: Aboriginal Resource and Development Services.

Westerman, T. 2004: Engagement of Indigenous clients in mental health services: What role do cultural differences play? *Australian e-Journal for the Advancement of Mental Health* 3. www.auseinet.com/journal/vol3iss3/westermaneditorial.pdf.

Zhao, Y., Guthridge, S., Magnus, A. and Vos, T. (2004). Burden of disease and injury in Aboriginal and non-Aboriginal populations in the Northern Territory. *Medical Journal of Australia* 180, 498–502.

Zubrick, S., Silburn, S., Lawrence, D., Mitrou, F., Dalby, R., Blair, E.M., Griffin, J., Milroy, H., De Maio, J.A., Cox, A. and Li, J. 2005. *The Western Australian Aboriginal Child Health Survey: The social and emotional wellbeing of Aboriginal children and young people*. Perth: Curtin University of Technology and Telethon Institute for Child Health Research.

# 27

# Hong Kong – Development of psychiatric services

## Ka Chee Yip

## THE EARLY YEARS OF PSYCHIATRIC CARE

Records of psychiatric care in Hong Kong can be traced back to 1875 when a temporary asylum was opened to admit non-Chinese patients. This temporary asylum was relocated in around 1880 and was finally replaced by the European Lunatic Asylum in 1885 (Medical Department, 1893). Later the Chinese Lunatic Asylum was built next to it and was opened in 1891. Overcrowding was a problem and in 1894 the Hong Kong Government arranged with the authorities in Canton to accept transfers of Chinese patients to the John Kerr Refuge for the Insane in Fong Tsuen, Canton (Medical Department, 1894). Non-Chinese patients were repatriated to their own countries. The European and the Chinese asylums merged in 1895. An Asylum Ordinance was enacted in 1906. In 1928 the term 'lunatic asylum' was substituted by 'mental hospital' in official reports. The main function of the hospital was to provide custodial care for disturbed mental patients until their transfer to mainland China or repatriation to their own countries. In the 1950s there was only one old and dilapidated mental hospital with 140 beds and the management of the patients was mainly custodial.

## THE DEVELOPMENT OF A MODERN PSYCHIATRIC SERVICE

In 1948 Dr P.M. Yap, a British trained psychiatrist, was appointed medical superintendent of the mental hospital and development of the public mental health service began to take shape. It was a centralized service with a senior specialist psychiatrist in charge of the overall planning, development and operation.

In the late 1940s and early 1950s the large influx of immigrants from mainland China led to rapid population increase, urbanization and changes in the traditional family structure. During the three decades from the 1960s to the 1980s there was great economic development. The rapid growth in population together with the changes in socio-economic situation gave rise to a variety of mental health problems and people's increased expectations on the provision of mental health care (Lo, 1976).

Various psychiatric facilities in Hong Kong were developed based on the British model. The provision of hospitals and outpatient facilities was largely the responsibility of the Government. The services were organized on a non-regional basis taking into consideration the needs and demands of the whole territory. A network of psychiatric hospitals, psychiatric wards in general hospitals, psychiatric centres, psychiatric clinics and psychiatric day hospitals were supported by various aftercare rehabilitation services. During the period from 1960 to the late 1980s shortage of psychiatric staff was a problem. The supply of doctors was limited until the latter part of the 1980s when there were medical graduates from a second medical school in Hong Kong.

In the 1970s the Government began to put emphasis on the rehabilitation of disabled persons and published the first Rehabilitation Program Plan in 1977. Facilities in the community such as halfway houses, hostels, shelter workshops, compassionate re-housing and long-stay care homes were provided at a faster pace in the 1980s and 1990s.

## PUBLIC PSYCHIATRIC INPATIENT SERVICE

In 1961, the first modern mental hospital, Castle Peak Hospital (1000 beds), was opened. There was an occupational therapy department in it and a multidisciplinary approach to patient care began emerging. The first psychiatric nursing school in the territory was also set up there. In the 1970s psychiatric units were set up in general hospital settings. In 1981 another large mental hospital, Kwai Chung Hospital with 1300 beds, was opened to cater for the increasing inpatient need. At that time large mental hospitals were still required because acceptance of the mentally ill was low and there was insufficient support in the community. Thereafter, additional psychiatric beds were found in general hospital settings only and no more stand-alone mental hospitals were built.

From 2000 to 2003 there was a reduction in hospital beds to around 0.7 per 1000 of the general population. This was achieved through the availability of more places in long-stay care homes and more discharges into the community through better services and support in the community.

A survey in mid-2000 of the length of stay of patients admitted to psychiatric inpatient facilities showed that 32 per cent were hospitalized for up to 90 days, 18 per cent were hospitalized for 91–365 days, 27 per cent were hospitalized for 1–4 years and 23 per cent were hospitalized for more than 4 years. The number of psychiatric hospital beds in the public sector as at 31 March 2002 was 4796. These beds were distributed in two mental hospitals and eight psychiatric units in general hospital settings (Hospital Authority, 2002).

## PUBLIC OUTPATIENT AND DAY HOSPITAL SERVICES

Several psychiatric outpatient clinics were set up in the 1960s and in the following 30 years over a dozen psychiatric centres (mental health centres)/clinics were set up at various locations in the territory to facilitate the care of patients in the community and they were well received by the patients and relatives because of convenience.

The number of psychiatric outpatient attendances in 1984 was 210 000 and by the end of March 2002 had reached 511 127. The outpatient facilities were available at 18 different locations in hospitals, clinics and centres by 31 March 2002 (Hospital Authority, 2002).

### An outpatient follow-up system for high-risk patients

Following a tragic incident in 1982 in which a schizophrenic patient stabbed over 30 people, a Priority Follow System with a central register of the involved patients was launched to enhance the follow-up care of the target group of severely mentally ill patients with histories of criminal violence. This also targeted those assessed to have a disposition to violence and kept them all engaged in treatment (Health and Welfare Branch, 1983).

## Day hospitals

This service was first provided in 1960s. Previously the planning ratio for psychiatric day hospital places was 0.1 per 1000 of the general population. With the move towards more community-based care, in a review in 1999, it was proposed to increase the day hospital places to 0.15 per 1000 of the general population. On 31 March 2002, there were 782 psychiatric day hospital places distributed at 14 different locations with total attendances of 180 764 in the year 2001/2002 (Hospital Authority, 2002).

## COMMUNITY PSYCHIATRIC SERVICES

The provision of psychiatric care outside mental hospitals in psychiatric centres (with outpatient clinic and day hospital) and psychiatric clinics started in the 1960s. In the 1970s, psychiatric units (with inpatient, outpatient and/or day hospital facilities) in general hospital settings were also established. The community psychiatric nursing service was set up in 1982. In the 1990s it was explicitly stated in the psychiatric service policy that it would shift from a previously more hospital-based to a more community-based service. Community psychiatric teams were first set up in 1994. On 31 March 2002 there were 90 community psychiatric nurses, and 54 320 home visits were made; this was more than a 2.5 times increase compared with the figure of just over 20 000 in 1992. This increase was mainly in the latter half of this period, reflecting the move towards enhancing community care.

A 24-hour psychiatric telephone advisory service run by the public psychiatric service was set up in 1984. It provided the public with quick and easily accessible information and practical advice on psychiatric problems. The Social Welfare Department and various non-governmental organizations also have telephone hot-line services for the general public on mental health issues.

## Psychiatric rehabilitation in the community

The Government Social Welfare Department and non-governmental organizations run many of the psychiatric rehabilitation services in the community. Social rehabilitation includes residential service with halfway houses, supported housing, supported hostels, long-stay care homes and care and attention homes; respite service; training and activity centres; support services such as medical, social services, family casework service, financial assistance, job placement service, support services provided by patients/relatives resource centres, home help services, community mental health links and aftercare service for clients discharged from halfway houses.

The community mental health links are attached to halfway houses or training and activity centres and the service is district based, making it more easily accessible and able to be proactive. The objectives of the links are to provide support for the mentally ill persons and their carers in their neighbourhood. As at early 2002 there were 25 community mental health links established, covering the whole territory. Vocational rehabilitation includes work-related training and supports are provided in vocational skills centres and sheltered workshops. There was on-the-job training for people with disabilities, supported employment and selective job placement.

## PSYCHIATRIC SUBSPECIALTIES

The bulk of psychiatric work was centred upon general adult psychiatry. The development of subspecialties has been slow due to resources and manpower constraints. By 1989 forensic psychiatry, consultation-liaison psychiatry and child psychiatry were the more developed subspecialties. In the 1990s the subspecialties substance misuse, psychiatric rehabilitation and psycho-geriatrics were developed. Mental handicap and psychotherapy are the subspecialties lagging behind in development as compared with other subspecialties. However, by the end of 2006, psychotherapy had been developed in each training unit/department.

## PSYCHIATRIC TRAINING

The Hong Kong Psychiatric Association was founded in 1967 with the aim of organizing scientific meetings and fostering relationships with overseas psychiatric colleges and associations. It became the Hong Kong College of Psychiatrists in 1990. The training of psychiatrists is now the joint responsibility of the Hong Kong College of Psychiatrists, the public psychiatric service and the psychiatric departments of the two medical schools. The public psychiatric service has always played an important role in providing in-service training for doctors. In the 1980s the accreditation visits by the Royal College of Psychiatrists helped to set the standard and requirements of training and supervision and a mechanism for the provision of training was set up. Starting from 2002, the Hong Kong College of Psychiatrists and the Royal College of Psychiatrists had joint accreditation visits to the training facilities in Hong Kong. By the end of this decade it is estimated that there will be one psychiatrist per 30 000 of the general population.

With the closure in 2002 of the nursing schools that were attached to mental hospitals, psychiatric nurses and other health care professionals are now trained in universities.

## MENTAL HEALTH LEGISLATION

The Asylum Ordinance was enacted in 1906. It was renamed the Mental Hospitals Ordinance in 1950. In 1962 the Mental Health Ordinance was enacted and replaced the Mental Hospitals Ordinance (Lo, 1988). Amendments were made in 1988, 1996 and 1997. In June 1997, the Mental Health (Amendment) Ordinance 1997 was enacted.

The Mental Health Ordinance consisted of five parts. Part I defined the various terms used in the ordinance. Part II covered the management of properties and affairs of mentally disordered persons. Part III covered the reception, detention and treatment of patients, and disposal options of persons concerned in criminal proceedings. Part IV covered the patient offenders, mental health review tribunal, guardianship and medical and dental treatment and Part V covered general provisions such as protection of patients and staff.

## RECENT AND FUTURE DEVELOPMENTS

Starting from 1994, psychiatric services evolved towards a decentralized and cluster-based service. When fully reformed, each cluster with a defined catchment area and population had a comprehensive range of inpatient, outpatient, day hospital and community-based services to facilitate patient accessibility and continuity of care as well as staff accountability and autonomy.

More emphasis was placed on care in the community and in the least restrictive environment possible and the number of inpatient psychiatric beds will be further reduced to below 0.7 beds per 1000 of the general population. The duration of each hospitalization was shortened. The social support networks, aftercare work, self-help/mutual help groups needed to be strengthened and there was to be further collaboration between service providers to achieve seamless care. Psychoeducation for patients and their families was becoming part of the 'standard care'.

General practitioners and family doctors are given the appropriate support and training and can then play a more important role in the care of patients with less serious psychiatric illnesses in the primary care setting. This will help in the issues of early intervention and stigmatization as well as the imbalance of psychiatric services in the primary and secondary care settings.

Prevention is an important direction. An elderly suicide prevention programme was launched in 2002 in which fast track clinics have been set up for the assessment and management of old people with suicidal tendency to tackle the high prevalence of suicides amongst the elderly. Another early intervention programme targeted first-episode psychotic patients with a view to preventing irreversible neurobiological and social problems through intervention at first presentation and early course of psychosis. Each patient in this group is offered prompt assessment and intensive treatment in a

low-stigma setting. In tertiary prevention, a programme has been launched to facilitate the early
integration of extended care psychiatric inpatients
into the community. This is known as the Extended-
care Patients Intensive Treatment, Early Diversion
and Rehabilitation Stepping Stone (EXITERS)
project. It is also a service direction that every
patient requiring rehabilitation should be offered
it as early as possible in the course of the illness to
minimize possible deterioration.

Other areas of development are quality improvement and incorporation of evidence-based practice into psychiatry. Process and outcome indicators
will continue to be identified and introduced
for quality assurance. A knowledge support system
called the electronic knowledge gateway is being
developed in the hospital authority to act as a
medium for exchanging information, experience
and opinion; to keep professionals updated with
the latest developments in their field; to provide
resources for continuing professional development; and to facilitate clinical decision-making
using the best evidence available.

To conclude, Hong Kong is developing a
community-based quality psychiatric service with
an appropriate balance of prevention, treatment
and rehabilitation in the primary and secondary
care settings. A better social support network with
more client empowerment still needs to be developed. The introduction of the practice of evidence-
based medicine in psychiatry is one of the important
means of improving quality.

The return of sovereignty in 1997 brings us
opportunities. In the colonial days traditional
Chinese medicine was not practised in the public
health care system but was practised in the private
sector by traditional Chinese medicine practitioners. It is not uncommon to see people taking herbal
medicines for problems of fatigue, neurasthenia,
insomnia, etc. Since 1997, it has been the policy of the
Government of the Hong Kong Special Administrative Region to encourage the development of traditional Chinese medicine. There is an opportunity for
the evaluation of the use of traditional Chinese medicine in psychiatry and to introduce those treatments found useful. There is also the opportunity
for close collaboration with health care organizations in mainland China in areas of psychiatric
training and patient care. Hong Kong may have the
chance to develop into a training centre for health
care professionals in China.

## REFERENCES

Health and Welfare Branch 1983: *Report of the Working Group on Ex-mental Patients with a History of Criminal Violence and Assessed Disposition to Violence*. Hong Kong: Hong Kong Government.

Hospital Authority 2002: *Hospital Authority Statistical Report 2001–2002*. Hong Kong: Hospital Authority.

Lo, W.H. 1976: Urbanization and psychiatric disorders – the Hong Kong scene. *Acta Psychiatrica Scandinavica* 54: 174–83.

Lo, W.H. 1988: Development of legislation for the mentally ill in Hong Kong. *Journal of Hong Kong Psychiatric Association* 8, 6–9.

Medical Department 1893: *Annual Report of the Medical Department*. Hong Kong.

Medical Department 1894: *Annual Report of the Medical Department*. Hong Kong.

# 28

# Cultural adaptation of cognitive therapy for Chinese peoples

## Roger MK Ng

## INTRODUCTION

Cognitive therapy is a well-researched treatment modality in the West, especially in North America (Prochaska and Norcross, 2003). However, the applicability of cognitive therapy in the non-Western world is less well documented. Only 6 per cent of humanity resides in North America and more than 20 per cent of all humans are Chinese (Triandis, 1996). There is a pressing need to understand the cultural relevance of cognitive therapy in the Chinese population, given the public health requirements for psychological therapies for common mental disorders, and to assist people to return to employment. This chapter attempts to identify the cultural adaptation in cognitive therapy for the Chinese population, from the perspective of a cognitive therapist practising in the public health sector in Hong Kong.

## CULTURAL CONTEXT OF THE THERAPEUTIC RELATIONSHIP

Chinese people are highly aware of social position and social hierarchy due to the moral concept of filial piety (Ho, 1996). The strong moral concept of filial piety establishes the importance of five cardinal relationships: king and officials, father and son, among brothers, husband and wife, among friends. Each relationship has a certain set of rules and obligations that govern intergenerational relationships, with stringent demands on how a son should serve his father and preserve family face. This respect of order and social position is important in maintaining social harmony in a densely populated country like China. The very encounter of therapist and patient in a therapeutic setting inevitably activates multiple cultural beliefs, such as: therapist as a superior, therapist expects obedience and respect from the patient, and listening without challenging the views of the superior (Gao *et al.*, 1996). A patient might appear overly compliant in the session and appear uninvolved in the session. Western therapists might find the passive behaviour frustrating as therapists expect more active collaboration from Chinese patients. Chinese patients seldom challenge hypotheses set up by the therapists even if they regard them as not personally valid.

People in a collectivistic culture are concerned with others' 'face' and public dignity, therefore they are likely to avoid conflict and avoid direct confrontation (Bond, 1991). Chinese people prefer to save the face of others (more than their own face) through the adoption of an obliging and avoiding style of management (Ting-Toomey *et al.*, 1991). Without special attention to such beliefs and respect for authority through listening, therapists may easily accept patients' agreement with hypotheses.

As the communicative pattern of Chinese people puts so much emphasis on listening to superiors and obedience to authority (Gao *et al.*, 1996), this belief can be geared to therapist advantage in the early phase of socialization into cognitive therapy. Chinese patients are likely to be attentive in listening but reticent about raising questions or misunderstandings; the therapists can assign patients with specific homework on summarizing what has been taught in the session and on giving negative feedback about the applicability of the model to his problem.

Therapists may also use the Confucian concept of '*jiao xue shang zhang*' (teachers and students both benefit from mutual exchange of ideas) and emphasis on the value of education to encourage patients to contribute to the learning process of cognitive therapy. Alternatively, if patients continue to avoid giving comments or feedback, therapists can offer such cultural hypotheses as 'You may be unwilling to tell me your feelings about the session because you think that it is not nice to challenge a teacher'.

Another important aid to facilitate talking from the patient is to notice and put up hypotheses about non-verbal behaviour. Chinese communication emphasizes the non-verbal rather than verbal aspects of communicative activity (Gao *et al.*, 1996). Meanings tend to reside in meta-messages: a hand movement, a smile and a shrug. Chinese expect people to anticipate others' needs or to know their feelings without asking or being told; to do so implies poor social skills or a character deficit (Gabrenya and Hwang, 1996). The importance of attention to non-verbal behaviour is also increasingly emphasized in recent literature of cognitive therapy (Safran and Muran, 2000). The therapist's ability to detect subtle non-verbal behaviour will enrich the therapeutic relationship.

Another important issue is the Chinese perception of the doctor/therapist–patient relationship. In a study of Chinese students, it was found that

friends were sought for psychological problems, with medical doctors preferred only for more physiological problems (Cheung, 1984). Doctors are expected to deal with medical problems and discussion of feelings with doctors is a challenging task for Chinese people, considering that they seldom disclose their own feelings even to their parents. There is a very sharp demarcation between close and casual friends in Chinese societies so that there is a greater disclosure of feelings and thoughts to in-groups (*zijiren*) than to the out-groups (*weiren*) (Gudykunst *et al.*, 1992). It also takes a longer time to develop trust among the Chinese (Zhang and Bond, 1993). Therefore, therapists might be considered not only as a superior but also as an out-group (*weiren*). Disclosure of feelings and thoughts to relationships other than friends is also a relatively new experience that requires time and patience on the part of the therapist. Leung and Lee (1996) also stated that therapists should expect a longer time for Chinese clients to confide and should refrain from being too intrusive in the initial sessions.

## COGNITIVE DISTORTIONS, MALADAPTIVE ASSUMPTIONS, ATTITUDES AND ATTRIBUTIONS

People with strong filial attitudes tend to be uncreative, passive and uncritical towards learning (Ho, 1996). They are more inclined to endorse fatalistic, superstitious and stereotyped beliefs, and are predisposed to be authoritarian, dogmatic and highly conformative. Ho coined the term 'cognitive conservatism' to describe these personality attributes. Special effort in cognitive therapy is required to encourage creativity in patients with strong filial piety orientation, for example, by relegating the responsibility of designing session-relevant homework to the patients, more liberal use of imagery techniques and design of behavioural experiments (Beck 1995).

Furthermore, Spasojevic and Alloy (2003) found that over-controlling parenting style was related to ruminative response style. Ruminative style mediated the relationship between this parental style and the number of major depressive episodes experienced by subjects during the follow-up period. Depressive rumination has been found to predict the duration and severity of depression (Roberts et al., 1998).

Depressed Chinese patients who were raised in typical Chinese families with strong emphasis on filial piety might be particularly prone to depressive rumination, so that active distraction tasks are useful to break streams of negative thoughts and improve problem-solving skills (Lyubomirsky and Nolen-Hoeksema, 1995).

Might personality be structured along cultural and ethnic lines? Chinese people have higher expectations of perfectionism in comparison with 'Caucasians' (Chang, 1998). Furthermore, Chang (1998) also reported that Asian American students reported more doubts about their actions, concerns about making mistakes, and greater parental expectations, and perceived more criticism from parents than Caucasian students. The two groups, however, did not differ significantly in personal standards and personal organization skills. Castro and Rice (2003) found that perfectionism, with high scores in 'doubts about actions' and concerns about 'making mistakes', is highly maladaptive. The results suggest that certain aspects of perfectionism may adversely affect psychological health, and these may be more important in a Chinese context with Chinese patients. Chang (1998) found that Asian Americans who scored high on perfectionism also reported more hopelessness and a higher suicidal potential. Chinese adolescents in Hong Kong also had more depressive symptoms compared with Western counterparts (Chan, 1995). It is therefore important to identify the maladaptive aspects of perfectionism in Chinese patients and to apply cognitive strategies (Beck, 1995), including cognitive continuum (to reduce the dichotomous view of success versus failure) and cost–benefit analysis of perfectionism over certain aspects of life (work and achievement) with relative neglect of other aspects (physical health or marital relationship). There has to be special emphasis given to Chinese patients that cognitive therapy is not intended to lower their aspirations or high personal standards but is to help them to have a more comprehensive

personal standard of excellence (including emotional and psychological wellbeing).

While individual societies in developed countries, such as the USA or UK, tend to attribute failures to internal causes, Chinese people predominantly prefer an external attribution for successes and internal attribution for failures (Crittenden, 1991). Chinese people were also more likely to attribute academic limitations to a lack of effort (Hess et al., 1987). This emphasis on effort is derived from a belief in human malleability and ability to improve, endorsed and advocated by Confucianism (Chen and Uttal, 1988). Chinese externality in the locus of control has been linked with poor psychological health (Chien, 1984; Chan, 1989; Lau and Leung, 1992). Use of a pie chart to obtain a more objective view of responsibility for failure (Beck, 1995) and reattribution of positive events to internal qualities are important strategies that we have found useful. Similar findings were reported in a study on group cognitive–behavioural therapy for Hong Kong Chinese (Wong et al., 2002).

Chinese people have a deep conviction about yuan – the belief that interpersonal outcomes are determined by fate or supernatural forces. Attributions based on yuan function as a defence mechanism to shield an individual from the negative emotions associated with negative interpersonal outcomes (Lee, 1995). However, there is also a tendency to attribute positive interpersonal outcomes to yuan, thereby weakening the self-esteem (Huang et al., 1983). In the author's experience, it is important to emphasize personal effort in the formation of yuan, as one can accumulate yuan through behaviour throughout life and can involve oneself in relationships to search out a suitable partner (Lee, 1995). The salient point here is to shift from a passive recipient of yuan to a more active modifier of yuan in both positive and negative relationship outcomes. Again, responsibility in negative relationship outcome can be translated into opportunity to learn and to change the future course of yuan. In certain circumstances (such as irretrievable loss), acceptance strategies in a mindfulness-based approach (Zegal et al., 2002) can be highly acceptable to Chinese patients who strongly endorse the concept of yuan.

## COGNITIVE AND BEHAVIOURAL STRATEGIES

Cognitive strategies such as dysfunctional thought records are used frequently in cognitive therapy to identify and challenge cognitive distortions (Beck, 1995). This is a particularly daunting task for Chinese patients because emotions like anger, joy and depression are seldom expressed in Chinese culture (Lin and Lin, 1981). By not showing sadness or joy, the Chinese avoid imposing their feelings on others and thereby maintain harmony (Bond, 1993). Considerable effort is required to first teach Chinese patients to label their emotion correctly (emotion chart) and to quantify their degree of emotion using an emotional intensity scale (Beck, 1995). Furthermore, it is necessary to address and challenge the cultural assumptions that lead the patient to fear imposing difficult feelings on the therapist or exposing him- or herself to shame.

Chinese psychiatric patients usually present with somatic complaints (Tsai and Chentsova-Dutton, 2002). Many patients complain of tiredness, dizziness and chronic pain and are commonly diagnosed as suffering from neurasthenia by Chinese psychiatrists. Kleinman (1982) found that most neurasthenia could be re-diagnosed as major depression. Draguns (1996) suggested that somatization might protect the sufferer from losing face if personal and private sentiments were redirected as bodily discomfort. Cheung (1984) also supported the theory that complaints of bodily discomfort and aches provided an appropriate problem for presentation in a health-oriented setting with no ambiguity or disapproval. In this respect, a cognitive therapist is well trained to explore the automatic thoughts and associated attributions around physical complaints.

Assertiveness in front of seniors is considered rude and impolite, which is in direct contrast to Western counterparts that emphasize autonomy and self-efficacy. Training in assertiveness skills in Chinese people requires considerable modification, as the Chinese emphasize compromise and negotiation in conflict situations (Gabrenya and Hwang, 1996). There is also an emphasis on saving others' 'face' in conflict situations, so that conflict resolution skills focus on compromise and exercising caution to avoid hurting the other party (Chiao, 1989). Sometimes, skills in selecting suitable intermediaries and mediators to minimize loss of face on both sides are taught in social skills training exercises.

## CONCLUSIONS

Recent local literature has supported the applicability of cognitive therapy in Chinese populations in various diagnoses, including generalized anxiety disorders (Zhang et al., 2002), prevention of mental problems in at-risk populations (Huang et al., 2001; Wong et al., 2002) and schizophrenia (Zhang et al., 1999; Ng et al., 2003). More rigorous and collaborative multicentre trials in greater China will provide more definitive conclusions about the effectiveness of cognitive therapy in a Chinese population.

## REFERENCES

Beck, J.S. 1995: *Cognitive Therapy: Basics and Beyond*. New York: Guilford Press.

Bond, M.H. 1991: *Beyond the Chinese Face: Insights from Psychology*. Hong Kong: Oxford University Press.

Bond, M.H. 1993: Emotions and their expression in Chinese culture. *Journal of Nonverbal Behavior* 17, 245–62.

Castro, J. and Rice, K.G. 2003: Perfectionism and ethnicity: implications for depressive symptoms and self-reported academic achievement. *Cultural Diversity and Ethnic Minority Psychology* 9, 64–78.

Chan, D.W. 1989: Dimensionality and adjustment: correlates of locus of control among Hong Kong Chinese. *Journal of Personality Assessment* 53, 145–60.

Chan, W.C. 1995: Depressive symptoms and coping strategies among Chinese adolescents in Hong Kong. *Journal of Youth and Adolescents* 24, 267–79.

Chang, E.C. 1998: Cultural differences, perfectionism, and suicidal risk in a college population: does social problem solving still matter? *Cognitive Therapy and Research* 22, 237–54.

Chen, C.S. and Uttal, D.H. 1988: Cultural values, parents' beliefs and children's achievement in the United States and China. *Human Development* 31, 351–58.

Cheung, F.M. 1984: Preferences in health seeking among Chinese students. *Culture, Medicine and Psychiatry* 8, 371–80.

Chiao, C. 1989: Chinese strategic behavior: some general principles. In Bolton, R. (ed.) *The Content, Constants and Variants.* New Haven: HRAF Press, 525–37.

Chien, M.F. 1984: The effect of teacher leadership style on adjustment of elementary school children. *Bulletin of Educational Psychology* 17, 99–120.

Crittenden, K.S. 1991: Asian self-effacement or feminine modesty? Attributional patterns of female university students in Taiwan. *Gender and Society* 5, 98–117.

Draguns, J.G. 1996: Abnormal behavior in Chinese societies: clinical, epidemiological and comparative studies. In Bond, M.H. (ed.) *Handbook of Chinese Psychology.* Hong Kong: Oxford University Press, 412–28.

Gabrenya, W.K. and Hwang, K.K. 1996: Chinese social interaction: harmony and hierarchy on the good earth. In Bond, M.H. (ed.) *Handbook of Chinese Psychology.* Hong Kong: Oxford University Press, 309–21.

Gao, G., Ting-Toomey, S. and Gudykunst, W.B. 1996: Chinese communication processes. In Bond, M.H. (ed.) *Handbook of Chinese Psychology.* Hong Kong: Oxford University Press, 280–93.

Gudykunst, W.B., Gao, G., Schmidt, K.L., Nishida, T., Bond, M.H., Lung, K., Wang, G. and Barraclough, R.A. 1992: The influence of individualism and collectivism on communication in in-group and out-group relationships. *Journal of Cross-Cultural Psychology* 23, 196–213.

Hess, R.D., Chang, C.M. and McDevitt, T.M. 1987: Cultural variations in family beliefs about children's performance in mathematics: comparison among People's Republic of China, Chinese Americans and Caucasian-American families. *Journal of Educational Psychology* 79, 179–88.

Ho, D.Y.F. 1996: Filial piety and its psychological consequences. In Bond, M.H. (ed.) *Handbook of Chinese Psychology.* Hong Kong: Oxford University Press, 155–65.

Huang, H.C., Hwang, K.K. and Ko, Y.H. 1983: Life stress, attribution style, social support and depression among university students. *Acta Psychologica Taiwanica* 25, 31–47.

Huang, X., Zhang, Y. and Yang, D. 2001: Chinese Taoist cognitive therapy in prevention of mental health problems of college students. *Chinese Mental Health Journal* 15, 243–46.

Kleinman, A. 1982: Neurasthenia and depression: a study of somatization and culture in China. *Culture, Medicine and Psychiatry* 6, 117–90.

Lau, S. and Leung, K. 1992: Relations with parents and school and Chinese adolescents' self-concept, delinquency, and academic performance. *British Journal of Educational Psychology* 62, 193–202.

Lee, R.P.L. 1995: Cultural tradition and stress management in modern society: learning from Hong Kong experience. In Lin, T.Y., Tseng, W.S. and Yeh, Y.S. (ed.) *Chinese Societies and Mental Health.* Hong Kong: Oxford University Press.

Leung, P.W.L. and Lee, P.W.H. 1996: Psychotherapy with the Chinese. In Bond, M.H. (ed.) *Handbook of Chinese Psychology.* Hong Kong: Oxford University Press, 441–56.

Lin, T.Y. and Lin, M.C. 1981: Love, denial and rejection: responses of Chinese families to mental illness. In Kleinman, A. and Lin, T.Y. (ed.) *Normal and Abnormal Behavior in Chinese Culture.* Dordrecht: D. Reidel, 387–401.

Lyubormirsky, S. and Nolen-Hoeksema, S. 1995. Effects of self-focused rumination on negative thinking and interpersonal problem solving. *Journal of Personality and Social Psychology* 69, 176–90.

Ng, R.M.K., Cheung, M. and Sun, L. 2003: Cognitive-behavioural therapy of psychosis: an overview and three case studies from Hong Kong. *Hong Kong Journal of Psychiatry* 13, 26–33.

Prochaska, J.O. and Norcross, J.C. (ed.) 2003: *Systems of Psychotherapy: a Transtheoretical Analysis* (5th edn). Pacific Grove, CA: Brooks/Cole.

Roberts, J.E., Gilboa, E. and Gotlib, I.H. 1998: Ruminative response style and vulnerability to episodes of dysphoria: gender, neuroticism and episode duration. *Cognitive Therapy and Research* 22, 401–23.

Safran, J.D. and Muran, J.C. 2000: *Negotiating the therapeutic alliance. A relational treatment guide.* New York: Guilford Press.

Spasojevic, J. and Alloy, N. 2003: Who becomes a ruminator? Developmental antecedents of ruminative response style. *Journal of Cognitive Psychotherapy: An International Quarterly* 16, 405–19.

Ting-Toomey, S., Gao, G., Trubsiky, P., Yang, Z., Kim, H., Lin, S. and Nishida, T. 1991: Culture, face maintenance, and styles of handling interpersonal conflict: a study in five cultures. *International Journal of Conflict Management* 2, 275–96.

Triandis, H.C. 1996: Foreword: Psychology moves East. In Bond, M.H. (ed.) *Handbook of Chinese Psychology.* Hong Kong: Oxford University Press, v–vii.

Tsai, J.L. and Chentsova-Dutton, Y. 2002: Understanding depression across cultures. In Gotlib I.H. and Hammen, C.L. (ed.) *Handbook of Depression.* New York: Guilford Press, 467–91.

Wong, D.F.K., Sun, S.Y.K., Tse, J. and Wong, F. 2002: Evaluating the outcomes of a cognitive-behavioural group intervention model for persons at risk of developing mental health problems in Hong Kong: a pretest-posttest study. *Research on Social Work Practice* 12, 534–45.

Zegal, Z.V., Williams, J.M.G. and Teasdale, J.D. 2002: *Mindfulness-based Cognitive Therapy.* New York: Guilford Press.

Zhang, J.X. and Bond, M.H. 1993: Target-based interpersonal trust. Cross-cultural comparison and its cognitive model. *Acta Psychologica Sinica* 2, 164–72.

Zhang, Z., Yao, S. and Fang, R. 1999: Controlled study on the role of cognitive psychotherapy in the remission of paranoid schizophrenia. *Chinese Mental Health Journal* 13, 174–75.

Zhang, Y., Young, D., Lee, S., Li, L., Zhang, H., Xiao, Z., Hao, W., Feng, Y., Zhou, H. and Chang, D.F. 2002: Chinese Taoist cognitive therapy in the treatment of generalized anxiety disorder in contemporary China. *Transcultural Psychiatry,* 39, 115–29.

# 29

# Psychiatric services in China – Guangzhou

## Veronica Pearson and Paul CW Lam

## INTRODUCTION

As is traditional in communist states, China has a system of central planning, which includes health and disability services. Every five years the central authorities produce a plan that is then passed down to the provincial and then lower levels of governance. They in their turn produce another plan that implements the principles, strategies and goals in the central plan in relation to their own particular circumstances. The framework of this chapter will be based on looking at developments in mental health services in the years since the Eighth Five Year Plan (Phillips and Pearson, 1994) was published in 1991 and particularly how this has been interpreted and implemented in one city, Guangzhou, which is classified as a 'model city' in disability issues.

There are several reasons for choosing Guangzhou. The author is very familiar with the mental health services there and is well acquainted with several key cadres who were willing to be interviewed for this chapter. Guangzhou shares the same Cantonese culture and language as Hong Kong and is of similar population, 6.7 million. Readers should bear in mind that China contains approximately one-quarter of the world's population and is a country of enormous geographical, economic and cultural diversity, especially in relation to the rural/urban divide. Inevitably, these diversities affect the provision of mental health services, making claims about mental health provision that are generalizable throughout China virtually impossible.

## CHANGES IN POLICY DIRECTIONS SINCE 1991

The Eighth Five Year Plan was the first in recent years to cover the health and welfare sector in any detail. Indeed, it was exciting because it put forward a coherent model for the community based treatment of mental illness that was to be tested in a number of urban and rural settings. It foundered on the usual rocks of lack of funding and properly trained staff. There is a discernible difference in philosophy between the Eighth Five Year Plan and the current Tenth Five Year Plan (All China Federation of the Disabled, 2001). The former emphasized monitoring mentally ill people at home (where most of them lived) via the 'guardianship team', taking medicine and ensuring that they did not 'cause trouble'. The biomedical perspective also dominated.

The current plan gives more recognition to the psycho-social model of understanding and treatment and is more concerned with helping people with a mental illness integrate and participate in normal community life. The overall goal is that they should also benefit from the economic and social developments that have taken place in recent years. Implementing these goals presents a very serious challenge.

## SERVICES IN GUANGZHOU

## Medical services

There are three psychiatric hospitals in Guangzhou. The largest and most prestigious – Fong Tsuen – with an official capacity of 1360 is run by the Bureau of Public Health and is also the oldest psychiatric hospital in China, having been established by an American medical missionary, John Kerr, in 1898. Fees are approximately RMB3000–4000 per month, which is about three times the average monthly household income in Guangzhou of RMB1225 in 2001 (Guangzhou Statistical Bureau, 2002). In the first month fees may be inflated by the addition of extra tests, examinations and medication. The second largest hospital, with a capacity of around 900 beds, is run by the Bureau of Civil Affairs. Originally, these hospitals were supposed to cater for poor people who could not pay fees, and for army veterans. However, with the increased pressure over the last 20 years for hospitals to become self-supporting the original mission has been greatly diluted. Monthly fees are around RMB1500. Finally, there is a private hospital, Bai Yun, with approximately 600 beds concentrating on psycho-geriatric patients. Fees at this hospital are lower than at the other two, around RMB1000. Thus the approximate total of psychiatric beds for a population of about 7 million people is 2860 or one bed per 2448 people.

Community-based services do not fill all service gaps. There are psychiatric outpatients services in every district but no day hospitals or day centres. Guardianship networks that are supposed to support the patient in the home consist largely of family members with occasional input from neighbours or local officials. Their major purpose is to stop the patient 'causing chaos' and the pressure falls on the family to do that. Some psychiatrists are willing to make home visits, or to hold fairly informal clinics in local community centres at very reasonable costs. Generally, the costs of outpatient treatment are low, especially in comparison with inpatient care. Psychotropic medication produced in China tends to be affordable, although imported medication is exorbitantly priced. Some family members, who cannot even afford the fees for an outpatient visit, will go to the pharmacy and purchase the medicine direct. Yet there are still some who can afford neither consultation nor medication and who are confined at home, sometimes in physical restraint.

## Community-based psycho-social services

### Vocational services

The issue of work is central to the Chinese psyche and the sense of positive individual personhood, contributing member of the community and fully paid-up citizen. Indeed, the Chinese Constitution (Article 42, 1982) enshrines the right and duty of every person to work. Work marks the graduation from child to adult status, particularly in a society where the separation from parents is far less well-defined than it tends to be in North America or Western Europe. The benefits of work do not only include wages and a job for life but also access to housing, social and medical insurance. Until the economic changes in the 1980s it was possible for most people with a mental illness to have a job because factories and other enterprises did not have to show a profit and deficits were bankrolled by the various levels of government. Thus nobody worried about how productive workers were, or if they needed medical treatment. Once a more rational economic model was introduced, managers became increasingly reluctant to employ people with a mental illness because they were seen as a liability for whom expensive medical treatment would have to be paid, possibly over a lifetime. Thus since the mid-1980s unemployment, particularly among younger people with a mental illness, has become a serious issue.

In Guangzhou enterprises with over 100 employees are supposed to have at least 1.5 per cent of staff that are classified as disabled. People with a mental illness would be the least preferred group. However, employers can avoid this requirement by paying 80 per cent of the average annual wage in Guangzhou for every person that they are under quota. This money is supposed to find its way, via the Department of Finance at national level, back to the city or district in which the enterprise is registered where it should be spent on services for people with a disability – at least in Guangzhou. The local Federation for the Disabled would very much prefer that enterprises simply employ people with a disability. There are tax benefits for enterprises who do employ their quota of people with a disability so another phenomenon is that managers pay a very minimum wage to workers with a disability but ask them to stay at home (Pearson, 1995; Wong, 1998).

The Bureau of Civil Affairs runs vocational workshops for people with a disability but these have never accepted people with a mental illness as clients. Likewise the Guangzhou branch of the Federation of the Disabled provides a job matching and placement service for people with a disability but this service is not available to those with a mental illness. People with a learning disability are included in both these services. The argument is that employers are not interested in taking on staff with a history of mental illness partly because of fear and partly because they are concerned that they will have to pay for extensive and expensive treatment in the future. Thus this exclusion seems to be based on a mixture of stigma and economic self-interest.

To overcome some of these discriminatory attitudes the Guangzhou branch of the Federation of the Disabled decided to build a purpose-built workshop for mentally ill people providing 200 places. Planning started in 2003 but the opening of the workshop was delayed by the complaints of residents in the neighbourhood who did not want such a facility close to their homes. It took some time for the cadres of the Federation for the Disabled to calm their fears and so the workshop did not admit its first 40 trainees until the summer of 2006. Their initial aim is to admit 100 trainees but they hope to expand this over time to 200. Their goal is to offer a variety of vocational opportunities including

supported employment, on-the-job training and other approaches that involve real work in real settings. A further, unexpected obstacle was also encountered. It has proven difficult to recruit trainees although there are more than enough people eligible for places. Parents have been reluctant to let their adult children attend the workshop, fearing that their child would not be able to tolerate the stress of activity mirroring the expectations of the workplace. The workshop is a centre of vocational rehabilitation of various kinds and is the first such resource in China for people with a mental illness. As such it is an important development and many people will be watching to see whether and how well it works. A mark of its importance is that Mr Deng Pufang (Chairman of the All China Federation of the Disabled and the son of the late Paramount Leader, Mr Deng Xiaoping) has agreed to officiate at the opening ceremony.

Providing services for people in rural areas has been both a priority and a major stumbling block. It is a national target of the Federation of the Disabled to provide rehabilitation farms to help mentally ill people in rural areas and also those urbanites who are chronically mentally ill and cannot survive in an industrial setting. The Guangzhou Federation of the Disabled has acquired two farms. One mainly grows vegetables and has around 20 trainees working there and the second is an orchard which is not yet in operation as a therapeutic farm. Similar problems to those that the workshop experienced have been encountered in that parents have been very hesitant to permit their adult children to go to live and work on a farm. Some of this reluctance is doubtless due to a desire to protect their children from stress, but some of it is probably an unwillingness to let their children be involved in work which is considered by most urbanites to be hard and inferior. In both the case of the workshop and the farms the Li Kang Resource Centre (see below) liaised with parents to educate them about the value of structured vocational and day programmes for their children. In the case of the therapeutic farms they organized several experiential camps for trainees. While parents acknowledged that their children became more independent after attending these camps, they were still reluctant to let them go to live and work on the farm for longer periods of time. This may well be an indication that independence from parents as a developmental goal is not given the same priority by parents in China as it would be in westernized countries.

## Accommodation services

The huge psychiatric hospitals that became places of permanent residence for thousands of patients in the UK never developed in China. Some Chinese psychiatric hospitals, especially those in the Ministry of Civil Affairs system, do have long-stay patients but on the whole the majority of people with a mental illness in China (about 90 per cent) live with family members (Pearson and Phillips, 1994). Chinese psychiatrists are aware of accommodation alternatives that have developed in other countries and there is some interest in exploring these possibilities in China. For instance, the national Tenth Five Year Plan included setting up half-way houses. When overtures were made at the district level in Guangzhou to develop a half-way house, there was a great deal of resistance from local cadres and residents who objected to having psychiatric patients living in their midst – a tale all too familiar internationally. The Federation of the Disabled decided to drop the initiative and concentrate on issues that were more achievable.

There was also some disquiet among cadres themselves that by introducing accommodation alternatives they would undermine family care which is currently strong and prevalent. The issue of funding is also important. It is expected that new services will be largely, if not completely, self-funding. It seems very likely that half-way houses or other types of accommodation would rapidly fill with people whose families could afford to keep them there, rather than residents being selected on the grounds of need. There are still some who find this idea distasteful and in contradiction of the best tenets of socialism.

## The Likang Family Resources Centre

The centre is based on a model developed in Hong Kong. The objectives are:

- To provide information, counselling, and other community-based rehabilitation support for mentally ill people and their families.

- To promote mental health education in order to strengthen prevention and treatment of mental illness in the community.

The services provided by the centre include a resource library, community mental health education, a family psycho-education programme, activity groups, individual and group counselling and professional training and consultation and recreational activities (Pearson and Lam, 2001; Lam, 2004). Programmes and activities are provided at little or no cost to participants in order to encourage maximum participation and to ensure no one is excluded on grounds of poverty.

This resource centre started in 1999 as a pioneer joint project between the Richmond Fellowship of Hong Kong (a Hong Kong-based non-governmental organization that provides community-based rehabilitation services for mentally ill people and their families) and the Guangzhou branch of the All China Federation for the Disabled. It was generously funded for five years by the Kadoorie Foundations. During the first five years a qualified social worker from Hong Kong was employed, along with two staff from Guangzhou. The major function of the Hong Kong social worker was to establish the programme and train Guangzhou people with the necessary skills to run it. The Likang Centre has been well received and was honoured by a visit from the Chairman of the national level of the All-China Federation of the Disabled, Mr Deng Pufang, thus giving the centre recognition at national level. While this service model was not explicitly written into the Tenth Five Year Plan at national level, the plan does emphasize work with caregivers and mentions 'multi-channel, multi-service, community based psycho-social approaches and social work elements'. This constitutes a major change in approach. Social work is not yet well defined in China but in this context may be taken to mean intervention 'not focused on medicine, using group work, case-work and psycho-education' (Dr Liang of the Guangzhou Federation of the Disabled, personal communication).

The Family Resource Centre Model was written into the Guangzhou Tenth Five Year Plan where there are now four Likang Centres in different districts, with staff from the original centre providing training and guidance to the three new ones. The original Likang Centre was handed over to the Guangzhou branch of the Federation of the Disabled to incorporate into their own administrative and financial systems in 2003. It is a measure of the success of the project that this transition has gone smoothly. There have been no staff cuts and permanent positions within the Federation structure have been allocated to the Guangzhou staff of the Likang Centre, ensuring their security of employment. The Richmond Fellowship of Hong Kong continues to have a role providing staff development and training.

## CONCLUSION

Since the 'opening up' of China, Guangzhou has benefited from its close proximity to Hong Kong in many ways, including the willingness of non-governmental organizations in Hong Kong to provide services and training to Guangzhou cadres in health and welfare matters. Thus, Guangzhou's development has been significantly faster than in many other areas of China. However, this does not necessarily make it representative. The problems of funding and lack of trained staff are neither easily nor quickly overcome. Despite national and local levels of planning, too much continues to rest on the chance of there being key personnel at local levels who care enough about people with a mental illness to take effective action in implementing and developing new goals and services, even when working within severe funding constraints.

## REFERENCES

All China Federation of the Disabled 2001: *Tenth Five Year Plan (Mental Illness)* (in Chinese). www.cdpf.org.cn (accessed 16 March 2004).

Guangzhou Statistical Bureau 2002: *Guangzhou Statistical Yearbook 2001.* Beijing: China Statistics Press.

Constitution of the People's Republic of China 1982: Beijing: Foreign Languages Press.

Lam, P.C.W. 2004: A comparative study of the experience of caring and the coping strategies used by families of adults with schizophrenia in Guangzhou and Hong Kong. PhD thesis, Department of Social Work and Social Administration, University of Hong Kong.

Pearson, V. 1995: *Mental Health Care in China: State Policies, Professional Services and Family Responsibilities.* London: Gaskell/New York: American Psychiatric Press.

Pearson, V. and Lam, P.C.W. 2001: On their own; caregivers in Guangzhou. In Lefley, H.P. and Johnson, D.L. (eds) *Family Interventions in Mental Illness; International Perspectives.* Estport, CT/London: Praeger, 171–84.

Pearson, V. and Phillips, M.R. 1994: The social context of psychiatric rehabilitation in China. *British Journal of Psychiatry* Suppl. 24: 11–18. Review.

Phillips, M.R. and Pearson, V. 1994: Future opportunities and challenges for the development of psychiatric rehabilitation in China. *British Journal of Psychiatry* Suppl. 24, 128–42.

Wong, L. 1998: *Marginalization and Social Welfare in China.* London: Routledge.

# 30

# European perspectives on cultural psychiatry

Christoph Lauber and Wulf Rössler

## INTRODUCTION

Diversity of mental health care in Europe reflects economic capacity and the extent each country is prepared to invest in mental health (Marusic, 2004). As a result, there are many disparities in the mental health of the populations in the different European countries as assessed by a variety of indicators of mental health (Agius *et al.*, 2005). Among others, there are variations of general menta0l health in terms of perceived wellbeing or psychological distress, amount and type of interventions, rates of death from suicide or due to substance use, mental illness-related diseases such as liver cirrhosis due to alcohol misuse, the proportion of people in the general population who recognize the symptoms of a given mental disorder, the percentage of psychiatrists who know and apply best practice guidelines for the identification and management of mental illness, and, finally, the proportion of medication needs met among people with mental illness. Thus,

writing about mental health services in Europe may end up as a country-by-country description. As McKee and Jacobson (2000) pointed out, 'any attempt to describe public health in Europe faces the twin problems of defining Europe and of dealing with the diversity of health and health systems it contains'.

Despite these caveats, this chapter aims to describe different aspects of mental health services and the respective research in favour of these systems. It gives an overview of the current state of development in European psychiatry, and presents the challenges facing European mental health services in the next years. The status of mental health care in Europe is presented to reflect the cultural values in society and in mental health care in Europe. These are likely to be more visible and discernible by readers from outside Europe, as to most Europeans the developments 'appear' to be driven by evidence and the interests of patients, yet it is undoubtedly the case that European nations express culture through their institutions and show their cultural values in the way priorities are set in public services. European approaches to cultural psychiatry have not always focused on race, ethnic group or culture of immigrants but on cultural influences from neighbouring countries, and sometimes from people of the same ethnic origin, but of different national origins.

## MENTAL HEALTH POLICY IN EUROPE

### The intentions

The World Health Report (World Health Organization, 2001) specifies that services are provided in the community where the patient lives. They include a variety of different facilities, among them general hospital psychiatric wards and long-term residential facilities. Moreover, services are fully co-ordinated among themselves and with other community health and social agencies. They are ambulatory rather than static, and also offer the possibility of home treatment, if appropriate. Interventions are targeted to prevent and minimize disabilities, and not only symptoms. Treatment and care are specific for the diagnosis and the general needs of the patient. There is a clear partnership with carers and families. Finally, there is clear legislation to support and make possible all the above (World Health Organization, 2001).

Since 2005, European mental health policy is additionally endorsed by the Mental Health Declaration for Europe and the respective Mental Health Action Plan. It was approved by the ministers of health of the 52 member states in the European region of the World Health Organization (WHO). It sets a clear policy direction for the development of mental health services in Europe for at least the next decade (Thornicroft and Rose, 2005). The recommendations to be realized in the member states include the fostering of mental wellbeing, social inclusion as well as the fight against stigmatization and discrimination of people with mental illness, the implementation of comprehensive mental health services, the provision of a quantitatively and qualitatively skilled workforce and, finally, the inclusion of users and caregivers in planning, developing and running mental health services (Thornicroft and Rose, 2005; World Health Organization, 2005a,b).

In Europe, mental health problems account for nearly 20 per cent of the total burden of ill-health and come second only to cardiovascular disease. The International Labour Organization (ILO) estimates the economic costs of mental health problems at a conservatively estimated 3–4 per cent of total European gross national product (GNP). They do not take into account negative effects of mental health on other aspects of health, for example, co-morbidity with physical illness and increased mortality. Adverse health consequences are only one element of the overall impact of mental health on society. Besides social exclusion and stigma due to mental illness, reduced employment opportunities and lost employment, absenteeism and sick leave, reduced performance at work, lost leisure opportunities, early retirement and premature mortality account for between 60 and 80 per cent of the costs of both schizophrenia and depression. These impact on those suffering with mental illness and also their family members and caregivers.

### The reality

In what context do these initiatives take place? As a first step when discussing mental health policy in Europe we should take a closer look at the economic and social development of European countries by looking, for example, at economic inequalities between countries reflected in respective GNPs per capita. The Swedish GNP (US$23 750), for example, exceeds 10 times Russia's GNP (US$2240). Consequently, there are vast differences in available resources to be allocated to health care. Other global indicators such as life expectancy or infant and child mortality make the inter-country contrasts in health even more evident (Feachem, 2000).

Although shared human rights legislation fosters greater harmonization of mental health practices, there remains great diversity in psychiatric practice between European countries (see Chapter 7). Differences exist in, for instance, funding and implementing a mental health policy, the level of public attitude and awareness of mental illnesses, (mental) health behaviour of the population and access to psychiatric care, the education of the professions involved in mental health care provision, diagnosing and treating psychiatric disorders, the equipment of mental health services, the epidemiology of particular diseases, in involving family members in care, and in empowering affected people to be involved in mental health service development (van Os and Neeleman, 1994).

Europe can be categorized into at least three parts: countries with mental health services mostly provided in asylums, those in a process of replacing asylums by a spectrum of mental health services and, finally, countries with a well-developed mental health system based on a pragmatic balance of community and hospital care (Thornicroft and Tansella, 2004). The deinstitutionalization process is advancing at different paces in different countries, again depending on the level of available resources (Fakhoury and Priebe, 2002). Costs were reported to be generally the same or even less for discharged patients living in the community (Rothbard and Kuno, 2000). Others have noted that deinstitutionalization has put too much of a focus on the locus of care, while little attention is given to the humaneness, effectiveness and quality of care (Geller, 2000). Most importantly, the emergence of managed care – shifting responsibilities of care for patients with severe mental illness from the public to the private sector – was suggested to have led to fears of undertreatment or lower-quality services because of the capitation system; this system led to agencies having a fixed amount of money per patient. The concern is that this system may reduce patient choice of treatment. McCulloch et al. (2000), however, expressed concern that, for community safety reasons, governments will adopt more conservative and safety-oriented care practices, which could only lead to further alienation and stigmatization of mentally ill people.

In contrast to deinstitutionalization, there has been increasing consideration of 'confinement' of some patients with severe mental illness in some countries. Forensic care is expanding in several countries, including Austria and the UK (Fakhoury and Priebe, 2002). In these countries, resources

for community care are relatively scarce, so these services are overloaded and too few specialized community mental health services exist.

Deinstitutionalized patients also seem to be facing community residents' opposition to their deinstitutionalization. Wright et al. (2000) noted that discharging patients into hostile communities may affect their self-concept, mental health status and success in adjusting to community life. The effects of deinstitutionalization depend on national traditions and socio-cultural context, the availability of resources and financial incentives as well as specific features of the given social welfare and health care systems (Rasanen et al., 2000; Silfverhielm and Kamis-Gould, 2000). As a result, deinstitutionalization varies across countries and seems to encompass policies ranging from having severely mentally ill patients in psychiatric units in general instead of mental hospitals, to having patients in the community in supported/supportive housing or in psychiatric service complexes away from the community.

In countries with advanced deinstitutionalization, the discussion currently focuses on ensuring that patients are integrated within the community and have access to employment and housing (Fakhoury and Priebe, 2002). Furthermore, most of this research has been confined to comparisons between different catchment areas and this does not help with comparisons between countries (Salvador-Carulla et al., 2005).

Though considerable regional differences may exist, Western Europe has accomplished by and large the transition from hospital-based psychiatry to community-oriented mental health care. In contrast, Eastern Europe – after 40 years under regimes whose totalitarianism is well reflected in the asylum-oriented organization of mental health care – is at best at the beginning of this process (Knapp et al., 2005). Thus, in these times Eastern European countries face an enormous task in reorganizing their mental health services. Whereas Western European countries spend on average 5 per cent of their health budget on mental health care, with Luxembourg, England and Sweden spending more than 10 per cent each, the mental health expenditures of Eastern European countries are fairly low. The lowest budgets are reported from Russia and the former satellite countries of the Soviet Union where mental health services were a low priority in the past. Albania and Russia spend less than 2 per cent and Slovakia 2 per cent of their health budgets on mental health (Knapp *et al.*, 2005). The economic funds available will have an effect on service provision, on locations in which services are provided, and on the skills and capacity of the workforce. The 'brain drain' of (mental) health professionals from Eastern to Western Europe maintains the difficult situation of (mental) health care in these countries, and impedes the progress they can make.

## Community care: the evidence

International studies of mental health care provision are relevant to investigate the extent of inequities within the European countries and to assess the needs for development of the health care systems of Eastern Europe. Empirical assessment of service systems is also required to verify to what extent policies of mental health services reform have been implemented in practice. Finally, comparison of mental health care systems between areas is important for research, providing a context for understanding why outcomes from evaluations of apparently similar interventions may differ between areas and countries (Burns and Priebe, 1996).

A number of studies have compared mental health care systems in various European regions in terms of inputs and processes (Gater *et al.*, 1995; Salize *et al.*, 1999; Sytema and Burgess, 1999), some of which will now be reported on.

In the Netherlands, intensive community-based care has increased five times more than hospital-based care was reduced. This contradicts the goals set in the Dutch mental health policy that aims at substituting outpatient and other community care for inpatient care and not at expanding mental health services (Pijl *et al.*, 2000). The current concern is that community mental health centres may have serviced new and less severely ill patients instead of patients with severe and persistent illnesses, a criticism known from the UK and the USA.

In Germany, a greater number of patients with mental illness live in institutionalized homes, but

with little access to the community and with little empowerment. Deinstitutionalization was reported to have led in many parts of the country to patients staying in renamed sections of hospitals or in homes for the disabled (von Cranach, 2000). A lack of community mental health teams and community psychiatric nursing, a shortage of social work back-up, and understaffed residential and nursing homes are some of the problems of deinstitutionalization in Germany (Richter and Nollau, 2000). Despite this, research has shown that in Germany a large number of former long-stay patients appear to be able to live in the community, albeit in highly staffed settings, with a significant decrease in time spent in hospital. Böcker *et al.* (2001) investigated mental health services in former East Germany. They found that in East Germany the policy of psychiatric reform had not yet been implemented as intended.

Becker *et al.* (2002) investigated urban mental health services in five Western European countries and found marked variations in service organization and pattern of use. In a study comparing Italy and Spain, great differences emerged in patterns of service provision and use between and within countries. In contrast to Northern Europe, high unemployment rates were not associated with high service utilization rates, but areas with large numbers of single-person households tended to have high service use. Most service utilization rates were substantially below those reported from Northern Europe. Spanish centres tended to have low rates of hospital service utilization despite limited development of community-based services. Trieste, with its strong emphasis on developing innovative community services, showed a distinctive pattern with low hospital bed use and high rates of day service use and of contacts in the community (Salvador-Carulla *et al.*, 2005).

In Greece, the existing number of community-based alternatives to inpatient psychiatric care is considered to still be inadequate to reduce admissions in public mental hospitals and to accommodate the yet-to-be deinstitutionalized long-stay patients (Madianos *et al.*, 2000). In Sweden, Silfverhielm and Kamis-Gould (2000) indicated that the insufficient reallocation of resources to establish community-based services has led to patients continuing to be hospitalized. The limited co-operation among the specialty mental health system, primary health care and local social services was reported to have unintended disincentives to serving consumers with multiple needs.

In Finland, patients from smaller counties with fewer resources are more likely to move to alternative community placements, whereas those in larger counties with more resources are more likely to be treated in hospitals (Rasanen et al., 2000). Large Finnish counties seem more able to afford continuous hospitalization and have less incentive to deinstitutionalize. Successful deinstitutionalization in Finland is argued to be dependent on the availability of alternative types of community placements with more and better trained staff providing community-based support.

An interesting study on pathways to care in Eastern Europe was published recently (Gater et al., 2005). It reported that direct access was the route for more than a third of new patients in six centres. Irrespective of diagnosis, GPs played a limited role in the pathways to psychiatric care. Only a small proportion of patients consulted GPs and the only treatment provided by GPs was sedatives and hypnotics. Antidepressants were prescribed to very few and were almost as likely to be given to those with schizophrenia as those with depression. This pattern may arise in part from the constraints imposed by prescribing regulations and by the limitations imposed by the 'positive' list; there may also be reservations of both patients and doctors to the use of 'strong' medicines (such as antidepressants or antipsychotics), with connotations of severe mental illness, in favour of 'mild' medicines (such as sedatives or hypnotics), which are less taboo. These patterns of prescribing are not unique; they do not differ greatly from those reported from several centres in the World Health Organization pathways study. Many factors contributed to this, including lack of training and experience in psychiatry in primary care, absence of incentives, poor contact between GPs and psychiatrists, availability of medication and regulations limiting the autonomy of GPs in managing mental disorders. If mental health is to be integrated into primary care, then an educational approach is more likely to succeed if this broader complex of factors is also addressed through the formal inclusion of mental health as a component of primary care and the further development and implementation of evidence-based national programmes for mental health (Gater et al., 2005).

## Hospital versus community-based mental health treatment

In recent years there has been a debate between those who are in favour of the provision of mental health treatment and care in hospitals, and those who prefer to use primarily or even exclusively community settings, in which the two forms of care are often seen as incompatible. There is no compelling argument and no scientific evidence favouring the use of hospital services alone. On the other hand, there is also no evidence that community services alone can provide satisfactory and comprehensive care. The overall evidence base and clinical experience support a balanced approach that incorporates elements of both hospital and community care (Thornicroft and Tansella, 2002).

Thornicroft and Tansella (2002) concluded that the lack of material resources severely constrains how mental health policy is translated into practice. The authors suggest a three-step model, with step A in areas with low level of resources (primary care with specialist back-up), step B with medium level of resources (mainstream mental health care) and step C in areas with high level of resources (specialized/differentiated mental health services). In low-resource areas it may be unrealistic to invest in any of the components described here as mainstream mental health care: outpatient/ambulatory clinics, community mental health teams and long-term community-based residential care. The focus will need to be upon primary mental health care with specialist back-up, where the main role for the relatively few specialist mental health staff is to support and train primary care staff, for example, in psychopharmacology. Areas that can afford a more differentiated model of care may first consolidate their mainstream mental health care, with the capacity of each service component decided as a balance between the known local needs, the resources available and the priorities of local stakeholders.

In general, as mental health systems develop away from an asylum-based model, the proportion of the total budget spent on the large asylums gradually decreases. In other words, new services outside hospital can only be provided by using extra resources (which is uncommon) or by using the resources that are transferred from the hospital sites and staff (which is the more usual case). Interestingly, the evidence from cost-effectiveness studies of deinstitutionalization and the provision of community mental health teams suggest that the quality of care is closely related to the expenditure on services, and overall community-based models of care are largely equivalent in cost to the services that they replace.

## EVIDENCE-BASED MENTAL HEALTH: IS THIS EUROPEAN REALITY?

### Treatment

European countries differ in terms of mental health service organization, but also regarding clinical parameters: the lack of reliable markers for psychiatric diagnoses has contributed to the continued use of 'nationalistic' diagnostic categories such as the Scandinavian 'reactive psychosis' and the French 'bouffée delirante'. Modified electroconvulsive therapy has fallen into disrepute in countries such as the Netherlands, Switzerland and Germany, whereas in Britain, Denmark, France and Bulgaria it continues to be widely used (van Os and Neeleman, 1994). Psychoanalytical theory (revolving around 'unconscious' conflicts) is popular among mental health workers in many countries, such as France, Germany and Switzerland, whereas ostensibly more scientific biological and behavioural principles are favoured in, for example, the UK (van Os et al., 1993). There are international differences in the indications and perceived therapeutic properties of drugs such as antipsychotic agents and a curious north–south divide in the annual per capita exposure to benzodiazepines. The German practice to treat relatively mild neurotic disorders on an inpatient basis in costly 'psychosomatic' hospitals

contrasts with efforts elsewhere to treat these conditions in the community (van Os and Neeleman, 1994).

The Americas are the mother- or father-land of evidence-based principles in general health care, whereas for mental health care it could be the UK that deserves this title. Without addressing the controversies about whether or not to practise evidence-based medicine (Miles et al., 2003), Cooper (2003) found in a meta-analysis of publications on evidence-based psychiatry and health care that, although evidence-based health care is now being promulgated as a rational basis for mental health planning in Britain, its contributions to service evaluation have been distinctly modest. Only 10 per cent of clinical trials and meta-analyses have been focused on effectiveness of services, and many reviews proved inconclusive. The current evidence-based approach is overly reliant on meta-analytic reviews, and is more applicable to specific treatments than to the care agencies that control their delivery.

A wide variety of community-based service models are in operation for people with mental health problems, following the deinstitutionalization movement of the last 30 years. Despite this shift, however, the evidence in their favour continues to be equivocal, while the specific nature of different service models is unclear (Burns et al., 2002). For example, although Marshall and Lockwood (2000) reviewed studies of assertive community treatment (ACT), they excluded studies of ACT as an alternative to hospital admission, or as a hospital diversion programme, or for those in crisis. However, those under the care of ACT were less likely to be admitted to hospital or to be lost to follow-up.

A systematic review has investigated the effectiveness of day care for individuals with severe mental disorders (de Girolamo and Bassi, 2004). Nine randomized controlled trials were evaluated for the effectiveness of acute day hospitals compared with usual hospital admissions. The authors found that a quarter to a third of hospitalized patients may be effectively and safely treated in a day hospital setting. Although there was no difference between the two groups in the overall number of hospital days, patients admitted to day hospital spent fewer days as inpatients and showed a faster improvement in mental state (but not in social functioning). Finally, day hospital care was cheaper than usual hospital care, for between 20 and 37 per cent of patients.

Only five randomized trials compare day care and ordinary outpatient care for patients aged 18–65 years, without a primary diagnosis of substance abuse or organic mental disorder (Marshall *et al.*, 2001). Two trials clearly showed superior effectiveness on psychiatric symptoms of day treatment programmes compared with outpatient care for patients with anxiety or depression resistant to treatment. However, there was no difference on any other outcome variable. On the other hand, comparing day care and outpatient treatment for the severely mentally ill did not ascertain any difference on any outcome variable (but day care seemed to be more expensive).

In a comprehensive review on the effectiveness of home treatment in terms of hospitalization and cost-effectiveness, Burns *et al.* (2001) reviewed 91 studies published in a 30-year span. Of these, 87 focused on psychotic patients and 56 were randomized trials. For studies comparing home treatment with usual hospital admission, there was on average a reduction of five days spent in hospital for each patient treated at home (no statistically significant difference). In contrast, for studies comparing home treatment with other types of community-based care, there was no difference in terms of days spent in hospital or with regard to other outcome variables. Regular home visits and taking responsibility for both the health and social needs of patients was also associated with a decrease in hospital days.

These meta-analyses show that once the initial enthusiasm for community care as a sort of 'magic box' has faded, there is growing awareness that community care 'is a service delivery vehicle'. It can allow treatment to be offered to a patient, but is not the treatment itself. This distinction is important, as the actual ingredients of treatment have been 'insufficiently emphasised' (Brunt and Hansson, 2002; de Girolamo and Fioritti, 2002).

An approach to assess the quality of mental health services was presented by Lasalvia *et al.* (2000). They assessed needs for care according to both patient and staff perspectives in a sample of

patients that includes the full spectrum of diagnoses of mental disorder. Patients and staff showed poor agreement on both the presence of a need and on whether or not a need had been met. Higher disability predicted a higher number of patient-rated needs, while higher disability, higher number of service contacts and patient unemployment predicted a higher number of staff-rated needs. Lower global function predicted higher disagreement in patients' and staff's ratings of needs. In general, staff tended to identify more needs in areas related to medical issues, while patients tended to report more needs in areas of everyday life. Disagreement between patient and staff opinions seems to be the rule rather than the exception, especially when provision of individualized mental health care is concerned. As patients and staff showed different perceptions of needs for care, multiple perspectives should be considered for planning and providing effective needs-led mental health care.

Inappropriate termination of contact with mental health services is considered another indicator of poor quality of mental health services (Young *et al.*, 2000). Thus varying levels of disengagement might be found for between 20 and 40 per cent of people who attend a community-based mental health service. Compared with patients who left treatment prematurely, patients who stayed were older, more likely to have a psychotic disorder, less likely to be married, more likely to be living in an institution, more satisfied with their relationships with friends and family, and less likely to have legal problems. However, on average outcomes improved both for patients who stayed and for patients who left. On the other hand, Lasalvia *et al.* (2000) found that lower age, less use of day care and less use of outpatient care in the previous year all increased the risk of dropping out of treatment. Premature termination of treatment was not associated with other socio-demographic characteristics, psychiatric history or diagnosis (except schizophrenia) and inpatient days or community care contact in the previous year.

## Employment

One of the most important developments in social psychiatry during the past years has been the emergence of more effective strategies of psycho-social treatment, with particular reference to the rehabilitation of patients with severe and persistent mental disorders. Programmes of supported employment have gained the most favourable reports (Drake *et al.*, 1999). Interest in the implementation and evaluation of supported employment programmes has grown contemporaneously in several countries, including Finland (Saloviita and Pirttimaa, 2000), Germany (Reker *et al.*, 2000) and Switzerland (Hoffmann *et al.*, 2003). The most systematic implementation and evaluation of such programmes has been carried out by one group in Rhode Island, USA (Drake *et al.*, 1999), where the authors have introduced innovative rehabilitation programmes based on manualized forms of psycho-social treatment, aimed at supporting job placement into the free labour market circuit, known as individual placement support (IPS). Outcome studies of supported employment programmes based on the IPS model have yielded impressive results. In a randomized controlled trial of IPS against enhanced vocational rehabilitation, 152 unemployed inner-city patients who expressed an interest in obtaining competitive jobs were followed up for 19 months. The IPS group became competitively employed significantly more often than the enhanced vocational rehabilitation group (61 per cent versus 9 per cent), whereas non-vocational outcomes were similarly improved for both groups. With regard to vocational rehabilitation, supported employment was more effective than vocational rehabilitation for patients suffering from a severe mental disorder who did want to work. The general implication of these findings is that people suffering from mental disorders who want to work should be offered a supported employment option. Commissioning agencies would be justified in encouraging vocational rehabilitation providers to develop more supported employment schemes. From a research perspective, the cost-effectiveness of supported employment should be examined in larger multicentre trials. Similar conclusions have been reached in a systematic review and meta-analysis for the Cochrane Collaboration (Crowther *et al.*, 2001). Supported employment was significantly more effective than pre-vocational training on primary outcome variables (number

of patients in competitive employment); for example, at 18 months 34 per cent of individuals in supported employment were employed versus 12 per cent in pre-vocational training.

Clients in supported employment also earned more and worked more hours per month than those in pre-vocational training. There was no evidence that pre-vocational training was more effective in helping clients to obtain competitive employment than standard community care. As with other forms of psycho-social treatment that originate from the USA, the issue of replicability in non-US settings needs to be kept in mind. In particular, it is not easy to predict whether the same results would be achieved in countries where the labour market is more protected, for example, in Europe, where workers have more rights and are partly protected by powerful worker unions, but access to jobs is more difficult and turnover proceeds at a slower pace and not according to the 'hire and fire' principle. Thus, this model is currently being replicated in a variety of settings outside the USA (e.g. in Europe) (de Girolamo and Fioritti 2002; Burns *et al.*, 2006).

## Housing

In the last few decades, in parallel with the closing of many mental hospitals around the world, large numbers of severely mentally ill patients have been relocated to a variety of non-hospital residential settings, called residential facilities. These include different types of accommodation such as 'group homes', 'intermediate facilities', 'wards in the community', 'boarding-and-care homes', 'supervised hostels' or 'sheltered apartments'. To date, no internationally agreed and precise taxonomy has been developed to classify residential facilities and identify their distinct functions for specific groups of patients with severe mental disorders. Different facility names (as indicated above) often correspond to identical settings, while sometimes facilities having similar names exhibit very different characteristics and pursue divergent objectives (de Girolamo and Bassi, 2004).

The most important longitudinal study providing data about patients resettled in residential facilities is the Team for the Assessment of Psychiatric Services (TAPS) project, carried out in the greater London area and assessing the five-year outcome of a representative cohort of 523 patients discharged from two mental hospitals to a variety of community residences (Leff and Trieman, 2000). Although there was no change in the patients' clinical state or in their problems of social behaviour, they gained domestic, community living skills and more freedom than in the previous hospital setting, they acquired friends, and they wanted to remain in their current state. In the framework of the same project, a specific analysis has recently focused on a subgroup of 61 long-stay psychiatric inpatients, initially regarded as unsuitable for community placement and followed up for five years (Trieman and Leff, 2002). Substantial improvements occurred in clinical and social functioning which enabled 29 patients (40 per cent of the study group) to be resettled in various residential facilities, gaining better access to community amenities and living more independently (de Girolamo and Bassi, 2004).

Violence risks of severely mentally ill patients may represent a significant problem for community resettlement. The TAPS study (Leff and Trieman, 2000) showed that violence and aggressiveness may drop in most residents as they become more and more familiar with their place of residence and feel comfortable in their living environment.

Current data on residents' turnover show that discharge to independent living is an infrequent event. In Italy, more than a third of residential facilities (37.7 per cent) did not discharge any patients and 31.5 per cent discharged only one or two patients during the course of an entire year (de Girolamo et al., 2002). Also in the five-year follow-up study, very low rates of turnover were shown for patients discharged to community residences. In general, even when optimal treatment is provided to all long-term patients, a substantial proportion of patients will remain and for many of them residential facilities will possibly be 'homes for life' (de Girolamo and Bassi, 2004).

An alternative to the dimensional sheltered housing model may be represented by a categorical 'supported housing' model. Within this model there are, on the one hand, high-cover residential facilities and, on the other hand, residential facilities with limited cover, and a flexible system of on-site support can allow a temporary increase in the quantity of required help in less intensive settings, when patients face a crisis. In the continuum model the system provides fixed levels of supervision and patients are expected to move around as they get better (or worse). In the supported housing model, apart from residential facilities with 24-hour support, the remaining facilities are organized according to flexible levels of supervision around 'usual' housing options, and staff are expected to move around according to the fluctuating needs of patients. For both models, a problem faced by the high-cover residential facilities may be the difficulty in providing individually centred and sensitive care. If mismatches occur between levels of dependency and levels of supervision (more often in the direction of too much supervision), there is the risk of decreasing functioning by over-provision and not presenting an optimal challenge.

An important implication of the supported housing model is that discharge to independent living should not necessarily be considered a (feasible) target. A substantial number of patients may remain indefinitely within the residential network, while other objectives (e.g. clinical stabilization, ensured compliance, quality of life (QOL) improvements, etc.) become the objective of the intervention. Longitudinal studies, using large, representative samples of residents, are needed in order to clarify the feasibility of this model on a large scale. However, QOL among patients living in residential facilities was generally better than QOL of patients living in traditional hospital settings, and residents are generally satisfied with their residential status (Leisse and Kallert, 2000). A methodological problem is that subjective and objective QOL are weakly correlated, and substantial improvements in living conditions may not be rapidly reflected in parallel improvements in subjective satisfaction.

The physical environment of health care facilities and its relationship with the satisfaction of residents (and staff) are seldom scrutinized. Several studies have highlighted that most residents attribute great importance to privacy, which was virtually non-existent in the former mental hospitals. This has significant and precise implications in terms of favoured architectural features, for example, the availability of single rooms, private bathrooms, etc. (de Girolamo and Bassi, 2004).

In conclusion, it may be difficult to establish precise standards of residential facility provision. The availability of residential places is negatively related to the number of community mental health centres and day centres, and is positively related to the number of beds in inpatient units. Housing needs assessments crucially depend on the range and quality of local services and cannot be separated from the functioning and dynamics of the total service system. Provision of residential facilities largely depends on another key variable: the extent of informal family support, which can substitute and replace the formal support granted by residential facilities. Thus, efforts are needed to identify acceptable ranges of residential facility places in all countries with a developed system of mental health care. Additional efforts will be necessary to clarify the need for residential facilities in those developing countries that are trying to overcome the traditional asylum system. Quantitative standards will have to be adapted to the specific local contexts and needs (de Girolamo and Bassi, 2004).

## INVOLVEMENT OF USERS AND RELATIVES IN MENTAL HEALTH SERVICES AND CARE

### Psychiatric patients, clients, (ex-)users or survivors of psychiatric services

Labelling the clients of mental health services as 'patients' is not always well received by those affected. User/survivor organizations refer most often to (ex-)users or service users or survivors of psychiatry. Although the term 'patients' is often retained in professional discourse, in this section patients, clients, people with mental disorders, (ex-) users and survivors of psychiatric services, will be referred to as users/survivors (after Hölling, 2001).

Users/survivors are often seen as passive utilizers of the health care system. They are confronted with a supply of medical services and they are allowed to show their satisfaction with it, retrospectively (Fleischmann, 2003). Professionals have difficulty in identifying users/survivors' priorities and have different views about desired outcomes. Lack of congruence between the views of users/survivors and providers is a concern, given that clinical outcomes are linked to users/survivors' perceptions that services meet their needs (Noble and Douglas, 2004). However, a systematic review of studies (Lasalvia et al., 2000) found that the majority of users/survivors attending mental health services had requests which they expressed when encouraged to do so.

Furthermore, better outcomes were associated with services meeting users/survivors' requests or acknowledging requests which could not be met (Allen et al., 2003; Fleischmann, 2003; Noble and Douglas, 2004). User/survivor satisfaction is highest in areas pertaining to staff and care discussions, and lowest in areas pertaining to information.

Users/survivors want good relationships with care providers, clear management plans, including preparations for discharge and follow-up, good co-ordination among services and contact with users/survivors who can provide peer support (Noble and Douglas, 2004). Although users/survivors are quite satisfied with their treatment in general, the single most common request was the users/survivors' 'desire to make decisions for themselves', namely to be informed and involved in decisions about their care, regardless of the type of service they attend (Siponen and Valimaki, 2003).

Users/survivors clearly do not reject medications categorically. Almost half indicated that they wanted medications and a similar number indicated benefit from medications, although many complained of forced administration and unwanted side-effects. They preferred benzodiazepines and ranked haloperidol as the least preferred option (Allen et al., 2003).

The majority reported adverse experiences with general hospital emergency rooms. One-fifth attributed their emergency contact to lack of access to more routine mental health care. These users/survivors stressed the development of alternatives to traditional emergency room services, the increased use of advance directives, more comfortable physical environments for waiting and treatment, increased use of peer support services, improved training of emergency staff to foster a more humanistic and person-centred approach, increased collaboration between practitioners and users/survivors, and improved discharge planning and post-discharge follow-up (Allen *et al.*, 2003).

In a survey about users/survivors' hope for psychiatric treatment (Fleischmann, 2003), 61 per cent of the users/survivors expected a pharmacological therapy. Most thought of psychopharmacotherapy with antidepressants (32 per cent), drugs against addiction (31 per cent) and tranquillizers (29 per cent). Only 10 per cent of the users/survivors anticipated receiving antipsychotics. Seventy-six per cent of the users/survivors expected a verbal psychotherapy. To consult a doctor was the immediate expectation among 69 per cent, followed by consulting a psychologist (60 per cent), nurses (58 per cent) and other users/survivors (56 per cent). Only 40 per cent of the users/survivors expect psychotherapy in the strict sense. Furthermore, privacy and recreation through walking are most mentioned (69 per cent), followed by relaxation (59 per cent), occupational therapy (55 per cent) and sports or exercise (54 per cent). Seventy-five per cent of the users/survivors want to be informed about the therapy and 69 per cent want to co-operate in their therapy planning. Only 21 per cent entrust the therapy entirely to their doctors. About one-third of the users/survivors expect a consultation with their relatives, the nurses and their family doctor. However, users/survivors' wishes to involve their families vary. Some users/survivors feel their family had been over- or under-involved in their care, and a third of users/survivors would not like to involve their family (Eisen *et al.*, 2002). Clearly, with multiple teams, and a greater reliance on non-medical health professionals in Europe, there is a tension between the wishes of service users and the direction of travel for services and modern mental health services.

In the 1990s, the European Network of (ex-) Users and Survivors of Psychiatry (ENUSP) was founded. ENUSP is an initiative to give users/survivors of psychiatric services a means to communicate, to exchange opinions, views and experiences in order to support each other in the personal, political and social struggle against expulsion, injustice and stigma in European countries. The European Network is against any unilateral approach to and stigmatization of mental and emotional distress, human suffering and unconventional behaviour. It should support users/survivors' autonomy and responsibility in making their own decisions (self-determination). ENUSP attempts to influence institutions that produce or bring about policy on a European level, concentrating on legislation and human rights issues, demedicalization of psychiatry and supporting alternative(s to) psychiatry (Hölling, 2001).

Furthermore, ENUSP decided to employ the term (ex-)users and survivors of psychiatry in order to provide a possibility of identification to the different groups and positions represented in these international non-governmental organizations. Those who identify as survivors of psychiatry distinguish themselves mainly by an antipsychiatric attitude and thus a radical criticism of the psychiatric system. Those who identify as users of psychiatry or mental health services are more orientated towards psychiatric reform and have also sometimes experienced psychiatric services as helpful. These different terms which users/survivors choose to identify themselves already reflect some of the differences in positions represented in the user/survivor movement (Hölling, 2001).

## The relatives' viewpoint

The importance of considering the needs of relatives who are carers has been recognized only in the last few years (Noble and Douglas, 2004). Between 40 and 60 per cent of the chronically mentally ill still live with their families. The clients of the system have the greatest experience in practical terms since they are the ones who have to deal with the reality resulting from any changes and improvements (and deterioration) in the mental health care system (Brand, 2001a). Studies examining relatives' wishes have uniformly demonstrated that family caregivers want more involvement in treatment planning, more information and support from mental health professionals, and help in communicating with service providers (Simpson and House, 2002).

Caregivers mentioned as most important understandable and sincere explanations to caregivers regarding the user/survivor's disease, support of the user/survivor's self-confidence and gains in confidence, psychotherapy for the user/survivor, and by no means psychopharmacological treatment (Spiessl *et al.*, 2004). From their point of view, gaps between expectations and satisfaction with inpatient care exist, especially regarding psychotherapy, information to caregivers about therapies, medication, side-effects and treatment progress, explanation to caregivers, support in dealing with the users/ survivors and information about the possibilities of rehabilitation after inpatient care.

Relatives are organized in the European Federation of Associations of Families of Mentally Ill People (EUFAMI) founded in 1990. The common ground of experience, burdens and visions tied the family members of people with mental illness together. They resolved to work together to help both themselves and the people they cared for. Today, EUFAMI is the representative body for 17 voluntary organizations throughout Europe which promotes the interests and wellbeing of people with a mental illness and their carers (Brand, 2001a). EUFAMI's principal aims are to achieve a continuous improvement throughout Europe in mental health, in the quality of care and welfare for people with a mental illness, and in the level of support for their family and friends; to enable the member associations to combine their efforts to act jointly at a European level; and, finally, to strengthen and assist the member associations in their efforts to improve health conditions in their own areas.

Thematic priorities identified by EUFAMI members as key activities include (a) representing families; (b) developing best practice; (c) prospect; (d) anti-stigma; and (e) strengthening member associations. EUFAMI particularly focuses on anti-stigma and discrimination issues; best professional practice; empowerment and self-help strategies. The policy of EUFAMI tries to secure better resources for health services and social care for people with mental illness and their carers, as it tries to ensure equality of legislation throughout Europe (Brand, 2001a,b).

## The interaction between users/survivors and mental health services

Over the last 20 years governments throughout Europe have sought to encourage users/survivors to play a more active role in the planning and delivery of health care. In Europe, the World Health Organization has highlighted the need to involve service users in the development and delivery of health care and legislation. This aims to strengthen service user initiatives that exist in several countries already (Crawford *et al.*, 2003). Users of mental health services have been at the forefront of attempts to change the structure and delivery of services and groups of service users who are actively involved in these issues throughout Europe. Support for user involvement has tended to be generated by policy-makers, and service managers and health care professionals may be reluctant to support plans for extending the involvement of service users (Crawford *et al.*, 2003). A study conducted in London found that more than half of the mental health providers feel that service users are insufficiently represented. Service providers employed a wide variety of different methods for involving users, but none met national standards for user involvement. Service providers stated that the main obstacle to user involvement was that users who took part were not representative of local users/survivors. In contrast, user/survivor groups identified staff resistance as a main obstacle to developing effective user involvement. Eighty per cent stated that they were not satisfied with current arrangements for user involvement and that staff needed training in order to better understand what meaningful user involvement signifies. Only 31 per cent of the NHS trusts in the UK currently provide this training (Crawford *et al.*, 2003).

Evidence from comparative studies of the effects of involving users in the delivery and evaluation of mental health services is rare. A systematic review identified five randomized controlled trials and seven other comparative studies (Simpson and House, 2002). Half of the studies considered involving users in managing cases. Involving users as employees of mental health services led to clients having greater satisfaction with personal circumstances and less hospitalization. Providers of services who had been trained by users had more positive attitudes toward users. Clients reported being less satisfied with services when interviewed by users. Simpson and House (2002) conclude that involving users with severe mental disorders in the delivery and evaluation of services is feasible. Users can be involved as employees, trainers or researchers without detrimental effect.

## Interaction between users/survivors and relatives

Congruence between the wishes of users/survivors and relatives is an issue. Although users/survivors and their relatives desire similar outcomes, they have different treatment preferences, with relatives much more in favour of hospitalization and more intensive and supportive interventions, whereas users/survivors prefer more independence. This applies to both emergency and longer-term care. Relatives assigned higher importance to the option of having compulsory admission and compulsory medication during a first psychotic episode, they prefer hospital-based to community care when users/survivors have a psychotic relapse, and they assign higher importance to safe and stable housing whilst users/survivors prefer more independent arrangements (Noble and Douglas, 2004).

## COUNTRY, CULTURE, ETHNIC GROUPS AND MENTAL HEALTH CARE

As pointed out by Bhugra (2002), medicine and the delivery of health care are cultural systems which reflect symbolic meanings anchored in the particular arrangements of social as well as clinical institutions where health care is delivered. The health care system is responsible for identifying those who are in need and dealing with the consequences of ill-health. This includes cultural aspects such as beliefs and attitudes towards mental health, mental illness, those afflicted, the respective treatments and institutions involved. Spiritual beliefs affect individual models of illness, for example,

whether they see illness as of spiritual, physical or psychological causation (Bhugra, 2002). These models determine help-seeking and pathways to care. In some settings religion allows people to see mental illness as an essential part of suffering and mentally ill patients may be revered. Clinicians must understand the cultural context of religious suffering and religious culture itself, as expressed through the individual's attitudes towards life, death, happiness and suffering (Rhi, 2001).

Only in the last decade of the twentieth century did governments in Europe become aware of the special needs of migrants and ethnic minority groups in terms of mental health service provision. There are only a few studies on this topic so far. The reason for this lack is unclear.

One obstacle for migrants to get mental health service provision might be the resources available in mental health services. In many European countries, access to services is via professional gatekeepers, mostly general practitioners (GPs). Barriers may arise from the GPs' lack of knowledge and cultural competence in dealing with migrant clients. This may be compounded by the migrants' own lack of knowledge of the health care system. 'Brokers', 'advocates' or 'mediators' thus have an important role to play in ensuring good access and appropriate referral (Watters and Ingleby, 2004). A further common problem is the rate of misdiagnosis among migrants. Haasen et al. (2000) reported from Germany a misdiagnosing rate of 19 per cent in Turkish migrants with mental illness as compared with 4 per cent among German-speaking people. Interestingly, the rate of misdiagnosis was not strongly correlated to poor second language proficiency. Thus, there are many other important cultural factors that interact in the process of diagnostic evaluation. In fact, younger age at migration, which was found to be a predictor for diagnostic agreement, may allow for stronger acculturation that is not expressed only by language proficiency. The authors concluded that this should lead to a more differentiated approach in resolving deficits in health care for migrants, where there is a definite tendency to see it only as a language problem. A third point to be mentioned here are difficulties that ethnic minorities can encounter in their proper countries. Overt or subtle discrimination of ethnic minorities by the ethnic majority is occasionally reported. For example, this is often reported by gypsies across Europe, Basques in Spain, Romanians in Hungary, Hungarians in Romania and from the Balkans. There is increasing evidence that discrimination can influence mental health outcomes (see Bhui, 2002; Bhui *et al.*, 2005), and therefore should be of public health importance.

## The role of the European Commission and the World Health Organization

The WHO European Ministerial Conference on Mental Health, held in Helsinki in January 2005, regarded the migrant population as a marginalized and vulnerable group that is at particular risk for mental health problems (World Health Organization, 2005a). Among the actions to consider, the conference called for specialized mental health services for this group. The European Commission Council Directive of January 2003 (European Commission, 2003) set out minimum standards with respect to health care. Nevertheless, in most EU countries, 'access to mental health care and specialist treatment for migrants is not widely available and not easily accessible for migrants who need special care' (Red Cross/EU Office, 2003). Finally, the European Commission has a central role in policy development. It recommends setting up level surveys on mental health across the EU especially among migrants to enable valid comparisons as very few data exist to allow comparisons on migrant mental health status across countries (European Communities, 2004). This should enable the Community to:

- improve information and knowledge for the development of public health,
- enhance the capability of responding rapidly and in a coordinated fashion to health threats, and
- promote health and prevent disease through addressing health determinants across all policies.

The existing network concerned with mental health in Europe, the European Network on Mental Health Policy, produced a framework and proposed key concepts and indicators relevant to good mental health (European Communities, 2004). A number of factors have been suggested as affecting the health of immigrants in their host country. These include: labour and economic instability, cultural and social marginalization, family estrangement, pressures to send money back to their families, racial discrimination and a lack of statutory documentation. These differences in migration patterns, the migration experience and the reception that immigrants receive as they try to settle mean that it is not possible to consider migrants as one homogeneous group with identical risks for poor mental health. Further research is needed to identify factors that may lead to an increased risk of mental ill-health or increased need for mental health services. Factors to explore include reasons for migration and distance from host culture (including religion, language etc., ability to develop mediating structures and legal status as a resident) (European Communities, 2004).

## Western Europe

After forcing citizens to emigrate, for example, in the nineteenth century to North and South America, Western European society itself is now faced with in-migration. Most countries in Western Europe have ethnic minorities, whether people immigrating from outside into a host country or people who are different from the ethnic majority in a country who have been settled for several generations. Within Europe there are very different patterns of migration. Northern European countries, such as the UK, the Netherlands, Germany and Sweden, have had a long experience of immigration throughout history, and especially immediately after World War II. In Southern European countries, such as Spain or Portugal, the immigration phenomenon is relatively recent (European Communities, 2004).

The composition of immigrant populations also varies from country to country. Three main groups of migrants can be identified in Europe: a considerable number of migrants come from former colonies such as from Asia in the UK, and from

African and Caribbean countries for other parts of Europe. People seeking employment are another substantial group of migrants: in Germany people from Turkey and in Switzerland Italian people. Finally, political refugees, for example, from South-East Asia (Vietnam, Cambodia), Africa (Rwanda) or south-eastern Europe (former Yugoslavia, Albania), immigrated to Western Europe. The last were mainly seeking asylum and contributed to a continuous change in the structure of the migrant population in the last few decades. However, trends in migration in Europe began to change a few decades ago as a result of changes in the economic, political and social realms.

European countries have been practising a policy of closing borders that has become even tougher in recent years. However, the policy of closed borders does not stop migration, but instead seems to create a new underclass of undocumented migrants who are – contrary to all declarations of human rights – inhumanely suppressed and highly exploited.

Migration has become a major political and social concern in Western European societies (Freeman, 1997; Hutchinson and Haasen, 2004c). Apart from two other countries, Switzerland has the highest rates of migrants (21.2 per cent) among the general population in Western Europe (Luxembourg 36.6 per cent; Liechtenstein 34.3 per cent), followed by Germany with 8.9 per cent and Austria with 8.7 per cent, respectively (Swiss Federal Statistical Office, 2005). The origin of the migrants, however, is specific for every host country: unlike in the UK and the Netherlands, where most migrants come from their former colonies, migrants in other countries mainly originate from Europe or Africa. Looking at the general population in the three major European countries – the UK, France and Germany – the following picture emerges: in the UK 92.4 per cent of the population are white and of the major ethnic minorities, 50.2 per cent are Asian and 27.1 per cent are black people; 4.1 per cent of the population are non-British citizens (2001 data; Office for National Statistics, 2005). In France 5.6 per cent of the population are not French, of whom 46.9 per cent are of European origin and 44.2 per cent from Africa. People from Maghrebian countries (Algeria, Tunisia,

Morocco) are the most predominant minority (34.5 per cent), followed by Portuguese people (16.7 per cent) (2002 data; Office Nationale de Statistique, 2004). Finally, in Germany 8.9 per cent of the general population are non-Germans, with people from Turkey (26.0 per cent) and the former Yugoslavia (15.2 per cent) as predominant minorities (2003 data; Federal Statistical Office of Germany (Statistisches Bundesamt Deutschland), 2003).

Since Ødegård's landmark study in the 1930s, migration is recognized as a risk factor for mental disorders (Ødegård, 1932; Hutchinson and Haasen, 2004b). Only in the last decade has psychiatry expanded its attention to migration based on reports of increased rates of mental illness, such as schizophrenia and other psychotic disorders among migrants and more recently among refugees and asylum seekers (Cantor-Graae et al., 2003; Hutchinson and Haasen, 2004a). Several studies on the utilization of mental health services reported that migrants are more likely to view services as inappropriate to their needs and are, therefore, likely to have longer duration of untreated illness and more adverse patterns of introduction to these services (Bhugra, 2002; Hutchinson and Haasen, 2004d).

Switzerland is in a particular situation: traditionally, Switzerland is one of the countries with the highest rate of foreign citizens in Europe. A further particularity is that it has no substantial non-white minority. From 1995 to 2001, about 20 per cent of the population living in Switzerland were non-Swiss citizens, with people from the former Yugoslavia and Italy as predominant minorities (between 20 and 25 per cent each; Swiss Federal Statistical Office, 2005). Thus, when speaking about migration, some countries such as the UK are mainly focusing on race and ethnicity and not on the country of origin, whereas others such as Germany or Switzerland are centring more on minorities defined by foreign nationality (Lay et al., 2005).

A paper from Switzerland (Baleydier et al., 2003) revealed that the probability of foreign patients consulting emergency psychiatry is higher compared with natives (odds ratio 1.44). Socio-demographic factors show significant differences between the foreigners and the Swiss population: immigrants are younger, more active and clustered to a familial structure; this pattern is not dissimilar from immigrants to most European countries. They are less often diagnosed with alcohol abuse (14.7 per cent for foreigners versus 23.9 per cent in the Swiss population), personality disorders (8.1 per cent versus 13 per cent), but more with affective (54.7 per cent versus 43 per cent) and anxiety disorders (18.4 per cent versus 12.3 per cent). Furthermore, the only statistically significant difference is the recommendation for short-term therapeutic interventions which are given more frequently to foreigners (15.5 per cent versus 11.3 per cent; Baleydier *et al.*, 2003).

Two papers shed light on the debate about cultural influence on psychoses among people of African-Caribbean ethnic origin living in the UK. An incidence study from Barbados found that the rates were far lower than those of the emigrant group, suggesting that environmental factors, as opposed to genetic factors, were important determinants (Mahy *et al.*, 1999). The outcome of psychotic illness is similar in the immigrant group to that in white Britons (Goater *et al.*, 1999); if anything, social outcomes and disability seemed better (see Chapter 4).

## Eastern Europe

Eastern Europe is now opening its borders to visitors and migrants, but there is little on the approach to working with black and minority ethnic groups, or indeed foreigners to the country. In part, in-migration has not been obvious, but also the lack of information reflects problems regarding the validity of official data in Eastern European countries. At the root of this problem was the central planning that accepted data as valid only if they confirmed planned accomplishments. This led to systematic bias in reporting. An even more problematic aspect of validity had to do with what was construed as evidence: for decades the conflation of fact and belief had not been prevented through independent peer review of research. Lastly, the culture of undertaking surveys and population studies was not evident in Eastern Europe; this made

the cultivation of research culture and methods in the region a major priority (Tomov, 2001). Accounts of health systems tend to be written from within a certain role, usually that of a researcher. Accounts coming from Eastern Europe, especially until about a decade ago, used to be compiled in an upbeat style and avoided analysis. This reflected the lack of field experience of their authors, usually health administrators, but also gave the flavour of the organizational culture of health bureaucracies in those times (Tomov, 2001).

Currently the countries from the eastern part of Europe simultaneously face both the ethical and the economic issues involved in psychiatric reforms. At the core of de-institutionalization is the ethical concern about the alienating effect of institutional life on those characteristics of the person, which enable self-governance and integrity. At the core of the economic argument for reforms is the capacity to demonstrate through evidence-based psychiatry that psychiatric interventions make a difference in terms of outcome, defined as a positive contribution to individual and public health (Tomov, 2001).

Communities with underserved populations are usually economically poor, isolated and in segmented areas with little or no sources of payment for health care. It might be that ethnic minorities are provided with fewer resources. Health care providers in poor areas treat a high number of underserved and underinsured individuals who lack the financial ability to pay out-of-pocket funds for uncovered health care services. This forces the primary care practitioner to relocate to areas that are more financially stable, although there may be a misdistribution and saturation of physicians in larger metropolitan areas. The socio-economic status of these populations results in behavioural health problems such as domestic violence, drug and alcohol addictions, and high-risk lifestyle behaviours in general.

The countries of Eastern Europe pressed by circumstance do not have much of a choice in sorting them out. As a result of constraints imposed by the economy and by the organizational culture of health systems, these countries have failed so far to embark on mental health reforms in the well-orchestrated way in which established democracies handle demands of change. Rather, while preoccupied with introducing paid services in general health care (usually by establishing health insurance and fee-for-service systems) they espouse beliefs that mental health is a small and unimportant segment of specialist care, or that psychiatric services are difficult to cost and hard to sell. This thinking usually results in decisions to postpone reforms in the mental health sector, or it leads to the introduction of packages of services in mental health, which do not cover chronic mental illness in that they fail to provide for teamwork and long-term inputs in community care. In particular, circumstances would not allow countries in Eastern Europe to concentrate on the systematic change of care delivery in the existing institutions, thus encouraging the staff into new methods of work and preparing for a later date when it will become possible to put into place a new organization designed to expedite the shift to community care (Tomov, 2001).

A growing concern in the Slovak Republic (a new member of the expanded European Union) adversely affecting community health is the issue of dealing with refugees of war and gypsies. These subgroups do not have and often do not seek access to medical care, health education and preventive medicine. Three principal barriers to reaching underserved populations in Slovakia include (1) cultural barriers, (2) communication deficiencies, and (3) poverty. The refugee problem emerged with the war in Yugoslavia in the last decade. Slovakia, north of the war-torn area, had a major influx of refugees. Social problems increased in the area of this ethno-demographic conflict: drug addictions, domestic violence and criminality have become endemic. These impoverished communities are worried about survival, not about addressing behavioural and physical health concerns. A similar problem exists with the gypsy population. This population group has historically stayed outside the community health system in whatever form and has not sought help for behavioural health concerns resulting from a cultural segregation from society. The problem of lack of availability of behavioural health services and health education has been aggravated by a perception in the subculture that societal concerns are not important to individuals. Therefore, the gypsy population does not attempt

to access or act on information on healthy behaviour and health care. The use of social marketing to improve receptiveness and acceptance of behavioural health services can be effective.

## South-Eastern Europe

The political and economic turmoil that occurred in south-eastern Europe in the last decade of the twentieth century left a legacy of physical damage to the infrastructure of the country. This aspect of the conflict has received considerable coverage in the media. However, surprisingly less has been reported about the effects of that turmoil on the health and the mental health of the people living in the region. War affects the self-perceived health, physical ability, and emotional and mental health of the entire population that is affected by war, especially younger age groups, those with lower education and lower income (Babic-Banaszak et al., 2002).

In an epidemiological study of Bosnian refugees resident in a camp in Croatia, a combination of post-traumatic stress disorder (PTSD) and depression was observed in 20 per cent of the population; this greatly increased the risk of psycho-social disability (Mollica et al., 1999). Thus, it seems unwise to draw any general inferences about the overall impact of war and displacement on the psychological health of whole populations. Personal vulnerability, the intensity, nature and 'dose' of traumas experienced, the cultural, religious and political context, and conditions in the post-traumatic environment combine in shaping psycho-social outcomes. Important recent findings are that co-morbidity of PTSD and depression may be particularly disabling (Mollica et al., 1999), and intrusive symptoms of PTSD may be the strongest predictor of health service utilization over time (Bramsen and van der Ploeg, 1999). Perhaps the greatest deficiency in the field is the paucity of systematic studies evaluating treatments and other psycho-social interventions. Passion and compassion have motivated clinicians working in these unpopular and stigmatized areas of interest; the future sustainability and development of these interests depend on identifying interventions that work (Silove, 2000; see Chapters 24, 25 and 26).

## Mental health and the legitimacy for asylum: a challenging situation

Political and socio-economic instability in and around Europe has significantly increased the number of refugees and asylum seekers arriving in European countries. Among all the changes a person can face during his or her life, few are so wide and complex as those that take place during migration. Practically everything changes that surrounds the emigrating person. These difficulties are accentuated when migration is accomplished under adverse conditions. In the case of refugees, this process is even more complex.

Different authors (Watters and Ingleby, 2004; Fassin and Rechtman, 2005) draw attention to the importance of a medical diagnosis as a rare avenue of legitimacy for asylum seekers at a time of significant decline in the numbers of asylum seekers being granted refugee status. The diagnosis of health and mental health problems in refugee populations is undertaken in a politically charged environment in which diagnosis could have a significant impact on crucial decisions regarding the right to stay (Watters and Ingleby, 2004).

For example, in southern European countries where there are relatively few asylum seekers (and low acceptance rates for those who do apply), and the main avenue of access is through irregular migration, there is likely to be little in the way of specialist mental health services (Watters and Ingleby, 2004). In countries with relatively large numbers of asylum seekers and where they are held in induction or accommodation centres while their claim is processed (for example, Germany), mental health care is likely to be delivered in these formal settings and distant from mainstream health care practices, and related quality and values. In countries where the emphasis is on the dispersal of asylum seekers so that no one part of the country is seen as having a disproportionate 'burden' (for example, in the UK), there are significant challenges in terms of the access to, and appropriateness of, mainstream services (Watters and Ingleby, 2004).

Two studies from the Netherlands found that lack of work, family issues and asylum procedure stress led to the highest risk of psychopathology among Iraqi refugees. The findings appeal to governments which seek to shorten the asylum procedures, allow asylum seekers to work, and give preference to family reunion. Mental health workers should recognize the impact of post-migration living problems and consider focusing their treatment on coping with these problems as well as addressing traumas from the past where these remain significant factors (Laban *et al.*, 2004, 2005; Murad *et al.*, 2004).

Brune *et al.* (2002) sought to determine the role of belief systems in the outcome of psychotherapy for traumatized refugees. The severity of traumatization was correlated with a more severe course of PTSD (and other post-traumatic disorders), while firm belief systems have been found to be a protective factor against post-traumatic disorders. A firm belief system was found to be an important predictor for a better therapy outcome (Brune *et al.*, 2002).

## Life expectancy

By 1990, the probability of people dying before the age of 65 if from the communist countries of Central and Eastern Europe was 70 per cent higher compared with Western Europe (Forster and Jozan, 1990; McKee and Shkolnikov, 2001). Men were especially susceptible to dying prematurely. Although men in all industrialized countries live shorter lives than women, in Eastern Europe the gap between the sexes was especially large. In 1990, the life expectancy of men living in the Soviet Union was only 64 years – nine years less than in Western Europe. Soviet women could expect to live to 74 years – 10 years longer than men and only six years less than women in Western Europe. The disadvantage in life expectancy relative to Western Europe was less for countries of Central and Eastern Europe, but even there the gap was six years for men and five years for women. Mortality was higher in Eastern Europe than in Western Europe for men and women alike, suggesting that some factors contributing to death were common to both sexes, whereas other factors especially disadvantaged men.

Considerable national diversity was also evident (McKee and Shkolnikov, 2001). A further division separates countries in Central and Eastern Europe that have seen marked improvements in health, such as Poland and the Czech Republic, from those that have not, such as Romania and Bulgaria (Forster and Jozan, 1990). Sex differences in life expectancy are especially large in Poland, Hungary, Russia and the European post-Soviet republics (Waldron, 1993). By 1997 mortality from all external causes in men before age 65 was five times lower in Western Europe than in the countries of the former Soviet Union; in Central and Eastern Europe it was double that in Western Europe. All causes of injury are more common in Eastern than in Western Europe (McKee and Shkolnikov, 2001).

Life expectancy is also influenced by ethnicity: in the period 1989–2000, ethnic differences in life expectancy between Estonians and Russians living in Estonia increased from 0.4 years to 6.1 years among men and from 0.6 years to 3.5 years among women. In 2000, Russians had a higher mortality than Estonians in all age groups and for almost all selected causes of death. The largest differences were found for some alcohol-related causes of death especially in 2000. Political and economic upheaval, increasing poverty, and alcohol consumption can be considered the main underlying causes of the widening ethnic mortality gap (Leinsalu et al., 2004).

# CONSEQUENCES OF ALCOHOL CONSUMPTION

Alcohol-related issues have been much debated in the discussion of mortality changes in transitional Russia since Gorbachev's alcohol reforms in 1985 (Shkolnikov et al., 2001). Evidently, the assumed crucial role of drinking in mortality changes in Russia has provoked much international medical attention to alcohol issues there. Much less attention has been paid to other transitional societies in Eastern Europe, although in some of these countries the level of alcohol consumption and the prevalence of alcohol-related harm may exceed that in the Russian Federation (Simpura et al., 1999). Moreover, in the three Baltic countries (as well as in Russia), the gap between the official recorded per capita consumption level and various alternative estimates has been wide indeed. In Russia, for instance, the official figures for the early 1990s varied by around 6 litres of pure alcohol per capita per year. Indirect measures based on the number of certain alcohol-related deaths have given estimates between 13 and 15 litres per capita. In addition, similar indirect estimation of the total consumption in Latvia indicates that the country would occupy the top-ranking position in the world's alcohol statistics with a figure of more than 15 litres per capita (Simpura et al., 1999).

Injuries and cardiovascular diseases account for a large part of the difference in mortality between Eastern and Western Europe, but several other causes, although less important numerically, are much more frequent in Eastern Europe than in Western Europe. These include various causes directly or indirectly associated with alcohol consumption. Direct causes include acute alcohol poisoning and cirrhosis; indirect causes include conditions such as stroke and pneumonia (McKee and Shkolnikov, 2001). High mortality from injuries, cardiovascular deaths, and acute alcohol poisoning is seen in countries where the drinking culture favours vodka. These countries also tend to have relatively low mortality from cirrhosis, possibly because death from other causes occurs before cirrhosis can develop. In southern parts of the region, however, in particular in a band stretching from Slovenia to Moldova, the acute effects of alcohol are less apparent (with the exception of deaths from road traffic accidents), but deaths from cirrhosis are extremely common. The reason for this is unclear. One possible explanation is found in the pattern of drinking, with many heavy drinkers drinking from early morning. Another is a low level of dietary micronutrients from fruit and vegetables, which could otherwise provide some protective effect. Finally, the consumption of home-made spirits is an additional risk factor for the development of alcohol-induced cirrhosis (see similar issues in South Asian countries in Chapter 21). Restrictions on the supply and sale of alcohol from illicit sources are needed urgently to reduce significantly the mortality from chronic liver disease (Szucs et al., 2005).

Other consequence of heavy alcohol consumption might not be forgotten: child-reported levels of emotional and physical abuse in Eastern Europe were closely related to parental alcohol overuse (Sebre et al., 2004). Moreover, Central European mortality rates for cancer sites related to alcohol have increased rapidly in recent decades (Bray et al., 2000).

The countries of Central and Eastern Europe display many similarities in both political history and measures of health such as overall life expectancy. When examined more closely, substantial differences emerge, some of which are going to be discussed here: the pattern of alcohol-related mortality in Poland and Hungary is quite different. In both countries, death rates increased in the 1960s and 1970s. In Poland, this increase stopped in 1980 and death rates have levelled out, with the exception of those in young women. In Hungary, rates have continued to climb, although the rate of increase decreased in the 1980s. This change coincides with the introduction of a policy, following the introduction of martial law, to reduce alcohol consumption (Varvasovsky et al., 1997).

Rates of problem drinking and of negative consequences of drinking were much higher in Russian men (35 per cent and 18 per cent, respectively) than in Czechs (19 per cent and 10 per cent) or Poles (14 per cent and 8 per cent). This contrasts with substantially lower mean annual intake of alcohol reported by Russian men (4.6 litres) than by Czech men (8.5 litres), and with low mean drinking frequency in Russia (67 drinking sessions per year, compared with 179 sessions among Czech men). However, Russians consumed the highest dose of alcohol per drinking session (means 71 g in Russians, 46 g in Czechs and 45 g in Poles), and had the highest prevalence of binge drinking. In women, the levels of alcohol-related problems and of drinking were low in all countries. In ecological and individual level analyses, indicators of binge drinking explained a substantial part of the differences in rates of problem drinking and negative consequences of drinking between the three countries. These data confirm high levels of

alcohol-related problems in Russia despite a low volume of drinking. The binge-drinking pattern partly explains this paradoxical finding (Bobak et al., 2004). Similar results are reported from Lithuania (Chenet et al., 2001).

A co-occurrence of stressful, possibly self-inflicted, life events and a related increase of alcohol use has been observed (Kubicka et al., 1995). One study investigated the alcohol consumption of 608 Prague women aged 20–49 years in 1987 and 1992, three years after the revolution that ended the 41 years of the Communist era in Czechoslovakia. The average yearly consumption of alcohol at follow-up increased between 1987 and 1992 from 3.6 litres to 4.8 litres. The percentage of heavier drinkers (with average daily consumption of over 20 g alcohol) increased from 7.2 per cent to 14.0 per cent. The women expressed increased tolerance of drunkenness in their attitudes to drinking. The consumption increase was mainly due to increased drinking frequency of spirits and to increased quantities of beer consumed per occasion. The consumption increase was largest in women working on a freelance basis, and the newly emerging self-employed women; economically inactive women did not increase their consumption. Women who reported a positive impact of the socio-political changes on their personal lives and an expansion of social contacts also reported larger than average consumption increases.

Alcohol is making a substantial contribution to the burden of disease and premature mortality in Bulgaria (Balabanova and McKee, 1999). In Bulgaria, overall 50.7 per cent of men and 13.6 per cent of women drink at least weekly (1997 figures). In both sexes, drinking is least common among the elderly and those living in villages. It is also less common among those with poor financial status. Muslims are less likely to drink than are orthodox Christians. Drinking is most common among those living in cities, with higher education and high incomes. Heavy drinking, defined as 80 g/day or more, is rare among women, but is reported by 18.2 per cent of men.

In the Baltic States, weekly alcohol consumption varied by country and sex. Age and income were the strongest and most consistent correlates of the likelihood of consuming alcohol weekly (McKee *et al.*, 2000). Approximately half the men and one in six women in the Baltic States reported consuming alcohol at least weekly (men: Estonia 61 per cent, Latvia 41 per cent, Lithuania 55 per cent; women: Estonia 26 per cent, Latvia 8 per cent, Lithuania 14 per cent). Within each country, this proportion decreased with age in both sexes, and increased with income in women. Ethnic differences were observed only in Estonia: drinking alcohol weekly was significantly lower in Russian than in Estonian ethnicity. In Lithuania, drinking was more common in highly educated men than in those with a low education level. Daily alcohol intake was higher in Estonia than in the other countries, as was the percentage of respondents drinking heavily.

## SUICIDE

The distribution of suicide mortality demonstrates large and persistent differences between European nations. Lithuania (69.0 per cent), Estonia (60.4 per cent), Latvia (58.4 per cent), Belarus (40.6 per cent), Ukraine (26.4 per cent), Poland (26.5 per cent) and Romania (16.5 per cent) had the most important perceptual increase in suicide rate between 1989 and 1994, while East Germany (27.1 per cent), Slovakia (20.9 per cent), Macedonia (18.3 per cent) and Hungary (15.1 per cent) showed a decrease in the same time period (Mäkinen, 2000).

The high-suicide, but unequal sex distribution group consisted of Belarus, Estonia, Latvia, Lithuania, Slovenia and Ukraine. Characterizing this group of countries was a higher-than-average suicide rate; men are more likely than women to commit suicide (called a high sex quota); and more suicides were of a younger compared to older age group (called a low age quota). The high-suicide, but unequal age distribution group consisted of Croatia, East Germany and Hungary. This group was distinguished from the first one by its relative lack of sex difference in suicide rates and more suicides in older compared with younger people. In 1994, East Germany demonstrated strongly declining suicide rates (Mäkinen, 2000).

The low-suicide, but unequal sex distribution group was made up of Poland, Romania and Slovakia. These countries showed a lower-than-average suicide rate together with a high sex quota and a low age quota. The low-suicide, but unequal age distribution group included Bulgaria, Czech Republic, Macedonia and former Yugoslavia (Serbia and Montenegro). The low-suicide, equal distribution group, including Albania, Armenia, Azerbaijan, Georgia, Tajikistan, Turkmenistan and Uzbekistan, demonstrated lower-than-average values of suicide rate. These countries are the former Soviet republics with less Russian influence, together with the only predominantly Muslim country of Europe (Mäkinen, 2000).

General trends of suicide mortality in Eastern Europe or in the 'newly independent states' of the former Soviet Union cannot be identified. The countries of the former Eastern Bloc could be divided into five groups on the basis of their suicide mortality profiles (the level of suicide and its age/sex distribution). However, all the countries studied have been going through similar transformations. From these results it is obvious that rapid transformations of society do not per se necessarily produce more suicide. An explanation of this could be the intermediate role of culture (reflected in the different suicide mortality profiles): similar social factors can lead to different outcomes in different environments.

There were large falls in the suicide rates in the former Soviet Union between 1984 and 1987. This was mainly attributed to Gorbachev's anti-alcohol campaign, a central aim of which was to increase taxes on alcohol. However, this was followed in some cases by even larger rises of taxes between 1986 and 1988. Changes in suicide rates have been more or less simultaneous with the great societal transformation. The most frequently proposed cause for the changes in suicide rates is alcohol consumption (Wasserman *et al.*, 1994). Other explanations include political developments and optimism or frustrated feelings associated with changes in general socio-economic circumstances, especially unemployment, the quality of medical services, changes in norms and values, and broken social relations (Mäkinen, 2000).

## ILLICIT DRUG ABUSE

Abuse of illicit drugs is an important mental health problem in Eastern Europe. Some of these countries already had a drug problem long before the political transitions of the 1980s. At that time, however, drug use patterns had their own specificity, were based on local resources (locally grown poppy and home-made stimulants) and the level of criminality was low. Pronounced social change has been associated with a rapid increase in both supply and demand for drugs, reinforced by wars in Central Asia, the Caucasian republics and in the Balkans (Moskalewicz, 2002). Some Eastern European countries such as Romania, Albania and Bulgaria have become target countries by virtue of lying at the junction of trafficking routes for illicit drugs. In the last few years they have become main drug storage centres and sites for the production of illicit drugs (Poznyak *et al.*, 2002).

Some general features can be reported for Eastern Europe: the common denominator for these countries is that drug abuse has increased remarkably in all of them during the last 10–12 years. This holds true especially for cannabis use, but also for heroin, cocaine and synthetic drugs (Moskalewicz, 2002). Cannabis is the drug most widely used in all Eastern European countries. In the Czech Republic, Slovakia and in Slovenia, mental health services cannot meet the new demand to treat people with substance use problems (Csemy *et al.*, 2002a; Flaker 2002). Civic associations partly took over the task and opened new facilities. Problems of funding these non-governmental organizations as well as acceptance of these services among the general population are reported. Especially in countries with low socio-economic power, such as Ukraine and Belarus, understaffed and underfunded public health services offered mainly short-term detoxification treatment, and the limited number of treatment slots for abstinence-oriented treatment was and is insufficient and unattractive to injecting drug users (Poznyak *et al.*, 2002).

In Romania, drug abuse practically did not exist before the transition period. However, a survey conducted in 2000 among adolescents across Romania showed that 5.2 per cent had already used drugs (Poznyak *et al.*, 2002). More than 8 per cent of 16-year-old high school students admitted cannabis use (Kovács and Antal, 1999). In another survey among students in Transylvania, lifetime prevalence approached 12 per cent. In this multi-ethnic part of Romania, prevalence of drug use among ethnic minorities, including a Hungarian minority, substantially exceeded the prevalence among students of Romanian origin (Kovács, 2001). In Hungary, the lifetime prevalence of illicit drugs was 6.4 per cent in 2001, while the proportion of habitual users was 2.3 per cent. The rate of consumption is highest among 18- to 24-year-old males living in the capital. Cannabis is the drug most widely used, but it is worth mentioning that cannabis users also take far more other illicit drugs than cannabis users in other European countries. This means that the concentration of drug use is higher in Hungary (Poznyak *et al.*, 2002). A recent survey reported that boys are more likely to use drugs than girls. Moreover, the risk of drug use was significantly higher in those children who reported a drug user in the family (Nyari *et al.*, 2005).

A report prepared by the Moldavian Ministry of Health estimates that the proportion of drug use among teenagers is about 12 per cent. The number of people treated at health institutions also indicates the extent of drug use. Between 1995 and 2000, the number of individuals treated for drug addiction had more than tripled. The patients are rarely older than 30 and patients are becoming younger: at the end of the 1990s the proportion of those under 25 was a little more than 80 per cent, in 2000 it was close to 90 per cent. The majority of the patients in treatment are male (88.8 per cent) (Elekes and Kovács, 2002).

The period of the last decade has been marked by an increase in drug use in the Czech Republic and in Slovakia. Seventeen per cent of adults in the Czech Republic and 12 per cent of the Slovaks report lifetime drug use. The respective figures are even higher for the population of adolescents. Thirty-five per cent of young Czechs and 19 per cent of young Slovaks used cannabis. Metamphetamine is the most misused substance among drug users in the Czech Republic, and heroin dominates in Slovakia (Csemy *et al.*, 2002b).

## STIGMATIZATION AND DISCRIMINATION AGAINST PEOPLE WITH MENTAL ILLNESS

### Mental health literacy

It is a common finding from all over the world that people with mental illness are stigmatized. This is often due to a lack of knowledge about their illness. Various campaigns against discrimination and stigmatization because of mental illness, especially schizophrenia, have been launched in the last few years (Sartorius, 1998; Crisp *et al.*, 2000). The general public has been the main target of these endeavours because its knowledge and beliefs about mental disorders and the awareness of different treatment options has repeatedly been shown to be low (Jorm *et al.*, 1997b; Lauber *et al.*, 2001, 2003b; Beck *et al.*, 2003; Addison and Thorpe, 2004). However, these campaigns are based on common sense rather than on sound research-based strategies.

The concept of 'mental health literacy' was introduced by Jorm *et al.* in 1997 (Jorm *et al.*, 1997a). It is defined as the ability to gain access to, understand and use information in ways that promote and maintain good mental health. It refers to knowledge and beliefs about mental disorders which aid their recognition, management or prevention, including the ability to recognize specific disorders; knowing how to seek mental health information; knowledge of risk factors and causes, of self-treatments and of professional help available; and attitudes that promote recognition and appropriate help-seeking. This definition is very broad and seems to be a summary of the knowledge mental health professionals should have about mental illness. Thus, it is at least questionable whether the public can be judged according to this definition or whether this definition inevitably must result in poor public mental health literacy.

### Some specific findings

Research has shown that the social distance to people with mental illness – that is, the relative willingness of one person to participate in relationships of varying degrees of intimacy with a person who has a stigmatized identity (Bowman, 1987) – is greater with people with schizophrenia than those with depression. Social distance is more pronounced among women, thus opposing the belief that they have generally less stigmatizing attitudes toward mental illness (Angermeyer *et al.*, 1998; Lauber *et al.*, in press). There is a considerable influence of cultural context on social distance. In the Italian-speaking part of Switzerland, greater social distance towards people with mental illness was reported.

People with mental illness cause emotional reactions as they are perceived to be 'unpredictable, frightening and threatening' (Link *et al.*, 1999). Negative emotional reactions were found to predict greater social distance. Perceived discrimination – the perception of how mentally ill people are stigmatized by 'others' – increases social distance.

A medical understanding of mental illness leads to greater social distance. Consequently, believing that a mental illness is an expression of a life crisis implies less social distance. These results suggest that more knowledge about mental illnesses, especially schizophrenia, may increase social distance. They may help to focus anti-stigma campaigns not only on transmission of knowledge, but also on integrating different approaches such as encouraging personal contacts and engaging with lay explanations of illness.

People with mental illness are faced with discrimination. This also resonates in the public's attitude to the civil rights of those affected. A representative public opinion survey from Switzerland (Lauber *et al.*, 2000) revealed that most people believe that people with mental illness should not be allowed to hold a driving licence, whereas withdrawal of the right to vote and a recommendation to abort in the case of pregnancy were rejected by the majority. The public acceptance of these restrictions depends on age, education and gender, but also on social distance and contact with people with mental illness. The cultural influence of the language region is significant; living in Italian- or French-speaking Switzerland is a significant predictor of the acceptance of restrictions.

A different picture emerges when studying the rejection or acceptance of compulsory admission. More than 70 per cent of the respondents displayed a positive attitude to compulsory admission (Lauber *et al.*, 2002). The mostly positive attitude to compulsory admission suggests that the public trust in psychiatry to deal with the assigned responsibility. Education, negative stereotypes and living in French-speaking Switzerland are predictors for accepting compulsory admission, whereas older age, extreme political opinion and rigid personality traits show an inverse effect. Negative emotions, anomie, social distance and contact with the mentally ill have no significant influence.

Two crucial questions are whether the lay public recognize mental illness and what treatment they recommend in the case of mental illness. This can be assessed by using vignettes. In the previously mentioned study, the depression vignette was correctly recognized by 39.8 per cent whereas 60.2 per cent of the respondents considered the person depicted as having a 'crisis' (Lauber *et al.*, 2003b). The schizophrenia vignette was correctly identified by 73.6 per cent of the interviewees. A positive attitude to psychopharmacology positively influenced the recognition of the two vignettes whereas a positive attitude to community psychiatry had the inverse effect. Moreover, for the depression vignette, previous contact with mentally ill people had a positive influence on the recognition. For the schizophrenia vignette instead, rigidity and interest in mass media had a negative influence. The low knowledge about mental disorders, particularly depression, confirms the importance and need to increase mental health literacy. Furthermore, professionals must openly discuss illness models with their patients, especially emphasizing the differences between illness and crisis. Psychologists, GPs, fresh air and psychiatrists were mostly proposed as being helpful in cases of mental illness. Among several psychiatric treatment approaches psychotherapy was favoured, while psychopharmacological treatment and electroconvulsive therapy were considered to be harmful. Treatment by a psychiatrist was regarded as being more helpful for individuals with schizophrenia than for those with depression. For a person experiencing a life crisis, treatment by a psychiatrist and psychological treatment were viewed as being harmful, and non-medical interventions were preferred. However, for people thought to be mentally ill, psychiatric and psychopharmacological treatments were recommended. The perception of whether a condition is considered to be an illness or a life crisis has significantly more influence on lay treatment proposals than the diagnosis in the vignette (Lauber *et al.*, 2001).

As to the perceived causes of mental illness, the study revealed that for more than half of the respondents (56.6 per cent) difficulties within the family or the partnership represent the causes of depression (Lauber *et al.*, 2003a). Occupational stress is the second most mentioned cause (32.7 per cent) whereas unspecified stress is in third place (19.9 per cent). Traumatic events (17.9 per cent), depressive disorder (14.1 per cent) and unspecified illnesses (11.6 per cent) follow. The respective causal attributions are mainly independent of demographic factors and thus generalizable for the population. The attributions are primarily shaped by psycho-social ideas about aetiology. Nevertheless, one-third of the interviewees held biological or disease-related beliefs about causes of depression. Illness-models cannot be neglected in the therapeutic relationship. In other European countries, but also overseas, researchers found identical or similar results.

## CONCLUDING REMARKS

The delivery of mental health services in Europe is generally of a high level. There are still noteworthy differences between countries, in particular a clear gap between western and eastern countries. European policy should focus on this discrepancy by supporting these countries with results from mental health service research. This would enable them to build up services that are both evidence-based and cost-effective. Research should focus on at least five topics, whereas the regional and local research foci depend on the level of mental health provision already achieved:

- Help-seeking behaviour and access to care for people with mental disorders.

- The better integration of users and relatives in mental health care.
- More effective treatment approaches for and rehabilitation of people with severe mental illness. Research is mainly under the influence of biological psychiatry, focused on acute symptoms and less on the evaluation of rehabilitation and long-term courses of mental illnesses (guidelines, cognitive–behavioural therapy, different types of psycho-pharmacological treatments).
- The provision of services for people with psychiatric disorders that have not so far been the main focus of psychiatric research. This includes special groups such as immigrants, homeless people, people with co-morbid mental and physical disorders, ethnic-specific care, gender differences including pregnancy and postnatal care, violence, self-harm, post-traumatic stress disorders (post-war psychiatry), old age psychiatry, lesbian and gay psychiatry, etc. Special issues such as quality of life for people with mental illness, their everyday (e.g. work) living and leisure situations, coercion (involuntary treatment, juridical coercion) and specific treatment approaches for people with long-term disabilities due to mental illness are increasing in Europe, mainly influenced by recent research findings from the USA.
- The integration and combination of neurobiological and neuropsychological research questions with health service research. This may close the gap between social and community psychiatry on the one side and biological psychiatry on the other.

## REFERENCES

Addison, S.J. and Thorpe, S.J. 2004: Factors involved in the formation of attitudes towards those who are mentally ill. *Social Psychiatry and Psychiatric Epidemiology* 39, 228–34.

Agius, M., Zaman, R., Singh, S., Gallagher, O., Jones, P.B., McGuire, P., Power, P., Craig, T., Bahn, S., Grech, A., Casha, C., Pace, C., Cassar, D., Blinc-Pesek, M., Avgustin, B.,

Gruber, E., Biocina, S.M., Andelic, J., Dinolova, R., Van os, J. and Lambert, M. 2005: Psychiatry in Europe. *British Journal of Psychiatry* 187, 92.

Allen, M.H., Carpenter, D., Sheets, J.L., Miccio, S. and Ross, R. 2003: What do consumers say they want and need during a psychiatric emergency? *Journal of Psychiatric Practice* 9, 39–58.

Angermeyer, M.C., Matschinger, H. and Holzinger, A. 1998: Gender and attitudes towards people with schizophrenia. Results of a representative survey in the Federal Republic of Germany. *International Journal of Social Psychiatry* 44, 107–16.

Babic-Banaszak, A., Kovacic, L., Kovacevic, L., Vuletic, G., Mujkic, A. and Ebling, Z. 2002: Impact of war on health related quality of life in Croatia: population study. *Croatian Medical Journal* 43, 396–402.

Balabanova, D. and McKee, M. 1999: Patterns of alcohol consumption in Bulgaria. *Alcohol and Alcoholism* 34, 622–28.

Baleydier, B., Damsa, C., Schutzbach, C., Stauffer, O. and Glauser, D. 2003: Comparison between Swiss and foreign patients' characteristics at the psychiatric emergencies department and the predictive factors of their management strategies. *L'Encéphale* 29, 205–12.

Beck, M., Matschinger, H. and Angermeyer, M.C. 2003: Social representations of major depression in West and East Germany – do differences still persist 11 years after reunification? *Social Psychiatry and Psychiatric Epidemiology* 38, 520–25.

Becker, T., Hulsmann, S., Knudsen H C., Martiny, K., Amaddeo, F., Herran, A., Knapp, M., Schene, A.H., Tansella, M., Thornicroft, G. and Vazquez-Barquero, J.L. 2002: Provision of services for people with schizophrenia in five European regions. *Social Psychiatry and Psychiatric Epidemiology* 37, 465–74.

Bhugra, D. 2002: Ethnic factors and service utilization. *Current Opinion in Psychiatry* 15, 201–204.

Bhui, K. (2002) *Racism and Mental Health.* London: Jessica Kingsley.

Bhui, K., Stansfeld, S., McKenzie, K., Karlsen, S., Nazroo, J. and Weich, S. (2005) Racial/ethnic discrimination and common mental disorders among workers: findings from the EMPIRIC Study of Ethnic Minority Groups in the United Kingdom. *American Journal of Public Health* 95, 496–501.

Bobak, M., Room, R., Pikhart, H., Kubinova, R., Malyutina, S., Pajak, A., Kurilovitch, S., Topor, R., Nikitin, Y. and Marmot, M. 2004: Contribution of drinking patterns to differences in rates of alcohol related problems between three urban populations. *Journal of Epidemiology and Community Health* 58, 238–42.

Böcker, F.M., Jeschke, F. and Brieger, P. 2001: Psychiatric care in Sachsen-Anhalt: a survey of institutions and services with the 'European Services Mapping Schedule' ESMS. *Psychiatrische Praxis* 28, 393–401.

Bowman, J.T. 1987: Attitudes toward disabled persons: social distance and work competence. *Journal of Rehabilitation* 53, 41–44.

Bramsen, I. and van der Ploeg, H.M. 1999: Use of medical and mental health care by World War II survivors in The Netherlands. *Journal of Traumatic Stress* 12, 243–61.

Brand, U. 2001a: European perspectives: a carer's view. *Acta Psychiatrica Scandinavica 104, Supplementum* 410: 96–101.

Brand U. 2001b: Mental health care in Germany: carers' perspectives. *Acta Psychiatrica Scandinavica 104, Supplementum* 410: 35–40.

Bray, I., Brennan, P. and Boffetta, P. 2000: Projections of alcohol- and tobacco-related cancer mortality in Central Europe. *International Journal of Cancer* 87, 122–28.

Brune, M., Haasen, C., Krausz, M., Yagdiran, O., Bustos, E. and Eisenman, D. 2002: Belief systems as coping factors for traumatized refugees: a pilot study. *European Psychiatry* 17, 451–58.

Brunt, D. and Hansson, L. 2002: A comparison of the psychosocial environment of two types of residences for persons with severe mental illness: small congregate community residences and psychiatric inpatient settings. *International Journal of Social Psychiatry* 48, 243–52.

Burns, T. and Priebe, S. 1996: Mental health care systems and their characteristics: a proposal. *Acta Psychiatrica Scandinavica* 94, 381–85.

Burns, T., Knapp, M., Catty, J., Healey, A., Henderson, J., Watt, H. and Wright, C. 2001: Home treatment for mental health problems: a systematic review. *Health Technology Assessment* 5, 1–139.

Burns, T., Catty, J., Watt, H., Wright, C., Knapp, M. and Henderson, J. 2002: International differences in home treatment for mental health problems. Results of a systematic review. *British Journal of Psychiatry* 181, 375–82.

Burns, T., Becker, T., Catty, J., Fioritti, A., Knapp, M., Lauber, C., Rössler, W., Tomov, T., van Busschbach, J., White, W., Wiersma, D. and the EQOLISE Group 2006: *Enhancing the Quality of Life and Independence of Persons Disabled by Severe Mental Illness through Supported Employment: The EQOLISE Study*. Final Report to European Commission – QLRT-2001-00683.

Cantor-Graae, E., Pedersen, C.B., McNeil, T.F. and Mortensen, P.B. 2003: Migration as a risk factor for schizophrenia: a Danish population-based cohort study. *British Journal of Psychiatry* 182, 117–22.

Chenet, L., Britton, A., Kalediene. R. and Petrauskiene, J. 2001: Daily variations in deaths in Lithuania: the possible contribution of binge drinking. *International Journal of Epidemiology* 30, 743–48.

Cooper, B. 2003: Evidence-based mental health policy: a critical appraisal. *British Journal of Psychiatry* 183, 105–13.

Crawford, M.J., Aldridge, T., Bhui, K., Rutter, D., Manley, C., Weaver, T., Tyrer, P. and Fulop, N. 2003: User involvement in the planning and delivery of mental health services: a cross-sectional survey of service users and providers. *Acta Psychiatrica Scandinavica* 107, 410–14.

Crisp, A.H., Gelder, M.G., Rix, S., Meltzer, H.I. and Rowlands, O.J. 2000: Stigmatisation of people with mental illnesses. *British Journal of Psychiatry* 177, 4–7.

Crowther, R., Marshall, M., Bond, G. and Huxley, P. 2001: Vocational rehabilitation for people with severe mental illness. *Cochrane Database of Systematic Review* CD003080.

Csemy, L., Kubick, A.L. and Nociar, A. 2002a: Drug scene in the Czech Republic and Slovakia during the period of transformation. *European Addiction Research* 8, 159–65.

Csemy, L., Kubicka, L. and Nociar, A. 2002b: Drug scene in the Czech Republic and Slovakia during the period of transformation. *European Addiction Research* 8, 159–65.

De Girolamo, G. and Bassi, M. 2004: Residential facilities as the new scenario of long-term psychiatric care. *Current Opinion in Psychiatry* 17, 275–81.

De Girolamo, G. and Fioritti, A. 2002: Public health and psychiatry: between evidence and hopes. *Current Opinion in Psychiatry* 15, 177–80.

De Girolamo, G., Picardi, A., Micciolo, R., Falloon, I., Fioritti, A. and Morosini, P. 2002: Residential care in Italy. National survey of non-hospital facilities. *British Journal of Psychiatry* 181, 220–25.

Drake, R.E., McHugo, G.J., Bebout, R.R., Becker, D.R., Harris, M., Bond, G.R. and Quimby, E. 1999: A randomized clinical trial of supported employment for inner-city patients with severe mental disorders. *Archives of General Psychiatry* 56, 627–33.

Eisen, S. V., Wilcox, M., Idiculla, T., Speredelozzi, A. and Dickey, B. 2002: Assessing consumer perceptions of inpatient psychiatric treatment: the perceptions of care survey. *Joint Commission Journal on Quality Improvement* 28, 510–26.

Elekes, Z. and Kovács, L. 2002: Old and new drug consumption habits in Hungary, Romania and Moldova. *European Addiction Research* 8, 166–69.

European Commission 2003: *Article 13(2), Council directive 2003/9/EC of 27 January 2003*. Laying down minimum standards for the reception of asylum-seekers; entered into force 6 February 2003. It applies to all EU member states, except Denmark and Ireland. http://www.unhcr.org.au/pdfs/Discussionpaper2006.pdf. Brussels: European Commission.

European Communities 2004: *The State of Mental Health in the European Union*. http://ec.europa.eu/health/ph_determinants/life_style/mental/docs/action_1997_2004_en.pdf. Brussels: European Commission.

Fakhoury, W. and Priebe, S. 2002: The process of deinstitutionalization: an international overview. *Current Opinion in Psychiatry* 15, 187–92.

Fassin, D. and Rechtman, R. 2005: An anthropological hybrid: the pragmatic arrangement of universalism and culturalism in French mental health. *Transcultural Psychiatry* 42, 347–66.

Feachem, R.G. 2000: Health systems: more evidence, more debate. *Bulletin of the World Health Organization* 78, 715.

Federal Statistical Office of Germany (Statistisches Bundesamt Deutschland). 2003: http://www.destatis.de/basis/d/bevoe/bevoetab4.htm (accessed 30 April 2004).

Flaker, V. 2002: Heroin use in Slovenia – a consequence or a vehicle of social changes. *European Addiction Research* 8, 170–76.

Fleischmann, H. 2003: What do psychiatric patients expect of inpatient psychiatric hospital treatment? *Psychiatrische Praxis* 30, S136–S139.

Forster, D.P. and Jozan, P. 1990: Health in Eastern Europe. *Lancet* 335, 458–60.

Freeman, G.P. 1997: Immigration as a source of political discontent and frustration in Western democracies. *Studies in Comparative International Development* 32, 42–64.

Gater, R., Amaddeo, F., Tansella, M., Jackson, G. and Goldberg, D. 1995: A comparison of community-based care for schizophrenia in south Verona and south Manchester. *British Journal of Psychiatry* 166, 344–52.

Gater, R., Jordanova, V., Maric, N., Alikaj, V., Bajs, M., Cavic, T., Dimitrov, H., Iosub, D., Mihal, A., Szalontay, A.S., Helmchen, H. and Sartorius, N. 2005: Pathways to psychiatric care in Eastern Europe. *British Journal of Psychiatry* 186, 529–35.

Geller, J.L. 2000: The last half-century of psychiatric services as reflected in psychiatric services. *Psychiatric Services* 51, 41–67.

Goater, N., King, M., Cole, E., Leavey, G., Johnson-Sabine, E., Blizard, R. and Hoar, A. 1999: Ethnicity and outcome of psychosis. *British Journal of Psychiatry* 175, 34–42.

Haasen, C., Yagdiran, O., Mass, R. and Krausz, M. 2000: Potential for misdiagnosis among Turkish migrants with psychotic disorders: a clinical controlled study in Germany. *Acta Psychiatrica Scandinavica* 101, 125–29.

Hoffmann, H., Kupper, Z., Zbinden, M. and Hirsbrunner, H.P. 2003: Predicting vocational functioning and outcome in schizophrenia outpatients attending a vocational rehabilitation program. *Social Psychiatry and Psychiatric Epidemiology* 38, 76–82.

Hölling, I. 2001: About the impossibility of a single (ex-)user and survivor of psychiatry position. *Acta Psychiatrica Scandinavica 104, Supplementum* 410: 102–106.

Hutchinson, G. and Haasen, C. 2004a: Migration and schizophrenia: the challenges for European psychiatry and implications for the future. *Social Psychiatry and Psychiatric Epidemiology* 39, 350–57.

Hutchinson, G. and Haasen, C. 2004b: Migration and schizophrenia: the challenges for European psychiatry and implications for the future. *Social Psychiatry and Psychiatric Epidemiology* 39: 350–57.

Hutchinson, G. and Haasen, C. 2004c: Migration and schizophrenia: the challenges for European psychiatry and implications for the future. *Social Psychiatry and Psychiatric Epidemiology* 39, 350–57.

Hutchinson, G. and Haasen, C. 2004d: Migration and schizophrenia: the challenges for European psychiatry and implications for the future. *Social Psychiatry and Psychiatric Epidemiology* 39, 350–57.

Jorm, A.F., Korten, A.E., Jacomb, P.A., Rodgers, B., Pollitt, P., Christensen, H. and Henderson, S. 1997a: Helpfulness of interventions for mental disorders: beliefs of health professionals compared with the general public. *British Journal of Psychiatry* 171, 233–37.

Jorm, A.F., Korten, A.E., Jacomb, P.A., Rodgers, B., Pollitt, P., Christensen, H. and Henderson, S. 1997b: Helpfulness of interventions for mental disorders: beliefs of health professionals compared with the general public. *British Journal of Psychiatry* 171, 233–37.

Knapp, M., McDaid, D., Mossialos, E. and Thornicroft, G. 2005: *Mental Health Policy and Practice across Europe.* Buckingham: Open University Press.

Kovács, L. 2001: *Drug Use in the Transylvanian Secondary School Population [Hungarian].* Symposium, Hungarian Academia of Sciences.

Kovács, L. and Antal, Á. 1999: Alcohol and drug use in the secondary school population of Cluj. *Addiction Hungary* 8, 186–208.

Kubicka, L., Csemy, L. and Kozeny, J. 1995: Prague women's drinking before and after the 'velvet revolution' of 1989: a longitudinal study. *Addiction* 90: 1471–78.

Laban, C.J, Gernaat, H.B., Komproe, I.H., Schreuders, B.A. and De Jong, J.T. 2004: Impact of a long asylum procedure on the prevalence of psychiatric disorders in Iraqi asylum seekers in the Netherlands. *Journal of Nervous and Mental Disease* 192, 843–51.

Laban, C.J., Gernaat, H.B., Komproe, I.H., Van, D.T. and De Jong, J.T. 2005: Postmigration living problems and common psychiatric disorders in Iraqi asylum seekers in the Netherlands. *Journal of Nervous and Mental Disease* 193, 825–32.

Lasalvia, A., Rugger, I., Mazzi, M.A. and Dall'agnola, R.B. 2000: The perception of needs for care in staff and patients in community-based mental health services. The South-Verona Outcome Project 3. *Acta Psychiatrica Scandinavica* 102, 366–75.

Lauber, C., Nordt, C., Sartorius, N., Falcato, L. and Rössler, W. 2000: Public acceptance of restrictions on mentally ill people. *Acta Psychiatrica Scandinavica Supplementum* 102, 26–32.

Lauber, C., Nordt, C., Falcato, L. and Rössler, W. 2001: Lay recommendations on how to treat mental disorders. *Social Psychiatry and Psychiatric Epidemiology* 36: 553–56.

Lauber, C., Nordt, C., Falcato, L. and Rössler, W. 2002: Public attitude to compulsory admission of mentally ill people. *Acta Psychiatrica Scandinavica* 105, 385–89.

Lauber, C., Falcato, L., Nordt, C. and Rössler, W. 2003a: Lay beliefs about causes of depression. *Acta Psychiatrica Scandinavica Supplementum* S96–99.

Lauber, C., Nordt, C., Falcato, L. and Rössler, W. 2003b: Do people recognise mental illness? Factors influencing mental health literacy. *European Archives of Psychiatry and Clinical Neuroscience* 253, 248–51.

Lauber, C., Nordt, C., Falcato, L. and Rössler, W. in press: Lay attitudes towards psychotropic drugs and their relationship to the recognition of mental illness. *Australian and New Zealand Journal of Psychiatry.*

Lay, B., Lauber, C. and Rössler, W. 2005: Are immigrants at a disadvantage in psychiatric in-patient care? *Acta Psychiatrica Scandinavica* 111, 358–66.

Leff, J. and Trieman, N. 2000: Long-stay patients discharged from psychiatric hospitals. Social and clinical outcomes after five years in the community. The TAPS Project 46. *British Journal of Psychiatry* 176, 217–23.

Leinsalu, M., Vagero, D. and Kunst, A.E. 2004: Increasing ethnic differences in mortality in Estonia after the collapse of the Soviet Union. *Journal of Epidemiology and Community Health* 58, 583–89.

Leisse, M. and Kallert, T.W. 2000: Social integration and the quality of life of schizophrenic patients in different types of complementary care. *European Psychiatry* 15, 450–60.

Link, B.G., Phelan, J.C., Bresnahan, M., Stueve, A. and Pescosolido, B.A. 1999: Public conceptions of mental illness: labels, causes, dangerousness, and social distance. *American Journal of Public Health* 89, 1328–33.

Madianos, M.G., Zacharakis, C. and Tsitsa, C. 2000: Utilization of psychiatric inpatient care in Greece: a nationwide study (1984–1996). *International Journal of Social Psychiatry* 46, 89–100.

Mahy, G.E., Mallett, R., Leff, J. and Bhugra, D. 1999: First-contact incidence rate of schizophrenia on Barbados. *British Journal of Psychiatry* 175, 28–33.

Mäkinen, I.H. 2000: Eastern European transition and suicide mortality. *Social Science and Medicine* 51, 1405–20.

Marshall, M. and Lockwood, A. 2000: Assertive community treatment for people with severe mental disorders. *Cochrane Database Systematic Review* CD001089.

Marshall, M., Crowther, R., Almaraz-Serrano, A., Creed, F., Sledge, W., Kluiter, H., Roberts, C., Hill, E., Wiersma, D., Bond, G.R., Huxley, P. and Tyrer, P. 2001: Systematic reviews of the effectiveness of day care for people with severe mental disorders: (1) acute day hospital versus admission; (2) vocational rehabilitation; (3) day hospital versus outpatient care. *Health Technology Assessments* 5, 1–75.

Marusic, A. 2004: Mental health in the enlarged European Union: need for relevant public mental health action. *British Journal of Psychiatry* 184, 450–51.

McCulloch, A., Muijen, M. and Harper, H. 2000: New developments in mental health policy in the United Kingdom. *International Journal of Law in Psychiatry* 23, 261–76.

McKee, M. and Jacobson, B. 2000: Public health in Europe. *Lancet* 356, 665–70.

McKee, M. and Shkolnikov, V. 2001: Understanding the toll of premature death among men in eastern Europe. *British Medical Journal* 323, 1051–55.

McKee, M., Pomerleau, J., Robertson, A., Pudule, I., Grinberga, D., Kadziauskiene, K., Abaravicius, A. and Vaask, S. 2000: Alcohol consumption in the Baltic Republics. *Journal of Epidemiology and Community Health* 54, 361–66.

Miles, A., Grey, J.E., Polychronis, A., Price, N. and Melchiorri, C. 2003: Current thinking in the evidence-based health care debate. *Journal of Evaluation in Clinical Practice* 9, 95–109.

Mollica, R.F., McInnes, K., Sarajlic, N., Lavelle, J., Sarajlic, I. and Massagli, M.P. 1999: Disability associated with psychiatric comorbidity and health status in Bosnian refugees living in Croatia. *Journal of the American Medical Association* 282, 433–39.

Moskalewicz, J. 2002: Drugs in countries of central and Eastern Europe. *European Addiction Research* 8, 157–58.

Murad, S.D., Joung, I.M., Verhulst, F.C., Mackenbach, J.P. and Crijnen, A.A. 2004: Determinants of self-reported emotional and behavioral problems in Turkish immigrant adolescents aged 11–18. *Social Psychiatry and Psychiatric Epidemiology* 39, 196–207.

Noble, L.M. and Douglas, B.C. 2004: What users and relatives want from mental health services. *Current Opinion in Psychiatry* 17, 289–96.

Nyari, T.A., Heredi, K. and Parker, L. 2005: Addictive behaviour of adolescents in secondary schools in Hungary. *European Addiction Research* 11, 38–43.

Ødegård, O. 1932: Emigration and insanity: a study of mental disease among Norwegian born population in Minnesota. *Acta Psychiatrica et Neurologica Scandinavica* 7, 1–206.

Office for National Statistics 2005: *Population Size.* London: Office for National Statistics.

Office Nationale de Statistique 2004: *Immigrant population in French metropolitan areas* [La population etrangere legale en France metropolitaine]. Office Nationale de Statistique. http://www.interieur gouvfr/rubriques/a/a4_publications/sejour2002/population pdf (accessed 30 April 2004).

Pijl, Y.J., Kluiter, H. and Wiersma, D. 2000: Change in Dutch mental health care: an evaluation. *Social Psychiatry and Psychiatric Epidemiology* 35, 402–407.

Poznyak, V.B., Pelipas, V.E., Vievski, A.N. and Miroshnichenko, L. 2002: Illicit drug use and its health consequences in

Belarus, Russian Federation and Ukraine: impact of transition. *European Addiction Research* 8, 184–89.

Rasanen, S., Hakko., H., Herva, A., Isohanni, M., Nieminen, P. and Moring, J. 2000: Community placement of long-stay psychiatric patients in northern Finland. *Psychiatric Services* 51, 383–85.

Red Cross/EU Office 2003: *Final report of the Conference on the EC Directive on Minimum Reception Standards for Asylum Seekers*. Brussels: Red Cross/EU Office.

Reker, T., Hornung, W.P., Schonauer, K. and Eikelmann, B. 2000: Long-term psychiatric patients in vocational rehabilitation programmes: a naturalistic follow-up study over 3 years. *Acta Psychiatrica Scandinavica* 101, 457–63.

Rhi, B.Y. 2001: Culture, spirituality, and mental health. The forgotten aspects of religion and health. *Psychiatric Clinics of North America* 24, 569–79.

Richter, R.A. and Nollau, M. 2000: Perspectives of psychiatric care in Leipzig – deinstitutionalization from the viewpoint of neurologist/psychiatrist in private practice and the work of a consortium of community psychiatric services. *Psychiatrische Praxis* 27, S95–S99.

Rothbard, A.B. and Kuno, E. 2000: The success of deinstitutionalization. Empirical findings from case studies on state hospital closures. *International Journal of Law in Psychiatry* 23, 329–44.

Salize, H.J., Kustner, B.M., Torres-Gonzalez, F., Reinhard, I., Estevez, J.F. and Rössler, W. 1999: Needs for care and effectiveness of mental health care provision for schizophrenic patients in two European regions: a comparison between Granada (Spain) and Mannheim (Germany). *Acta Psychiatrica Scandinavica* 100, 328–34.

Saloviita, L. and Pirttimaa, R. 2000: The arrival of supported employment in Finland. *International Journal of Rehabilitation Research* 23, 145–47.

Salvador-Carulla, L., Tibaldi, G., Johnson, S., Scala, E., Romero, C. and Munizza, C. 2005: Patterns of mental health service utilisation in Italy and Spain – an investigation using the European Service Mapping Schedule. *Social Psychiatry and Psychiatric Epidemiology* 4, 149–59.

Sartorius N. 1998: Stigma: what can psychiatrists do about it? *Lancet* 352, 1058–59.

Sebre, S., Sprugevica, I., Novotni, A., Bonevski, D., Pakalniskiene, V., Popescu, D., Turchina, T., Friedrich, W. and Lewis, O. 2004: Cross-cultural comparisons of child-reported emotional and physical abuse: rates, risk factors and psychosocial symptoms. *Child Abuse and Neglect* 28, 113–27.

Shkolnikov, V., McKee, M. and Leon, D.A. 2001: Changes in life expectancy in Russia in the mid-1990s. *Lancet* 357, 917–21.

Silfverhielm, H. and Kamis-Gould, E. 2000: The Swedish mental health system. Past, present, and future. *International Journal of Law in Psychiatry* 23, 293–307.

Silove, D. 2000: Trauma and forced relocation. *Current Opinion in Psychiatry* 13, 231–36.

Simpson, E.L. and House, A.O. 2002: Involving users in the delivery and evaluation of mental health services: systematic review. *British Medical Journal* 325, 1265.

Simpura, J., Tigerstedt, C., Hanhinen, S., Lagerspetz, M., Leifman, H., Moskalewicz, J. and Torronen, J. 1999: Alcohol misuse as a health and social issue in the Baltic Sea region. A summary of findings from the Baltica Study. *Alcohol and Alcoholism* 34, 805–23.

Siponen, U. and Valimaki, M. 2003: Patients' satisfaction with outpatient psychiatric care. *Journal of Psychiatric and Mental Health Nursing* 10, 129–35.

Spiessl, H., Schmid, R., Vukovich, A. and Cording, C. 2004: [Expectations and satisfaction from relatives of psychiatric patients in inpatient treatment]. *Nervenarzt* 75, 475–82.

Swiss Federal Statistical Office 2005: *Population Size and Developmental Perspectives* [Bevölkerungsstand und entwicklung]. Neuchâtel: Swiss Federal Statistical Office.

Sytema, S. and Burgess, P. 1999: Continuity of care and readmission in two service systems: a comparative Victorian and Groningen case-register study. *Acta Psychiatrica Scandinavica* 100, 212–19.

Szucs, S., Sarvary, A., McKee, M. and Adany R. 2005: Could the high level of cirrhosis in central and Eastern Europe be due partly to the quality of alcohol consumed? An exploratory investigation. *Addiction* 100: 536–42.

Thornicroft, G. and Rose, D. 2005: Mental health in Europe. *British Medical Journal* 330, 613–14.

Thornicroft, G. and Tansella, M. 2002: Balancing community-based and hospital-based mental health care. *World Psychiatry* 1, 84–90.

Thornicroft, G. and Tansella, M. 2004: Components of a modern mental health service: a pragmatic balance of community and hospital care: overview of systematic evidence. *British Journal of Psychiatry* 185, 283–90.

Tomov, T. 2001: Mental health reforms in Eastern Europe. *Acta Psychiatrica Scandinavica* 104, Supplementum 410: 21–26.

Trieman, N. and Leff, J. 2002: Long-term outcome of long-stay psychiatric in-patients considered unsuitable to live in the community. TAPS Project 44. *British Journal of Psychiatry* 181, 428–32.

Van Os, J. and Neeleman, J. 1994: Caring for mentally ill people. *British Medical Journal* 309, 1218–21.

Van Os, J., Galdos, P., Lewis, G., Bourgeois, M. and Mann, A. 1993: Schizophrenia sans frontieres: concepts of schizophrenia among French and British psychiatrists. *British Medical Journal* 307, 489–92.

Varvasovsky, Z., Bain, C. and McKee, M. 1997: Deaths from cirrhosis in Poland and Hungary: the impact of different alcohol policies during the 1980s. *Journal of Epidemiology and Community Health* 51, 167–71.

Von Cranach, M. 2000: Housing for psychiatric patients inside and outside of hospitals. *Psychiatrische Praxis* 27, S59–S63.

Waldron, I. 1993: Recent trends in sex mortality ratios for adults in developed countries. *Social Science and Medicine* 36, 451–62.

Wasserman, D., Varnik, A. and Eklund, G. 1994: Male suicides and alcohol consumption in the former USSR. *Acta Psychiatrica Scandinavica* 89, 306–13.

Watters, C. and Ingleby, D. 2004: Locations of care: meeting the mental health and social care needs of refugees in Europe. *International Journal of Law in Psychiatry* 27, 549–70.

World Health Organization 2001: *The World Health Report, 2001. Mental Health: New Understanding, New Hope.* Geneva: World Health Organization.

World Health Organization 2005a: *Mental Health Action Plan for Europe.* Copenhagen: World Health Organization.

World Health Organization 2005b: *Mental Health Declaration for Europe.* Copenhagen: World Health Organization.

Wright, E.R., Gronfein, W.P. and Owens, T.J. 2000: Deinstitutionalization, social rejection, and the self-esteem of former mental patients. *Journal of Health and Social Behaviour* 41, 68–90.

Young, A.S., Grusky, O., Jordan, D. and Belin, T.R. 2000: Routine outcome monitoring in a public mental health system: the impact of patients who leave care. *Psychiatric Services* 51, 85–91.

# 31

# Mental health and cultural psychiatry in the Caribbean

## Robert Kohn

## INTRODUCTION

The Caribbean is a region of the Americas consisting of the Caribbean Sea, its islands and the surrounding coasts. Also known as the West Indies, the Caribbean is organized into 28 territories including sovereign states, overseas departments and dependencies (Table 31.1). Three of the territories are on mainland South America: French Guiana, Guyana and Suriname. Four languages are spoken in the region: English, Spanish, French and Dutch. Most of the population originated from African slave descendants.

The only surviving indigenous people of the Caribbean are the Carib. Although they were virtually exterminated during the colonial period they survived on the islands of Dominica, Saint Vincent, Saint Lucia and Trinidad. Those who mixed with African slaves on Saint Vincent were known as Black Caribs and were deported and became the descendants of the Garifuna found in Belize. The largest population of Caribs is found in Dominica, where there are about 3000. The Dominican Republic's population is estimated to be 60 per cent part-indigenous. On the South American continent Suriname, Guyana and French Guiana have sizeable Amerindian indigenous populations, ranging from 3 to 9 per cent.

The economies of the territories in the region vary widely, reflecting and reflected by marked differences in the percentage of the population under the age of 15, life expectancy and literacy rates (Table 31.2). As a result, the contribution of neuropsychiatric disorders in the Caribbean to disability adjusted life years (DALYs) also varies widely, from 9.1 per cent in Haiti, the poorest country in the Western Hemisphere, to 26.4 per cent in Jamaica (Table 31.3). This variability is a reflection of early mortality and the high prevalence of infectious diseases, including HIV/AIDS in the poorer countries. In Haiti, as well as some of the other countries, the contribution of HIV/AIDs (21.2 per cent) alone exceeds the total contribution of neuropsychological problems to DALYs (World Health Organization, 2006).

## PREVALENCE OF PSYCHIATRIC DISORDERS

The only community-based prevalence studies of psychiatric disorders are from Puerto Rico, where studies of both adults and adolescents and children have been conducted. Individuals aged 10–20 years comprise about 30 per cent of the population of the Caribbean. Among children aged 4–17 years,

**Table 31.1** *Language, ethnicity and nationality of Caribbean countries*

| Country | Language | Dependency | Ethnicity | Other languages |
|---|---|---|---|---|
| Anguilla | English | UK | 90% African descent | Patois (Creole English) |
| Antigua and Barbuda | English | Independent | Mostly African descent | Papiamento (Creole) |
| Aruba | Dutch | Netherlands | Mixed | Portuguese |
| Bahamas | English | Independent | 56% African descent; 34% white | Bajan, an English dialect |
| Barbados | English | Independent | 90% African descent | Patois |
| Bermuda | English | UK | 85% African descent | |
| Cayman Islands | English | UK | 83% African descent | |
| Cuba | Spanish | Independent | 51% Mulatto; 37% white; 11% black | Patois (Creole French) |
| Dominica | English | Independent | 90% African descent | |
| Dominican Republic | Spanish | Independent | 75% Mulatto | Creole (French) |
| French Guiana | French | France | 66% Creole (mixed black–white) | |
| Grenada | English | Independent | 80% African descent | |
| Guadeloupe | French | France | 75% Black or Mulatto | |
| Guyana | English | Independent | 45% East Indian; 43% African descent | Haitian Creole |
| Haiti | French | Independent | 95% African descent | Patois (Jamaican Creole) |
| Jamaica | English | Independent | 90% African descent | |
| Martinique | French | France | 90% Mixed African descent | |
| Montserrat | English | UK | Mostly Mixed Irish and African descent | Papiamentu (Creole), |
| Netherlands Antilles | Dutch | Netherlands | 85% Mixed African descent | English |
| Puerto Rico | Spanish | USA | Mostly mixed European–Amerindian | |
| Saint Kitts and Nevis | English | Independent | 90% African descent | Patois (Creole French) |
| Saint Lucia | English | Independent | 90% African descent | |
| Saint Vincent and Grenadines | English | Independent | 66% African descent; 19% mixed | |
| Suriname | Dutch | Independent | 37% East Indian | Sranang Tongo |
| Trinidad and Tobago | English | Independent | 40% North Indian; 40% African descent | Creole English |
| Turks and Caicos Islands | English | UK | | |
| Virgin Islands (UK) | English | UK | | |
| Virgin Islands (USA) | English | USA | | |

Aruba uses spelling that is closer to Spanish, whereas the other islands tried to stay closer to their roots in that respect. As a result, some words may have more than one way of spelling them, for example Papiamento and Papiamentu.

**Table 31.2** Demographic data of Caribbean countries

| Country | Population (thousands) | Urban population (%) | Age <15 (%) | Age >60 (%) | Literacy (%) | Life expectancy at birth (years) | Suicide (%) | Homicide (%) |
|---|---|---|---|---|---|---|---|---|
| Anguilla | 131 | 100 | 16.0 | 9.6 | 95.4 | 77.1 | – | – |
| Antigua and Barbuda | 69 | 38.4 | 19.0 | 5.4 | 88.5 | 71.9 | 0.6 | 4.8 |
| Aruba | 72 | 44.7 | 14.0 | 16.9 | 97.0 | 79.1 | – | – |
| Bahamas | 323 | 90.0 | 26.4 | 9.3 | 95.8 | 71.1 | 1.2 | 16.4 |
| Barbados | 270 | 52.9 | 17.8 | 13.2 | 99.7 | 75.8 | 2.3 | 10.5 |
| Bermuda | 65 | 100 | 12.8 | 17.1 | 98.5 | 77.8 | 7.4 | 3.3 |
| Cayman Islands | 44 | 100 | 14.2 | 12.2 | 98.0 | 80.0 | 2.1 | 4.3 |
| Cuba | 11 269 | 76.0 | 17.9 | 15.3 | 97.3 | 78.0 | 18.1 | 7.0 |
| Dominica | 69 | 72.2 | 18.6 | 10.4 | – | 74.7 | 3.0 | 3.8 |
| Dominican Republic | 8895 | 60.1 | 30.4 | 6.3 | 85.5 | 68.0 | 3.3 | 11.1 |
| French Guiana | 187 | 75.6 | 32.1 | 6.4 | 83.0 | 75.7 | – | – |
| Grenada | 90 | 42.2 | 22.8 | 4.7 | 98.0 | 64.5 | 1.1 | 1.6 |
| Guadeloupe | 448 | 99.8 | 23.3 | 13.8 | 90.1 | 78.9 | 8.7 | 1.4 |
| Guyana | 751 | 38.8 | 34.7 | 6.0 | 99.0 | 64.4 | 11.2 | 5.8 |
| Haiti | 8528 | 46.4 | 36.4 | 5.6 | 54.8 | 68.6 | 0.9 | 18.6 |
| Jamaica | 2651 | 52.2 | 29.3 | 10.2 | 88.7 | 70.9 | 0.1 | 0.2 |
| Martinique | 396 | 96.2 | 20.2 | 16.8 | 98.0 | 79.1 | 9.4 | 2.7 |
| Montserrat | 9 | 13.8 | 15.0 | 13.8 | 97.0 | 78.7 | – | 5.6 |
| Netherlands Antilles | 183 | 70.1 | 21.5 | 14.0 | 96.9 | 76.5 | – | – |
| Puerto Rico | 3955 | 97.5 | 20.9 | 16.9 | 94.6 | 76.5 | 7.2 | 18.7 |
| Saint Kitts and Nevis | 39 | 31.9 | 19.1 | 10.5 | 97.3 | 72.2 | 4.9 | 13.0 |
| Saint Lucia | 161 | 31.3 | 27.0 | 9.7 | 81.5 | 72.8 | 7.1 | 20.1 |
| Saint Vincent and Grenadines | 119 | 60.5 | 27.3 | 8.9 | 96.0 | 71.6 | 6.0 | 11.0 |
| Suriname | 449 | 77.2 | 28.0 | 9.0 | 93.0 | 69.7 | 11.5 | 3.0 |
| Trinidad and Tobago | 1305 | 76.2 | 20.1 | 10.8 | 98.8 | 70.0 | 12.6 | 10.5 |
| Turks and Caicos Islands | 21 | 47.4 | 21.4 | 6.2 | 98.5 | 74.5 | 6.4 | 8.7 |
| Virgin Islands (UK) | 23 | 65.4 | 4.0 | 8.1 | 98.2 | 76.5 | 2.6 | 10.5 |
| Virgin Islands (USA) | 112 | 94.1 | 22.7 | 16.6 | – | 79.0 | 3.3 | 28.8 |

Source: Pan American Health Organization website (www.paho.org) based on most recent data available as of 2004.

**Table 31.3**  *Percentage of DALYs attributed to neuropsychiatric causes and HIV/AIDS 2002 among Caribbean countries*

| Country | DALY (%) | |
| --- | --- | --- |
|  | Psychiatric | HIV/AIDS |
| Antigua and Barbuda | 22.1 | 2.3 |
| Bahamas | 22.5 | 13.2 |
| Barbados | 23.9 | 7.1 |
| Cuba | 25.1 | 0.2 |
| Dominica | 24.8 | 1.2 |
| Dominican Republic | 19.3 | 13.5 |
| Grenada | 18.5 | 2.1 |
| Guyana | 16.6 | 18.1 |
| Haiti | 9.1 | 21.2 |
| Jamaica | 26.4 | 6.5 |
| Saint Kitts and Nevis | 24.8 | 1.0 |
| Saint Lucia | 24.8 | 1.4 |
| Saint Vincent and the Grenadines | 21.7 | 5.4 |
| Suriname | 19.2 | 7.0 |
| Trinidad and Tobago | 17.5 | 19.3 |

DALY, disability adjusted life years.

**Table 31.4**  *One-year prevalence of DSM-IV diagnoses in Puerto Rican children aged 4–17 years*

| Diagnosis (DSM-IV/DISC-IV) | Rate (%) | |
| --- | --- | --- |
|  | Without impairment criteria | With impairment criteria |
| Major depression | 3.0 | 1.4 |
| Dysthymic | 0.5 | 0.5 |
| Social phobia | 2.5 | 1.5 |
| Separation anxiety | 3.1 | 1.5 |
| Panic | 0.5 | 0.1 |
| Generalized anxiety | 2.2 | 1.0 |
| Post-traumatic stress | 0.8 | 0.1 |
| Attention deficit hyperactivity disorder | 8.0 | 3.7 |
| Conduct disorder | 2.0 | 1.3 |
| Oppositional defiant disorder | 5.5 | 3.4 |
| Alcohol abuse/ dependence | 0.8 | 0.4 |
| Nicotine dependence | 0.8 | 0.3 |
| Marijuana abuse dependence | 0.7 | 0.2 |
| Any diagnosis | 16.4 | 6.9 |

DSM, *Diagnostic and Statistical Manual of Mental Disorders*; DISC, Diagnostic Interview Schedule for Children.
Source: Canino *et al.* (2004).

16.4 per cent met *Diagnostic and Statistical Manual of Mental Disorders* (DSM-IV) criteria using the Diagnostic Interview Schedule for Children (DISC-IV) without considering impairment; 6.9 per cent had at least one disorder when impairment was taken into account (Table 31.4). The most prevalent disorders were attention deficit hyperactivity disorder (8.0 per cent) and oppositional defiant disorder (5.5 per cent) (Canino *et al.*, 2004).

More recently, classroom surveys in nine countries were undertaken to include 15 695 adolescents aged 10–18 years; the countries included Antigua, the Bahamas, Barbados, British Virgin Islands, Dominica, Grenada, Guyana, Jamaica and Saint Lucia (Halcón *et al.*, 2003). One in six students saw themselves as sad, angry or irritable, with nearly half wondering if anything was worth while. Eleven per cent of the males and 12.8 per cent of the females had attempted suicide. Physical abuse was reported by 15.9 per cent of adolescents, primarily at home; 10.0 per cent of adolescents reported sexual abuse, mainly by other teens or adults outside the home. Most (65.9 per cent) had not had sexual intercourse; however,

of those who had, a quarter of the females and over 50 per cent of males had had sexual intercourse prior to the age of 10. Exposure to violence was common, with 20 per cent of the males carrying weapons in school, and two out of five having thoughts of hurting or killing someone. One-fifth of the males and nearly 13 per cent of females had belonged to gangs. Most striking was that one in six in the English-speaking Caribbean did not believe they would live to age 25.

Disorders among adults were studied in 1984 using the Diagnostic Interview Schedule (DIS) based on DSM-III criteria (Canino *et al.*, 1987). The six-month prevalence among those aged 18–64 years old was 16.0 per cent (Table 31.5). Alcohol use disorders were the most prevalent overall and among men. Among women, agoraphobia had the highest prevalence rate.

**Table 31.5**  *Six-month and lifetime prevalence of DSM-III/DIS disorders in adults aged 18–64*

| Disorder | Six-month | | | Lifetime | | |
|---|---|---|---|---|---|---|
| | Total | Male | Female | Total | Male | Female |
| Any disorder | 16.0 | 18.7 | 13.4 | 28.1 | 34.0 | 22.8 |
| Manic episode | 0.3 | 0.3 | 0.3 | 0.5 | 0.7 | 0.4 |
| Major depressive | 3.0 | 2.4 | 3.3 | 4.6 | 3.5 | 5.5 |
| Dysthymia | | | | 4.7 | 1.6 | 7.6 |
| Social phobia | 1.1 | 1.1 | 1.1 | 1.6 | 1.5 | 1.6 |
| Simple phobia | 4.4 | 3.4 | 5.3 | 8.6 | 7.6 | 9.6 |
| Agoraphobia | 3.9 | 2.4 | 5.4 | 6.9 | 4.9 | 8.7 |
| Panic disorder | 1.1 | 1.2 | 0.9 | 1.7 | 1.6 | 1.9 |
| Obsessive–compulsive | 1.8 | 1.3 | 2.3 | 3.2 | 3.3 | 3.1 |
| Somatization | 0.7 | 0.7 | 0.6 | 0.7 | 0.7 | 0.7 |
| Schizophrenic disorders | 1.7 | 2.1 | 1.3 | 1.8 | 2.2 | 1.4 |
| Alcohol abuse/dependence | 4.9 | 10.0 | 0.5 | 12.6 | 24.6 | 2.0 |

DSM, *Diagnostic and Statistical Manual of Mental Disorders*; DIS, Diagnostic Interview Schedule.
Source: Canino *et al.* (1987).

**Table 31.6**  *Rate of lifetime substance use by age in Dominican Republic, Haiti and Jamaica (per cent)*

| | Marijuana | Cocaine | Crack | Opiates | Inhalants | Stimulants | Alcohol | Tobacco |
|---|---|---|---|---|---|---|---|---|
| Dominican Republic | | | | | | | | |
| 12–14 | 0.6 | 0.2 | 0.0 | | 5.5 | 4.1 | 43.3 | 2.8 |
| 15–19 | 0.7 | 0.6 | 0.3 | | 3.2 | 6.6 | 66.3 | 8.3 |
| 20–24 | 3.5 | 2.3 | 0.2 | | 3.1 | 10.6 | 69.5 | 20.0 |
| 25–29 | 3.2 | 2.4 | 0.0 | | 1.8 | 7.6 | 74.3 | 25.6 |
| 30–34 | 1.2 | 0.0 | 0.0 | | 1.3 | 5.1 | 73.3 | 29.9 |
| 35–39 | 2.3 | 0.7 | 0.0 | | 0.2 | 3.9 | 67.8 | 36.2 |
| 40–45 | 2.0 | 0.4 | 0.0 | | 1.1 | 6.3 | 66.5 | 43.0 |
| Haiti | | | | | | | | |
| 12–14 | 0.7 | 0.0 | 0.0 | | 3.4 | | 46.6 | 3.4 |
| 15–18 | 1.2 | 0.6 | 0.3 | | 3.8 | | 54.0 | 11.8 |
| 19–24 | 2.9 | 0.6 | 0.4 | | 2.9 | | 62.7 | 21.0 |
| 25–29 | 4.0 | 1.1 | 0.5 | | 2.1 | | 59.6 | 28.6 |
| 30–34 | 5.1 | 1.8 | 0.4 | | 2.6 | | 58.4 | 33.2 |
| 35–39 | 4.8 | 0.0 | 0.0 | | 4.3 | | 62.4 | 37.0 |
| 40–44 | 0.9 | 1.3 | 0.0 | | 3.6 | | 55.4 | 46.2 |
| Jamaica | | | | | | | | |
| Less 20 | 9.4 | 0.0 | 0.4 | 0.4 | 1.0 | | 53.4 | 11.5 |
| 20–29 | 25.1 | 0.4 | 0.6 | 0.9 | 1.1 | | 80.7 | 30.7 |
| 30–39 | 25.7 | 0.2 | 1.1 | 1.0 | 0.9 | | 84.3 | 44.8 |
| 40+ | 14.1 | 0.0 | 0.2 | 0.8 | 0.3 | | 78.6 | 43.6 |

Community-based surveys of lifetime drug use have been conducted in Jamaica, Haiti and the Dominican Republic. These were published in 1989 (National Council on Drug Abuse, 1989), 1991 (Arellano *et al.*, 1991) and 1992 (Jutkowitz *et al.*, 1992) respectively (Table 31.6). These surveys showed a high rate of marijuana use in all age groups in Jamaica, and a high rate of inhalant use in

Haiti and the Dominican Republic. In Haiti and the Dominican Republic, marijuana use initially occurs on average in the twenties, later than alcohol and tobacco use (Jutkowitz and Eu, 1994). Nearly half of all adolescents had experimented with alcohol during their lifetime. It is not known, however, if these studies are still representative of those countries. A 1999 survey of high school students in Jamaica found that 10.2 per cent used marijuana, 2.2 per cent used cocaine, 1.5 per cent used heroin, and 1.2 per cent used opium (Soyibo and Lee, 1999). In students sampled aged 11 years and over, 8 per cent had ever used cannabis in the Bahamas (Smart and Patterson, 1990). In addition, it is unlikely that these estimates are translatable to the rest of the territories.

A recent study of lifetime tobacco smoking among high school students found much lower rates in the Dominican Republic (3.2 per cent), in contrast to Central American countries (6.2–25.5 per cent) (Vittetoe et al., 2002). Halcón et al. (2003) also inquired about substance use and found much lower rates, although this was for current use: 1.4 per cent tobacco; alcohol 3.9 per cent females and 7.9 per cent males; marijuana 1.2 per cent females and 2.3 per cent males; and steroids 1.4 per cent females and 3.2 per cent males. One-fifth reported problems related to drinking or drugs.

## SERVICE UTILIZATION

Little is known about mental health service utilization. A study conducted in Trinidad and Tobago suggested that psychiatrists were not utilizing newer psychotropic drugs, in particular serotonin reuptake inhibitors to treat depression (Moore et al., 2002). In Puerto Rico, which has well-established mental health services, 76 per cent of those with alcohol use disorders, 70.0 per cent with major depression and 9.7 per cent with non-affective psychosis did not receive treatment (Kohn et al., 2005). It may be assumed that the treatment gap is greater and levels of treatment of mental disorders are even lower in much of the Caribbean.

Mental health literacy was examined in Dominica (Kohn et al., 2000) and it was shown that the community had difficulty in identifying depression, hyperactivity and alcoholism as mental illness or even serious problems. In addition, community leaders, for example teachers and police, had less knowledge about mental illnesses than the general population. Although the World Health Organization Mental Health Atlas (2005) provides insights into the availability of mental health resources in the Caribbean (Table 31.7), these resources vary widely between countries.

**Table 31.7**   *Selected results from countries that provided data for the World Health Organization Project Atlas*

| Country | Percentage of health care budget | Psychiatric beds/10 000 | Psychiatrists/ 100 000 | Psychologists/ 100 000 | Social workers/ 100 000 | Psychiatric nurses/ 100 000 |
|---|---|---|---|---|---|---|
| Antigua and Barbuda | 3.0 | 17.9 | 2.0 | 3.0 | | 4.5 |
| Bahamas | 11.0 | 12.0 | 4.7 | 3.0 | 3.7 | 21.6 |
| Barbados | 12.0 | 23.5 | 34.0 | 0.7 | 1.9 | 186.0 |
| Cuba | | 8.8 | 9.8 | 7.9 | 16.0 | 2.7 |
| Dominican Republic | | 0.4 | 1.8 | 14.0 | | 1.0 |
| Grenada | 10.0 | 10.8 | 1.0 | 1.0 | 3.0 | 5.4 |
| Guyana | | 3.0 | 0.2 | 0.0 | 0.4 | 0.6 |
| Jamaica | 5.0 | 4.0 | 0.7 | 0.1 | 0.4 | 8.0 |
| Saint Lucia | 4.0 | 10.7 | 1.3 | 0.0 | 0.7 | 2.6 |
| Saint Vincent and Grenadines | 4.6 | 10.6 | 0.9 | 1.8 | 2.7 | 14.2 |
| Suriname | 4.2 | 8.4 | 1.4 | 0.2 | 0.4 | 15.0 |
| Trinidad and Tobago | | 9.5 | 1.0 | 0.3 | 1.6 | 11.5 |

In addition, these data do not provide a full picture of the mental health needs in the community. The psychiatric consequences of high rates of physical violence in community settings have not been examined. Although it is an issue in many of the territories (Halcón *et al.*, 2003), it is of particular concern in Jamaica where 33 per cent of students aged 9–17 have been exposed to violence, as have 60 per cent of their family members (Gardner *et al.*, 2003). Similarly, in Haiti over 60 per cent of adults reported a history of childhood maltreatment (Martsolf, 2004; Kutcher *et al.*, 2005).

Another challenge to the Caribbean population is the growing exposure to serious natural disasters that may result in mental health problems, malnutrition and exposure to violence (Bravo *et al.*, 1990; Sattler *et al.*, 2002; Avery, 2003; Kutcher *et al.*, 2005; Stair and Pottinger, 2005). Improved surveillance and service planning for mental health services in the Caribbean are needed, as well as better public health promotion to address the growing issues of violence, HIV/AIDS and substance use among the younger population. These will all increase the future mental health burden.

## REFERENCES

Arellano, R., Garcia, J. and Jutkowitz, J. 1991: *National Study of Drug Prevalence and Attitudes Towards Drug Use in Haiti, Revised Final Report*. Arlington, VA: Development Associates for US Agency for International Development/Bureau for Research and Development/Narcotics Awareness and Education Project.

Avery, J.G. 2003: The aftermath of a disaster. Recovery following the volcanic eruptions in Montserrat, West Indies. *West Indian Medical Journal* 52, 131–35.

Bravo, M., Rubio-Stipec, M., Canino, G.J., Woodbury, M.A. and Ribera, J.C. 1990: The psychological sequelae of disaster stress prospectively and retrospectively evaluated. *American Journal of Community Psychology* 18, 661–80.

Canino, G.J., Bird, H.R., Shrout, P.E., Rubio-Stipec, M., Bravo, M., Martinez, R., Sesman, M. and Guevara, L.M. 1987: The prevalence of specific psychiatric disorders in Puerto Rico. *Archives of General Psychiatry* 44, 727–35.

Canino, G., Shrout, P.E., Rubio-Stipec, M., Bird, H.R., Bravo, M., Ramirez, R., Chavez, L., Alegria, M., Bauermeister, J.J., Hohmann, A., Ribera, J., Garcia, P. and Martinez-Taboas, A.

2004: The DSM-IV rates of child and adolescent disorders in Puerto Rico: prevalence, correlates, service use, and the effects of impairment. *Archives of General Psychiatry* 61, 85–93.

Halcón, L., Blum, R.W., Beuhring, T., Pate, E., Campbell-Forrester, S. and Venema, A. 2003: Adolescent health in the Caribbean: a regional portrait. *American Journal of Public Health* 93, 1851–57.

Gardner, J.M., Powell, C.A., Thomas, J.A. and Millard, D. 2003: Perceptions and experiences of violence among secondary school students in urban Jamaica. *Revista Panamericana de Salud Pública* 14, 97–103.

Jutkowitz, J.M. and Eu, H. 1994: Drug prevalence in Latin American and Caribbean countries: a cross national analysis. *Drug Education, Prevention and Policy* 1, 199–252.

Jutkowitz, J.M., Eu, H., Leavy, M., Pagan, L., Kunhart, I. and Valleyron, J. 1992: *Survey on Drug Prevalence and Attitudes in Dominican Republic*. Arlington, VA: Development Associates for US Agency for International Development/Bureau for Research and Development/Narcotics Awareness and Education Project.

Kohn, R., Sharma, D., Camilleri, C.P. and Levav, I. 2000: Attitudes towards mental illness in the Commonwealth of Dominica. *Revista Panamericana de Salud Pública* 7, 148–54.

Kohn, R., Levav, I., de Almeida, J.M., Vicente, B., Andrade, L., Caraveo-Anduaga, J.J., Saxena, S. and Saraceno, B. 2005: Mental disorders in Latin America and the Caribbean: a public health priority. *Revista Panamericana de Salud Pública* 18, 229–40.

Kutcher, S., Chehil, S. and Roberts, T. 2005: An integrated program to train local health care providers to meet post-disaster mental health needs. *Revista Panamericana de Salud Pública* 18, 338–45.

Martsolf, D.S. 2004: Childhood maltreatment and mental and physical health in Haitian adults. *Journal of Nursing Scholarship* 36, 293–99.

Moore, S., Jaime, L.K., Maharajh, H., Ramtahal, I., Reid, S., Ramsewak, F.S. and Maharaj, M. 2002: The prescribing of psychotropic drugs in mental health services in Trinidad. *Revista Panamericana de Salud Pública* 12, 207–14.

National Council on Drug Abuse 1989: *Drug use in Jamaican Households, 1987*. Kingston, Jamaica: National Council on Drug Abuse.

Sattler, D.N., Preston, A.J., Kaiser, C.F., Olivera, V.E., Valdez, J. and Schlueter, S. 2002: Hurricane Georges: a cross-national study examining preparedness, resource loss, and psychological distress in the U.S. Virgin Islands, Puerto Rico, Dominican Republic, and the United States. *Journal of Trauma Stress* 15, 339–50.

Smart, R.G. and Patterson, S.D. 1990: Comparison of alcohol, tobacco, and illicit drug use among students and delinquents in the Bahamas. *Bulletin of the Pan American Health Organization* 24, 39–45.

Soyibo, K. and Lee, M.G. 1999: Use of illicit drugs among high-school students in Jamaica. *Bulletin of the World Health Organization* 77, 258–62.

Stair, A.G. and Pottinger, A.M. 2005: Disaster preparedness and management in the Caribbean the need for psychological support. *West Indian Medical Journal* 54, 165–66.

Vittetoe, K., Lopez, M.F., Delva, J., Wagner, F. and Anthony, J.C. 2002: Panama, Centro America, y Republica Dominicana Research Group. Behavioral problems and tobacco use among adolescents in Central America and the Dominican Republic. *Revista Panamericana de Salud Pública* 11, 76–82.

World Health Organization 2005: *Mental Health Atlas.* Geneva: World Health Organization.

World Health Organization 2006: *WHO Statistical Information System (whosis).* http://www3.who.int/whosis/menu.cfm (accessed June 2006).

# 32

# Understanding mental illness in the English-speaking Caribbean

Gerard Hutchinson

## INTRODUCTION

The English-speaking Caribbean, formerly known as the West Indies, is an archipelago of islands situated just east of the American continent stretching from Jamaica on the western point of the northern Antillean range to Trinidad and Tobago on the southern tip.

The Caribbean as a whole forms a link between North and South America, with Cuba being the closest land mass to Jamaica and Venezuela the closest to Trinidad. The distance between Jamaica and Trinidad, for example, is in excess of 1600 km (1000 miles) and belies the perception of a close geographic bond between the islands. The factor that unites these islands in fact is their history of colonization by Britain (Lewis, 1968) and the cross-fertilization of cultures and peoples from Europe, Africa and Asia who journeyed to these islands. This followed Columbus' landmark journeys in the late fifteenth century and the subsequent Atlantic slave trade and movement of indentured labourers from India.

This history has led to a culturally and ethnically heterogeneous people who continue to struggle to define their own identity as distinct from that defined for them by their former colonizers and the influences of their own ancestral traditions. The relevance of this is that even in the post-Independence era, most of the social structures and institutions established in the islands are derived from the antecedent British models. While the nationals of the English-speaking Caribbean recognize their uniqueness and their diversity, it seems that they remain unclear as to how this diversity fits into a scheme of larger regional identity (Smith, 1965). Mental health services and treatment models are no exceptions to this and the mental health laws that govern the English-speaking Caribbean are derived from British law, in spite of the burgeoning cultural influence of North America on the region (Patterson, 2004).

Epidemiological data regarding the distribution and determinants of mental illness in the Caribbean are primarily available through the various Ministries of Health which collate these as part of their regulatory or supervisory function for health care in most of the islands (see Chapter 31). This responsibility is based on membership of the Pan American Health Organization (PAHO) and, by extension, the World Health Organization (WHO). This facilitates the recording and compilation of national statistics that allow for the production of status documents such as the *Health of the Americas* document produced by PAHO for comparison between member states. The national data would usually come from those patients who have been admitted to hospital or who have made contact with the public mental health service and therefore may not always reflect the reality of the mental health landscape of the country concerned, particularly for mental illness where there may be some stigma attached to accessing public mental health treatment. Another difficulty is the disparity in the training and diagnostic rubric used by most clinicians (the *Diagnostic and Statistical Manual of Mental Disorders*, DSM-IV) and the official recording classification of the WHO, the *International Classification of Diseases* (ICD-10).

Another challenge facing mental health epidemiology in the Caribbean is the sometimes sharp and even antipathic delineation between the public and the private sectors. Information from the private treatment sectors is vital to understanding the real nature of population pathology, especially as one would expect that the private sector patients would be of higher socio-economic and educational standing. This distinction often deludes observers into thinking that mental health disorders are the preserve of the poor and dispossessed and while the incidence and prevalence of some disorders would be higher in that demographic, the pathology of the higher income earners is frequently underreported. This is perhaps particularly relevant to the non-psychotic disorders as many people may experience significant pathology but remain functional because of their psycho-social and economic buffers. Other populations such as prisons, children's homes, homeless shelters and old age homes are not naturally included in the epidemiologic surveys and again represent a large reservoir of psychopathology.

## CURRENT STATISTICS

### Severe mental illness: psychosis

It is interesting that the study of psychotic illness in general and schizophrenia in particular has taken on a special significance in the Caribbean because of the reports of markedly increased rates for these disorders in the Caribbean migrant population living in Britain (Sharpley *et al.*, 2001). There have now been four completed incidence studies of schizophrenia in the Caribbean (Hickling and Rodgers-Johnson, 1995; Bhugra *et al.*, 1996; Mahy *et al.*, 1999; Selten *et al.*, 2005). These represent studies in Jamaica, Trinidad, Barbados and Suriname and all reflect the need to establish the rates of psychosis in the sending populations of the Caribbean. The findings consistently indicate that the incidence of schizophrenia (between 2/10 000 and 4/10 000) is not elevated in the Caribbean and is well within the range of those reported for the native populations of Britain and Holland as well as, more generally, within the range of those reported by the World Health Organization. This in one sense confirms the hypothesis that the incidence of schizophrenia, if narrowly defined, is relatively constant around the world if the estimates and confidence intervals are interpreted conservatively (see Kirkbride *et al.*, 2006, for an alternative view based on recent data showing geographical variations of incident schizophrenia and psychosis in the UK). An age-corrected prevalence rate for schizophrenia was also calculated for Jamaica (Hickling and Rodgers-Johnson, 1994). At 3.1/1000, this rate was within the range of other studies reported by the World Health Organization.

The prevalence rate for schizophrenia in Dominica was reported by Kay (1992) as 11.8 per 1000 in a case register study using diagnoses of the 9th Edition of the *International Classification of Diseases* (ICD-9) and 7.8 per 100 000 using the *Diagnostic and Statistical Manual of Mental Disorders*, Edition III (DSM-III) diagnostic criteria. These rates are somewhat higher than the Jamaican prevalence rate although they are in the same range as that of the native white population in the UK (8.7/1000 reported by Cochrane and Bal, 1989). Caution is urged in the interpretation of prevalence rates from the very small Caribbean islands with populations under 50 000, as there is significant migration of people from the smaller island states of the Caribbean to other larger Caribbean territories and other parts of the world, thereby considerably contracting the denominator population used for the calculation of prevalence rates.

There have been no comprehensive incidence studies done with regard to bipolar disorders. However, data from Trinidad indicate that there is a 0.8 per 1000 admission rate for affective psychoses

(Neehall, 1991) and data from Jamaica estimate an age-corrected prevalence rate of 0.16 per 1000 for the same condition (Hickling and Rodgers-Johnson, 1995). Unfortunately, the gender and ethnic distributions of psychoses are still not entirely clarified. In the multi-ethnic Caribbean, there is some evidence that people of African descent are more likely to present with psychotic illness, while those of Indian origin are more likely to have non-psychotic illnesses in general and depression specifically (Hutchinson *et al.*, 2003a). The ethnic distribution of excessive alcohol, cannabis and cocaine use may also be instructive in this context. This needs to be investigated as a means of determining the potential relevance and significance of these findings.

The role of cannabis demands some clarification. Studies undertaken in the 1970s in Jamaica pointed to an association between cannabis and mania (Beaubrun and Knight, 1973; Harding and Knight, 1973). It is now more generally thought to be an environmental risk factor for schizophrenia, for earlier onset or for precipitating an onset in the presence of other risk factors, but not sufficient or necessary to cause psychosis alone. Still others believe that there is a specific phenomenological entity – cannabis-related psychosis – that has the propensity to exist independently even after cannabis use has ceased. The widely pervasive use of cannabis makes it somewhat difficult to distinguish whether psychotic symptoms that have been precipitated by cannabis use are due to its toxic effects on the brain or whether they are a product of the interaction between a genetic vulnerability and the use of the drug. Nevertheless we seem well placed in the region to answer this burning question for world psychiatry.

The epidemiological characteristics of disorders such as schizoaffective disorder and delusional disorder are also not well known in the region. This is also applicable to the occurrence of brief psychotic episodes, schizophreniform disorder and late onset psychoses.

## Depression

Several studies have addressed the problem of co-morbid depression with physical illness in the Caribbean with rates in those populations ranging from 25 to 45 per cent. Populations studied include those with systemic lupus erythematosus, attendees at primary care clinics, haematological disease and acute medical admissions (Hutchinson *et al.*, 1996, 2003b). There has also been the validation of the Zung scale for Trinidadian and Jamaican populations (Maharaj *et al.*, 2005). Community prevalence of depression remains unknown, though one recent study suggests that it is in the range of 14 per cent in Trinidad (Bandhan *et al.*, 2005) which is higher than the 11 per cent reported for a family practice population also in Trinidad (Maharaj, 2005). The impact of untreated depression remains unknown, particularly with regard to rates of homicide and suicide. The former is rising all over the Caribbean and the latter is high in the multi-ethnic countries of Trinidad, Guyana and Suriname. The differences in presentation between bipolar and unipolar depression, the role of alcohol dependence in the evolution of depressive disorders and the likelihood that anxiety disorders and depressive disorders are commonly entwined all need to be confirmed and reported in the Caribbean context.

The available evidence supports the established international dictum that women are more likely to be depressed or at least present with depressive syndromes more commonly than men, but certainly more work is needed to estimate more accurately the determinants of this phenomenon in the Caribbean, where women have traditionally played strong roles in the nurturing and management of families (Lewis, 1968). Disorders such as post-partum depression and depression in late life have also not been reported in the region and very little is known about their epidemiology.

## Anxiety disorders

Whenever public education forums are hosted in Trinidad, these are always overrun by a large number of people claiming to satisfy criteria for the diagnosis of anxiety disorders. Whether this is an exaggeration of the current preoccupation with being stressed or represents a true picture of pathology is unknown. However, generalized anxiety disorders and panic disorder, judging from the anecdotally observed prescribing patterns for antidepressants and benzodiazepines, do seem to have a high prevalence in the region. Because anxiety is a natural human experience and likely to increase in times of social and cultural unease, the distinction between this and pathological anxiety is sometimes difficult in the light of the rapid changes occurring in regional and international affairs. However, GPs and cardiologists, for example, are especially likely to see patients who might be suffering from these anxiety disorders and for this reason alone there should be closer collaboration between psychiatry and these other medical disciplines. Other anxiety disorders such as obsessive–compulsive disorder and social anxiety disorder are also likely to exist in ways that might surprise most clinicians, and this is one of the ways in which psychiatric disorders can adversely affect family life and economic productivity without coming to the notice of the mental health and indeed the medical services.

There is some indication that the prevalence of these disorders is increasing in Trinidad while not being so common in other Caribbean countries. However it may be that they are not being recognized as illnesses by those experiencing the symptoms, who may be seeking solace and indirect treatment through church and other community activities. This also needs to be investigated.

In recent years there has been increased frequency of hurricane-related damage and other natural disasters in the region; consequently a local epidemiology of post-traumatic stress dis-order is also needed. The way in which this diagnosis affects the response to these natural disasters and the subsequent recovery is in urgent need of investigation. Identification of vulnerability factors and determination of the qualities of resilience that produce best responses to these unpredictable natural events are vital to understand. This know-ledge can then be used in relief efforts. The best and most cost-effective treatments can only be determined if there is an accurate establishment of symptom targets and outcomes based on this analysis.

## Dementia

While the demographic shift that has resulted in the exponential growth of the over-65 populations in many developed countries has been less marked in the Caribbean region, improvements in life expectancy and declines in fertility have seen increases in the relative percentage of those living in the over-65 age range all over the region and certainly for the larger territories, life expectancy is now well into the mid-70s. This has resulted in a proliferation of geriatric nursing homes, especially in Trinidad, and in greater awareness and prevalence of both Alzheimer's disease and vascular dementia. The latter may be due in part to high rates of hypertension and diabetes mellitus in our populations. This is a natural epidemic that has yet to reach the notice of the policy-makers but will certainly demand increasing attention in the years ahead. Issues such as the development of geriatric services, appropriate screening instruments, levels of impairment, investment in caregiver support, regulation of geriatric homes and treatment services for the elderly all require urgent attention (Eldemire, 1996). Trials of anti-dementia drugs are also certain to become very important in the coming years.

There is also a need to distinguish between vascular dementia and Alzheimer's disease, in terms of both phenomenology and outcome in Caribbean populations. Initial studies suggest that Alzheimer's disease, for example, may be a disease that is far more common in the Western world. Hendrie et al. (2004) showed that there is a gradient of risk that is lowest in Africa, intermediate in the Caribbean and greatest in North America among people of African origin. This suggests that environmental factors acting in concert with increasing urbanization or some other environmental factor may be increasing the risk of Alzheimer's disease in genetically similar populations. The relationship of dementia to depression and neurological disorders such as Parkinson's disease is not well known; nor is its occurrence in the aftermath of cerebrovascular accidents, which have a high prevalence in the Caribbean.

## Suicide and homicide

Overall suicide rates for Jamaica (Abel and Hickling, 2004), Barbados (Mahy, 1987) and Trinidad (Hutchinson and Simeon, 1997) are estimated at 2.3/100 000, 5.2/100 000 and 12.3/100 000 respectively. Suicide remains a major problem for the multi-ethnic Caribbean countries such as Trinidad and Tobago, Guyana and Suriname. These are all countries with relatively high numbers of Hindu religious adherents. This has been postulated as one of the major reasons for the disparity between these countries and the rest of the region (Ameerali, 2002). For example, a study from Trinidad (Hutchinson *et al.*, 1991) indicated that of 270 deaths by suicide between 1986 to 1990, 54 per cent were in people of East Indian origin and 42 per cent in people of African origin; the rate of suicide in East Indian females outnumbered the rate for African women by a ratio of 2:1. However, the reasons for the higher rate of suicide among East Indians may be more complex than issues of religion or culture. Access to poisons through agricultural activity may also be a contributing factor as well as higher levels of alcohol abuse perhaps masking untreated depression (Hutchinson *et al.*, 1999; see also Chapter 21).

Self-harm behaviour is on the rise throughout the region, particularly the ingestion of tablets by women and more pungent chemicals by men. Another recent trend is a growing incidence of self-mutilation or cutting among adolescents and young adults. As yet there are no studies that have addressed these empirically but in Trinidad, for example, at least three people are admitted every day to the nations' hospitals in the context of deliberate self-harm. The typical epidemiological pattern of more females than males engaging in non-fatal deliberate self-harm with the reverse being true for fatal self-harm is likely to be due to males using more lethal methods; however, the occurrence of non-intentional suicide in response to relationship conflict and a subsequent impulsive self-harming response has also not been well studied. Self-immolation is also seen in these populations, again primarily among those who are Hindus. The poisons most favoured are paraquat and lanate.

Homicide is also a growing problem throughout the region, with rising rates in most Caribbean countries. With access to guns increasing this is also becoming a public health problem and the role of underlying psychiatric and neurocognitive disorders has not yet been fully explored. Depression, attention deficit hyperactivity disorders (ADHD), minor learning disabilities causing poor educational achievement and substance abuse are among other factors are likely to impact on this phenomenon. Anger management, conflict resolution skills and impulse control are all necessarily implicated here in dealing with this burgeoning problem likely to have a negative impact on the development potential of the Caribbean. The ongoing drug trafficking trade and the growing inequality between the rich and the poor demand collaboration with other disciplines so that workable solutions can be identified and implemented before the development potential is permanently derailed.

## Substance abuse

Substance abuse remains possibly the single greatest contributor to psycho-social morbidity in the region. The impact on mental health service utilization, either indirectly through psychosis, depression and other psychiatric disorders or directly in the rehabilitative treatment process, places a high demand on limited resources. The wider societal impact on issues such as domestic violence, criminal behaviour, road traffic and other accidents and decreased economic productivity must also be quantified and investigated. The problems related to alcohol use may be different in their archaeology than those related to cannabis and cocaine use but the impact is consistently negative and profound. The Caribbean Epidemiology Centre (CAREC) has begun to monitor trends in substance use across the region and the need for preventive strategies and the efficacy of current rehabilitative options need to be urgently documented.

## Personality disorders

With increasing information available, it is becoming increasingly obvious that people with personality disorders may be living in the community undiagnosed. Increasing rates of violence, self-mutilation and foundering relationships all lend support to this possibility in this almost completely unexplored area in the Caribbean. While it has not been empirically studied, the anecdotal evidence suggests that diagnoses of borderline personality disorders are being made with increasing frequency. The relationship to anxiety disorders in women and substance abuse and mood disorders in men remains unreported. Another emerging trend is the diagnosis of eating disorders, particularly bulimia nervosa. In addition, research into this area may provide us with a lens through which we can view the presence, if it exists, of the Caribbean personality and how it is evolving in the face of globalization and models of urban development. The currently accepted cluster distribution of personality disorders is undergoing re-evaluation for the next iteration of DSM and ICD. In the context of culture, it is clear this whole field needs exploration, and specifically the classification needs revised for use in the Caribbean.

## HIV/AIDS

With rates of HIV infection in the Caribbean second only to sub-Saharan Africa, there is a significant connection with mental health problems (Calleja *et al.*, 2002). Patients with psychiatric illness are at increased risk of HIV infection and individuals who are HIV positive are likely to develop HIV-related psychiatric illnesses such as dementia and mood disorders. Other populations at high risk for HIV infection include the homeless and substance abusers, who are also likely to have serious mental health co-morbidity. These are all important in the Caribbean context and require a concerted epidemiological effort to understand the impact of HIV on mental health in the Caribbean.

## UPDATED AND COMPREHENSIVE RECORDING SYSTEMS/REGISTRIES

The foregoing underlines the need for consistent recording and diagnostic systems in the Caribbean that will allow for accurate epidemiological understanding of the mental health problems in the region. There is also a strong case to be made for a large-scale community-based epidemiological study of all mental illnesses so that prevalence data and the associated risk factors can be obtained and documented. It will also serve to direct treatment and training needs. This is fundamental to the development of relevant and more effective services as

well as identifying the economic burden of these disorders in the Caribbean on both the afflicted and their caregivers. It will also allow for a better appreciation of the community perception of mental illness and the pathways through which communities negotiate mental distress.

It is almost universally accepted that the traditional and religious healers are the first contact for most people with psychopathology but perhaps it is because the symptoms are not recognized as illness or indeed not recognized at all. Service contact studies are also useful but do not fully reflect the true nature of the population pathology and the perception of mental health services in the population so that access and utilization of services can be better understood. This is especially relevant in terms of the public perceptions of the efficacy of psychiatric treatments, the confidentiality associated with the use of services and responsiveness of the services to their needs.

The broader approach to epidemiological data collection would also facilitate better regional planning and sharing and distribution of resources. Evidence-based and needs analysis are crucial to the best practice models, and without adequate information, planning will be futile. This also applies to training needs, particularly as they apply to allied mental health professions and subspecialties within psychiatry. For example, there is a gaping shortage of forensic and child and adolescent psychiatrists. These projects will be fundamental toward developing the trajectory of the future direction of mental health activity in the Caribbean and provide a haven for research activity for decades.

## Aetiology

Certainly no genetic epidemiology studies have been conducted to establish the genetic aetiology of mental illnesses in the Caribbean. The oft-repeated mantras of unstable early family life, childhood abuse and lack of appropriate mentoring may all apply but we still do not understand the way in which genes and environment interact to express mental illness as psychopathologies in the Caribbean. The populations of the Caribbean, because of their extraordinary ethnic and cultural variation, would provide very appropriate samples for research studies to disentangle the effects of genes and the environment on the presentation of mental illness. A combination of molecular and behavioural genetics would be very useful in this process of identifying the way in which our genetic inheritance has contributed to the landscape of psychopathology. That would also allow for more accurate comparisons with other countries and regions. For example, Bhugra *et al.* (2003) compared the occurrence of pregnancy and birth complications in patients with schizophrenia in London and Trinidad and found essentially no difference between the British and the Trinidadian groups. This further discounted the notion that an excess of pregnancy and birth complications could account for the increased rates of psychosis among the Caribbean population in Britain.

In order to better understand diasporic patterns of behaviour and how these cause tensions or indeed provide protection against mental health distress, more of these comparisons could be undertaken. However, an agenda that is informed by our own priorities rather than those that elucidate pathological mechanisms in the migration destinations of our populations would be a welcome change. Understanding aetiology is, of course, central to the development of preventive strat-egies and collaborations with agencies and institutions that support and regulate education, family and community support; housing and social ser-vices may also be vital in this process. The role of substance abuse has already been mentioned in this context.

Improvements in neuroimaging resources and more active encouragement of an unbiased neuroscientific agenda would be necessary to establish a new basis for planning and policy of mental health and other services. The region is not optimally served in this area either in terms of diagnostics and services for neuropsychiatric disorders or in terms of research that combines genes, brain imaging and social risk factors in an integrated agenda. Other useful research strategies could include merging interests in economics, psychology, sociology and history in order to better understand our position in the world and how to best improve our resilience and diminish our vulnerabilities.

The role of social influences in the epidemiology of mental illness has also not been sufficiently studied. These include issues such as overcrowded housing, internal migration, urbanization and unemployment. The specific role of protective factors such as religion, community integration and family support also need to be documented. Clinical trials of medication and other interventions are also needed to clarify the best use of resources in the treatment of the mentally ill.

## REFERENCES

Abel, W. and Hickling, F.W. 2004: *Suicide Rates in Jamaica 1998–2003.* Kingston. (Unpublished MS.)

Ameerali, D.P. 2002: Intra-country variation of suicide rates in Trinidad and Tobago. Doctor of Medicine research thesis, University of the West Indies.

Bandhan, T., Chastanet, Y., Emmanuel, A., Regobert, J., Subramian, B., Yogi, D., PoonKing, C. and Hutchinson, G. 2005: The prevalence of selected vascular risk factors in a community setting in Trinidad. *West Indian Medical Journal* 54, S78.

Beaubrun, M.H. and Knight, F. 1973: Psychiatric assessment of 30 chronic users of cannabis and 30 matched controls. *American Journal of Psychiatry* 130, 309–11.

Bhugra, D., Hilwig, M., Hossein, B., Marceau, H., Neehall, J., Leff, J., Mallett, R. and Der, G. 1996: First-contact incidence rates of schizophrenia in Trinidad in a one-year follow-up. *British Journal of Psychiatry* 169, 587–92.

Bhugra, D., Hutchinson, G., Hilwig, M., Hossein, B., Neehall, J.E. and Murray, R.M. 2003: Pregnancy and birth complications in schizophrenia. Comparison between Trinidad and London. *West Indian Medical Journal* 52, 124–26.

Calleja, J.M., Walker, N., Cuchi, P., Llazzari, S., Ghys, P.D. and Zacaria, F. 2002: Status of the HIV/AIDS epidemic and methods to monitor it in the Latin American and Caribbean region. *AIDS* 16, S3–S12.

Cochrane, R. and Bal, S. 1989: Mental hospital admission rates of immigrants to England. *Social Psychiatry and Psychiatric Epidemiology* 24, 2–11.

Eldemire, D. 1996: Level of impairment in the Jamaican elderly and the issues of screening levels, caregiving support systems, carepersons and female burden. *Molecular and Chemical Neuropathology* 28, 115–20.

Harding, T. and Knight, F. 1973: Marihuana modified mania. *Archives of General Psychiatry* 29, 635–37.

Hendrie, H.C., Hall, K.S., Ogunniyi, A. and Gao, S. 2004: Alzheimer's disease, genes and environment: the value of international studies. *Canadian Journal of Psychiatry* 49, 92–99.

Hickling, F.W. and Rodgers-Johnson, P. 1994: The prevalence of schizophrenia and affective disorders in Jamaica. *West Indian Medical Journal* 44, S29.

Hickling, F.W. and Rodgers-Johnson, P. 1995: The incidence of first contact schizophrenia in Jamaica. *British Journal of Psychiatry* 167, 193–96.

Hutchinson, G. and Simeon, D.T. 1997: Suicide in Trinidad and Tobago, associations with measures of social distress. *International Journal of Social Psychiatry* 43, 269–75.

Hutchinson, G., Daisley, H., Simmonds, V. and Gordon, A. 1991: Suicide by poisoning: a preliminary epidemiological report. *West Indian Medical Journal* 40, 69–73.

Hutchinson, G., Neehall, J.E. and Simeon, D.T. 1996: Psychiatric disorders in systemic lupus erythematosus. *West Indian Medical Journal* 45, 48–50.

Hutchinson, G., Daisley, H., Simeon D.T., Simmons, V., Shetty. M. and Lynn, D. 1999: High rates of paraquat induced suicide in southern Trinidad, *Suicide and Life Threatening Behaviour* 29, 186–91.

Hutchinson, G., Ramcharan, C. and Ghany, K. 2003a: Gender and ethnic differences in first admissions to a psychiatric unit in Trinidad. *West Indian Medical Journal* 52, 300–303.

Hutchinson, G., Kodali, S., Bruce, C. and Thomas, C. 2003b: Depressive symptoms among acute adult medical admissions to a general hospital. *West Indian Medical Journal* 52, S51.

Kay, R.W. 1992: Prevalence and incidence of schizophrenia in Afro-Caribbeans. *British Journal of Psychiatry* 160, 421.

Kirkbride, J.B., Fearon, P., Morgan, C., Dazzan, P., Morgan, K., Tarrant, J. and Lloyd, T. 2006: Heterogeneity in incidence rates of schizophrenia and other psychotic syndromes: findings from the 3-center AeSOP study. *Archives of General Psychiatry* 63, 250–58.

Lewis, G.K. 1968: *The Growth of the Modern West Indies*. New York: Monthly Review Press.

Maharaj, R.G. 2005: The prevalence of depression among family practice patients in north west Trinidad. *West Indian Medical Journal* 54, S61.

Maharaj, R.G., Reid, S. and Misir, A. 2005: Validation of an interviewer applied modified Zung scale for detecting depression in a West Indian population. *West Indian Medical Journal* 54, S61.

Mahy, G. 1987: Completed suicide in Barbados. *West Indian Medical Journal* 36, 91–94.

Mahy, G.E., Mallett, R., Leff, J. and Bhugra, D. 1999: First-contact incidence rate of schizophrenia in Barbados. *British Journal of Psychiatry* 175, 28–33.

Neehall, J. 1991: An analysis of psychiatric in-patient admissions from a defined geographic catchment area over a one year period. *West Indian Medical Journal* 40, 16–21.

Patterson, O. 2004: Ecumenical America: global culture and the American Cosmos. In Bolland, O.N. (ed.) *The Birth of Caribbean Civilisation*. Kingston: Ian Randle, 633–651.

Selten, J.P., Zeyl, C., Dwarkasing, R., Kumsden, V., Kahn, R.S. and Van Harten, P.N. 2005: First-contact incidence of schizophrenia in Suriname. *British Journal of Psychiatry* 186, 74–75.

Sharpley, M., Hutchinson, G., McKenzie, K.J. and Murray, R.M. 2001: Understanding the excess of psychosis among the African Caribbean population in England. Review of the current hypotheses. *British Journal of Psychiatry* 178, S60–68.

Smith, M.G. 1965: *The Plural Society of the British West Indies*. Berkeley: University of California Press.

# Epilogue: In search of the way of tea

## Kamaldeep Bhui and Dinesh Bhugra

The evaluation of services in cultural psychiatry and the evolution of national policies to address the limitations of conventional mental health care are rare. One approach adopted in the policy framework in the UK is to modify pathways into and out of care and into recovery, as well as to engage local communities in care processes. The Pathways To Care approach has arisen largely in the context of statutory service development and therefore focuses largely on the system from within and on constraints from without. It documents the movement of individuals from the community to primary care and then into specialist, or secondary care. It then documents routes through different levels of specialist care and notes the importance of particular filters and pathways as if these were natural and inexorable pathways into and through mental health care services (Figure 1).

The consideration of pathways to care has often neglected the factors and services that operate before statutory care is sought, or when people have disengaged from statutory care (level 1 and filter 1). As has been noted throughout this volume, pre-statutory services or non-professional care is potentially important because intervention here may decrease the number of people needing and using the statutory sector. It is worth bearing in mind that of all people who enter the professional sector of services, only a small proportion become long-term users of services. Therefore, the statutory sector makes a small and significant contribution to care for mental distress, but consumes a disproportionate amount of the allocated resources.

The conventional pathways model addresses statutory levels of care from community to inpatient care but overlooks the voluntary and the folk and popular sectors of care. Furthermore, the existing policy frameworks tend to take a disease model of mental health problems, to assume seeking care means that an individual suffers with a particular mental health problem which requires a particular intervention, that will be identically effective irrespective of nation and cultural origins. Reconceptualization of this model has already been undertaken (Bhui and Bhugra, 2002). There has been little work, however, on pathways prior to contact with statutory services and these are crucial for care choices to be offered and for choices to be utilized. Furthermore, a Pathways to Care approach contains, as its cornerstone, an illness rather than a disease model of mental distress and recovery. Due to the substantial shift in values within mental health care, it is worth emphasizing that the challenge of culturally capable care provision raises fundamental questions about what constitutes mental health and wellbeing, and therefore what it means to provide mental health care for all populations.

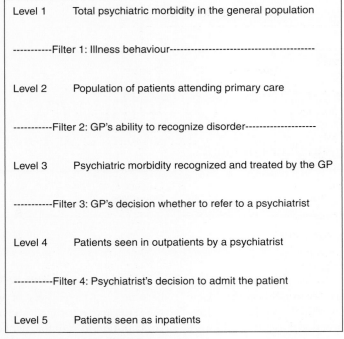

Figure 1    *Conventional pathways map.*

## PATHWAYS TO RECOVERY

Figure 2 outlines a pathway from distress in the community into statutory care. Most people display self-regulation processes to manage distress. When they encounter stress, they find internal and external resources to deal with it. They first use their own coping mechanisms and only turn to the family/community or folk sector if personal coping proves insufficient. Of course, not everybody takes one clear pathway, and extreme situations can lead to people skipping stages or using multiple sources and sectors of help at the same time.

What is important about this model is that the direction of travel goes both ways. Though a person may move down the pathway if the stress they are under is greater than their resources, a person moves back up the pathway when resources (whether personal, family, community, non-statutory or statutory) mitigate the stress. Hence this can be considered a pathway to recovery or through care rather than to care. The focus of

services using this model is to move a person, if at all possible, to a lower level of care provision.

Less than 1 per cent of those distressed ever see someone in statutory services. The vast majority of mental health problems are dealt with in the community by the community. If the architecture of services reflected this model of care, it may be possible to capitalize on community and folk care paradigms and to decrease the reliance on statutory care. It could unlock potential in the community to decrease the rates of presentation to statutory services of people with mental illness. Such an approach would allow services to refocus their efforts to be consistent with communities to promote recovery.

In order to keep people at lower (non-statutory) levels of care, a variety of interventions, including prevention and education as well as community-based and treatment models, will be required. This will offer maximum choice to those in distress. It will minimize disabilities due to chronic inattention and facilitate early intervention, sanctioning community, folk and popular sectors of

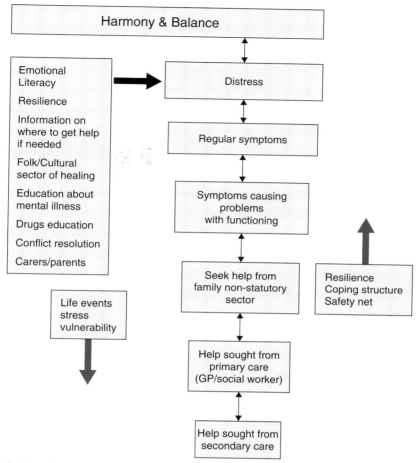

Figure 2 *A pathway from distress in the community into statutory care.*

health care and the voluntary agencies in their role in health promotion and prevention, and in intervention. It could also offer choice at a primary care level when help is sought from a GP or practice nurse or others; these professionals need not automatically refer into the statutory health care system but may refer out into the community. An understanding of communities and culture is therefore vitally important for recovery and public health. This has traditionally been the cornerstone of practice among cultural and transcultural mental health professionals, but this textbook and the discourse within suggest a broader range of actors should now be engaged, to include practitioners alongside experts in public

health, philosophy, social sciences, service development and policy.

*Culture and Mental Health* synthesizes the knowledge and experiences of people all over the world to achieve harmony and balance in life. Ogden (2006) proposes that

*(Psychoanalytic) teaching at best opens a space for thinking and dreaming in situations in which the (understandable) impulse is to close that space. To fill that space as a teacher is to preach, to proselytize, to perpetuate dogma; not to fill it is to create conditions in which one may become open to previously inconceivable possibilities.*

This textbook helps students open up a space and to 'dream', with us, with each other and with service users in order to bring about a real shift in the quality of life and wellbeing of people. This textbook also brings together policy-makers, managers, practitioners and researchers to address misfortune and human suffering through any means that can be harnessed at international, national, local, organizational and individual levels. This textbook emphasizes healing and recovery through person-centred and personal, and indigenous systems of recovery related to culture and personality, biology and society. Communication and expression of deep aspects of the cultural self, and of connections between the conscious and collective world reveal what is benevolent and nurturing and essential for recovery and wellbeing (Bhui and Bhugra, 2004). In such a spirit, at the XIIth World Congress of Psychiatry, in Yokohama, Dr Sen Shoshitsu (2002) proposed peacefulness and mental harmony through the healing world of the 'way of tea'. The tea ceremony was proposed to be a way of respectfully relating to each other, and to be a ritual that contains all the essential elements of caring, sharing and appreciating what is nurturing in our lives and what is not. We hope that you enjoy the many tastes and varieties of tea found within *Culture and Mental Health: A Comprehensive Textbook.*

## REFERENCES

Bhui, K. and Bhugra, D. 2002: Mental illness in black and Asian ethnic minorities: pathways to care and outcomes. *Advances in Psychiatric Treatment* 8, 26–33.

Bhui, K. and Bhugra, D. 2004: Communication with patients from other cultures: the place of explanatory models. *Advances in Psychiatric Treatment* 10, 474–78.

Ogden, T. 2006: On teaching psychoanalysis. *International Journal of Psychoanalysis* 87, 1069–86.

Shoshitsu, S. 2002: Peacefulness through a bowl of tea – the healing world of the way of tea. Plenary lecture 26 August 2002 at XIIth World Congress of Psychiatry in Yokohama. Plenary Lecture Booklet, 16.

# Index

Bold references indicate figures and tables